The Failing Heart

The Failing Heart

Editors

Naranjan S. Dhalla, Ph.D.
Distinguished Professor and Director
MRC Group in Experimental Cardiology
Division of Cardiovascular Sciences
Faculty of Medicine, University of Manitoba
St. Boniface General Hospital Research Centre
Winnipeg, Canada

Robert E. Beamish, M.D., F.R.C.P.C.
Professor Emeritus
Division of Cardiovascular Sciences
Faculty of Medicine, University of Manitoba
St. Boniface General Hospital Research Centre
Winnipeg, Canada

Nobuakira Takeda, M.D., Ph.D.
Associate Professor
Department of Internal Medicine
Aoto Hospital
Jikei University School of Medicine
Tokyo, Japan

Makoto Nagano, M.D., Ph.D.
Professor Emeritus
Jikei University School of Medicine
Tokyo, Japan

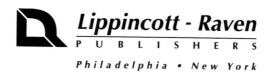

Lippincott - Raven
P U B L I S H E R S
Philadelphia • New York

Lippincott-Raven Publishers, 227 East Washington Square, Philadelphia, Pennsylvania 19106

Made in the United States of America

Library of Congress Cataloging-in-Publication Data

The failing heart / editors, Naranjan S. Dhalla . . . [et al.].
    p. cm.
  Proceedings of the International Conference on Heart Failure, held in Winnipeg, Canada, May 20–23, 1994.
  Includes bibliographical references and index.
  ISBN 0-7817-0311-5 (hard cover)
  1. Heart failure—Congresses. I. Dhalla, Naranjan S.
II. International Conference on Heart Failure 1994 : Winnipeg, Man.)
  [DNLM: 1. Heart Failure, Congestive—physiopathology—congresses.
2. Heart Failure, Congestive—therapy—congresses. 3. Myocardial—Infarction—physiopathology—therapy—congresses. 4. Heart Ventricle—pathology—congresses. 5. Renin-Angiotensin System—physiology—congresses. WG 370 F1605 1995]
RC685.C53F35   1995
616.1′29—dc20
DNLM/DLC
for Library of Congress   95-19810
                                         CIP

9 8 7 6 5 4 3 2 1

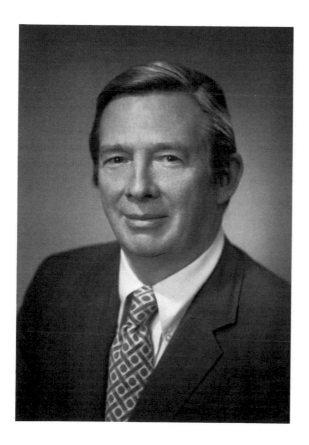

Robert E. Olson, M.D., Ph.D, Tampa, FL, USA

This book is dedicated to Robert E. Olson, who, during the early 1950s, outlined the concept that heart failure is due to either a defect in the process of energy production or a defect in the process of energy utilization. This hypothesis stimulated worldwide research concerning the metabolic status of the failing heart under both clinical and experimental conditions and resulted in our current understanding of heart function in health and disease. Dr. Naranjan S. Dhalla is particularly grateful to Professor Olson for his continued advice and support since his postdoctoral training (1966–68) at the St. Louis University.

Contents

Part I. Pathophysiologic and Clinical Considerations

vii

Part II. Ventricular Remodeling and the Renin-Angiotensin System

Part III. Treatment of Heart Failure

Contributing Authors

Margaret L. Ackman,
B.Sc.(Pharm), Pharm. D.
Research Fellow
Division of Cardiology
University of Alberta Hospitals
EPICORE Centre
2C2 Mackenzie Centre
Edmonton, Alberta T6G 2R7
Canada

Nasir Afzal, M.D., Ph.D.
Resident
Department of Pathology
University of Manitoba
Health Sciences Centre
820 Sherbrook Street
Winnipeg, Manitoba R2N 3J1
Canada

Moses Agbanyo, Ph.D.
Research Associate
Department of Internal Medicine
  (Cardiology)
University of Manitoba
Health Sciences Centre
700 William Avenue
Winnipeg, Manitoba R3E 0Z3
Canada

Piero Anversa, M.D.
Professor of Medicine and
Director, Cardiovascular Research
  Institute
Department of Medicine
New York Medical College
Vosburgh Pavilion, 302A
Valhalla, New York 10595
United States

Junichi Azuma, M.D.
Professor
Department of Clinical Evaluation of
  Medicines and Therapeutics
Faculty of Pharmaceutical Sciences
Osaka University
1-6 Yamada-oka,
Suita, Osaka 565
Japan

Kenneth M. Baker, M.D.
Staff Scientist
Weis Center for Research
Geisinger Clinic
100 North Academy Avenue
Danville, Pennsylvania 17822–2611
United States

Marion E. Barnes, M.Sc.
Research Associate
Department of Medicine
University of Alberta
EPICORE Centre
2C2 Mackenzie Centre
Edmonton, Alberta, T6G 2R7
Canada

Robert E. Beamish, M.D.,
  F.R.C.P.C.
Professor Emeritus
Division of Cardiovascular Sciences
Faculty of Medicine
University of Manitoba
St. Boniface General Hospital
  Research Centre
351 Taché Avenue
Winnipeg, Manitoba R2H 2A6
Canada

Palmira Bernocchi, Ph.D.
Fondazione Clinica del Lavoro
Centro di Fisiopatologia
   Cardiovascolare "S. Maugeri"
Via Pinidolo, 23
25064 Gussago, Brescia
Italy

Baikunth Bharadwaj, M.D.,
  F.R.C.S.(C.)
Professor and Head
Division of Thoracic and
   Cardiovascular Surgery
Foothills Hospital
1403 29th Street NW
Calgary, Alberta T2N 2T9
Canada

Martial G. Bourassa, M.D.
Medical Director
Montreal Heart Institute
5000 Belanger Street
Montreal, Quebec H1T 1C8
Canada

Alberto Braghiroli, M.D.
Chief Assistant
Division of Pulmonary Disease
"Clinica del Lavoro" Foundation
Medical Center of Rehabilitation
Via Revislate 13
I-28010 Veruno (NO)
Italy

Anna Cargnoni, B.S., Ph.D.
Researcher
Centro di Fisiopatologia
   Cardiovascolare "S. Maugeri"
Fondazione Clinica del Lavoro
Via Pinidolo, 23
25064 Gussago, Brescia
Italy

Claudio Ceconi, M.D.
Spedali Civili
P. le Spedali Civili, 1
25123 Brescia
Italy

Kanu Chatterjee, M.D., (Lond),
  F.R.C.P. (Edin), F.A.C.C.,
  F.C.C.P., F.A.C.P.
Professor of Medicine and
  Lucie Stern Professor of
  Cardiology
Division of Cardiology
Moffitt-Long Hospital
University of California at San
  Francisco
505 Parnassus Avenue 1186-M
San Francisco, California 94143
United States

Ray C.-J. Chiu, M.D., Ph.D.
Professor and Chairman
Department of Cardiovascular and
  Thoracic Surgery
McGill University
The Montreal General Hospital
1650 Cedar Avenue, Room C9.169
Montreal, Quebec H3G 1A4
Canada

Horacio E. Cingolani, M.D.
Director of the Cardiovascular
  Research Center
Department of Physiology
Centro de Investigaciones
  Cardiovasculares
Facultad de Medicina
Calle 60 y 120
1900 La Plata
Buenos Aires
Argentina

**Jack P. M. Cleutjens, Ph.D.,
Dr. Ir.**
Department of Pathology
Cardiovascular Research Center
Maastricht
University of Limburg
P.O. Box 616
6200 MD Maastricht
The Netherlands

Jay N. Cohn, M.D.
Professor of Medicine and
Head, Cardiovascular Division
Department of Medicine
University of Minnesota Medical
School
420 Delaware Street, SE
Minneapolis, Minnesota 55455
United States

Roberta Confortini, M.D.
Cattedra di Cardiologia
Spedali Civili di Brescia
P. le Spedali Civili, 1
25123 Brescia
Italy

Mat J.A.P. Daemen, M.D., Ph.D.
Associate Professor
Department of Pathology
Cardiovascular Research Institute
Maastricht
University of Limburg
P.O. Box 616
6200 MD Maastricht
The Netherlands

Francis Darkwa, M.D.
Department of Pharmacology and
Therapeutics
University of Manitoba
Health Sciences Centre
700 William Avenue
Winnipeg, Manitoba R3E 0Z3
Canada

Federica de Giuli, M.D.
Fondazione Clinica del Lavoro
Centro di Fisiopatologia
Cardiovascolare "S. Maugeri"
Via Pinidolo, 23
25064 Gussago, Brescia
Italy

Teresa DeMarco, M.D., F.A.C.C.
Associate Clinical Professor of
Medicine
Division of Cardiology
Moffitt-Long Hospital
University of California at San
Francisco
505 Parnassus Avenue, 1186-M
San Francisco, California 94143
United States

Roxanne Deslauriers, B.Sc., Ph.D.
Group Leader and Senior Research
Officer
Department of Biosystems
Institute for Biodiagnostics
National Research Council Canada
435 Ellice Avenue
Winnipeg, Manitoba R3B 1Y6
Canada

Naranjan S. Dhalla, Ph.D.
Distinguished Professor and
Director, MRC Group in
Experimental Cardiology
Division of Cardiovascular Sciences
Faculty of Medicine
University of Manitoba
St. Boniface General Hospital
Research Centre
351 Taché Avenue
Winnipeg, Manitoba R2H 2A6
Canada

Ian M. C. Dixon, B.Sc., M.Sc., Ph.D.
Assistant Professor
Department of Physiology
Division of Cardiovascular Sciences
Faculty of Medicine
University of Manitoba
St. Boniface General Hospital
  Research Centre
351 Taché Avenue
Winnipeg, Manitoba R2H 2A6
Canada

John C. Docherty, B.Sc., Ph.D.
Associate Research Officer
Department of Biosystems
Institute for Biodiagnostics
National Research Council Canada
435 Ellice Avenue
Winnipeg, Manitoba R3B 1Y6
Canada

Claudio F. Donner, M.D., F.C.C.P.
Chief
Division of Pulmonary Disease
"Clinica del Lavoro" Foundation
Medical Center of Rehabilitation
Via Revislate 13
I-28010 Veruno (NO)
Italy

David E. Dostal, Ph.D.
Associate Scientist
Weis Center for Research
Geisinger Clinic
100 North Academy Avenue
Danville, Pennsylvania 17822–2611
United States

Masao Endoh, M.D., Ph.D.
Professor
Department of Pharmacology
Yamagata University School of
  Medicine
2-2-2 Iida-nishi
Yamagata 990-23
Japan

Gloria R. Engel, M.D.
Assistant Professor of Medicine and
  Cardiology
Department of Medicine
Loma Linda University Medical
  Center
11234 Anderson Street
Loma Linda, California 92354
United States

Roberto Ferrari, M.D., Ph.D.
Professor of Cardiology
Universita' Degli Studi di Brescia
c/o Spedali Civili
P. le Spedali Civili, 1
25123 Brescia
Italy

Gary S. Francis, M.D.
Professor
Department of Medicine
University of Minnesota Medical
  School
Box 508
420 Delaware Street, SE
Minneapolis, Minnesota 55455
United States

A. Martin Gerdes, Ph.D.
Professor and Chair
Department of Anatomy and
  Structural Biology
University of South Dakota School of
  Medicine
414 E. Clark Street
Vermillion, South Dakota 57069
United States

Amerigo Giordano, M.D.
Divisione di Cardiologia
Fondazione Clinica del Lavoro
Via Pinidolo, 23
25064 Gussago, Brescia
Italy

Leonard S. Golfman, Ph.D.
Division of Cardiovascular Sciences
Faculty of Medicine
University of Manitoba
St. Boniface General Hospital
*   Research Centre*
351 Taché Avenue
Winnipeg, Manitoba R2H 2A6
Canada

J. B. Gupta, Ph.D.
Director
Cardiovascular Research Laboratory
Ranbury Research Laboratory
New Delhi
India

Haruo Hanawa, M.D.
First Department of Internal Medicine
Niigata University School of Medicine
Asahimachi 1-754
Niigata 951
Japan

Gerd Hasenfuss, M.D.
Assistant Professor
Department of Cardiology and
*   Angiology*
University of Freiburg
Hugstetter Strasse 55
79106 Freiburg
Germany

Tomoji Hata, M.D.
Assistant Professor
Department of Bioclimatology and
*   Medicine*
Medical Institute of Bioregulation
Kyushu University
4546 Tsurumihara
Beppu, Oita 874
Japan

J. Thomas Heywood, M.D.
Associate Professor of Medicine and
*   Director, Cardiomyopathy Service*
Department of Medicine
Loma Linda University Medical
*   Center*
11234 Anderson Street
Loma Linda, California 92354
United States

Satoru Hirono, M.D.
First Department of Internal Medicine
Niigata University School of Medicine
Asahimachi 1-754
Niigata 951
Japan

Christian Holubarsch, M.D.
Professor
Department of Cardiology and
*   Angiology*
University of Freiburg
Hugstetter Strasse 55
79106 Freiburg
Germany

Hiroyuki Hosono, M.D.
First Department of Internal Medicine
Niigata University School of Medicine
Asahimachi 1-754
Niigata 951
Japan

Tohru Izumi, M.D.
Professor
First Department of Internal Medicine
Niigata University
Asahimachi 1-754
Niigata 951
Japan

Bodh I. Jugdutt, M.B.Ch.B.,
  M.Sc., F.R.C.P.C., F.A.C.C.
Professor
Department of Medicine
University of Alberta Hospitals
2C2 Mackenzie Center
8440-112 Street
Edmonton, Alberta T6G 2R7
Canada

Hanjörg Just, M.D.
Professor
Department of Cardiology and
  Angiology
University of Freiburg
Hugstetter Strasse 55
79106 Freiburg
Germany

Jawahar Kalra, M.D., Ph.D.,
  F.R.C.P.(C.)
Professor and Head
Department of Pathology
College of Medicine
University of Saskatchewan
107 Wiggins Road
Saskatoon, Saskatchewan S7N 5E5
Canada

Yumi Katano, Ph.D.
Associate Professor
Department of Pharmacology
Yamagata University School of
  Medicine
2-2-2 Iida-nishi
Yamagata 990-23
Japan

Youichi Kawabata, Ph.D.
Postgraduate Student
Department of Pharmacology
Yamagata University School of
  Medicine
2-2-2 Iida-nishi
Yamagata 990-23
Japan

Scott E. Kellerman, M.D.
Department of Pediatrics
Rainbow Babies and Childrens
  Hospital
2074 Abington Road
Cleveland, Ohio 44106
United States

Jagdish C. Khatter, M.Sc., Ph.D.
Associate Professor
Departments of Internal Medicine
  (Cardiology) and Pharmacology
  and Therapeutics
University of Manitoba
Health Sciences Centre
700 William Avenue
Winnipeg, Manitoba R3E 0Z3
Canada

Irwin Klein, M.D.
Professor of Medicine and Cell
  Biology
Chief, Division of Endocrinology
Departments of Medicine and
  Endocrinology
North Shore University Hospital
Cornell University Medical College
300 Community Drive
Manhasset, New York 11030
United States

John Klemperer, M.D.
Resident in Surgery
Department of Surgery
New York Hospital
Cornell University Medical College
525 East 68th Street
New York, New York 10021
United States

Makoto Kodama, M.D.
First Department of Internal Medicine
Niigata University School of Medicine
Asahimachi 1-754
Niigata 951
Japan

Bodo Kretschmann
Department of Cardiology and
    Angiology
University of Freiburg
Hugstetter Strasse 55
79106 Freiburg
Germany

Marrick L. Kukin, M.D., F.A.C.C.
Assistant Professor of Medicine
Director, Coronary Care Unit
Director, Heart Failure Program
Arthur Ross Scholar in
    Cardiovascular Medicine
Cardiovascular Institute
Mount Sinai Medical Center
One Gustave Levy Place
Box 1030
New York, New York 10029-6574
United States

Valerie V. Kupriyanov, B.Sc., Ph.D.
Associate Research Officer
Department of Biosystems
Institute for Biodiagnostics
National Research Council Canada
435 Ellice Avenue
Winnipeg, Manitoba R3B 1Y6
Canada

Haruhiko Kuwano, M.D.
First Department of Internal Medicine
Niigata University School of Medicine
Asahimachi 1-754
Niigata 951
Japan

Sylvain Lareau, B.Sc., Ph.D.
President
Instruments Anateck, Inc.
279 rue Essiambre
Gatineau, Quebec J8R 1V1
Canada

Paul Lee, M.Sc.
Department of Physiology
College of Medicine
University of Saskatchewan
107 Wiggins Road
Saskatoon, Saskatchewan S7N 5E5
Canada

**Frans H.H. Leenen, M.D., Ph.D.,
    F.R.C.P.C.**
Professor, Medicine and
    Pharmacology
Hypertension Unit
University of Ottawa Heart Institute
1053 Carling Avenue
Ottawa, Ontario K1Y 4E9
Canada

Peng Li, M.D.
Assistant Professor
Department of Medicine
New York Medical College
Vosburgh Pavilion, 302A
Valhalla, New York 10595
United States

Naoki Makino, M.D.
Associate Professor
Department of Bioclimatology and
  Medicine
Medical Institute of Bioregulation
Kyushu University
4546 Tsurumihara
Beppu, Oita 874
Japan

Michael M. Mannino, M.D.
Instructor in Medicine
Department of Cardiology
The Mount Sinai Hospital
One Gustave L. Levy Place
New York, New York 10029-6574
United States

Kathleen A. Mansour, M.D.
Assistant Professor of Medicine
Department of Medicine (Cardiology)
Emory University
1264 Clifton Road, N.E.
Atlanta, Georgia 30322
United States

S.V. Mantha, Ph.D.
Clinical Assistant Professor
  (Research)
Department of Pathology
College of Medicine
University of Saskatchewan
107 Wiggins Road
Saskatoon, Saskatchewan S7N 5E5
Canada

Hirosuke Matsui, M.D.
Assistant Professor
Department of Bioclimatology and
  Medicine
Medical Institute of Bioregulation
Kyushu University
4546 Tsurumihara
Beppu, Oita 874
Japan

Anna Mazzoletti, M.D.
Cattedra di Cardiologia
Spedali Civili di Brescia
P. le Spedali Civili, 1
25123 Brescia
Italy

Kenneth McDonald, M.D.
Assistant Professor
Department of Medicine
University of Minnesota
Box 508
420 Delaware Street, SE
Minneapolis, Minnesota 55455
United States

Mark E. McGovern, M.D.,
  F.A.C.C., F.A.C.P.
Executive Director
Cardiovascular Clinical Research,
  Atherosclerosis
Department of Cardiovascular
  Clinical Research and Development
Bristol-Myers Squibb Company
Pharmaceutical Research Institute
P.O. Box 4000
Princeton, New Jersey 08540
United States

Robert S. McKelvie, B.Sc., M.Sc.,
  M.D., F.R.C.P.(C.)
Associate Professor of Medicine and
  Career Scientist of the Ontario
  Ministry of Health
Department of Medicine
Division of Cardiology
McMaster University
Hamilton General Hospital
237 Barton Street East
Hamilton, Ontario L8L 2X2
Canada

Davendra Mehta, M.D., M.R.C.P.,
Ph.D., F.A.C.C.
Assistant Professor
Department of Medicine
Mount Sinai Hospital of the City
University of New York
One Gustave L. Levy Place
New York, New York 10029
United States

Markus Meyer, M.D.
Department of Cardiology and
Angiology
University of Freiburg
Hugstetter Strasse 55
79106 Freiburg
Germany

Yoshio Misawa, M.D., Ph.D.
Associate Professor
Department of Thoracic and
Cardiovascular Surgery
Jichi Medical School
3311-1 Yakushiji
Minamikawachi
Tochigi 329-04
Japan

Terrence J. Montague, M.D.
Professor of Medicine and
Director of Cardiology
Division of Cardiology
University of Alberta Hospitals
EPICORE Centre
2C2 Mackenzie Centre
Edmonton, Alberta T6G 2R7
Canada

Abel E. Moreyra, M.D.
Associate Professor of Medicine
Department of Medicine
Division of Cardiology
University of Medicine and Dentistry
of New Jersey
Robert Wood Johnson Medical School
CN19 Room 582
New Brunswick, New Jersey 08903
United States

James P. Morgan, M.D., Ph.D.
Associate Professor of Medicine
Harvard Medical School; and
Chief, Cardiovascular Division
Beth Israel Hospital
330 Brookline Avenue
Boston, Massachusetts 02215
United States

Susana M. Mosca, Ph.D.
Established Investigator of the
CONICET
Department of Physiology
Centro de Investigaciones
Cardiovasculares
Facultad de Medicina
Calle 60 y 120
1900 La Plata
Buenos Aires
Argentina

Makoto Nagano, M.D., Ph.D.
Professor Emeritus
Jikei University School of Medicine
Shibuya-ku
Ebisu 3-31-6
Tokyo 150
Japan

Kaie M. Ojamaa, Ph.D.
Assistant Professor of Cell Biology
Departments of Medicine and
Endocrinology
North Shore University Hospital
Cornell University Medical College
300 Community Drive
Manhasset, New York 11030
United States

Giorgio Olivetti, M.D.
Professor
Department of Medicine
New York Medical College
Vosburgh Pavilion, 302A
Valhalla, New York 10595
United States

Cristina Opasich, M.D.
Fondazione Clinica del Lavoro
Centro di Montescano
27040 Montescano, Pavia
Italy

Satoru Otsuji, M.D., Ph.D.
Staff of the Department of Cardiology
The Center for Adult Diseases, Osaka
1-3-3 Nakamichi
Higashinari-ku
Osaka 537
Japan

Evasio Pasini, M.D.
Fondazione Clinica del Lavoro
Centro di Fisiopatologia
Cardiovascolare "S. Maugeri"
Via Pinidolo 23
25064 Gussago, Brescia
Italy

Robert C.J.J. Passier, Ph.D.
Department of Pharmacology
Cardiovascular Research Institute
Maastricht
University of Limburg
Universiteitssingel 50
6200 MD Maastricht
The Netherlands

Burkert Pieske, M.D.
Department of Cardiology and
Angiology
University of Freiburg
Hugstetter Strasse 55
79106 Freiburg
Germany

Kailash Prasad, M.D., Ph.D.,
F.R.C.P.(C.)
Professor
Department of Physiology
College of Medicine
University of Saskatchewan
107 Wiggins Road
Saskatoon, Saskatchewan S7N 5E5
Canada

Federico Quaini, M.D.
Associate Professor
New York Medical College
Vosburgh Pavilion, 302A
Valhalla, New York 10595
United States

Anna Ratajska, Ph.D.
Department of Anatomy
University of Iowa
51 Newton Road
Iowa City, Iowa 52242
United States

Thorsten Ruf, M.D.
Department of Cardiology and
Angiology
University of Freiburg
Hugstetter Strasse 55
79106 Freiburg
Germany

Marcel Ruzicka, M.D., Ph.D.
Research Fellow
Hypertension Unit
University of Ottawa Heart Institute
1053 Carling Avenue
Ottawa, Ontario K1Y 4E9
Canada

Carlo Sacco, M.D.
Assistant
Division of Pulmonary Disease
"Clinica del Lavoro" Foundation
Medical Center of Rehabilitation
Via Revislate 13
I-28010 Veruno (NO)
Italy

Tomás A. Salerno, M.D., M.Sc.
Professor and Chairman
Department of Cardiothoracic
Surgery
State University of New York at
Buffalo
100 High Street
Buffalo, New York 14203
United States

Laura Saward, B.Sc.
Department of Physiology
Division of Cardiovascular Sciences
Faculty of Medicine
University of Manitoba
St. Boniface General Hospital
Research Centre
351 Taché Avenue
Winnipeg, Manitoba R2H 2A6
Canada

Stephen W. Schaffer, Ph.D.
Professor
Department of Pharmacology
University of South Alabama
College of Medicine
Mobile, Alabama 36688
United States

Klaus Schlotthauer, M.D.
Department of Cardiology and
Angiology
University of Freiburg
Hugstetter Strasse 55
79106 Freiburg
Germany

Stephan Schmidt-Schweda, M.D.
Department of Cardiology and
Angiology
University of Freiburg
Hugstetter Strasse 55
79106 Freiburg
Germany

Douglas D. Schocken, M.D.
Professor and Director
Division of Cardiology
Department of Internal Medicine
University of South Florida
12901 Bruce B. Downs Boulevard
Tampa, Florida 33612
United States

Nobuhiko Shibata, M.D., Ph.D.
Chief
Department of Cardiology
The Center for Adult Diseases, Osaka
1-3-3 Nakamichi
Higashinari-ku
Osaka 537
Japan

Steven N. Singh, M.D.
Staff Cardiologist
Department of Medicine
Veterans Affairs Medical Center
Room 1E301
50 Irving Street, NW
Washington, DC 20422; and
Associate Professor of Medicine and
  Pharmacology
Georgetown University
3800 Reservoir Road, NW
Washington, DC 20007
United States

Jos F.M. Smits, Ph.D.
Professor
Department of Pharmacology
Cardiovascular Research Institute
  Maastricht
University of Limburg
Universiteitssingel 50
6200 MD Maastricht
The Netherlands

R. John Solaro, Ph.D.
Professor and Head
Departments of Physiology and
  Biophysics
The University of Illinois at Chicago
College of Medicine
835 South Wolcott Avenue (M/C 901)
Chicago, Illinois 60612-7342
United States

Edmund H. Sonnenblick, M.D.
Olson Professor of Medicine
Department of Medicine
The Albert Einstein College of
  Medicine
1300 Morris Park Avenue
Bronx, New York 10461
United States

Laura C. Stewart, B.Sc., M.Sc.,
  Ph.D.
Assistant Research Officer
Department of Biosystems
Institute for Biodiagnostics
National Research Center Canada
435 Ellice Avenue
Winnipeg, Manitoba R3B 1Y6
Canada

Masahiro Sugano, M.D.
Assistant Professor
Department of Bioclimatology and
  Medicine
Medical Institute of Bioregulation
Kyushu University
4546 Tsurumihara
Beppu, Oita 874
Japan

Yao Sun, M.D., Ph.D.
Assistant Professor of Medicine
Division of Cardiology
University of Missouri Health
  Sciences Center
Room MA432 Medical Science
  Building
Columbia, Missouri 65212
United States

Sachiyo Taguchi
Department of Bioclimatology and
  Medicine
Medical Institute of Bioregulation
Kyushu University
4546 Tsurumihara
Beppu, Oita 874
Japan

Nobuakira Takeda, M.D., Ph.D.
Associate Professor
Department of Internal Medicine
Aoto Hospital
Jikei University School of Medicine
Aoto 6-41-2
Katsushika-ku
Tokyo 125
Japan

Koon K. Teo, M.B.B.Ch., Ph.D.
Associate Professor of Medicine
Department of Medicine
University of Alberta
EPICORE Centre
2C2 Mackenzie Centre
Edmonton, Alberta T6G 2R7
Canada

Ganghong Tian, M.Sc., Ph.D.
Junior Research Officer
Department of Biosystems
Institute for Biodiagnostics
National Research Council Canada
435 Ellice Avenue
Winnipeg, Manitoba R3B 1Y6
Canada

Takashi Tsuda, M.D.
First Department of Internal Medicine
Niigata University School of Medicine
Asahimachi 1-754
Niigata 951
Japan

Suresh C. Tyagi, Ph.D.
Assistant Professor
Division of Cardiology
University of Missouri Health
   Sciences Center
Room MA432 Medical Science
   Building
Columbia, Missouri 65212
United States

Karl T. Weber, M.D.
Professor of Medicine
Division of Cardiology
University of Missouri Health
   Sciences Center
Room MA432 Medical Health
   Sciences Building
Columbia, Missouri 65212
United States

**E. Douglas Wigle, M.D.,
   F.R.C.P.(C.), F.A.C.P., F.A.C.C.**
Professor
Department of Medicine
Division of Cardiology
University of Toronto
The Toronto Hospital
General Division
200 Elizabeth Street
Toronto, Ontario M5G 2C4
Canada

Randall G. Williams, M.D.
Director
Coronary Care Unit
Royal Alexandra Hospital
6227 Royal Alexandra Hospital
10240 Kingsway Avenue
Edmonton, Alberta T5H 3V9; and
Lecturer
Department of Medicine
Division of Cardiology
University of Alberta Hospitals
2C2 Mackenzie Centre
Edmonton, Alberta T6G 2R7
Canada

Takashi Yanaga, M.D.
Professor
Department of Bioclimatology and
   Medicine
Medical Institute of Bioregulation
Kyushu University
4546 Tsurumihara
Beppu, Oita 874
Japan

Lorraine Yau, B.Sc.
Department of Physiology
Division of Cardiovascular Sciences
Faculty of Medicine
University of Manitoba
St. Boniface General Hospital
  Research Centre
351 Taché Avenue
Winnipeg, Manitoba R2H 2A6
Canada

Salim Yusuf, M.B.B.S., D. Phil.,
  F.R.C.P.(U.K.), F.R.C.P.C.,
  F.A.C.C.
Professor of Medicine
Director, Division of Cardiology
Department of Medicine
McMaster University
Hamilton General Hospital
237 Barton Street East
Hamilton, Ontario L8L 2X2
Canada

Peter Zahradka, Ph.D.
Assistant Professor
Department of Physiology
Division of Cardiovascular Sciences
Faculty of Medicine
University of Manitoba
St. Boniface General Hospital
  Research Centre
351 Taché Avenue
Winnipeg, Manitoba R2H 2A6
Canada

Preface

The heart was recognized as a pump in the Hippocratic era and Harvey described its circulation in 1628. In the following centuries, great progress was made in understanding the structure and function of the heart when it performs its task adequately, in health or disease. Knowledge of its performance when it becomes inadequate and fails to meet the requirements of the body it inhabits developed slowly. As Paul Wood observed, "The mechanism, and even the definition, of heart failure have been debated for over a century, and are still a source of controversy." The "backward-failure" concept was expressed by James Hope in 1832 but gave way to James Mackenzie's 1913 "forward-failure" hypothesis. In recent decades, the development of cardiac catheterization, sophisticated imaging devices, and new biochemical and metabolic assessments have increased our understanding of the heart but not enough to prevent the extensive morbidity and mortality of heart failure.

In 1992, the World Health Organization identified heart disease as the leading cause of death world-wide. Ironically, this harvest of death continues despite the great progress in prevention and treatment that has occurred during the past several decades. One of the reasons for this paradox is that control or eradication of several deadly diseases has spared many only to reach the age where heart disease becomes more frequent. As life expectancy lengthens, the incidence of heart disease increases and the heart, handicapped by disease, is unable to meet the demands of the body. This state of heart failure is characterized by impaired cardiac contraction, neuroendocrine changes, and exercise intolerance. As medical and surgical advances have increased survival of heart disease, the number of patients who live long enough to develop heart failure has also increased. It is now said that the only kind of heart disease that is not diminishing is heart failure. The "golden age of cardiology" is giving way to "the decade of heart failure."

In an effort to meet the challenge of the increasing incidence of heart failure, the International Conference on Heart Failure was held in Winnipeg, Canada in 1994. The purpose of the meeting was to bring together leading basic scientists and clinicians to improve knowledge of the pathophysiology and treatment of heart failure. The conference resulted in a synthesis of state-of-the-art information in molecular biology, cellular physiology, and structure-function relationships in the cardiovascular system in health and disease.

This book presents some selected papers that describe fundamental mechanisms underlying heart failure, and the medical and surgical approaches to its prevention and treatment. These chapters have been organized in three sections: Pathophysiologic and Clinical Considerations, Ventricular Remodeling and Renin-Angiotensin System, and Treatment of Heart Failure. This book will be of interest to clinical and experimental cardiologists.

Naranjan S. Dhalla
Robert E. Beamish
Makoto Nagano
Nobuakira Takeda

Acknowledgments

Thank you to Dr. Howard Morgan, Chairman of the Council on Molecular and Cellular Cardiology of the International Society and Federation of Cardiology for the sponsorship of this symposium. The collaboration of the Japanese Working Group on Cardiac Structure and Metabolism in this event is gratefully acknowledged. The help of Susan Zettler for the preparation of this book is highly appreciated. Special thanks to Lisa S. Berger and the editorial staff at Lippincott-Raven Publishers for their patience, interest, and hard work in assembling this volume.

We are grateful to the following institutions and corporations, both North American and Japanese, for their generous donations in support of the International Conference on Heart Failure, Winnipeg, Canada (May 20–23, 1994), as well as publication of this book: Banyu Pharmaceutical Co. Ltd.; Bayer Yakuhin Ltd.; Beckman Instruments (Canada) Ltd.; Boots Pharmaceutical; Bristol Myers Squibb Company; Bristol Myers Squibb Canada; Burroughs Wellcome Inc.; Calo International Ltd.; Chugai Pharmaceutical Co. Ltd.; Ciba-Geigy (Japan) Ltd.; Ciba-Geigy Canada Ltd.; Daiichi Pharmaceutical Co. Ltd.; Dainippon Pharmaceutical Co. Ltd.; Department of Cardiology, St. Boniface General Hospital; Department of Physiology, University of Manitoba; Eli Lily Canada Inc.; Faculty of Medicine, University of Manitoba; Fujisawa Canada Inc.; Fujisawa Pharmaceutical Co. Ltd.; Health Sciences Centre Research Foundation; Heart & Stroke Foundation of Manitoba; International Society and Federation of Cardiology–Council on Molecular and Cellular Cardiology; Japan Heart Foundation; Kaken Pharmaceutical Co. Ltd.; Kowa Shinyaku Co. Ltd.; Kuramoto Memorial Hospital; Kyowa Hakkou Kogyo Co. Ltd.; Manitoba Health Research Council; Marion Merrel Dow Canada; Medical Research Council of Canada; Medtronic of Canada Ltd.; Merck Frosst Canada Inc.; Miles Canada Inc.; Nippon Shinyaku Co. Ltd.; Ono Pharmaceutical Co. Ltd.; Otsuka Pharmaceutical Co. Ltd.; Parke-Davis; The Paul H. T. Thorlakson Foundation; Pfizer Canada Inc.; Pfizer Pharmaceuticals Inc.; Rhone-Poulenc Rorer Canada Inc.; Sandoz Canada Inc.; Sankyo Co. Ltd.; Searle Canada Inc.; Servier Canada Inc.; Shionogi Co. Ltd.; St. Boniface General Hospital Research Foundation; Sumitomo Co. Ltd.; Takeda Chemical Industries Co. Ltd.; Tanabe Seiyaku Co. Ltd.; Thomas Sill Foundation; Toray Medical Co. Ltd.; Warner Lambert Canada Inc.; Yoshitomi Pharmaceutical Industries Ltd.; Zeneca Pharma Inc.; and Zeria Pharmaceutical Co. Ltd.

The Failing Heart

The Failing Heart, edited by N. S. Dhalla,
R. E. Beamish, N. Takeda, and M. Nagano.
Lippincott-Raven Publishers, Philadelphia © 1995.

1

Demographic and Clinical Predictors of One-Year Outcome in Patients with Left Ventricular Dysfunction and/or Congestive Heart Failure: Results from the Studies of Left Ventricular Dysfunction Registry

Martial G. Bourassa

Montreal Heart Institute, Montreal, Quebec, H1T 1C8 Canada

Between 2.5 and 3 million people suffer from chronic congestive heart failure (CHF) in North America, and over 400,000 new cases are diagnosed each year (1–3). The incidence of CHF has more than doubled during the last two decades, to a large extent because of the increased life expectancy of the population. The Framingham study estimates indicate that the prevalence of heart failure increases progressively with age, from about 1% in those aged 50 to 59 years, to a prevalence of about 10% in persons 80 to 89 years (4,5). Both the prevalence and the incidence of new onset of heart failure approximately double with each decade of age (4,5). At virtually all ages, in the Framingham study, the incidence in men exceeds that in women (4,5). The incidence of heart failure is also greater in Whites than in Blacks (6). This is very likely because of a higher incidence of coronary heart disease in men than in women, and in Whites than in Blacks.

The prognosis of patients with CHF is grim (1,2,7–9). Approximately 20% die within the first year after diagnosis and between 10% and 20%, depending on severity of disease, subsequently die each year. Five-year survival is usually less than 50%. At least one-third of patients with CHF are hospitalized each year, and between 15% and 20% are hospitalized multiple times each year (8). Congestive heart failure is also responsible for countless visits to physicians' offices annually. Again, the Framingham study has shown that the prognosis of CHF is poorer in women than in men (4,5). More recently, Gillum suggested that Blacks with CHF also have a poorer prognosis than Whites (10).

The Studies of Left Ventricular Dysfunction (SOLVD) Registry was undertaken to assess the clinical characteristics and the natural course of consecutive unselected patients with left ventricular dysfunction (LVD) and/or CHF (11). A total of 6,273

1

patients were enrolled over a period of 14 months from 18 of the 23 clinical sites participating in the SOLVD trials. Of these 6,273 patients, roughly 86% were Whites, 11% were Blacks, and 3% were from other racial groups; 74% were men and 26% were women. Demographic, clinical, and laboratory data were obtained at baseline and at 1 year, vital status was available for 99% of patients and information on hospital admissions for 96%. This large, recent, hospital-based databank offers a unique opportunity to study the distribution of demographic and clinical features in patients with LVD and/or CHF and the influence of these factors on mortality and hospitalization at 1-year follow-up.

DISTRUBUTION OF DEMOGRAPHIC AND CLINICAL CHARACTERISTICS IN PATIENTS WITH LEFT VENTRICULAR DYSFUNCTION AND/OR CONGESTIVE HEART FAILURE

Age

The mean age was 62 ± 12 years in the SOLVD Registry, and about 60 % of the patients were 60 years of age or older. As indicated in the Framingham study (4,5), the incidence of LVD and/or CHF increased markedly with age. It practically doubled with each decade up to age 65, reaching a plateau between ages 65 and 75 and progressively declining afterward. At all ages, except for the 55-to-64 decade, Blacks with LVD and/or CHF were significantly younger than Whites (Fig. 1). Women were significantly older than men (not shown).

Etiology of Left Ventricular Dysfunction and/or Congestive Heart Failure

In contrast to the Framingham study (4,5), ischemic heart disease was the underlying etiology in approximately 70% of the Registry population, whereas hypertensive heart disease was considered to be primarily involved in only 7%. An idi-

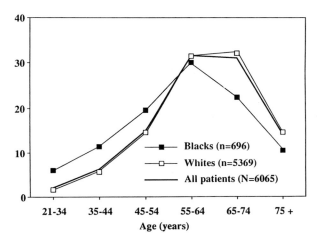

FIG. 1. Distribution of LVD and/or CHF by age.

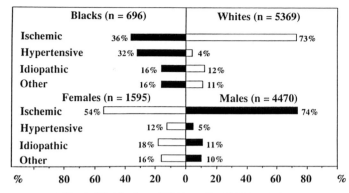

FIG. 2. Distribution of LVD and/or CHF by etiology.

opathic dilated cardiomyopathy was responsible for 13% of cases, and other etiologies, such as valvular heart disease and secondary cardiomyopathies, were responsible for 11%.

There were striking differences in the etiology of LVD and/or CHF among Blacks and Whites, and among men and women (Fig. 2). Seventy-three percent of Whites had an ischemic etiology versus only 36% of Blacks. Four percent of Whites had a hypertensive condition versus 32% of Blacks. Seventy-four percent of men had an ischemic etiology versus 54% of women, and 5% of men had hypertensive heart disease versus 12% of women (Fig. 2). Idiopathic dilated cardiomyopathy and other etiologies were also slightly more frequent in Blacks and in women (Fig. 2).

Ejection Fraction

Mean ejection fraction (EF) was $31 \pm 9\%$ in the SOLVD Registry. The severity of LVD (i.e., the reduction in EF) was similar among Blacks and Whites and among men and women (Fig. 3).

Hypertension and Diabetes Mellitus

Hypertension was present in 68% of Blacks versus 40% of Whites, and almost one-third of Blacks with LVD and/or CHF suffered from diabetes mellitus versus 22% of Whites (Fig. 4A). Hypertension and diabetes mellitus were also significantly more frequent in women than in men with LVD and/or CHF (Fig. 4B).

PREDICTORS OF CLINICAL EVENTS AT 1 YEAR

The total 1-year mortality was 18% in the SOLVD Registry. Slightly over half of these patients died of progressive CHF, and roughly 80% of the other deaths were of

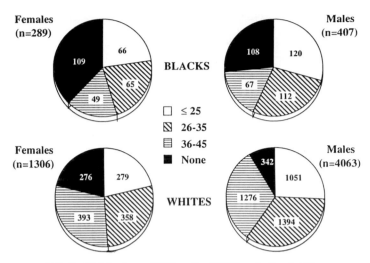

FIG. 3. Distribution of LVD and/or CHF by ejection fraction.

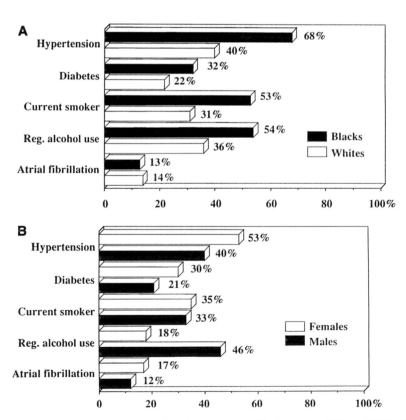

FIG. 4. (**A**) Distribution of LVD and/or CHF by risk factors: Blacks versus Whites. (**B**) Distribution of LVD and/or CHF by risk factors: females versus males.

cardiovascular origin. Nineteen percent of the patients were hospitalized for CHF, and 27% either died or were hospitalized for CHF during the first year of follow-up.

Several variables such as age, gender, race, etiology, EF, diabetes mellitus, hypertension, and atrial fibrillation influenced the rates of mortality and hospitalization at 1 year in the SOLVD Registry.

Age

Age markedly influenced all follow-up events at 1 year, including total mortality, mortality related to CHF, hospitalizations for CHF, and deaths or hospitalizations for CHF (Fig. 5). For all endpoints, the rate of events was relatively low in patients less than 55 years of age, and increased steadily thereafter. Patients 75 years of age or older often had more than twice the rate of younger patients.

Gender

Women had higher rates for all events than men: 22% total mortality rate versus 17% for men, 12% CHF mortality rate versus 9% for men, 22% CHF hospitalizations versus 17% for men, and 33% deaths or CHF hospitalizations versus 25% for men (Fig. 6A).

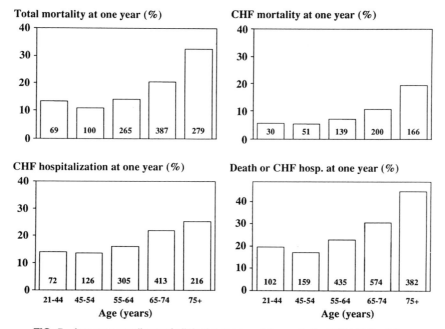

FIG. 5. Age as a predictor of clinical outcome at 1 year in the SOLVD Registry.

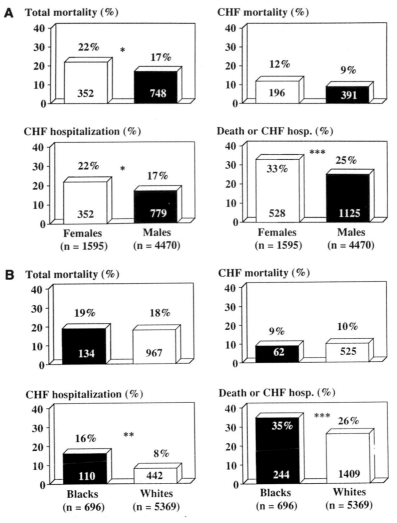

FIG. 6. **(A)** Gender as a predictor of clinical outcome at 1 year in the SOLVD Registry. **(B)** Race as a predictor of clinical outcome at 1 year in the SOLVD Registry. *p<0.05; **p<0.01; ***p<0.001.

Race

Total mortality, cardiovascular mortality, and mortality rates associated with progressive CHF were similar among Blacks and Whites in the SOLVD Registry. However, twice as many Blacks were hospitalized for CHF during this period: 16% versus 8%. When the endpoints of death or hospitalization for CHF were combined, Blacks had a higher rate of these events than Whites: 35% versus 26% (Fig. 6B).

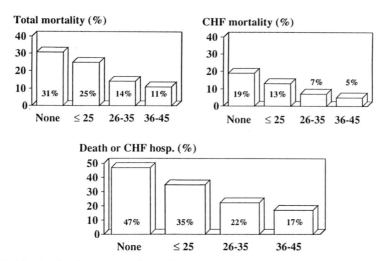

FIG. 7. Ejection fraction as a predictor of clinical outcome at 1 year in the SOLVD Registry.

Ejection Fraction

Total mortality rates and the incidence of deaths or hospital admissions for CHF increased markedly with decreasing EF (Fig. 7). Patients with an EF of 25% or less had more than twice the rate of events of patients with an EF between 36% and 45%. However, patients enrolled in the Registry not on the basis of an EF but because of a hospital discharge diagnosis of CHF with radiologic evidence of pulmonary congestion had the highest event rates at 1 year.

Etiology

The rates of total mortality, CHF mortality, and death or CHF hospitalizations at 1 year did not appear to be directly influenced by the origin of heart failure (Fig. 8).

Diabetes Mellitus, Hypertension, and Atrial Fibrillation

The presence of diabetes mellitus, atrial fibrillation, and, to a lesser extent, hypertension was a significant determinant of mortality and/or hospitalization rates in these patients with LVD and/or CHF (Fig. 9). The higher frequency of diabetes and hypertension in minorities and in women probably explains, to some extent, the higher rate of events at 1 year in these subgroups.

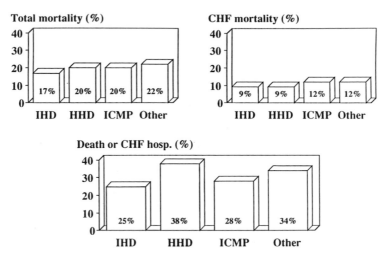

FIG. 8. Etiology of LVD and/or CHF as a predictor of clinical outcome at 1 year in the SOLVD Registry. IHD, ischemic heart disease; HHD, hypertensive heart disease; ICMP, idiopathic cardiomyopathy.

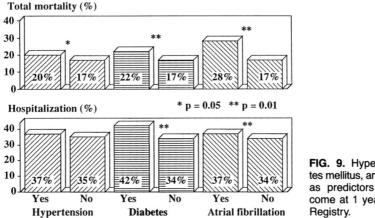

FIG. 9. Hypertension, diabetes mellitus, and atrial fibrillation as predictors of clinical outcome at 1 year in the SOLVD Registry.

LOG-RANK TESTS OF DIFFERENCES AND ODDS RATIOS

The strongest predictors of mortality and mortality or CHF hospitalization in the SOLVD Registry were, in a decreasing order of importance, age ≥65, EF <35%, presence of atrial fibrillation and diabetes mellitus, female gender, and ischemic etiology of heart failure (Table 1). Black race and a history of hypertension were not predictive of mortality at 1 year, but they were significantly related to an increased number of CHF hospitalizations.

TABLE 1. *Log-rank tests of differences in survival curves and odds ratios for selected variables in the SOLVD Registry*

Variable	Death		CHF hospitalization		Death or CHF hospitalization	
	Chi square	Odds ratio	Chi square	Odds ratio	Chi square	Odds ratio
Age (≥65 vs. <65)	230.1***	1.48***	63.6***	1.31***	247.9***	1.44***
Sex (M/F)	22.2***	0.70***	13.6**	0.75**	38.6***	0.67***
Race (W/B)	2.9	0.91	47.9***	1.33***	10.7***	1.09
Ejection fraction (<35% vs. ≥35%)	100.1***	1.56***	78.3***	1.64***	148.0***	1.66***
Atrial fibrillation (Y/N)	41.9***	1.81***	14.1**	1.39*	52.2***	1.76***
Diabetes mellitus (Y/N)	19.3***	1.37***	50.4***	1.78***	60.9***	1.63***
Etiology of CHF (ischemic vs. others)	8.1†	1.11**	41.3***	1.14***	33.1***	1.14***
Hypertension (Y/N)	2.3	1.14	9.0*	1.27*	11.5**	1.24**

Reprinted from Bourassa et al. (6), Table 2, with permission from the *Journal of the American College of Cardiology.*
p value: †*p*<0.05; *p*<0.01; **p*<0.001; ***p*<0.0001.
CHF, congestive heart failure; M, male; F, female; W, White; B, Black; Y, yes; N, no.

A multivariate analysis in patients with ischemic heart disease (roughly 70% of the SOLVD Registry population) selected age ≥65, EF <35%, female gender, and presence of diabetes mellitus and atrial fibrillation as independently related to death and death or CHF hospitalization at 1 year in the SOLVD Registry (6).

Prevention of Left Ventricular Dysfunction and/or Congestive Heart Failure

The SOLVD treatment and prevention trials have shown that an angiotensin-converting enzyme (ACE) inhibitor, enalapril, significantly reduces mortality and CHF hospitalizations in patients with overt CHF and prevents the occurrence of CHF and hospitalizations for CHF in patients with asymptomatic LVD (8,12). Although they were not prestated subgroup analyses in the SOLVD trials, there was no evidence in these studies that older patients, minorities, and women benefit more from ACE inhibitors than do their counterparts (8,12).

CONCLUSIONS

In summary, older patients, women, and minorities have an increased incidence of LVD and/or CHF and a poorer prognosis when these conditions are present. Left ventricular dysfunction and/or CHF should be treated aggressively in these sub-groups.

SUMMARY

The SOLVD Registry was undertaken to assess the demographic and clinical characteristics and the natural course of consecutive unselected patients with LVD and/or CHF. A total of 6,273 patients (11% Blacks and 26% women) were enrolled over a period of 14 months, and followed up for vital status and hospital admissions at 1 year. The incidence of LVD and/or CHF increased markedly with age; women with LVD and/or CHF were older than men, and Whites were older than Blacks. An ischemic etiology of LVD and/or CHF was present in 73% of Whites versus 36% of Blacks, and in 74% of men versus 54% of women, whereas hypertensive heart disease was the underlying cause in 4% of Whites versus 36% of Blacks, and in 5% of men versus 12% of women. Hypertension and diabetes mellitus were more frequent in Blacks and in women. Total mortality and mortality or CHF hospitalization at 1 year were strongly related to increasing age, female gender, decreasing EF, and the presence of diabetes mellitus and atrial fibrillation. Race was not related to mortality, but Blacks had a higher rate of CHF hospitalizations. Thus, older patients, women, and minorities have an increased incidence of LVD and/or CHF and a poorer prognosis when these conditions are present. Left ventricular dysfunction and/or CHF should be treated aggressively in these subgroups.

REFERENCES

1. Smith WM. Epidemiology of congestive heart failure. *Am J Cardiol* 1985;55:3A–8A.
2. Yusuf S, Thom T, Abbott RD. Changes in hypertension treatment and in congestive heart failure mortality in the United States. *Hypertension* 1989;13:174–179.
3. Brophy JM. Epidemiology of congestive heart failure: Canadian data from 1970 to 1989. *Can J Cardiol* 1992;8:495–498.
4. McKee PA, Castelli WP, McNamara PM, Kannel WB. The natural history of congestive heart failure: the Framingham study. *N Engl J Med* 1971;285:1441–1446.
5. Kannel WB, Bélanger AJ. Epidemiology of heart failure. *Am Heart J* 1991;121:951–957.
6. Bourassa MG, Gurné O, Bangdiwala SI, et al. Natural history and patterns of current practice in heart failure. *J Am Coll Cardiol* 1993;22:14A–19A.
7. Massie BM, Conway M. Survival of patients with congestive heart failure: past, present, and future prospects. *Circulation* 1987;75(suppl IV):IV-11–IV-19.
8. The SOLVD Investigators. Effects of enalapril on survival in patients with reduced left ventricular ejection fraction and congestive heart failure. *N Engl J Med* 1991;325:293–302.
9. The CONSENSUS Clinical Trial Study Group. Effects of enalapril on mortality in severe congestive heart failure: results of the Cooperative North Scandinavian Enalapril Survival Study (CONSENSUS). *N Engl J Med* 1987;316:1429–1435.
10. Gillum RT. Heart failure in the United States 1970–1985. *Am Heart J* 1987;113:1043–1045.
11. Bangdiwala SI, Weiner DH, Bourassa MG, Friesinger GC, Ghali JK, Yusuf S. Studies of Left Ventricular Dysfunction (SOLVD) Registry: rationale, design, methods and description of baseline characteristics. *Am J Cardiol* 1992;70:347–353.
12. The SOLVD Investigators. Effect of enalapril on mortality and the development of heart failure in asymptomatic patients with reduced left ventricular ejection fractions. *N Engl J Med* 1992;327:685–691.

The Failing Heart, edited by N. S. Dhalla,
R. E. Beamish, N. Takeda, and M. Nagano.
Lippincott-Raven Publishers, Philadelphia © 1995.

2

Atrial Fibrillation and Congestive Heart Failure

J. Thomas Heywood and *Gloria R. Engel

*Cardiomyopathy Service and *Department of Medicine,
Loma Linda University Medical Center, Loma Linda, California 92354 United States*

Congestive heart failure (CHF) and atrial fibrillation (AF), as two of the most frequently encountered disease entities in adult clinical medicine, often coexist and complicate the management of each other. Drugs effective in rate control have negative inotropic effects which may limit their usefulness when heart failure is present. Antiarrhythmic drugs commonly used to restore and maintain sinus rhythm appear to increase mortality in patients with decreased left ventricular systolic function. Therefore, the management of AF, both acutely and chronically, in the presence of CHF differs significantly from the management in patients with normal systolic function.

EPIDEMIOLOGY

Atrial fibrillation is the most common arrhythmia requiring therapy (1). In younger individuals AF is uncommon; about 0.4% of the population will have this dysrhythmia, whereas the prevalence increases to 2% to 4% in those over age 70. In the presence of cardiovascular disease, the prevalence increases to about 4% and has been reported to be as high as 40% in patients with overt CHF (2).

The Framingham study found that the most likely precursors to AF were cardiac failure and rheumatic heart disease (3). In men with cardiac failure followed for 2 years, 42.4% developed chronic and 33.6% developed transient AF, with risk ratios of 8.5 and 8.2, respectively. In women with cardiac failure followed for the same period, 45.1% developed chronic and 42.9% developed acute AF with corresponding risk ratios of 13.7 and 20.4. In contrast, hypertensive heart disease conveys a risk ratio for AF of about 4 in all groups (3). The Reykjavik study found that the overall prevalence of chronic AF was 276 per 100,000 in persons aged 32 to 64 years. In 14 years of follow-up of patients with chronic AF, 36% had CHF compared with only 2% of controls without AF (4).

MECHANISM

The precise mechanism of AF is unknown, but histopathological features found in patients with this dysrhythmia have been well described (5,6). Ischemia, valvular dysfunction, ventricular dysfunction, and direct myocyte toxins increase left and right atrial pressure. Over time, this leads to atrial dilatation and fibrosis within the atrial wall (7). Sinus node disease and dysfunction are frequently found at autopsy in those with AF; so failure of the normal sinus mechanism may be an integral feature of the dysrhythmia (8). In general, AF can result when orderly electrical propagation no longer occurs through the atria because of fibrosis and scarring and the depolarization wave front fractionates because of areas of fibrotic tissue (9). (See Fig. 1.)

Prognosis

In patients referred for cardiac transplantation, mortality is increased when AF is present, compared with patients in sinus rhythm. Middlekauff et al. found a decreased 1-year actuarial survival in AF versus sinus rhythm—52% versus 71% in patients with severe heart failure referred for transplant evaluation (10). The sudden-death-free survival is 69% in the same patient population with AF, compared with 82% in patients with sinus rhythm. Multivariate analysis has shown that the presence of AF in patients aged 17 to 73 with idiopathic dilated cardiomyopathy

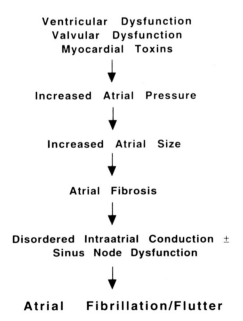

FIG. 1. Pathogenesis of atrial fibrillation/flutter.

followed for 4 years increases the probability of death from both CHF and sudden death (11).

The incidence of stroke is greater in patients with chronic AF when it complicates new-onset CHF with a relative risk of 2.6. This risk is greater than that conferred by age, hypertension, or even a history of previous thromboembolism (12).

Patients with both AF and CHF have decreased exercise capacity as determined by decreased maximum $\dot{V}O_2$, compared with patients with lone AF. At the same time, patients with lone AF have equally decreased capacity, compared with age-matched controls with sinus rhythm (13). On the other hand, in a study by Atwood et al. (14), the functional capacity of patients with lone AF was compared with age-matched controls in sinus rhythm. They found that the exercise limitation had more to do with the cardiac disease than with AF per se.

Acute Restoration of Sinus Rhythm in Atrial Fibrillation

Acute restoration of sinus rhythm is necessary when the sudden onset of AF or atrial flutter produces CHF (15). In a minority of patients, loss of the sinus mechanism and atrial transport produces a significant reduction in cardiac output and systemic blood pressure (16,17). This scenario is especially likely when left ventricular hypertrophy is present, and adequate filling depends on atrial contraction. Left ventricular hypertrophy delays ventricular relaxation, reducing early diastolic filling so that a major portion of filling occurs with atrial systole (18). The loss of atrial contraction with AF in this setting can be poorly tolerated. A second mechanism is the tachycardia freqently associated with the acute onset of AF which can produce ischemia, shorten ventricular filling, and raise end-diastolic pressures. Emergency cardioversion is the treatment of choice in patients in whom acute AF has produced clinical and hemodynamic deterioration (15).

Acute Control of Ventricular Response in Atrial Fibrillation or Flutter

Digoxin

For the majority of patients with the acute onset of AF, even in the setting of chronic CHF, the dysrhythmia results in mild-to-moderate symptoms of increased shortness of breath, fatigue, palpitations, or chest discomfort. Heart rate control is not so urgent and can be obtained pharmacologically rather than through cardioversion. Digoxin has many theoretical and practical advantages in this setting (19). Various preparations of digitalis glycosides have been available for over 200 years to slow ventricular response in AF, so clinicians have great experience with this agent (20). Its beneficial effect on left ventricular function makes it an even more appropriate choice for heart rate control in the setting of systolic dysfunction (21,22). When given acutely, however, up to 9 hours are required to achieve a significant reduction in heart rate, and toxicity with this agent is neither infrequent nor benign (23–25). Many different regimens exist for the administration of digoxin. For patients not currently taking the agent, 0.5 mg are given intravenously, followed by 0.25 mg every 2 to 4 hours until the heart rate falls consistently below 90 to 100 beats per minute or 1.5 to 2.0 mg have been given in a 24-hour period. Although approximately 50% of patients return to sinus rhythm when hospitalized for an acute episode of AF with the administration of digoxin, this same effect is seen with placebo (26,27).

Beta-adrenergic Blocking Agents

Although beta-adrenergic receptor blockers, especially given intravenously, have been extensively used for heart rate control in AF, they should be used very cautiously, if at all, when CHF is present. Acute exacerbations of heart failure have been reported with the administration of intravenous beta antagonists (28). Moreover, when there is significant left ventricular dysfunction (LVD), these agents can result in reduction in ejection fraction (EF) and elevation in pulmonary artery wedge pressure. Iskandrian et al. (29) reported that 10 to 16 mg/min of esmolol reduced the EF from 27% to 21% in patients with LVD. The wedge pressure rose from 11 to 15 mmHg as well. Shettigar et al. (30) studied the effect of combining esmolol and digoxin for the acute control of heart rate in AF. A significant reduction in heart rate occurred within 20 minutes with this combination. Seven patients had evidence of LVD at the initiation of the trial (EF 18–61%), and this became transiently worse in one patient. Hypotension is a significant side effect of esmolol (31). Beta-antagonists may be better tolerated in the setting of heart failure with diastolic dysfunction, but there is not enough clinical information about their use in this setting to recommend them when clinical heart failure is present.

Calcium Channel Blocking Agents

Calcium channel blockers, specifically verapamil and diltiazem, impede conduction across the atrioventricular node and thus have been studied for heart rate control in AF. Evaluating the effects of calcium channel blockers on left ventricular function is complex because they can simultaneously impair contractility, reduce afterload, and produce reflex sympathetic simulation (32). Thus, classical measures of left ventricular function such as changes in maximum dp/dt are actually composites of these effects when calcium channel blockers are given. Böhm et al. (33) attempted to minimize these interactions by placing papillary muscle excised from patients undergoing transplant or mitral valve replacement in physiologic solutions into which various calcium channel blockers were added (33). Changes in contractile force could be measured directly in this way. They reported that on an equimolar basis, nifedipine had the greatest negative inotropic effect, followed by verapamil. Diltiazem had about one-third the reduction of verapamil, and the newer dihydropyridine calcium channel blockers had almost negligible negative inotropic

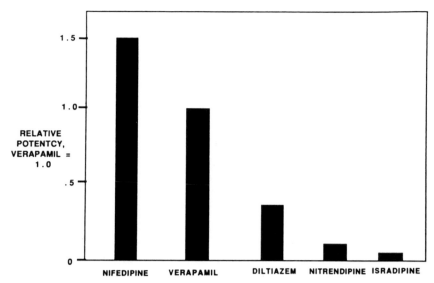

FIG. 2. Equimolar amounts of various calcium antagonists were placed in a solution bathing papill-ary muscles obtained from patients undergoing mitral valve replacement. The relative effects of each agent on myocardial contraction are shown. Data from Böhm et al. (33); figure reprinted from Heywood JT. Calcium antagonists and left ventricular function. *Am J Cardiol* 1991;68:52C–57C.

effects. However, the dihydropyridines are not useful for the treatment of AF be-cause of their minimal effects on atrioventricular (AV) node conduction (Fig. 2).

There are only limited data about the use of verapamil in patients with impaired left ventricular systolic function, with or without AF. Ferlinz and Citron (34) gave 0.1 mg/kg intravenous verapamil to patients undergoing cardiac catheterization. Average EF rose from 29% to 37% with a concomitant fall in systemic vascular resistance. Left ventricular diastolic pressure was unchanged, although right atrial pressure rose significantly. Chew et al. (35) administered a larger bolus (0.145 mg/kg) followed by an infusion to a diverse group of patients with acute myocardial infarction and symptomatic coronary artery disease. Of the 25 patients in this study, three had mean wedge pressure >20 mmHg and EF <35%. These three patients deteriorated clinically and hemodynamically with the drug infusion. There are other isolated reports of CHF developing after verapamil administration (36,37).

Although diltiazem reduces contractility (38), there is evidence that it can be administered in the setting of ventricular dysfunction without causing hemodynamic compromise (39). We evaluated the effects of intravenous diltiazem in nine patients with AF with rapid ventricular response complicated by CHF (40). A pulmonary artery catheter was placed prior to the administration of 0.25 mg/kg diltiazem given over 2 minutes. Average heart rate fell from 142 to 114 beats per minute with eight of the nine patients responding to this treatment. Systemic vascular resistance de-clined from a mean of 1,838 to 1,464 dynes/s/cm^{-5} ($p = 0.02$), whereas the wedge

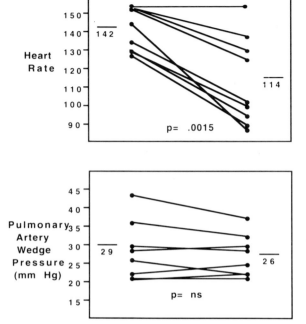

FIG. 3. Effect of intravenous diltiazem on heart rate and pulmonary artery wedge pressure in nine patients presenting with AF and rapid ventricular response and CHF; mean EF 34% (range 15–65). Data from Heywood et al. (40).

pressure was not significantly different with diltiazem (Fig. 3). No patient had an exacerbation of heart failure with diltiazem.

A multicenter, placebo-controlled trial has evaluated the safety and efficacy of acute intravenous diltiazem again in patients with rapid AF and CHF (41). In this study of 37 patients, 21 of 22 patients responded to diltiazem with a 20% reduction in heart rate, compared with none of the patients receiving placebo initially. No patient developed worsening heart failure with diltiazem, and 54% reported improvement in their symptoms, compared with none of the patients with placebo. Four patients receiving diltiazem became hypotensive, which resolved without pharmacologic intervention.

In summary, experience is very limited with either verapamil or diltiazem in the treatment of AF with rapid ventricular response complicated by CHF. A minority of patients with decompensated left ventricular function can worsen clinically with verapamil; however, this drug has not been evaluated specifically in the setting of rapid AF and CHF. Patients who present with CHF secondary to diastolic dysfunction would most likely improve with verapamil because of rate control and improved relaxation (42). There are more clinical data with diltiazem in this setting, but the data are limited to fewer than 50 patients.

Chronic Control of Ventricular Response in Atrial Fibrillation or Flutter

Digoxin

As in the acute management of rapid ventricular response, digoxin has primacy of place for chronic heart rate control of AF. Digoxin frequently provides adequate heart rate control at rest. Unfortunately, heart rate control is not so successful during exercise. Digoxin reduces ventricular response by directly reducing conduction through the AV node as well as by enhancing vagal tone (43). With exercise, vagal tone is withdrawn, and there is rapid increase of heart rate when digoxin alone is used for rate control. Roth et al. found that 66% of the total increase in heart rate occurred after only 1 minute of exercise when digoxin alone was used for heart rate control (44). This response would seemingly be accentuated in CHF because sympathetic tone as reflected by circulating norepinephrine levels is higher than in patients with normal left ventricular systolic function (45). Since digoxin produces improvements in exercise performance and EF and reduces the rate of rehospitalization in patients with heart failure, however, it should be included in the management of heart rate in AF complicated by CHF (22). The effect of digoxin on long-term survival in heart failure is not clear, but is being evaluated in the Digoxin Investigator Group trial, the results of which should be available in 1996.

Calcium Channel Blocking Agents

Although calcium channel blockers are very useful for the acute management of ventricular response in AF, even when it is complicated by CHF, their use in chronic rate control in this setting is problematic. Verapamil, because of its significant negative inotropic effects, can cause acute deterioration of hemodynamics and thus should be used very cautiously, if at all, in the setting of systolic dysfunction and CHF (35,46). Diltiazem, although well tolerated acutely, has been shown to worsen mortality when used in patients with roentgenographic pulmonary edema following a myocardial infarction (47). Although these data cannot be generalized to all patients with CHF, this safety concern for the long-term use of diltiazem should not be ignored (48,49). In the absence of data proving the safety of diltiazem in this setting, its long-term use should be avoided in the setting of heart failure and AF.

Beta-adrenergic Blocking Agents

Many studies have demonstrated the effectiveness of beta-adrenergic blocking agents for chronic heart rate control in AF (50,51). These agents traditionally have been thought to be contraindicated in patients with significant LVD. Data are rapidly accumulating, however, which challenge this view. In the Beta Blocker Heart Attack Trial (BHAT), propranolol reduced the risk of sudden death by almost 50%

in the group with some clinical signs of CHF, whereas there was no significant reduction in sudden death in those without failure (52). Many small trials have reported clinical improvement with beta blockers with improvement in functional status and EF (53,54). The largest trial to date, Metoprolol in Dilated Cardiomyopathy, also demonstrated an improvement in EF and a reduced need for transplantation in patients given beta blockers (55). Although the study was unblinded, it was a large, placebo-controlled multicenter trial whose results were concordant with other trials (Figs. 4 and 5).

Beta blockers are not as useful for the acute control of AF with rapid ventricular response because they must be used in dosage ranges that produce significant acute reductions in ventricular function (29). When beta blockers are given for the treatment of CHF alone, however, the initial doses are very small and are increased very gradually (55). Given in this way, the majority of patients with idiopathic dilated CHF tolerate beta-antagonists, with substantial improvement in a minority. The safety data from multiple beta blocker trials in heart failure and from the BHAT trial are much more impressive than for calcium channel blockers for the same population. Therefore, based on clinical evidence, there is much firmer support for the use of beta blockers for heart rate control in AF with heart failure than for calcium channel blockers. Indeed, even digoxin, although universally used in this setting, has not been shown to be safe.

In our cardiomyopathy clinic we have used beta blockers for AF and chronic rate control in patients. Beta blockers are generally well tolerated, although an occasional patient feels unwell with them, at which point they are stopped. The usual

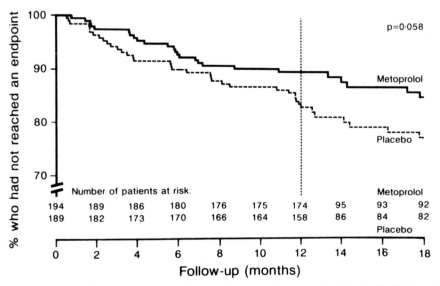

FIG. 4. Likelihood of reaching an endpoint, death, or need for transplantation in the Metoprolol in Dilated Cardiomyopathy Study. From Waagstein et al. (55).

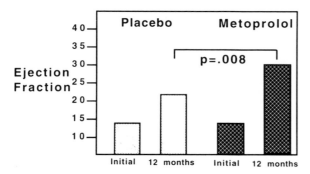

FIG. 5. Effects of metoprolol on EF in patients with initial EF less than 20% after 12 months of therapy; *p* value refers to difference in EF at 12 months between the placebo and metoprolol group. From Waagstein et al. (Metoprolol in Dilated Cardiomyopathy Trial) (55).

initial dose is 6.25 mg of metoprolol given twice a day with a doubling of the dose every week after a careful evaluation of the patient for appropriate heart rate, blood pressure, signs and symptoms of CHF, and overall tolerance of the medication. The target dose is 50 mg twice or three times a day (55). Beta blockers should be used in conjunction with digoxin rather than replacing it. In addition, we have seen similar improvement of EF in patients with AF to that which has been reported in CHF patients in sinus rhythm placed on metoprolol.

Nonpharmacologic Means of Rate Control

Atrioventricular node ablation and modification is now available as a nonpharmacologic means of heart rate control (56–58). This electrophysiologic technique produces either complete AV block requiring placement of a permanent pacemaker or selective ablation of the slow pathway so that heart rate is controlled in AF without the need for permanent pacing (59). This technique has a high success rate and a low complication rate (57). It has been employed in patients with CHF with AF safely with actual long-term improvement in cardiac function following the ablation and subsequent heart rate control (58,60,61). Scheinmann and his group report that hospitalization rates decline substantially for patients with difficult-to-control AF who undergo this procedure (62). Currently it is unclear what the precise role of this new and evolving technology will be. In its current form, however, it should be considered strongly for patients in whom heart rate control is difficult with digoxin alone and who have contraindications to beta blockers. Certainly some physicians will be reluctant to prescribe beta blockers for patients with heart failure, and some patients will be intolerant of beta blockers. Atrioventricular node modification then becomes the preferred option when digoxin alone is inadequate for heart rate control (Fig. 6).

Beyond simply controlling the heart rate, in some cases atrial flutter can be terminated and sinus rhythm restored by delivery of radio frequency energy to the right atrium (63). This technique is still relatively new and there are few data about

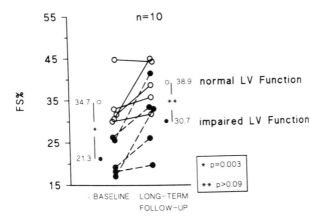

FIG. 6. Change in fractional shortening reported by Heinz et al. following AV node ablation in AF and atrial flutter. Long-term follow-up was a mean of 49 days after the ablation. From Heinz et al. (60).

patients who have CHF. Atrial flutter can be especially difficult to control medically, however, so if this technique proves to be effective in the long term, it will be especially appealing.

Antiarrhythmic Therapy for Maintenance of Sinus Rhythm in the Setting of Congestive Heart Failure

Because LVD so often precedes the development of AF, the issue of the safety and effectiveness of antiarrhthymic agents in this setting is germane. The development of AF is eight times more likely when the syndrome of CHF is present (4). Atrial fibrillation itself limits exercise tolerance, and the restoration of sinus rhythm has been demonstrated to improve indices of exercise performance and ventricular performance (64,65). Restoration of sinus rhythm also may reduce the risk of thromboembolic complications seen with both AF and CHF. For all of these reasons, clinicians often work diligently to restore sinus rhythm in the setting of CHF. What are the risks and benefits of antiarrhythmic therapy for AF when LVD is present?

Type IA Agents

Quinidine has been used since the early part of the twentieth century to restore and maintain sinus rhythm after an episode of AF (66). In unselected individuals, quinidine increases the likelihood that sinus rhythm will be maintained for a year from 25% to approximately 50% (67). On the other hand, it has been long appreciated that quinidine can produce life-threatening ventricular dysrhythmias, especially torsades de pointes, although the risk of this was thought to be small in patients with AF. A meta-analysis reported by Coplen et al. (67) demonstrated that mortality was, on average, three times higher in individuals given quinidine versus nothing

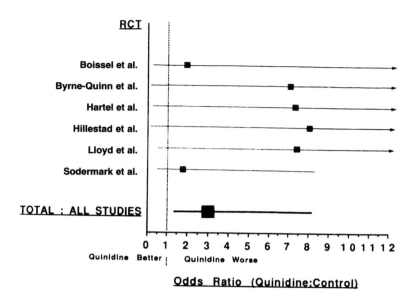

FIG. 7. Odds ratios for total mortality in six randomized trials comparing quinidine with a control group. For the pooled data, the mortality rate was three times higher with quinidine. From Coplen et al. (67).

for their AF (Fig. 7). There has been much criticism of their analysis, but it is clear that of the studies they collected, at least 1% to 2% of the patients either died or had a life-threatening ventricular dysrhythmia during the first week of their quinidine therapy. This finding was not seen in the groups not given quinidine. In a retrospective analysis of their data on stroke in AF, the Stroke Prevention in Atrial Fibrillation investigators found that antiarrhythmic therapy, in the presence of LVD, increased the risk of death by 3.3 times (68).

These findings, coupled with the well-known adverse effect that antiarrhythmic therapy produced in the Cardiac Arrhythmia Suppression Trial (CAST), indicate that antiarrhythmic agents, especially quinidine, should be used with great caution in the setting of LVD (69). Quinidine should not be started in the outpatient setting in patients with LVD. Many (but not all) of the proarrhythmic events occur early, especially during the conversion to sinus rhythm. It is clear that the long-term safety of quinidine is *not* proven for the maintenance of sinus rhythm in the context of CHF. Patients should have very strong clinical indications for conversion to or maintenance of sinus rhythm to warrant the inconvenience of hospitalization for drug initiation and the small but real risk of long-term therapy with quinidine. In general, this drug should be avoided when LVD is present.

Procainamide is also useful for restoration of sinus rhythm and has mild negative inotropic effects (70–72). Still, torsades is seen with procainamide, and the same precautions advised for quinidine should be taken. Disopyramide is more effective than placebo in maintaining sinus rhythm following direct-current cardioversion

(73). Unfortunately, it has significant negative inotropic effects and can produce ventricular proarrhythmic events (74). Its use in the setting of CHF has been disappointing (75). For these reasons, it should not be used to maintain sinus rhythm in the setting of CHF.

Type IC Agents

There is less experience with the newer type IC agents for the maintenance of sinus rhythm. Flecainide is effective in this regard, but it causes considerable depression of left ventricular function even when the EF is in the 35% to 40% range (76–78). Encainide appears to have fewer negative effects on ventricular function than does flecainide. The results of the CAST study with a clear increase in mortality in the groups given flecainide or encainide, indicate that chronic use of these agents for maintenance of sinus rhythm in patients with decreased ventricular function has not been proven to be safe and is most likely detrimental, and so should be avoided (69,79,80).

Several studies have demonstrated the usefulness of propafenone for the acute conversion of AF to sinus rhythm and its maintenance following direct-current cardioversion (77,81). These studies specifically excluded patients with CHF. In a large trial using various antiarrhythmic agents for the control of ventricular arrhythmias, propafenone induced new heart failure in 4.7% and worsened existing failure in 9.3% (82). This last study was limited to a 2-week period, so long-term effects of propafenone on ventricular function are unknown. Because of the effects on ventricular function and well-described proarrhythmic effects, which are likely to be poorly tolerated in the presence of ventricular dysfunction, propafenone should probably be used infrequently for maintenance of sinus rhythm in existing heart failure (79).

Type III Agents

Sotolol is a racemic compound consisting of d-sotolol with type III antiarrhythmic properties and l-sotolol, a beta antagonist. It has been used extensively for the control of ventricular dysrhythmias and appears to have a favorable effect on mortality (83). Its use in AF and atrial flutter has been more limited (84). Juul-Möller et al. (85) found that it was as effective as quinidine for the maintenance of sinus rhythm following cardioversion but with a much better side-effect profile. Nonetheless, there was at least one episode of severe proarrhythmia with sotolol. The potential for proarrhythmia with this drug is underscored by the fact that a recent trial of oral d-sotolol to prevent sudden death in patients with CHF and history of myocardial infarction was stopped because of increased mortality in the d-sotolol group. Thus, the long-term safety of sotolol in patients with ventricular dysfunction remains in doubt. This fact, coupled with the negative inotropic effect of sotolol, will limit the usefulness of this agent for AF in this group of patients (86).

For years, amiodarone has been the drug of last resort for difficult-to-control ventricular and atrial dysrhythmias. It is expensive and can produce significant, even life-threatening, side effects, such as marked photosensitivity, hepatitis and cirrhosis, and pulmonary toxicity (87). These effects are more pronounced at higher dosages of the drug, rather than the 200 mg/d dose that is the typical treatment for atrial arrhythmias (88). On the other hand, amiodarone seems to maintain some individuals in sinus rhythm when other drugs have failed. Gosselink et al. (89) gave an average of 200 mg/d of amiodarone to 89 patients who had failed to remain in sinus rhythm despite a trial of at least one antiarrhythmic agent. On an actuarial basis, 53% remained in sinus rhythm for 3 years. Of note, 14 of the subjects had severe CHF. Amiodarone did not exacerbate their heart function clinically, and 13 remained in sinus rhythm. One patient died due to progressive heart failure during the study.

Amiodarone can produce proarrhythymias, but these appear to be unusual (90,91). Gosselink et al. (89) started their patients on amiodarone in the outpatient setting with only one death from CHF and no sudden deaths. A recently completed trial from Argentina, in which amiodarone was given to patients with heart failure, demonstrated a reduction in risk of mortality of 28% (Fig. 8) (92). However, a double-blind trial from the United States, in which amiodarone or placebo was given to patients with mild-to-moderate heart failure, showed no change in mortal-

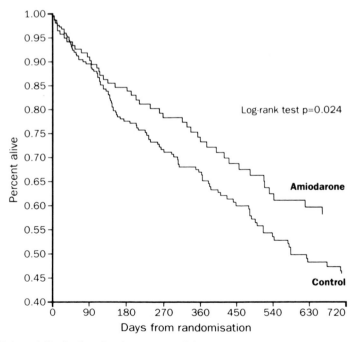

FIG. 8. Total mortality for the placebo group and the group given amiodarone (target dose 300 mg/d) in the GESICA trial. From Doval et al. (92).

ity (93). It is as yet unclear whether amiodarone improves mortality in patients with significant ventricular impairment, but, unlike so many other agents, it does not appear to worsen mortality. A randomized double-blind large-scale trial using amiodarone, which would examine both the efficacy of the drug and quantify adverse events in AF, has not been done (94).

Surgical techniques have been introduced, such as the maze procedure and the corridor procedure, which interrupt atrial reentry and restore sinus rhythm (95–97). As yet, these procedures have been reported on about 100 individuals. In most, sinus rhythm is restored, albeit a significant minority require pacemaker or single antiarrhythmic therapy to maintain sinus rhythm. Importantly, the atrial transport mechanism still functions, although its adequacy remains undetermined (97).

This is a remarkable achievement for individuals who have failed multiple drug attempts to maintain sinus rhythm. Lengthy follow-up data, however, are still lacking and are urgently needed before this procedure could be recommended to more than a small minority of patients with AF and heart failure. The issue of heart failure is especially germane because a significant minority of these patients develop marked fluid retention following the procedure, presumably on the basis of impaired production of atrial natriuretic hormones (95).

Rapid Atrial Fibrillation/Flutter Producing Congestive Heart Failure: Tachycardia-induced Cardiomyopathy

Classically, CHF has been viewed as a risk factor for the development of AF. Interestingly, there are a growing number of reports that long-standing AF, especially with poorly controlled ventricular response, can result in CHF (60,98,99). For several decades there have been reports of clinical heart failure resulting from incessant, rapid atrial arrhythmias, and more importantly, improvement of cardiac function if the heart rate could be controlled (100). Most of these early studies described patients with AV nodal reentrant tachycardias rather than AF (101,102).

Grogan et al. (99) reported a series of ten patients presenting with symptoms and signs of heart failure who were found to be in AF with rapid ventricular response. These patients had initial EFs of 12% to 30%. After controlling ventricular rate (and in half the cases, restoring sinus rhythm), all patients' symptoms had resolved, and EFs improved to 40% to 64% (Fig. 9). Similar improvement in ventricular function and clinical status has been reported by employing AV node ablation when ventricular response cannot be controlled pharmacologically (60).

If adequate rate control in AF can result in improved ventricular function for patients with heart failure, how should this be achieved? Based on the preceding discussion, an effort should be made to maintain sinus rhythm. Cardioversion is indicated when LVD complicates AF because of exercise improvement with return of sinus rhythm and increased risk of stroke with fibrillation (68). When the duration of fibrillation increases, however, and especially when it exceeds 1 year, the likelihood of prolonged sinus rhythm is reduced (103).

Pt.	Age (yr) & Sex	Initial NYHA Functional Class	Initial Heart Rate (beats/min)	Initial Ejection Fraction (%)	Follow-Up Heart Rate (beats/min)	Follow-Up Rhythm	Follow-Up Ejection Fraction (%)	Follow-Up Type of Treatment*	Follow-Up Duration (mos.)
1	22 F	III	175	25	66	AF	52	Amiodarone (digoxin, enalapril)	30
2	36 M	IV	140	29	50	SR	52	DC cardioversion (digoxin, quinidine)	22
3	38 M	III	180	12†	50	AF	40	DC cardioversion (digoxin, quinidine, nifedipine)	35
4	53 F	III	120	28	70	SR	61	DC cardioversion (digoxin, enalapril)	30
5	55 F	IV	150	20	80	SR	54	Amiodarone (digoxin, lisinopril)	56
6	58 M	III	150	24	60	AF	52	Digoxin, encainide (diltiazem, captopril, α-methyldopa)	14
7	60 F	III	140	28	50	AF	50	Amiodarone (diltiazem)	44
8	60 M	IV	130	23†	50	SR	64	DC cardioversion (digoxin, lisinopril, flecainide)	30
9	61 M	III	140	25	60	SR	50	Amiodarone (captopril, digoxin)	3
10	80 F	II	120	30	70	AF	60	Digoxin, propranolol	21

*Primary treatment that led to ventricular rate control or conversion to sinus rhythm is noted; other cardiac medications (with exception of diuretics) used at time of follow-up are in parentheses.
†Ejection fraction determined by ventriculography, rather than echocardiography.
AF = atrial fibrillation; DC = direct-current; NYHA = New York Heart Association; SR = sinus rhythm.

FIG. 9. Clinical characteristics, treatment, and outcome of ten patients with very rapid AF initially thought to have dilated cardiomyopathy, but who improved markedly with heart rate control. From Grogan et al. (99).

If cardioversion fails, amiodarone may be tried. Its reduced rate of proarrhythmic events, low-dose requirement for atrial dysrhythmias, and perhaps mortality benefit in CHF argue for this role. This agent may not cause reversion to sinus regimen by itself, so patients may require electrical cardioversion (89). A reasonable dose is 600 mg/d for 1 month and then 200 mg/d. Cardioversion can be done about 6 weeks after starting the drug. Several studies in heart failure have begun therapy with these doses in an outpatient setting. Although amiodarone is not completely free of proarrhythmic events, the rate appears low enough that this approach seems reasonable.

A significant proportion of patients, however, will not remain in sinus rhythm, even with amiodarone. How should the heart rate be controlled? Digoxin and beta blocker slowly titrated to produce a resting heart rate of 60 to 70 beats a minute are preferred for reasons stated previously. Alternatively, AV node ablation can be performed, either in patients intolerant of beta blockers or in those who have inadequate rate control despite them. Warfarin should be used in patients who do not show significant contraindications for its use.

SUMMARY

After years of neglect, the most common clinically significant arrhythmia, AF, is becoming the object of intense study. Only a few years ago, management consisted

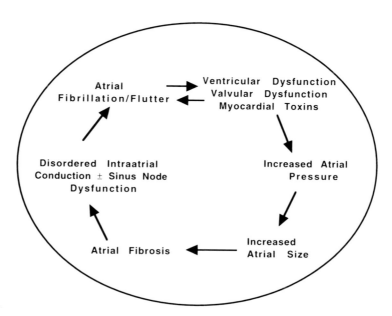

FIG. 10. The relationship between AF and CHF is more complex than thought initially. It is now clear that rapid AF per se can cause heart failure. More importantly, long-term heart rate control can reverse LVD in some cases.

of the almost reflexive combination of digoxin and quinidine. Now, large clinical trials have demonstrated new concepts—that the incidence of stroke can be reduced substantially in AF, while quinidine may be actually more harmful than beneficial. This is especially true in patients with heart failure. Heart failure and AF have a close and fascinating relationship. When one is present, the other is more likely to develop, and each one complicates the management of the other. Still, the presence of either can present unique opportunities only recently recognized. Namely, if both heart failure and AF are present, either can be aggressively treated, and both conditions may benefit. Skillful management of AF in the presence of heart failure can result in marked improvement in symptoms and patient well-being (Fig. 10).

REFERENCES

1. Podrid PJ, Falk RH. Pathology of atrial fibrillation: insights for autopsy studies. In: Falk RH, Podrid PJ, eds. *Atrial fibrillation: mechanisms and management*. New York: Raven Press; 1992:1–14.
2. Alpert JS, Petersen P, Godtfredsen J. Atrial fibrillation: natural history, complications and management. *Annu Rev Med* 1988;39:41–52.
3. Kannel WB, Abbott RD, Savage DD, McNamara PM. Coronary heart disease and atrial fibrillation: the Framingham study. *Am Heart J* 1983;106:389–396.
4. Önundarson PT, Thorgeirsson G, Jonmundsson E, Sigfusson N, Hardarson T. Chronic atrial fibrillation—epidemiologic features and 14 year follow-up: a case control study. *Eur Heart J* 1987; 8:521–527.
5. Davies MJ, Pomerance A. Pathology of atrial fibrillation in man. *Br Heart J* 1972;34:520–525.
6. Davies MJ, Anderson RH, Becker AE. Pathology of atrial arrhythmias. In: *The conduction system of the heart*. London: Butterworths; 1983:205–215.
7. Bharati S, Lev M. Histology of the normal and diseased atrium. In: Falk RH, Podrid PJ, eds. *Atrial fibrillation: mechanisms and management*. New York: Raven Press; 1992:15–39.
8. Waldo AL. Mechanisms of atrial fibrillation, atrial flutter and ectopic atrial tachycardia—a brief review. *Circulation* 1987;75:III-37–III-40.
9. Moe GK, Abildskov JA. Atrial fibrillation as a self sustaining arrhythmia independent of focal discharge. *Am Heart J* 1959;58:59–70.
10. Middlekauff HR, Stevenson WG, Stevenson LW. Prognostic significance of atrial fibrillation in advanced heart failure—a study of 390 patients. *Circulation* 1991;84:40–48.
11. Hofmann T, Meinertz T, Kasper W, et al. Mode of death in idiopathic dilated cardiomyopathy: a multivariate analysis of prognostic determinants. *Am Heart J* 1988;116:1455–1463.
12. The Stroke Prevention in Atrial Fibrillation Investigators. Predictors of thromboembolism in atrial fibrillation: I. Clinical features of patients at risk. *Ann Intern Med* 1992;116:1–7.
13. Ueshima K, Myers J, Ribisl PM, et al. Hemodynamic determinants of exercise capacity in chronic atrial fibrillation. *Am Heart J* 1993;125:1301–1305.
14. Atwood JE, Myers J, Sullivan M, et al. Maximal exercise testing and gas exchange in patients with chronic atrial fibrillation *J Am Coll Cardiol* 1988;11:508–513.
15. Podrid PJ, Falk RH. Management of atrial fibrillation—an overview. In: Falk RH, Podrid PJ, eds. *Atrial fibrillation: mechanism and management*. New York: Raven Press; 1992:400.
16. Linderer T, Chatterjee K, Parmley WW. Influence of atrial systole on the Frank-Starling relation and the end-diastolic pressure-diameter relation of the left ventricle. *Circulation* 1983;67:1045–1053.
17. Love JC, Haffajee CI, Gore JM, Alpert JS. Reversibility of hypotension and shock by atrial or atrio-ventricular sequential pacing in patients with right ventricular infarction. *Am Heart J* 1984; 108:5–13.
18. Lorell BH, Grossman W. Cardiac hypertrophy: consequences for diastole. *J Am Coll Cardiol* 1987; 9:1189–1193.
19. Meijler FL. An "account" of digitalis and atrial fibrillation. *J Am Coll Cardiol* 1985;5:60A–68A.
20. Ferriar J. An essay on the medical properties of digitalis purpurea. In: *Medical histories and reflections*. London: Cadell and Davies; 1810:281–344.

21. Cattell M, Gold H. The influence of digitalis glucosides on the force of contraction of mammalian cardiac muscle. *J Pharm Exp Ther* 1938;62:116–125.
22. Captopril Digoxin Multicenter Research Group. Comparative effects of therapy with captopril and digoxin in patients with mild to moderate heart failure. *JAMA* 1988;259:539–544.
23. Roberts SA, Diaz C, Nolan PE, et al. Effectiveness and costs of digoxin treatment for atrial fibrillation and flutter. *Am J Cardiol* 1993;72:567–573.
24. Fisch C, Knoebel SB. Digitalis cardiotoxicity. *J Am Coll Cardiol* 1985;5:91A–98A.
25. Beller GA, Smith TW, Abelmann WH, Haber E, Hood WB. Digitalis intoxication: a prospective clinical study with serum level correlations. *N Engl J Med* 1971;284:989–997.
26. Falk RH, Knowlton AA, Bernard SA, Gotlieb NE, Battinelli NJ. Digoxin for converting recent-onset atrial fibrillation to sinus rhythm. A randomized, double-blinded trial. *Ann Intern Med* 1987; 106:503–506.
27. Rawles JM, Metcalfe MJ, Jennings K. Time of occurrence, duration, and ventricular rate of paroxysmal atrial fibrillation: the effect of digoxin. *Br Heart J* 1990;63:225–227.
28. Epstein SE, Braunwald E. The effect of β-adrenergic blockade on patterns of urinary sodium excretion: studies in normal subjects and in patients with heart disease. *Ann Intern Med* 1966; 65: 20–27.
29. Iskandrian AS, Bemis CE, Hakki AH, et al. Effects of esmolol on patients with left ventricular dysfunction. *J Am Coll Cardiol* 1986;8:225–231.
30. Shettigar UR, Toole JG, Appunn DO. Combined use of esmolol and digoxin in the acute treatment of atrial fibrillation or flutter. *Am Heart J* 1993;126:368–374.
31. The Esmolol Multicenter Study Research Group. Efficacy and safety of esmolol vs propranolol in the treatment of supraventricular tachyarrhythmias: a multicenter double-blind clinical trial. *Am Heart J* 1985;110:913–922.
32. Francis GS. Calcium channel blockers and congestive heart failure. *Circulation* 1991;83:336–338.
33. Böhm M, Schwinger RHG, Erdmann E. Different cardiodepressant potency of various calcium antagonists in human myocardium. *Am J Cardiol* 1990;65:1039–1041.
34. Ferlinz J, Citron PD. Hemodynamic and myocardial performance characteristics after verapamil use in congestive heart failure. *Am J Cardiol* 1983;51:1339–1345.
35. Chew CYC, Hecht HS, Collett JT, McAllister RG, Singh BN. Influence of severity of ventricular dysfunction on hemodynamic responses to intravenously administered verapamil in ischemic heart disease. *Am J Cardiol* 1981;47:917–922.
36. Platia EV, Michelson EL, Porterfield JK, Das G. Esmolol versus verapamil in the acute treatment of atrial fibrillation or atrial flutter. *Am J Cardiol* 1989;63:925–929.
37. Mohindra SK. Long-acting verapamil and heart failure [Letter]. *JAMA* 1989;261:994.
38. Murikami T, Hess OM, Krayenbühl HP. Left ventricular function before and after diltiazem in patients with coronary artery disease. *J Am Coll Cardiol* 1985;5:723–730.
39. Walsh RW, Porter CB, Starling MR, O'Rourke RA. Beneficial hemodynamic effects of intravenous and oral diltiazem in severe congestive heart failure. *J Am Coll Cardiol* 1984;3:1044–1050.
40. Heywood JT, Graham B, Marais GE, Jutzy KR. Effects of intravenous diltiazem on rapid atrial fibrillation accompanied by congestive heart failure. *Am J Cardiol* 1991;67:1150–1152.
41. Goldenberg IF, Lewis WR, Dias VC, Heywood JT, Pedersen WR. Intravenous diltiazem for the treatment of patients with atrial fibrillation or flutter and moderate to severe congestive heart failure. *Am J Cardiol* 1994;74:884–889.
42. Setaro JF, Zaret BL, Schulman DS, Black HR, Soufer R. Usefulness of verapamil for congestive heart failure associated with abnormal left ventricular diastolic filling and normal left ventricular systolic performance. *Am J Cardiol* 1990;66:981–986.
43. Hoffman BF, Singer DH. Effects of digitalis on electrical activity of cardiac fibers. *Prog Cardiovasc Dis* 1964;7:226–265.
44. Roth A, Harrison E, Mitani G, Cohen J, Rahimtoola SH, Elkayam U. Efficacy and safety of medium- and high-dose diltiazem alone and in combination with digoxin for control of heart rate at rest and during exercise in patients with chronic atrial fibrillation. *Circulation* 1986;73:316–324.
45. Cohn JN, Levine TB, Olivari MT, et al. Plasma norepinephrine as a guide to prognosis in patients with chronic congestive heart failure. *N Engl J Med* 1984;311:819–823.
46. Ferlinz J, Gallo CT. Responses of patients in heart failure to long-term oral verapamil administration. *Circulation* 1984;70:II-305 (abst).
47. The Multicenter Diltiazem Postinfarction Trial Research Group. The effect of diltiazem on mortality and reinfarction after myocardial infarction. *N Engl J Med* 1988;319:385–392.

48. Figulla HR, Rechenberg JV, Wiegand V, Soballa R, Kreuzer H. Beneficial effects of long-term diltiazem treatment in dilated cardiomyopathy. *J Am Coll Cardiol* 1989;13:653–658.
49. Packer M, Kessler PD, Lee WH. Calcium-channel blockade in the management of severe chronic congestive heart failure: a bridge too far. *Circulation* 1987;75:V-56–V-64.
50. Atwood JE, Sullivan M, Forbes S, et al. Effect of beta-adrenergic blockade on exercise performance in patients with chronic atrial fibrillation. *J Am Coll Cardiol* 1987;10:314–320.
51. Matsuda M, Matsuda Y, Yamagishi T, et al. Effects of digoxin, propranolol, and verapamil on exercise in patients with chronic isolated atrial fibrillation. *Cardiovasc Res* 1991;25:453–457.
52. Chadda K, Goldstein S, Byington R, Curb JD. Effect of propranolol after acute myocardial infarction in patients with congestive heart failure. *Circulation* 1986;73:503–510.
53. Waagstein F, Caidahl K, Wallentin I, Bergh CH, Hjalmarson Å. Long-term β-blockade in dilated cardiomyopathy: effects of short- and long-term metoprolol treatment followed by withdrawal and readministration of metoprolol. *Circulation* 1989;80:551–563.
54. Engelmeier RS, O'Connell JB, Walsh R, Rad N, Scanlon PJ, Gunnar RM. Improvement in symptoms and exercise tolerance by metoprolol in patients with dilated cardiomyopathy: a double-blind, randomized, placebo-controlled trial. *Circulation* 1985;72:536–546.
55. Waagstein F, Bristow MR, Swedberg K, et al., for the Metoprolol in Dilated Cardimyopathy Trial Study Group. Beneficial effects of metoprolol in idiopathic dilated cardiomyopathy. *Lancet* 1993; 342:1441–1446.
56. Scheinman MM, Laks MM, diMarco J, Plumb V. Current role of catheter ablative procedures in patients with cardiac arrhythmias; a report for health professionals from the Subcommittee on Electrocardiography and Electrophysiology, American Heart Association. *Circulation* 1991;83: 2146–2153.
57. Yeung-Lai-Wah JA, Alison JF, Lonegran L, Mohama R, Leather R, Kerr CR. High success rate of atrioventricular node ablation with radiofrequency energy. *J Am Coll Cardiol* 1991;18:1753–1758.
58. Kay GN, Bubien RS, Epstein AE, Plum VJ. Effect of catheter ablation of the atrioventricular junction on quality of life and exercise tolerance in paroxysmal atrial fibrillation. *Am J Cardiol* 1988;62:741–744.
59. Fleck RP, Chen PS, Boyce K, Ross R, Dittrich HC, Feld GK. Radiofrequency modification of atrioventricular conduction by selective ablation of the low posterior septal right atrium in a patient with atrial fibrillation and a rapid ventricular response. *PACE* 1993;16:377–381.
60. Heinz G, Siostrzonek P, Kreiner G, Gössinger H. Improvement in left ventricular systolic function after successful radiofrequency His bundle ablation for drug refractory, chronic atrial fibrillation and recurrent atrial flutter. *Am J Cardiol* 1992;69:489–492.
61. Twidale N, Sutton K, Bartlett L, et al. Effects on cardiac performance of atrioventricular node catheter ablation using radiofrequency current for drug-refractory atrial arrhythmias. *PACE* 1993; 16:1275–1284.
62. Fitzpatrick AP, Kourouyan HD, Siu A, Lesh MD, Griffin JC, Scheinmann MM. Quality of life and outcomes after radiofrequency His bundle catheter ablation and permanent pacemaker implantation. *J Am Coll Cardiol* 1994;23:350A.
63. Feld GK, Fleck P, Chen P-S, et al. Radiofrequency catheter ablation for the treatment of human type 1 atrial flutter: identification of a critical zone in the reentrant circuit by endocardial mapping techniques. *Circulation* 1992;86:1233–1240.
64. Atwood JE, Myers J, Sullivan M, et al. The effect of cardioversion on maximal exercise capacity in patients with chronic atrial fibrillation. *Am Heart J* 1989;118:913–918.
65. Van Gelder IC, Crijns HJGM, Blanksma PK, et al. Time course of hemodynamic changes and improvement of exercise after cardioversion of chronic atrial fibrillation unassociated with cardiac valve disease. *Am J Cardiol* 1993;72:560–566.
66. Frey W. Weitere Erfährungen mit Chinidin bei absoluter Herzunregelmässigkeit. *Berlin Klin Wochenschr* 1918;55:849–853.
67. Coplen SE, Antman EM, Berlin JA, Hewitt P, Chalmers TC. Efficacy and safety of quinidine therapy for maintenance of sinus rhythm after cardioversion; a meta-analysis of randomized control trials. *Circulation* 1990;82:1106–1116.
68. Flaker GC, Blackshear JL, McBride R, Kronmal RA, Halperin JL, Hart RG (The Stroke Prevention in Atrial Fibrillation Investigators). Antiarrhythmic drug therapy and cardiac mortality in atrial fibrillation. *J Am Coll Cardiol* 1992;20:527–532.
69. The Cardiac Arrhythmia Suppression Trial. Mortality and morbidity in patients receiving encainide, flecainide or placebo. *N Engl J Med* 1991;324:781–788.
70. Fenster PE, Comess KA, Marsh R, Katzenberg C, Hager WD. Conversion of atrial fibrillation to sinus rhythm by acute intravenous procainamide infusion. *Am Heart J* 1983;106:501–504.

71. Halpern SW, Ellrodt G, Singh BN, Mandel WJ. Efficacy of intravenous procainamide infusion in converting atrial fibrillation to sinus rhythm: relation to left atrial size. *Br Heart J* 1980;44:589–595.
72. Angelakos ET, Hastings EP. The influence of quinidine and procainamide of myocardial contractility in vivo. *Am J Cardiol* 1960;5:791–798.
73. Karlson BW, Torstensson I, Åbjörn C, Jansson S-O, Peterson L-E. Disopryramide in the maintenance of sinus rhythm after electroconversion of atrial fibrillation. A placebo-controlled one-year follow-up study. *Eur Heart J* 1988;9:284–290.
74. Hoffmeister HM, Hepp A, Seipel L. Negative inotropic effect of class I antiarrhythmic drugs: comparison of flecainide with disopyramide and quinidine. *Eur Heart J* 1987:8:1126–1132.
75. Podrid PJ, Schoeneberger A, Lown B. Congestive heart failure caused by oral disopyramide. *N Engl J Med* 1980;302:614–617.
76. Van Gelder IC, Crijns HJ, Van Gilst WH, Van Wijk LM, Hamer HPM, Lie KI. Efficacy and safety of flecainide acetate in the maintenance of sinus rhythm after electrical cardioversion of chronic atrial fibrillation or atrial flutter. *Am J Cardiol* 1989;64:1317–1321.
77. Kingma JH, Suttorp MJ. Acute pharmacologic conversion of atrial fibrillation and flutter: the role of flecainide, propafenone, and verapamil. *Am J Cardiol* 1992;70:56A–61A.
78. de Paola AAV, Horowitz LN, Morganroth J, et al. Influence of left ventricular dysfunction on flecainide therapy. *J Am Coll Cardiol* 1987;9:163–168.
79. Marcus FI. The hazards of using type 1C antiarrhythmic drugs for the treatment of paroxysmal atrial fibrillation. *Am J Cardiol* 1990;66:366–367.
80. Feld GF, Chen P-S, Nicod P, Fleck RP, Meyer D. Possible atrial proarrhthymic effects of class 1C antiarrhythmic drugs. *Am J Cardiol* 1990;66:378–383.
81. Reimold SC, Cantillon CO, Friedman PL, Antman EM. Propafenone versus sotalol for suppression of recurrent symptomatic atrial fibrillation. *Am J Cardiol* 1993;71:558–563.
82. Ravid S, Podrid PJ, Lampert S, Lown B. Congestive heart failure induced by six of the newer antiarrhythmic drugs. *J Am Coll Cardiol* 1989;14:1326–1330.
83. Mason JW, for the Electrophysiologic Study versus Electrocardiographic Monitoring Investigators. A comparison of seven antiarrhythmic drugs in patients with ventricular tachyarrhythmias. *N Engl J Med* 1993;329:452–458.
84. Suttrorp MJ, Kingma JH, Peels HOJ, et al. Effectiveness of sotalol in preventing supraventricular tachyarrhythmias shortly after coronary artery bypass grafting. *Am J Cardiol* 1991;68:1163–1169.
85. Juul-Möller S, Edvardsson N, Rehnqvist-Ahlberg N. Sotalol versus quinidine for the maintenance of sinus rhythm after direct current conversion of atrial fibrillation. *Circulation* 1990;82:1932–1939.
86. Alboni P, Razzolini R, Scarfo S, et al. Hemodynamic effects of oral sotalol during both sinus rhythm and atrial fibrillation. *J Am Coll Cardiol* 1993;22:1373–1377.
87. Zipes DP, Prystowsky EN, Heger IJ. Amiodarone: electrophysiologic actions, pharmacokinetics and clinical effects. *J Am Coll Cardiol* 1984;3:1059–1071.
88. Dusman RE, Stanton MS, Miles WM, et al. Clinical features of amiodarone-induced pulmonary toxicity. *Circulation* 1990;82:51–59.
89. Gosselink ATM, Crijns HJGM, Van Gelder IC, Hillige H, Wiesfeld ACP, Lie KI. Low-dose amiodarone for maintenance of sinus rhythm after cardioversion of atrial fibrillation or flutter. *JAMA* 1992;267:3289–3293.
90. Faber TS, Zehender M, Van de Loo A, Hohnloser S, Just H. Torsade de pointes complicating drug treatment of low-malignant forms of arrhythmia: four case reports. *Clin Cardiol* 1994;17:197–202.
91. Keren A, Tzivoni D, Gottlieb S, Benhorin J, Stern S. Atypical ventricular tachycardia (torsades de pointes) induced by amiodarone. *Chest* 1982;81:384–386.
92. Doval HC, Nul DR, Grancelli HO, Perrone SV, Bortman GR, Curiel R, for Grupo de Estudio de la Sobrevida en la Insuficiencia Cardiaca en Argentina (GESICA). Randomised trial of low-dose amiodarone in severe congestive heart failure. *Lancet* 1994;344:493–498.
93. Singh SN, Fletcher RD, Fisher SG, et al., and the CHF STAT Investigators. Results of the congestive heart failure survival trial of antiarrhythmic therapy. *Circulation* 1994;90:I-546.
94. Middlekauff HR, Wiener I, Saxon LA, Stevenson WG. Low-dose amiodarone for atrial fibrillation: time for a prospective study? *Ann Intern Med* 1992;116:1017–1020.
95. Cox JL, Schuessler RB, D'Agostino HJ, et al. The surgical treatment of atrial fibrillation. *J Thorac Cardiovasc Surg* 1991;101:569–583.

96. Defauw JJ, van Hemel NM, Vermeulen FE, Kingma JH, Verrostte JM, Guiraudon GM. Short-term results of the "corridor operation" for drug-refractory paroxysmal atrial fibrillation. *Circulation* 1988;78:II-43.
97. McCarthy PM, Castle LW, Maloney JD, et al. Initial experience with the maze procedure for atrial fibrillation. *J Thorac Cardiovasc Surg* 1993;105:1077–1087.
98. Phillips E, Levine SA. Auricular fibrillation without other evidence of heart disease: a cause of reversible heart failure. *Am J Med* 1949;7:478–489.
99. Grogan M, Smith HC, Gersh BJ, Wood DL. Left ventricular dysfunction due to atrial fibrillation in patients initially believed to have idiopathic dilated cardiomyopathy. *Am J Cardiol* 1992;69:1570–1573.
100. Coleman HN, Taylor RR, Pool PE, et al. Congestive heart failure following chronic tachycardia. *Am Heart J* 1971;81:790–798.
101. McLaran CH, Gersh BJ, Sugrue DD, Hammill SC, Seward JB, Holmes DR. Tachycardia induced myocardial dysfunction: A reversible phenomenon? *Br Heart J* 1985;53:323–327.
102. Packer DL, Bardy GH, Worley SJ, et al. Tachycardia-induced cardiomyopathy: a reversible form of left ventricular dysfunction. *Am J Cardiol* 1986;57:563–570.
103. Brodsky MA, Allen BJ, Capparelli EV, Luckett CR, Morton R, Henry WL. Factors determining maintenance of sinus rhythm after chronic atrial fibrillation with left atrial dilatation. *Am J Cardiol* 1989;63:1065–1068.

The Failing Heart, edited by N. S. Dhalla,
R. E. Beamish, N. Takeda, and M. Nagano.
Lippincott-Raven Publishers, Philadelphia © 1995.

3

Sudden Death and Arrhythmias Complicating Heart Failure

Steven N. Singh

Department of Medicine, Veterans Affairs Medical Center and Department of Medicine, Georgetown University, Washington, DC 20007 United States

Congestive heart failure (CHF) has been a major worldwide health care problem, affecting more than 3 million people in the United States alone, and accounts for 200,000 deaths annually (1). Close to half a million new cases are diagnosed each year, a major cause of excessive hospitalization. The annual budget applied toward the care of these patients is in excess of $8 billion. Despite recent advances in therapeutic strategies, the prognosis of patients with heart failure remains poor with a 5-year survival rate of about 25% in men and 38% in women (2). The annual mortality ranges between 12% and 15%, with approximately one-half of all deaths described as sudden, the rest being from pump failure (Table 1).

Not all sudden death is from a tachyarrhythmia, however. Luu et al. (3) studied 21 patients with advanced CHF who suffered cardiac arrests while awaiting transplantations (Fig. 1). Sixty-two percent of these patients had bradyarrhythmias or electromechanical dissociation, while only 30% had ventricular tachycardia or fibrillation. Thus, antiarrhythmic treatment with conventional agents will only have an effect, if any, in one-third of patients with aborted cardiac arrest and advanced CHF. Perhaps these figures do not apply to patients with lesser forms of heart failure where tachyarrhythmia genesis may be more applicable to their dying suddenly. It is of interest to note that even though ventricular arrhythmia is an important prognostic indicator, and a risk factor for premature death, especially in patients with heart failure, there is some concern that such arrhythmia will only predict cardiovascular mortality and not sudden death (4). In other words, the arrhythmia is an expression of a "dying ventricle." In the Vasodilator–Heart Failure Trials (VHeFT I and II), patients with higher exercise oxygen consumption, higher ejection fraction (EF), and lower plasma epinephrine levels had a lower percentage of deaths from pump failure (5).

Ventricular arrhythmias documented with ambulatory ECG recordings are an extremely common finding in patients with CHF. They express themselves as single premature ventricular contractions (PVCs), pairs, or nonsustained ventricular tach-

TABLE 1. *Mortality in congestive heart failure*

	(n)	One-year mortality (%)	Sudden death (%)
VHeFT I (37)	642	12	45
VHeFT II (32)	804	15	50
CHF STAT (23)	674	15	49

Numbers within parentheses indicate the references from which data were taken.
VHeFT, Vasodilator Heart Failure study; CHF STAT, Congestive Heart Failure Survival Trial of Antiarrhythmic Therapy.

ycardia (≥consecutive PVCs but<30 seconds). In a large study of patients with heart failure, 60% had ≥30 PVC/h and 62% had at least one event of nonsustained ventricular tachycardia (6). Table 2 summarizes the prevalence of ventricular arrhythmias in CHF.

The cellular mechanisms responsible for abnormal rhythm disturbances in the failing myocardium include triggered activity (after-potentials), enhanced automaticity, and reentry (Table 3) (7). The failing myocardium is usually hypertrophied, leading to an increased action potential duration with prolongation of repolarization, which may increase the likelihood of an after-potential. Moreover, because of cardiac dilatation, stretch-regulated channels will predispose to an excessive inward current and decreased outward current leading to triggered activity and subsequent arrhythmias. Reentry is perhaps the most common mechanism involved with arrhythmogenesis (Fig. 2 on page 36).

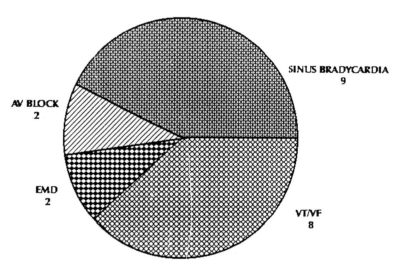

FIG. 1. Pie chart of initial rhythm of 21 cardiac arrests. Adapted with permission from Luu et al. (3). AV, atrio-ventricular; EMD, electromechanical dissociation; VT/VF, ventricular tachycardia/ventricular fibrillation.

TABLE 2. *Prevalence of ventricular arrhythmias in congestive heart failure*

	(n)	% with ≥10 PVC/h	% with ventricular tachycardia events
VHeFT I (37)	642	66	29
VHeFT II (32)	804	66	28
PROMISE (28)	1,088	60	60

VHeFT, Vasodilator Heart Failure Trial; PROMISE, Prospective, Randomized, Milrinone Survival Evaluation Trial.

METHODS TO EVALUATE VENTRICULAR ARRHYTHMIAS

Ambulatory ECG recordings have been the gold standard in quantifying ventricular arrhythmia density and have been used to gauge the successful or adverse effects of antiarrhythmic agents. Even though this technique can be equated to electrophysiologic testing (discussed next) in monitoring a high-risk population, such equality should be interpreted with caution, because the comparison was made in a very selective group of patients, with only 20% having had a cardiac arrest (8). Certainly ambulatory ECG is extremely helpful in symptomatic individuals in order to document objectively reasons for symptomatology.

The signal-averaged electrocardiogram is a noninvasive technique that allows a prediction of susceptible patients for a major arrhythmic event. When it is positive, especially in the presence of a left ventricular aneurysm, left ventricular dysfunction (LVD), and high PVC density, it has an excellent positive predictive value of either a spontaneous or electrophysiologically inducible sustained ventricular arrhythmia (9). It is a very good screening test for patients at high risk for a cardiac arrest and aids the physician in determining whether an aggressive approach to the patient might be necessary.

Electrophysiologic testing is reserved for patients presenting with a lethal arrhythmia, such as sustained ventricular tachycardia or an aborted cardiac arrest. Most of these patients have structural heart disease and reduced ejection fraction (EF) or CHF. This technique is used to guide antiarrhythmic therapy and has the potential of predicting outcome. In patients with advanced heart failure presenting

TABLE 3. *Cellular mechanisms of arrhythmias*

Mechanism	Requirements	Example
Triggered activity		
Early after-potential	↓ outward K^+ current	Quinidine toxicity
Late after-potential	↑ intracellular Ca^{2+}	Digitalis toxicity
Enhanced automaticity	↑ catecholamines	Ischemia
	↓ outward K^+	Hypokalemia
	↑ Ca^{2+} current	
Reentry	Slow conduction	Common variety of sustained ventricular
	Unidirectional block	tachycardia inducible with electro-
	Two pathways	physiologic testing

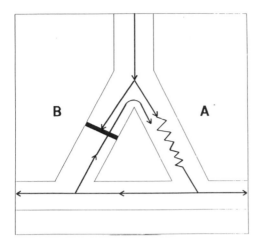

FIG. 2. Reentry occurs when impluse is blocked in pathway B, and conduction is slowed in pathway A, allowing enough time for pathway B to recover and conduct in a retrograde manner.

without significant arrhythmias, the yield of producing an electrophysiologically induced sustained arrhythmia is limited, especially in the setting of nonischemic cardiomyopathy (10).

TREATMENT

Because of the additional risk that ventricular arrhythmias pose to patients in heart failure, attempts to suppress such arrhythmias with the classical antiarrhythmic agents have been made. In order to keep it simple and structured, the studies involving the four different classes of antiarrhythmic agents are discussed (Table 4). The class I agents block sodium channels, interfering with depolarization and prolonging conduction velocity. In the Cardiac Arrhythmia Suppression Trial, drugs such as encainide and flecainide, despite their ability to suppress the arrhythmia,

TABLE 4. *Classification of antiarrhythmic drugs*

Class I: Sodium channel blockers (membrane stabilizers, depress depolarization)	
IA	Disopyramide, procainamide, quinidine
IB	Lidocaine, mexiletine, phenytoin, tocainide
IC	Encainide, flecainide, propafenone
Class II: Beta blockers (block beta-adrenergic receptors)	Propranolol, acebutolol, metoprolol
Class III: Potassium channel blockers (prolong repolarization)	Amiodarone, bretylium, sotalol
Class IV: Calcium channel blockers (block membrane calcium channels)	Diltiazem, nifedipine, verapamil

TABLE 5. *Effect by class*

Class	LVFx	Antiarrhythmic activity	Proarrhythmia
IA	↓	+ +	+ + +
IB	−	+ +	+
IC	↓	+ + + +	+ + + +
II	↑ ↓ −	+	−
III	↑ ↓ −	+ + + +	+
IV	↓	−	−

LVFx, left ventricular function; ↓, decrease in LV function; ↑, increase in LV function; −, no change; +, magnitude of strength of effect (arbitrary).

were harmful, with increases in both sudden and nonsudden deaths (11). It is well known that these agents depress left ventricular function and may lead to heart failure (12). It should be noted that there is an inverse relationship between left ventricular function, arrhythmia suppression, and toxicity (13). Simply stated, in the presence of heart failure, potent sodium channel blockers must be used with caution to avoid worsening heart failure and arrhythmia aggravation. Some sodium channel blockers (e.g., mexiletine) have little or no effect on left ventricular performance, with very little arrhythmia aggravation potential (14,15). Table 5 summarizes these various agents with respect to left ventricular function and antiarrhythmic and proarrhythmic activities.

Beta blockers (class II) improve survival, reducing sudden deaths and deaths from all causes, especially in the first 2 years after a myocardial infarction. This reduction in sudden death may be unrelated to PVC suppression and perhaps is related to the elevation of ventricular fibrillation threshold (16). The reduction in mortality is even more evident in the group with LVD (17). Chadda et al. (17), analyzing the data from the Beta Blocker Heart Atrial Trial (BHAT), found a strikingly differential response in both sudden and cardiovascular deaths, comparing the groups with and without heart failure. Moreover, Lichstein et al. (18) analyzed the relationship between beta blockers and left ventricular function and the chance of developing CHF. Those patients with the worst EF (<30%) who were on beta blockers had a much better outcome than those without such treatment. It appears that these agents provide better protection in patients with nonischemic cardiomyopathy. The Beta Blocker Survival Trial (BEST) is about to be initiated and will be randomizing patients in heart failure to beta blocker or placebo using angiotensin-converting enzyme inhibitors as background therapy.

There has been renewed interest in the class III antiarrhythmic agents, or potassium channel blockers. These compounds prolong repolarization and are considered antifibrillatory even though they may suppress ventricular tachycardia. The worst side effect of the class III agents is torsades de pointes, a pleomorphic ventricular tachycardia that may degenerate into ventricular fibrillation. This arrhythmia is usually bradycardia-dependent and occurs especially in the presence of heart failure and hypokalemia. Because of prolonged repolarization, calcium fluxes into the cardiac myocyte may be enhanced, leading to increased contractility, perhaps a desired effect in low-output states (19). A class III agent with the additional property of a beta blocker, dl sotalol, does not seem to affect adversely left ventricular performance (20). In the Electrophysiological Study versus Electrocardiographic Monitoring Study (ESVEM), with a mean EF of 32% for all patients, dl sotalol not only was best in protecting against inducible sustained arrhythmia, compared with six other antiarrhythmic agents, but also was significantly associated with less recurrence of spontaneous lethal arrhythmias (21). Because there was no control group, it would be difficult to judge its effect on survival.

The class III agent that has been studied most extensively is amiodarone. Even though its activity on suppression of arrhythmia is clear, the efficacy on survival is variable (22). Recently, the GESICA trial, involving patients with CHF, showed that amiodarone, compared with a control group, reduced not only sudden death and cardiovascular deaths, but also deaths from all causes (23). The Congestive Heart Failure Survival Trial of Antiarrhythmic Therapy (CHF STAT) has been completed, and the results will be available in the fall of 1995 (24).

Arrhythmias generated from automatic and triggered mechanisms may be calcium-mediated. Unfortunately, when calcium channel blockers (class IV) were tested in high-risk patients (i.e., those with CHF and prior myocardial infarction), these compounds tended to be harmful (25–27). Two vasoselective calcium channel blockers, amlodipine and felodipine, are being tested prospectively on a large scale in patients with heart failure.

The use of contractility agents in patients with heart failure has been a subject of great debate and interest. Despite their capabilities of increasing cardiac performance and exercise times, they have a propensity to increase cardiac arrhythmias and sudden death, and all-cause mortality (6,28). After 200 years, the use of digitalis is still in question. The Digoxin Investigator Group (DIG) study is currently randomizing patients on background angiotensin-converting enzyme inhibitors to either digoxin or placebo, the endpoint being death from all causes.

The angiotensin-converting enzyme inhibitors have undoubtedly been shown to improve survival in patients with heart failure and even in those with reduced EF (29,30). Although the Survival and Ventricular Enlargement Study (SAVE) and Survival of Left Ventricular Dysfunction (SOLVD) studies have shown no significant reductions in sudden death rates, the Vasodilator Heart Failure Trial (VHeFT II) showed that enalapril, compared with hydralazine-isosorbide combination, decreased sudden death (31). Moreover, in this study, ventricular tachycardia events were reduced over time (32). From these observations, it is reasonable to conclude that the angiotensin-converting enzyme inhibitors have the ability to decrease sudden arrhythmic deaths, perhaps by preventing deterioration of left ventricular function.

Antiplatelet agents, such as sulfurpyrazone and aspirin, will decrease sudden death (33,34). Such protection certainly relates to reduction in injury that might have led eventually to an arrhythmic substrate.

In the Coronary Artery Surgery Study (CASS), patients that were randomized to bypass surgery, compared with medically treated counterparts, had a decreased incidence of sudden death (35).

TABLE 6. *Guide to the use of pharmacologic agents in congestive heart failure*

Agents	Usage		
	Definite	Possible	Avoid
Contractility		* (short-term)	* (long-term)
Vasodilators	*		
Antiarrhythmics		*	
Beta blockers		*	
Calcium channel blockers			*
Antiplatelet/thrombotic agents	*		

*, recommended use.

Devices such as the Automatic Internal Defibrillation Cardioverter (AIDC) and Programmable Cardioverter Defibrillator (PCD) will reduce sudden death rates dramatically in patients whose arrhythmias cannot be controlled by pharmacologic means (36). These devices also have been used successfully as a bridge for cardiac transplantation. It is worthy to note that almost 60% of patients with these devices are on concomitant antiarrhythmic agents. The benefit in reducing deaths from all causes is still in question. The Canadian Implantable Device Study (CIDS) and the Antiarrhythmic versus Implantable Device (AVID) studies are comparing drugs to these devices on mortality rates.

SUMMARY

Congestive heart failure is associated with frequent ventricular arrhythmias, which act as a marker for a poorer prognosis. Attempts should be made to optimize therapy with antiplatelet agents, angiotensin-converting enzyme inhibitors, and cautious use of beta blockers. Contractility agents other than digoxin, at least for the moment, should be avoided on a long-term basis. Calcium channel blockers are contraindicated until the results of the vasoselective agent (felodipine, amlodipine) become available. Therapy with antiarrhythmic agents should be individualized. Table 6 summarizes a practical guide to the usage of various pharmacologic agents in CHF. Subsets of patients may benefit from implantable devices. Despite these endeavors, the prognosis of patients with CHF remains poor.

REFERENCES

1. Garg R, Packer M, Pitt B, Yusuf S. Heart failure in the 1990's: evolution of a major public health problem in cardiovascular medicine. *J Am Coll Cardiol* 1993;22[Suppl A]:3A–5A.
2. Ho K, Pinsky J, Kannel W, Levy D. The epidemiology of heart failure: the Framingham Study. *J Am Coll Cardiol* 1993;22[Suppl A]:6A–13A.
3. Luu M, Stevenson WG, Stevenson LW, Baron K, Waldein S. Diverse mechanisms of unexpected cardiac arrest in advanced heart failure. *Circulation* 1989;80:1675–1680.
4. Massie B, Francis G, Tandon P, Anderson S, Demets D, Packer M, on behalf of the PROMISE investigators. Asymptomatic ventricular arrhythmias do not identify patients with severe heart failure at risk for sudden death. *J Am Coll Cardiol* 1993;21[Suppl]:459A.

5. Cohn JN, Johnson GR, Shabetai R, et al. Ejection fraction, peak exercise oxygen consumption, cardiothoracic ratio, ventricular arrhythmias and plasma norepinephrine as determinants of prognosis in heart failure. *Circulation* 1993;87[Suppl VI]:VI-5–VI-16.
6. Packer M, Carver SR, Rodenheffer RJ, et al. Effect of oral milrinone on mortality in severe chronic heart failure. *N Engl J Med* 1991;325:1468–1475.
7. Aronson RS, Ming Z. Cellular mechanisms of arrhythmias in hypertrophied and failing myocardium. *Circulation* 1993;82[Suppl VII]:VII-76–VII-83.
8. Mason JW. A comparison of electrophysiologic testing with Holter monitoring to predict antiarrhythmic drug-efficacy for ventricular tachyarrhythmias. *N Engl J Med* 1993;329:445–451.
9. Simson M. Signal-averaged electrocardiography. In D. Zipes and J. Jalife: *Cardiac electrophysiology from cell to bedside.* Philadelphia: WB Saunders, 1990;807.
10. Stevenson WG, Stevenson LW, Weiss J, Tillisch JG. Inducible ventricular arrhythmias and sudden death during vasodilator therapy of severe heart failure. *Am Heart J* 1988:116:1447–1454.
11. CAST Investigators. Preliminary report: effect of encainide and flecainide on mortality in a randomized trial of arrhythmia suppression after myocardial infarction. *N Engl J Med* 1989;321:406–412.
12. Gottlieb SS, Kukin ML, Yushak M, Medina N, Packer M. Adverse hemodynamic and clinical effects of encainide in severe chronic heart failure. *Ann Intern Med* 1989;110:505–509.
13. Pratt CM, Eaton T, Francis M, et al. The inverse relationship between baseline left ventricular ejection fraction and outcome of antiarrhythmic therapy: dangerous imbalance in the risk-benefit ratio. *Am Heart J* 1989;118:433–440.
14. Singh S, Klein R, Eisenberg B, et al. Long term effect of mexiletine on left ventricular function and relation to suppression ventricular arrhythmia. *Am J Cardiol* 1990;66:1222–1227.
15. Dhein S, Muller A, Gerwin R, Klaus W. Comparative study on the proarrhythmic effects of some antiarrhythmic agents. *Circulation* 1993;87:617–630.
16. Ryden L, Ariniego R, Ainman K, et al. A double blind trial of metoprolol in acute myocardial infarction: effects on ventricular tachyarrhythmia. *N Engl J Med* 1983;308:614–618.
17. Chadda K, Goldstein S, Byington R, Curb JB. Effect of propranolol after acute myocardial infarction in patients with congestive heart failure. *Circulation* 1986;73(3):503–510.
18. Lichstein E, Hager D, Gregory JJ, Fleiss JL, Rolnitzky LM, Bigger JT. Relation between beta-adrenergic blocker use, various correlates of left ventricular function and the chance of developing congestive heart failure. *J Am Coll Cardiol* 1990;16:1327–1332.
19. Cingolani HE, Wiedman RT, Lynch JJ, et al. Negative lusitropic effect of DP 201-106 and E4031. Possible role of prolonging action potential duration. *J Mol Cell Cardiol* 1990;22:1025–1034.
20. Singh SN, Chen Y, Cohen A, et al. Relation between ventricular function and antiarrhythmic responses to sotalol. *Am J Cardiol* 1989;64:943–945.
21. Mason JW. A comparison of severe antiarrhythmic drugs in patients with ventricular tachyarrhythmia. *N Engl J Med* 1993;329:452–458.
22. Singh SN, Bennett BH. Ventricular arrhythmias associated with congestive heart failure: the role for amiodarone. *J Clin Pharmacol* 1991;31:1109–1111.
23. Nul RD, Doval H, Grancelli H, Perrone S, Bortman G, Curiel R. Amiodarone reduces mortality in severe congestive heart failure. *Circulation* 1993;88[Suppl I]:603.
24. Singh SN, Fletcher R, Fisher S, et al., and the CHF STAT investigators. Veterans Affairs Congestive Heart Failure Anitarrhythmic Trial. *Am J Cardiol* 1993;72:99F–102F.
25. Elkayman U, Mehra A, Vasquez J, Weber L, Rahimtoola S. A prospective randomized, double blind crossover study to compare the efficacy and safety of chronic nifedipine therapy with that of isosorbide dinitrate and their combination in the treatment of chronic congestive heart failure. *Circulation* 1990;82:1954–1961.
26. The Danish Study Group on Verapamil in Myocardial Infarction. Effect of verapamil on mortality and major events after acute myocardial infarction (The Danish Verapamil Trial II—DAVIT II). *Am J Cardiol* 1990;66:779–785.
27. The Multicenter Diltiazem Postinfarction Trial Research Group. The effect of diltiazem on mortality and reinfarction after myocardial infarction. *N Engl J Med* 1988;319(7):385–392.
28. Yusuf S, Teo K. Inotropic agents increase mortality in patients with congestive heart failure. *Circulation* 1990;[Suppl]:III-673(Abst).
29. Pfeffer MA, Braunwald E, Moyé LA, et al. Effect of captopril on mortality and morbidity in patients with left ventricular dysfunction after myocardial infarction. *N Engl J Med* 1992;327:669–677.
30. SOLVD Investigators. Effect of enalapril on survival in patients with reduced left ventricular ejection fractions and congestive heart failure. *N Engl J Med* 1991;325:293–302.

31. Cohn JN, Johnson G, Ziesihe S, et al. A comparison of enalapril with hydralazine-isosorbide dinitrate in the treatment of chronic congestive heart failure. *N Engl J Med* 1991;325:303–310.
32. Fletcher RD, Cintron GB, Johnson G, Orndoff J, Carson P, Cohn JN, for the V-HeFT II VA Cooperative Studies Group. Enalapril decreases prevalence of ventricular tachycardia in patients with chronic congestive heart failure. *Circulation* 1993;87[Suppl VI]:VI-49–VI-55.
33. The Anturane Reinfarction Trial Research Group. Sulfinpyrazone in the prevention of cardiac death after myocardial infarction. *N Engl J Med* 1978;298:289–295.
34. ISIS 2 (Second International Study of Infarction Survival) Collaborative Group. Randomized trial of intravenous streptokinase, oral aspirin both or neither among 17,187 cases of suspected myocardial infarction. *Lancet* 1988;ii:349–360.
35. Holmes DR, Davis K, Gersh BJ, Mock MB, Pettinger MB, and participants in the Coronary Artery Surgery Study. Risk factor profiles of patients with sudden death and death from other cardiac causes: a report from the Coronary Artery Surgery Study (CASS). *J Am Coll Cardiol* 1989;13(3): 524–530.
36. Winkle RA, Mead RH, Ruder MA, et al. Longterm outcome with the automatic implantable cardioverter defibrillator. *J Am Coll Cardiol* 1989;13:1353–1361.
37. Cohn SN, Archibald DG, Franciosa SA, et al. Effects of vasodilator therapy on mortality in chronic congestive heart failure: a result of a Veterans Affairs Cooperative Study (V-HeFT). *N Engl J Med* 1986;314:1547–1552.

The Failing Heart, edited by N. S. Dhalla,
R. E. Beamish, N. Takeda, and M. Nagano.
Lippincott-Raven Publishers, Philadelphia © 1995.

4

Coronary Heart Disease, Heart Failure, and Angiotensin-Converting Enzyme Inhibitors: Insights for Primary Prevention

Terrence J. Montague, Marion E. Barnes, Margaret L. Ackman,
*Randall G. Williams, and Koon K. Teo

*The Epidemiology Coordinating and Research Centre (EPICORE), Department of Medicine,
Division of Cardiology, University of Alberta Hospitals, Edmonton, Alberta T6G 2R7
Canada; and *Royal Alexandra Hospital, Edmonton, Alberta T5H 3V9 Canada*

CORONARY HEART DISEASE AND CONGESTIVE HEART FAILURE: EPIDEMIOLOGY

In a recent overview of left ventricular dysfunction (LVD) and congestive heart failure (CHF), the prevalence of CHF was estimated at 1% of the entire population of North America. In the same review it was also suggested that the primary prevention of CHF could largely be accomplished by the abolition of atherosclerotic coronary heart disease (CHD) (1). This latter opinion was formed from clinical experience in the Heart Function Clinic of the University of Alberta Hospitals (1) and from participation in large clinical trials of CHF (2–4). In these settings, CHD was the designated etiology of the CHF syndrome in about three-fourths of all patients (1–4).

The clinical burden of CHD in CHF has also been apparent in the recent trials (2,3). For example, in the prevention arm of the Studies of Left Ventricular Dysfunction (SOLVD), cardiovascular causes for hospitalization accounted for 71% of all hospitalizations during the first year of the trial (3). Of these, new or worsening CHF accounted for 28% of the admissions. Acute ischemic events, however, manifest as new or worsening angina, acute myocardial infarction, or need for coronary artery bypass surgery, accounted for 23% of the admissions (3).

ANGIOTENSIN-CONVERTING ENZYME INHIBITORS AND HEART FAILURE

In the summer of 1994, angiotensin-converting enzyme (ACE) inhibitors were the only proven efficacious therapy in patients with severe LVD and CHF. Their first demonstration of efficacy was in the Cooperative North Scandinavian Enalapril Survival Study (CONSENSUS) of enalapril in patients with severe heart failure (5). In this study, published in 1987, there was a 40% reduction in overall mortality, and the trial was stopped prematurely because of this marked survival benefit (5).

Interestingly, based on clinical analysis, the CONSENSUS investigators suggested that the principal contribution to mortality reduction among the CHF patients was due to retardation of progression of heart failure (5). Retrospective analysis of the life-table curves from CONSENSUS also supports this opinion, revealing the beneficial effect of enalapril to be evident immediately from the onset of the trial (4). This was very similar to the immediate beneficial effects of ACE inhibitors on heart failure endpoints subsequently reported in the SOLVD (2,3) and the Survival and Ventricular Enlargement (SAVE) (6) trials. In these latter trials, patients with fewer severe symptoms of CHF were studied (2,3,6).

Thus, in all of the initial trials of patients with severe LVD, and irrespective of symptomatic CHF status, there was a consistent, and immediate, benefit on clinical heart failure events from ACE inhibitors (2,3,5,6). The effect sizes were, however, greater in the more severely ill patient subgroups (2,3,6). In the very ill patients of CONSENSUS, the reduction in mortality was greater than 40% (5). In contrast, in SAVE, where the patients had all suffered acute myocardial infarctions but clinical CHF was not an entry requirement, there was an overall 22% reduction in heart failure hospitalizations (6). A similar, on average 20% reduction in CHF events, including hospitalization for, and mortality from, new (3) or worsening heart failure (2), was seen in the SOLVD trials.

There was another consistent, and clinically important, finding in the SOLVD and SAVE trials—a marked reduction in acute ischemic events among the patients receiving ACE inhibitors. In contrast to the beneficial effect of ACE inhibition on heart failure events, however, the reductions in the incidence of unstable angina, acute myocardial infarction, and sudden death did not become apparent immediately at the onset of the trials. Rather, the beneficial ACE inhibitor effect on ischemic events was not manifest until several months after the trials had begun (2,3,6,7).

The temporal differences in the late onset of the beneficial anti-ischemic effects, compared with the rapid benefit on heart failure events, suggest that the inhibition of the ACE was affecting at least two clinically important pathophysiologic pathways in the SOLVD and SAVE patients (2,3,6,7). The early impact on heart failure progression is due possibly to ACE inhibition effects on the excessively stimulated neurohumoral axis of the CHF patients; the protracted time course of the anti-ischemic effects is more in keeping with a much slower process, such as atherosclerosis retardation or regression.

Recently, further relevant data have become available. In the Acute Infarction Ramipril Efficacy (AIRE) trial of patients with CHD and severe LVD, there was a slight, immediately apparent, decreased mortality of the ACE inhibitor–treated subjects, compared with the control subjects, and a more marked reduction of mortality beginning at 12 months (8). These findings also support a temporally biphasic impact on pathophysiologic pathways in patients with CHD and CHF receiving ACE inhibitors (8).

In contrast, the CONSENSUS II trial of early enalapril use in patients with acute myocardial infarction did not show any reduction in mortality in the treated group (9). This trial, however, may have had insufficient power to reliably detect an anti-failure benefit in a consecutive sample of infarction patients unselected for severe left ventricular damage (9). Moreover, CONSENSUS II lasted only 6 months, not long enough to reliably define the anti-ischemic effects of ACE inhibition (9).

ANTISCLEROSIS AND ANGIOTENSIN-CONVERTING ENZYME INHIBITORS IN OTHER SETTINGS

The time course of the presumed anti-ischemic, and likely antiatherogenic or antisclerotic, effects of ACE inhibition in patients with CHF and CHD is similar to the delayed separation of placebo and interventional groups in the primary and secondary CHD prevention trials of lipid-lowering therapy (10–12). For example, in the Helsinki Heart Study, the placebo and gemfibrozil patient groups did not differ in CHD event rates for 3 years, but became increasingly divergent, with increasingly greater beneficial effect, thereafter for at least 8 years (10). Similarly, in the Program of Surgical Correction for the Hyperlipidemias, the therapeutic efficacy of the intervention was not apparent for 4 years, but became increasingly more beneficial with time thereafter (11).

More recently, studies of patients with diabetes have demonstrated similarly delayed, but therapeutically beneficial, effects of intense glycemic control (13,14) and ACE inhibition (15) on sclerosis in many vascular beds, including the kidneys, eyes, and nerves. This work has supported the hypothesis that the mesenchymal cells and the epithelial cells of the glomerulus respond with positive growth to messages from several stimuli, including hyperglycemia, with a resultant increase in extracellular matrix substance, hypertrophy, and proliferation, and that this growth can be retarded or reversed with appropriate interventions (16).

At the University of Alberta (Canada), a similar approach with regard to coronary atherosclerosis has been proposed (Fig. 1) (17,18). In particular, we recognized the ACE protein catalyst, which can also be characterized as kininase II, was responsible not only for catalyzing the conversion of angiotensin I to angiotensin II, but also for rendering bradykinin an inactive product. Therefore, we reasoned, blockade of the ACE enzyme would cause a decrease in angiotensin II, with a resultant decrease in the vasoconstrictor, proliferative, and hypertrophic effects of angiotensin II (17,18). Blockade of the kininase activity would also result in vasodilatory, antiproliferative, antihypertrophic, and possibly anticoagulant, effects through enhancement of the availability of bradykinin to endothelial cells and the nitric oxide pathway (17,18).

Presently, several clinical trials are evaluating whether ACE inhibition can produce atherosclerosis retardation and regression in a general population of CHD patients (19). We are actively involved in the Heart Outcome Prevention Evaluation (HOPE) (20) and Simvastatin/Enalapril Coronary Atherosclerosis Regression Trial (SCAT) (17). Both studies are 2×2 factorial, randomized clinical trials of ACE

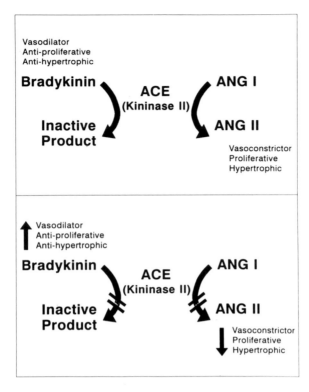

FIG. 1. In the top panel, the actions of angiotensin-converting enzyme (ACE), or kininase II, are represented diagrammatically. The presence of ACE facilitates the conversion of bradykinin to its inactive product and also catalyses the conversion of angiotensin I to angiotensin II, resulting in vasoconstriction, proliferation, and hypertrophy of smooth-muscle and endothelial cells. The bottom panel illustrates the biologically positive effects of blocking this enzyme, both at the endothelial and the smooth-muscle cell levels.

inhibitors, in conjunction with antioxidants (20) and powerful lipid-lowering therapy (17), respectively. Both will be completed and reported within the next several years.

THE FUTURE

Because CHD is such an overwhelming etiologic and pathophysiologic factor in CHF, it seems appropriate that agents proven to be efficacious in secondary prevention of CHD would also be effective in CHF. Beta blockers seem particularly attractive. There is, at least theoretical, concern in using negative inotropic medications, such as some beta blockers, in patients with CHF. Their promise, however, outweighs this concern, and they deserve a proper trial. Hopefully, this will be mounted in the near future.

Losartan, a direct blocker of angiotensin II receptors, is another agent that has been developed with promise of efficacy for CHF patients (21). Whether losartan will have as great an effect size on heart failure endpoints as ACE inhibition, however, remains unknown. As well, it is equally uncertain whether losartan, or other direct angiotensin II receptor blockers, will have any anti-ischemic efficacy in CHF patients because these drugs lack the kininase inhibition effects of ACE inhibitors (Fig. 1). Considering the large etiologic and clinical importance of CHD and CHD events in patients with CHF, this latter concern is not academic. Nonetheless, this group of agents may be useful in patients intolerant of ACE inhibitors because of side effects such as persistent cough.

Are there other effective management strategies for CHF in addition to development of additional efficacious medical therapies? One clinical approach we have been developing over the past several years is the intensive outpatient care of CHF. In the Heart Function Clinic of the University of Alberta Hospitals, we apply a multidisciplinary approach to CHF management (1). The Clinic's principles include optimal use of efficacious medications, participation in viable clinical trials, and foci on the outpatient setting and home care (1).

The short-term results from the Clinic indicate that such an approach improves quality of life for all patients and probably prolongs life for patients with minimal, mild, and moderate symptoms. For example, the survival of Heart Function Clinic patients with mild or moderate symptoms of CHF is greater than 90% at 24 months (unpublished data). The future for very sick CHF patients, however, remains grim. Even with intensive care, these patients continue to face a very high mortality risk.

In summary, CHF and CHD are enormous public health problems. The only presently proven efficacious agents for the secondary prevention of CHF—ACE inhibitors—were discovered, somewhat serendipitously, to also offer promise for the primary prevention of CHF by reducing the principal etiology—CHD. Used in conjunction with other emerging therapies for atherosclerosis regression and retardation, they offer promise that the primary prevention of CHF may well become a reality in the near future (1).

SUMMARY

Recent clinical trials have confirmed CHD as the dominant cause of CHF and acute ischemic events to be as common as worsening failure among CHF patients. The SOLVD and the SAVE trials have also demonstrated marked reductions in all ischemic events in patients taking ACE inhibitors. The reductions in acute ischemic events in SOLVD and SAVE became apparent only after 6 months of therapy, but then increased continuously. This delayed impact on CHD events resembles results from the cholesterol-lowering CHD trials and the antisclerotic effects in recent trials of intensive glycemic control and ACE inhibition in diabetics. These anti-ischemic and antisclerotic effects of ACE inhibitors may be related to enhanced endothelial cell function and retarded smooth-muscle cell migration and proliferation within arterial and glomerular intima. Currently, SCAT and HOPE are testing whether these effects are applicable to broad CHD populations. Thus, clinical trials of ACE inhibition in the secondary prevention of CHF have provided unique pathophysiologic insights and promise of efficacious therapy for the primary prevention of CHD. Further confirmatory studies are required and underway.

REFERENCES

1. Teo KK, Ignaszewski AP, Gutierrez R, Hill KL, et al. The contemporary medical management of left ventricular dysfunction and congestive heart failure. *Can J Cardiol* 1992;8:611–619.
2. The SOLVD Investigators. Effect of enalapril on survival in patients with reduced left ventricular ejection fractions and congestive heart failure. *N Engl J Med* 1991;325:293–302.
3. The SOLVD Investigators. Effect of enalapril on mortality and development of heart failure in asymptomatic patients with reduced left ventricular ejection fractions. *N Engl J Med* 1992;327:685–691.
4. The Digitalis Investigation Group. Rationale, design, implementation and baseline characteristics of patients in the DIG trial: a large, simple trial to evaluate the effect of digitalis on mortality in heart failure. *Controlled Clin Trials* (in press).
5. The CONSENSUS Trial Group. Effect of enalapril on mortality in severe congestive heart failure: results of the Cooperative North Scandinavian Enalapril Survival Study (CONSENSUS). *N Engl J Med* 1987;316:1429–1435.
6. Pfeffer M, Braunwald E, Moyé LA, et al., on behalf of the SAVE investigators. Effect of captopril on mortality and morbidity in patients with left ventricular dysfunction after myocardial infarction: results of the Survival and Ventricular Enlargement Trial. *N Engl J Med* 1992;327:669–677.
7. Yusuf S, Pepine CJ, Garces C, et al. Effect of enalapril on myocardial infarction and unstable angina in patients with low ejection fractions. *Lancet* 1992;340:1173–1178.
8. The Acute Infarction Ramipril Efficacy (AIRE) Study Investigators. Effect of ramipril on mortality and morbidity of survivals of acute myocardial infarction with clinical evidence of heart failure. *Lancet* 1993;342:821–828.
9. Swedberg K, Held P, Kjekshus J, Rasmussen K, Ryden L, Wedel H, on behalf of the CONSENSUS II Study Group. Effects of the early administration of enalapril on mortality in patients with acute myocardial infarction. Results of the Cooperative North Scandinavian Enalapril Survival Study II. *N Engl J Med* 1992;327:678–683.
10. Frick ME, Elo O, Haapa K, et al. Helsinki heart study: primary-prevention trial with gemfibrozil in middle-aged men with dyslipidemia: safety of treatment, changes of risk factors and incidence of coronary heart disease. *N Engl J Med* 1987;317:1237–1245.
11. Buchwald H, Varco R, Matts JP, Long JM, et al., for the POSCH Group. Effect of partial ileal bypass surgery on mortality and morbidity from coronary heart disease in patients with hypercholesterolemia. Report of the program on the surgical control of the hyperlipidemias (POSCH). *N Engl J Med* 1990;323:946–955.
12. Montague T, Tsuyuki R, Burton J, Williams R, Dzavik V, Teo K. Prevention and regression of coronary atherosclerosis. Is it safe and efficacious therapy? *Chest* 1994;105:718–726.
13. Reichard P, Nilsson BY, Rosenqvist U. The effect of long-term intensified insulin treatment on the development of microvascular complications of diabetes mellitus. *N Engl J Med* 1993;329:304–309.
14. The Diabetes Control and Complications Trial Research Group. The effect of intensive treatment of diabetes on the development and progression of long-term diabetes mellitus. *N Engl J Med* 1993;329:977–986.
15. Lewis E, Hunsicker LG, Bain RP, Rohde RD, for the Collaborative Study Group. The effect of angiotensin-converting-enzyme inhibition on diabetic mephropathy. *N Engl J Med* 1993;329:1456–1462.
16. Fogo A, Ichikawa I. Evidence for the central role of glomerular growth promoters in the development of sclerosis. *Semin Nephrol* 1989;9(4):329–342.
17. Teo KK, Burton JR, Buller C, Plante S, Yokoyama S, Montague TJ, on behalf of the SCAT Investigators. Rationale and design features of a clinical trial examining the effects of cholesterol lowering and angiotensin converting enzyme inhibition on coronary artherosclerosis. *Controlled Clin Trials* [submitted].
18. Montague TJ, Yusuf S, Tsuyuki RT, Teo KK. Importance of preventing ischemia in patients with congestive heart failure. *Can J Cardiol* 1993;9[Suppl F]:39F–43F.
19. Lonn EM, Yusuf S, Jha P, et al. The emerging role of angiotensin-converting enzyme inhibitors in cardiac and vascular protection. *Circulation* 1994;90(4):2056–2069.
20. The Canadian Cardiovascular Collaboration for the Heart Outcomes Prevention Evaluation (HOPE) Trial. Protocol of a trial to evaluate ramipril and vitamin E on clinically important vascular end points in high risk patients. Medical Research Council and Hoechst Ltd., Canada, 1993 [unpublished document].
21. Eberhardt RT, Kevak RM, Kang PM, Frishman WH. Angiotensin II receptor blockade: an innovative approach to cardiovascular pharmacotherapy. *J Clin Pharmacol* 1993;33:1023–1038.

The Failing Heart, edited by N. S. Dhalla,
R. E. Beamish, N. Takeda, and M. Nagano.
Lippincott-Raven Publishers, Philadelphia © 1995.

5

Postinfarcted Heart Failure Is Weakened by Supplementation of Eicosapentaenoic Acid

Nobuhiko Shibata and Satoru Otsuji

Department of Cardiology, The Center for Adult Diseases, Osaka, 537 Japan

How progression of the infarcted lesion is inhibited to salvage the infarcted myocardia is the most critical problem for prevention of the postinfarcted heart failure. Thus, we have undertaken biochemical and histological analysis in canine experimentally infarcted myocardia. In this study, we found that lipoxygenase metabolites of arachidonic acid (AA), such as 5- or 12-hydroxyeicosatetraenoic acids (HETEs), were produced only in the infarcted myocardia. In addition, these metabolites from AA have been well known to have strong biological activites, such as promoting inflammation and/or producing allergic reaction, and so on.

On the other hand, it has been well established that eicosapentaenoic acid (EPA), an n-3 polyunsaturated fatty acid (PUSFA), competes with AA to be incorporated into phospholipids in plasma membranes. After an appropriate stimulation, phospholipids that have incorporated EPA produce lipoxygenase and cyclooxygenase products of EPA. The biological activities of the lipoxygenase and cyclooxygenase products of EPA, however, are much fewer than those of the respective products of AA(1). Thus, attempts have been made to use EPA to inhibit progression of myocardial infarction and to prevent onset of the postinfarcted heart failure.

MATERIALS AND METHODS

Feeding Diets

Adult mongrel dogs (10–12 kg) were fed a standard diet (30 g/kg body weight/d) prepared by Oriental Yeast Co. The content of EPA in the diet was negligible. The ten dogs in the EPA group were fed the same standard diet, which had been supplemented with EPA ester (100 mg/kg body weight/d), kindly supplied by Nihon Suisan-Mochida Pharmaceutical Co. Dogs were fed for 8 weeks before coronary ligation.

Inducing Experimental Myocardial Infarction

Dogs were anesthetized by intravenous injection of thiopental (20 mg/kg), intubated, and artificially ventilated with room air via a Harvard respirator. Under ECG monitoring, thoracotomy was performed at the fifth intercostal space, the pericardium was opened, and the heart was exposed. The circumflex coronary artery was isolated from the fat and ligated 0.5 cm distal to its origin. After confirming ST segment elevation in ECG, the thoracic cage was closed. Electrocardiographic monitoring was maintained until the dogs recovered consciousness. The dogs then lay in the recovery room until they were killed and their hearts were excised, 72 hours after coronary ligation.

Estimation of Ventricular Arrhythmia in the Early Phase of Myocardial Infarction

In another 15 dogs fed with an EPA-rich diet, it was also estimated whether EPA-feeding would protect ischemia-induced ventricular arrhythmia in the early phase (within 3 hours) after the experimental myocardial infarction. In this experiment, the dogs were observed continuously, using Holter ECG monitoring (lead II) after the coronary ligation. Thereafter, the hearts were excised and biochemically analyzed. The degrees of arrhythmia were assayed by counting the number of ventricular extrabeats (VEBs), including those occurring as tachycardia (VT, seven or more consecutive ventricular extrasystoles at a rate faster than the normal sinus rhythm) and the incidence and total duration of all episodes of VT and ventricular fibrillation (Vf). In addition, the severity of arrhythmias was assessed quantitatively by an "arrhythmia score" on a hierarchical scale of 0 to 8 during occlusion, as described by Curtis et al. (2). The value 0 was given for 0 to 49 VEBs only; 1, for 50 to 499 VEBs only; 2, for >500 VEBs, or one spontaneously reversible episode of VT or Vf; 3, for more than one spontaneously reversible episode of VT/Vf, or one or more episode of nonspontaneously reversible VT/Vf lasting less than 60 seconds; 4, for VT/Vf episodes lasting 60 to 120 seconds; 5, for VT/Vf episodes lasting more than 120 seconds; 6, for irreversible Vf causing death within 15 to 240 minutes after coronary ligation; 7, for fatal Vf within 4 to 15 minutes; and 8, for fatal Vf within 4 minutes.

Digitalis-induced arrhythmias were also evaluated immediately after the coronary artery ligation in five dogs from each group. The administration of digitalis after coronary occlusion is assumed to enhance the elevation of the intracellular cytoplasma free Ca^{2+}, which is thought to be the principle cause of the inotropic effect of digitalis glycosides on the heart. The time of onset of VT or Vf was measured in five dogs with EPA supplementation and compared with five control dogs. The entire protocol followed the local ethical standards for the treatment of animals in our hospital.

Fatty Acid Composition of Platelet-cell Membrane and Microsomes from Noninfarcted and Infarcted Myocardium

Because EPA is believed to be incorporated into the cardiomyocyte membrane as well as those of platelets, we used the latter to estimate the incorporation of EPA into cell membranes. Platelets were used because purified membrane fractions were easily obtained. Platelets were isolated from peripheral blood immediately prior to coronary artery ligation. Cell membrane fractions were obtained using the method employed by Minkes et al. (3). Isolated heart preparations were separated into the infarcted area at the top of the posterior papillary muscle, indicating the presence of myocardial necrosis induced by coronary occlusion, and the noninfarcted area (the root area of anterior papillary muscle indicating the absence of myocardial necrosis). Microsomal vesicles were obtained from each area by sucrose gradient centrifugation, as described by Jones and Besch (4). The lipid component of the membranes was extracted with Folch's solution and the fatty acid composition was analyzed by gas chromatography (5,6).

Estimation of the Chemotactic Activities of Neutrophils

To estimate the chemotactic activities of neutrophils, blood was drawn from the femoral vein before and 72 hours after coronary ligation. Neutrophils were isolated by the Ficoll gradient method using Histopaque 1077 and 1119. Neutrophils were then suspended in Hanks balanced salt solution (pH 7.4) at a concentration of 3×10^6/ml. Chemotactic activities of neutrophils were measured with a blind well chamber by the method of Boyden (7), with minor modifications. As a chemotaxin, 200 μl of LTB4 was placed in the lower chamber at a concentration of 10^{-10} to 10^{-6} M, and 200 μl of the suspended neutrophils were placed in the upper chamber. A millipore filter (pore size: 5 μm) was inserted between the chambers and incubated at 37°C for 60 min. After the filter was fixed and stained with hematoxylin, we estimated the number of neutrophils that had migrated to the lower surface of the filter.

Quantification of Ultimate Infarct Size

The schemic or infarcted area was measured by the method employed by Fishbein et al. (8). Briefly, after 72 hours of coronary ligation, 30 ml of 0.5% Evans blue dye was injected through the femoral vein to stain the nonischemic area. Left ventricles of excised hearts were sectioned horizontally from the cardiac base to the apex in 1-cm intervals. Each section was subdivided into two horizontal sections. The apical half of the subdivided section was used for measurement of biochemical parameters, and the basal half was used for evaluation of the ultimate infarct size.

The basal halves of the myocardial slices were incubated with 1.5% triphenyl tetrazolium chloride at 37°C for 10 min to stain the noninfarcted area. After transferring the sections to tracing paper, the areas of infarcted and ischemic portions and of the left ventricular wall were calculated using a planimeter.

Measurement of Amount of Arachidonic Acid Lipoxygenase Products, Especially Hydroxyeicosanoid, in Myocardium

We measured the amount of HETEs to estimate AA lipoxygenase products in infarcted myocardium (9). Pieces of infarcted myocardium were obtained from the aforementioned area, and pieces of noninfarcted myocardium were obtained from the root of the anterior papillary muscle. The myocardial pieces (0.50-g wet weight) were homogenized in 5 volumes of 50-mM potassium-phosphate buffer (pH 7.0), with prostaglandin B2 (PGB_2, 100 ng in 0.2 ml of methanol) added as an internal standard. The eicosanoids were extracted with ethylacetate by shaking, followed by centrifugation. The homogenate was centrifuged at 3,300 g for 5 min. The supernatant was concentrated to fewer than 50 μl by evaporation under a stream of nitrogen gas and was then dissolved in 100 μl of pure methanol. Aliquots were analyzed for HETE and PGB by reverse-phase high-performance liquid chromatography (RP-HPLC) by using a column packed with Nucleosil C_{18} (4.6×150 mm). The solvent system consisted of methanol-water-acetic acid (65:35, 0.1 v/v). Detection was performed with an ultraviolet detector operating at 235 nm for HETE and 280 nm for PGB_2. The amount of HETE was calculated from the ratio of the peak height to that of PGB_2. Respective peaks corresponding to 12-, 5-, and 15-HETE were separated by HPLC and identified by gas chromatography mass spectrometry (GC-MS). Because it was always present in the greater amounts, the level of 12-HETE was used to represent the lipoxygenase products of AA in infarcted myocardium.

Measurement of Myelooxidase Activity of Infarcted Myocardium

To evaluate the extent of neutrophilic infiltration into the infarcted myocardium, we measured the neutrophil-specific myeloperoxidase (MPO) activities by an adaptation of the method of Bradley et al. (10), according to the procedure of Bednar et al. (11). Briefly, the serial myocardial pieces (0.20 g) were homogenized in 10 vol of 50-mM phosphate buffer (pH 6.8) to which hexadodecyl-trimethyl ammonium bromide had been added to 0.5%. The mixture was then centrifuged at 100,000 g for 15 min at 4°C. A 100-μl aliquot of the supernatant was added to 2.9 ml of 50-mM phosphate buffer containing 0.167 mg/ml o-dianisidine dihydrochloride and 0.0005% $H_2 O_2$. The reaction was analyzed spectrophotometrically at 460 nm. The results were expressed as units (U) of MPO/0.1 g wet tissue, where 1 U of MPO activity is defined as that which degrades 1 μmol of peroxide/min at 25°C.

Estimation of Ischemic Myocardial Injury

The extent of ischemic myocardial injury was estimated by measuring the activities of creatine kinase (CK) remaining in the myocardium at the center of the ischemic area. Myocardial pieces (0.25–0.50 g) obtained from infarcted and noninfarcted areas were suspended in 25 vol of extraction solution (0.25 M sucrose, 1 mM EDTA, 0.1 mM beta-mercaptoethanol) and homogenized with a Polytron homogenizer. After centrifugation at 16,000 g, the CK activity of the supernatant was then assayed spectrophotometrically with a commercial kit (Iatron Laboratries).

Measurement of dp/dt in the Left Ventricle

To estimate the contractile function of the left ventricle, dp/dt was measured with a tip transducer, which was inserted through the left carotid artery just before the animal was killed, and it was then connected to a polygraphic analyzer (Nihon-Koden Co.).

Histological Examination

After measuring the infarcted and noninfarcted areas, myocardial slices were fixed in 10% formalin and stained with hematoxylin and eosin. The extent of neutrophilic infiltration and tissue lysis was then compared with the ratio of EPA/AA in the platelet membrane.

Measurement of $(Ca^{2+}\text{-}Mg^{2+})$-ATPase, and NADPH Cytochrome-C Reductase Activities in Myocardial Microsomes

In the study estimating effects of TPA-feeding for ventricular arrhythmias, activities of microsomal $(Ca^{2+}\text{-}Mg^{2+})$-ATPase, $(Na^{+}\text{-}K^{+})$-ATPase, and NADPH cytochrome-C reductase from infarcted and noninfarcted myocardium were measured to examine changes in cellular membrane ion-transport proteins. The $(Ca^{2+}\text{-}Mg^{2+})$-ATPase activity was determined by a modified method of Itoh et al. (12). The reaction mixture contained 30 to 40 mg of myocardial microsomes, 50 mM of Tris-HCl (pH 7.2), 20 mM of NaN (an inhibitor of mitochondrial ATPase), 0.1 mM of ouabain (an inhibitor of $(Na^{+}\text{-}K^{+})$-ATPase), 1 mM of adenosine triphosphate (ATP), and the desired submicromolar free Ca^{2+} concentrations, adjusted by addition of Ca^{2+}-EGTA buffer. The association constants for Ca^{2+}-EGTA and Ca^{2+}-ATP at a pH of 7.2 were 6.8×10 and 8.5×10, respectively (13). The reaction was initiated by adding ATP and terminated by adding ice-cold trichloroacetic acid (TCA) after an incubation at 37°C for 30 min. The mixture was then centrifuged. The inorganic phosphate (Pi) concentration within the supernatant was determined by the method of Youngberg and Youngberg (14). The $(Ca^{2+}\text{-}Mg^{2+})$-ATPase activity was calculated by subtracting the values obtained with BGTA alone from those with Ca^{2+} and BGTA. The (Na^+-K^+)-ATPase activity was measured by a similar method (12), except for a different composition of reaction medium that consisted of 3 to 4 μg of myocardial microsomes, 50 mM of Tris-HCl (pH 7.2), 110 mM of NaCl, 15 mM of KCl, 5 mM of NaN_3, 0.5 mM of EGTA, 4 mM of $MgCl_2$ and 1 mM of ATP. The NADPH cytochrome-C reductase activity of the marker enzyme of sarcoplasmic reticulum (SR) was also determined (15).

Data Analysis

Data are presented as mean ± SEM. Student's test or Wilcoxon test was used to analyze continuous variables. The frequency of events was compared by the chi-square test. P values of <0.05 were considered to be statistically significant.

Results

Fatty Acid Composition of Total Phospholipids from Cell Membrane Fractions after Eicosapentaenoic Acid Supplementation

We examined the fatty acid composition of the platelet membranes and microsomes from noninfarcted and infarcted myocardium to ensure that dietary supplementation with EPA significantly replaced AA. Figure 1 shows the phospholipid fatty acid composition of the total phospholipids from the platelet membrane and myocardial microsomes of noninfarcted and infarcted myocardium. In the EPA-supplemented group, levels of linoleic acid and AA, which are n-6 PUFAs, tended to account for a lower percentage of the total phospholipids within not only platelet-cell membranes but also myocardial microsomes. In contrast, levels of EPA and docosahexaenoic acid (DHA), which are n-3 PUFAs, in the aforementioned membranous vesicles from cells were increased significantly. Consequently, the EPA/AA and n-3/n-6 PUFA ratios were markedly higher in the EPA-supplemented group than in the control group. The ratio of EPA/AA in the control versus the EPA group was $7 \pm 1\%$ versus $37 \pm 5\%$ within platelet-cell membranes, $3 \pm 1\%$ versus $12 \pm 5\%$ in noninfarcted myocardial microsomes, and $2 \pm 1\%$ versus $8 \pm 2\%$ in infarcted myocardial microsomes, respectively (p <0.01). Additionally, in the EPA group, the EPA/AA and n-3/n-6 PUFA ratios in the myocardial microsomes did not differ between the noninfarcted and infarcted areas. These findings suggested that dietary EPA competes efficiently with AA for incorporation into myocardial microsomes.

Arrhythmias following Coronary Ligation

Ventricular arrhythmias that developed within 3 hours after coronary ligation were analyzed using a Holter monitor. As shown in Fig. 2A, the total number of

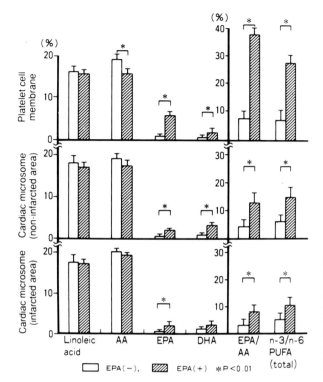

FIG. 1. The fatty acid in phospholipid composition of platelet-cell membrane and cardiac microsomal fraction. The ratio of EPA to AA and n-3 to n-6 PUFA is presented. Each bar represents the mean ± SEM. EPA(−), control group; EPA(+), EPA-treated group; DHA, docosahexaenoic acid.

VEBs was significantly higher in the control than in the EPA-treated group (393 ± 115 vs. 221 ± 98: control group vs. EPA group, $p < 0.05$). There was no difference, however, in the incidence of Vf between the two groups (control group: 2/10; EPA group: 2/10, NS; see Fig. 2B). We then analyzed the severity of the ventricular arrhythmias using the arrhythmia score, which is of particular value in aiding statistical evaluation when a low incidence of VT and/or Vf precludes comparisons of the duration of episodes. Consequently, the arrhythmia score obtained within 3 hours following coronary ligation was significantly reduced by EPA supplementation during occlusion (3.6 ± 1.2 vs. 2.2 ± 0.8, control vs. EPA, $p < 0.05$; see Fig. 2C). These findings indicated that arrhythmic vulnerability found in the early stage after coronary occlusion was attenuated under the EPA supplementation.

All animals given digitalis in the control group to induce arrhythmias developed VT or Vf after about 10 to 15 min. All animals in the EPA-supplemented group, however, required more than 25 min after the administration of digitalis to develop VT or Vf (Fig. 3). These results indicated that the toxic effect of digitalis is suppressed in the EPA-supplemented group, suggesting that the incorporation of EPA into myocardial microsomes prevents the toxic accumulation of cytosolic Ca^{2+}, which may subsequently increase after the administration of digitalis.

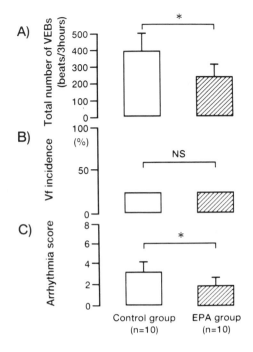

FIG. 2. A comparison of total numbers of (**A**) ventricular extrabeats (VEBs), (**B**) percent incidence of ventricular fibrillation (Vf), and (**C**) arrhythmia score after coronary ligation between the control and EPA groups; *, $p < 0.01$.

Chemotactic Activities of Neutrophils

Figure 4 shows the changes of the chemotactic activities of neutrophils before and 72 hours after coronary ligation. The chemotactic activities of neutrophils were examined at various concentrations of LTB4. The data show that (a) the chemotactic activities of the neutrophils in both groups increased as the concentration of LTB4 increased from 10^{-10} M to 10^{-6} M; (b) in both groups, the chemotactic activities of neutrophils were enhanced after coronary ligation; (c) the maximal activity was observed in neutrophils from control dogs at 72 hours after coronary ligation, while

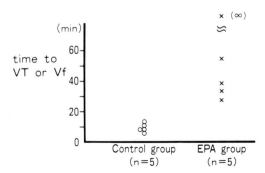

FIG. 3. The antiarrythmic effects of EPA on digitalis-induced ventricular tachycardia (VT) and ventricular fibrillation (Vf) after coronary artery ligation.

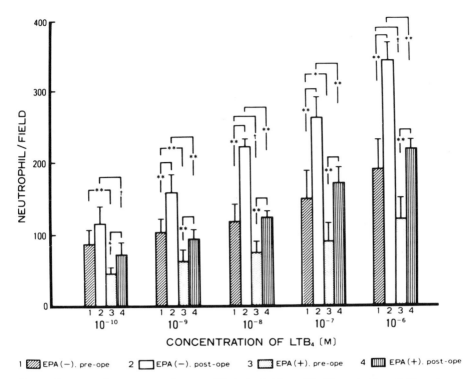

FIG. 4. Chemotactic response of neutrophils to leukotriene B4. Chemotactic activities of neutrophils were measured according to Boyden's method. Each bar represents the mean ± SEM. EPA (−), control group; EPA (+), EPA-treated group; pre-ope, neutrophils isolated before coronary ligation; post-ope, neutrophils isolated 72 hours after coronary ligation; +, $p < 0.05$; *, $p < 0.02$; **, $p < 0.01$.

the minimal activity was observed in neutrophils from EPA-treated dogs before surgery; and (d) the chemotactic activity of neutrophils from EPA-treated dogs was significantly lower than that of neutrophils from control dogs at all chemotaxin concentrations, both before and after coronary ligation (e.g., after coronary ligation, the neutrophil activity in the EPA-treated group was about 66% of that in the control at an LTB4 concentration of 10^{-6} M; $p < 0.01$). These results suggest that after treatment with EPA, the chemotactic activities of neutrophils are significantly suppressed, regardless of the ligation of the coronary artery.

Area at Risk and Infarct Size

Table 1 shows the effect of supplemental dietary EPA on the size of the area at risk and of the myocardial infarct. Dietary EPA significantly reduced the ultimate size of the infarcted area (IA), as compared to the control, whether expressed as a

TABLE 1. *Ratios of area at risk and infarct to left ventricular mass of control and EPA group at 72 hours permanent coronary ligation*

	Control	EPA group
AR/LV	49.3 ± 2.1	43.2 ± 6.9#
IA/LV	29.2 ± 0.5	17.6 ± 4.0*
IA/AR	59.3 ± 9.9	40.4 ± 5.8*

Data are expressed as percent.
#, NS; *p <0.01 control vs. EPA group.
AR, area at risk; IA, area at infarct; LV, left ventricular mass.

percent of the entire left ventricle (IA/LV, 29.2 ± 0.5% vs. 17.6 ± 4.0%, control vs. EPA group, *p* <0.01) or as a percent of the area at risk did not significantly differ between the two groups (expressed as a percent of the entire left ventricle, 49.3 ± 2.1% vs. 43.2 ± 6.9%, control vs. EPA group). These findings suggest that EPA supplementation inhibits the progression of ischemic myocardial injury.

Creatin Kinase (CK) and 12-Hydroxyeicosatetraenoic Acid Content, and Myeloperoxidase Activity in the Infarcted Myocardium

Figure 5 shows the CK content (as an indication of myocardial damage in the control and EPA-treated groups). In the control group, the amount of CK remaining in the infarcted myocardium was 17.0 ± 6.4% of that found in the noninfarcted

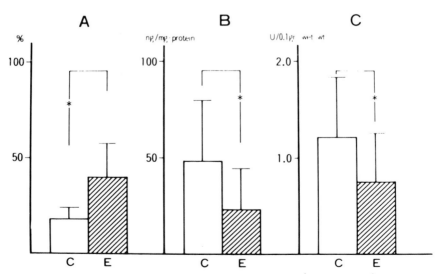

FIG. 5. (A) Creatin kinase content, **(B)** 12-HETE content, and **(C)** MPO activities in infarcted myocardium of the control group and the EPA-treated group at 72 hours after coronary ligation. C, control group; E, EPA-treated group. Each value represents the mean ± SEM; *p* <0.05.

myocardium, which was significantly lower than that of the EPA-treated group ($43.8 \pm 30.7\%$, $p <0.05$). This suggests that CK release was suppressed in the EPA-treated group as compared with the control.

The 12-HETE content in infarcted myocardium in the control group was 48.9 ± 32.0 ng/mg protein, which was significantly higher than that in the EPA-treated group (20.0 ± 19.0 ng/mg protein, $p <0.05$). This suggests that EPA reduces the production of 12-HETE (and other lipoxygenase products of AA) in infarcted myocardium.

The MPO activity in infarcted myocardium in the control group was 1.22 ± 0.55 U/0.1 g wet tissue, which was significantly higher than that found in the EPA-treated group (0.68 ± 0.25 U/0.1 g wet tissue, $p <0.05$). This suggests that EPA reduces the infiltration of neutrophils into the infarcted myocardium.

The representative relationship between myocardial injury produced by ischemia associated with the infiltration of neutrophils and the EPA/AA ratio in platelet membranes is shown in Fig. 6. The infiltration of neutrophils and tissue lysis were both suppressed as the EPA/AA ratio increased.

Contractile Function of the Left Ventricle

Contractile functions of the left ventricles in both groups were estimated by measuring the dp/dt of the left ventricle. The positive peak dp/dt in the EPA-treated group was 1408 ± 156 mmHg/sec^2, which was significantly higher than that in the control group (933 ± 115 mmHg/sec^2; $p <0.01$). This suggests that postinfarcted left ventricular systolic function was preserved better in the EPA-treated group than in the control group.

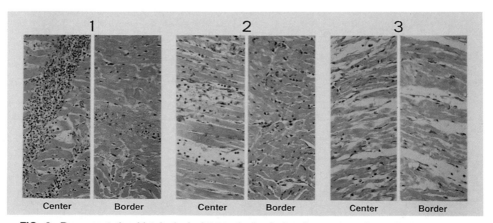

FIG. 6. Representative histological pictures in the ischemic center and marginal area at 72 hours after permanent coronary ligation in the EPA-treated group, compared with the ratio of AA and EPA levels in the platelet membranes. The EPA/AA ratio of the platelet membranes was 0.16 in panel 1, 0.23 in panel 2, and 0.63 in panel 3.

$(Ca^{2+}\text{-}Mg^{2+})$-ATPase and $(Na^{+}\text{-}K^{+})$-ATPase Activities in Myocardial Microsomal Vesicles

The Ca^{2+} and Na^{+} pump function in myocardial microsomal vesicles was estimated by measuring the ATPase activities of ion-transport proteins in cell membranes. In microsomal vesicles from noninfarcted and infarcted myocardium, the activities of NADPH-dependent cytochrome-C reductase, a marker enzyme of SR, were the same between the EPA and control groups (Table 2, *upper*). These vesicular samples thus represent myocardial microsomal vesicles. Figure 7 shows the $(Ca^{2+}\text{-}Mg^{2+})$-ATPase activities in microsomal vesicles from noninfarcted myocardium of both EPA-supplemented and control subjects. The enzyme activity increased in proportion to the Ca^{2+} concentrations in both the control and EPA-supplemented dogs. The Km value, calculated from the double reciprocal plot, was approximately 4.0×10^{-3} (M) for both groups. In contrast, the apparent V_{max} per milligram of protein in the EPA-supplemented group was significantly higher than that in the control group (149.3 vs. 90.7 nmol/mg/min, respectively). As shown in Table 2 (*middle-left*), similar values were also obtained in noninfarcted myocardium from another six dogs for the mean apparent V_{max} (140.5 ± 19.1 vs. 94.8 ± 28.9 nmol/mg/min, EPA vs. control group, $p < 0.01$). In noninfarcted myocardium, however, the Km values of the $(Ca^{2+}\text{-}Mg^{2+})$-ATPase activity in microsomes in both groups were not significantly different ($[4.0 \pm 1.0] \times 10^{-8}$ vs. $[3.9 \pm 1.0] \times 10^{-8}$ (M); EPA vs. control, respectively; NS, Table 2, *middle*). As shown in Table 2 (*middle, right column*) the $(Ca^{2+}\text{-}Mg^{2+})$-ATPase activity in microsomal vesicles from infarcted myocardium of each group also revealed results similar to those in noninfarcted myocardium. That is, apparent V_{max} in the EPA group was significantly higher than that in the control group, but values of Km did not differ (130.9 ± 18.4 vs. 90.2 ± 26.4 nmol/mg/min; EPA vs. control, $p < 0.01$).

In the EPA-treated group, the apparent V_{max} value did not differ between the noninfarcted and infarcted areas (140.5 ± 19.1 vs. 130.9 ± 18.4 nmol/mg/min, re-

TABLE 2. NADPH cytochrome-C reductase, $(Ca^{2+}\text{-}Mg^{2+})$-ATPase, and $(Na^{+}\text{-}K^{+})$-ATPase activities in noninfarcted and infarcted myocardial microsomes

	Noninfarcted area (n = 6)		Infarcted area (n = 6)	
NADPH cytochrome C reductase	V_{max} (nmol/mg/min)		V_{max} (nmol/mg/min)	
EPA(+)	341 ± 68		322 ± 54	
EPA(−)	360 ± 109		348 ± 78	
$(Ca^{2+}\text{-}Mg^{2+})$-ATPase	V_{max}	Km (M)	V_{max}	Km (M)
EPA(+)	$140.5 \pm 19.1^{*}$	$(4.0 \pm 1.0) \times 10^{-8}$	$130.9 \pm 18.4^{*}$	$(2.5 \pm 0.9) \times 10^{-8}$
EPA(−)	$94.8 \pm 28.9^{*}$	$(3.9 \pm 1.0) \times 10^{-8}$	$90.2 \pm 26.4^{*}$	$(2.5 \pm 0.7) \times 10^{-8}$
$(Na^{+}\text{-}K^{+})$-ATPase	V_{max}	IC_{50} by ouabain (M)	V_{max}	IC_{50} by ouabain (M)
EPA(+)	1997 ± 742	$(5.4 \pm 1.3) \times 10^{-7}$	1213 ± 218	$(5.6 \pm 1.5) \times 10^{-7}$
EPA(−)	2033 ± 342	$(5.6 \pm 1.3) \times 10^{-7}$	1270 ± 310	$(5.0 \pm 1.2) \times 10^{-7}$

Specific activities are expressed as nmol/mg/min at 37°C.
$^{*}p < 0.01$, EPA vs. control group.
EPA(+), EPA-treated group; EPA(−), control group.

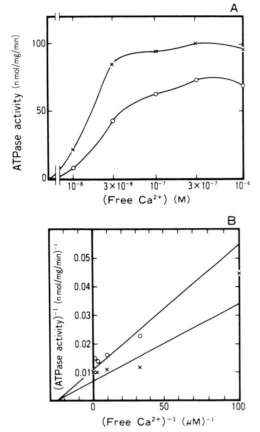

FIG. 7. **(A)** The comparison of the $(Ca^{2+}-Mg^{2+})$-ATPase activity on the free Ca^{2+} concentrations of cardiac microsomal vesicles from noninfarcted myocardium of both EPA (x) and control groups (o). Enzymatic activity was determined at the indicated free Ca^{2+} concentrations. Values are means after four experiments. The reaction medium followed was the same as those in the text. **(B)** Double reciprocal plot of part **A.**

spectively; NS), but the values in the control group were significantly lower than those in the EPA group. In addition, the values of Km from the noninfarcted myocardium were significantly higher than those from the infarcted area irrespective of the EPA treatment.

The $(Ca^{2+}-Mg^{2+})$-ATPase activity was inhibited in a dose-dependent manner by trifluoperazine (TFP), a calmodulin inhibitor, indicating that calmodulin is responsible for Ca^{2+}-dependent enzymatic activity (Fig. 8).

These findings also suggested that EPA-dependent increase of $(Ca^{2+}-Mg^{2+})$-ATPase activity within myocardial microsomes from either noninfarcted or infarcted myocardium results from increased levels of the enzyme, without alterations in its properties.

The $(Na^{+}-K^{+})$-ATPase activity within microsomal vesicles from noninfarcted and infarcted myocardium of both EPA and control groups was inhibited in a dose-dependent fashion by ouabain. The ouabain concentration leading to 50% inhibition

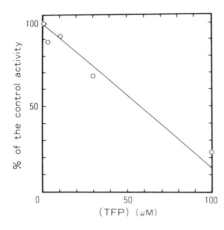

FIG. 8. The effect of trifluoroperazine (TFP) (a calmodulin antagonist) on $(Ca^{2+}\text{-}Mg^{2+})$-ATPase activity in cardiac microsomal fractions from noninfarcted area. The enzyme activity was estimated at a free Ca^{2+} concentration of 0.1 μM using Ca-EGTA buffer.

(IC_{50}) was similar in both groups, being approximately 5×10^{-7} (M) (Table 2, *lower*). These results suggest that the $(Na^+\text{-}K^+)$-ATPase activity remains unchanged after the incorporation of EPA into myocardial microsomes.

Discussion

The data demonstrate that supplemental dietary EPA for 8 weeks resulted in a significant reduction in infarcted myocardial damage induced by 72 hours of coronary ligation, as evidenced by a higher content of CK in the infarcted area, and a higher value of the peak positive dp/dt.

Our data also showed that after feeding with EPA (a) infiltration of neutrophils into the infarcted myocardium was suppressed; (b) the amount of 12-HETE, a chemotactic and/or neutrophil activating factor produced from AA in ischemic myocardium via a lipoxygenase pathway, was decreased; and (c) the chemotactic activities of neutrophils were depressed.

Our data indicate that EPA supplementation produces a decrease in neutrophilic infiltration into the ischemic myocardium. This decrease is the result of a reduction in the motility of neutrophils and a decrease in the production of lipoxygenase metabolites derived from AA in the infarcted myocardium. These effects may result from an increase of the EPA/AA ratio in the plasma membranes of various cells, including cardiomyocytes as well as neutrophils.

Based on these results, it is concluded that feeding with an EPA-rich diet for at least 2 months prior to the onset of myocardial infarction inhibits development of the infarcted lesion, leading to attenuation of the postinfarcted heart failure.

Furthermore, in this article it was shown that EPA-feeding prior to the onset of myocardial infarction reduced significantly the severity of ventricular arrhythmias induced by ischemia. To search its mechanism, we assayed the Ca^{2+} and Na^+

pump functions by measuring the activities of $(Ca^{2+}-Mg^{2+})$-ATPase and (Na^+-K^+)-ATPase in myocardial microsomes. The latter also serves as a marker enzyme of plasma membrane.

The activity of NaDPH-dependent cytochrome-C reductase, a marker of SR activity, was also measured and revealed a significant activity indicating that the obtained microsomal vesicles may contain plasma membrane as well as SR. In the results, we noted an increase in the enzymatic activity of $(Ca^{2+}-Mg^{2+})$-ATPase in the EPA-supplemented group. These results suggested that EPA is incorporated into myocardial microsomes and leads to stabilization of the myocardial membrane by modulating ion-transport proteins, such as $(Ca^{2+}-Mg^{2+})$-ATPase. The effects of this membrane modification may decrease intracellular Ca^{2+} overload during the early phase of infarction compared with the control group, and thereby reduce the severity of ischemic-mediated ventricular arrhythmias.

To evaluate how acute ischemia affects the fatty acid composition of myocardial microsomes and subsequently affect the function of the Ca^{2+} as well as Na^+ pump functions in myocardial membrane, we examined the heart preparations separated into infarcted and noninfarcted areas in both the control and the EPA groups. There were no measurable differences between the infarcted and noninfarcted areas with respect to fatty acid composition except that EPA/AA and n-3/n-6 PUFA ratios were significantly higher in the EPA group. Both areas in the EPA group contained significantly increased levels of $(Ca^{2+}-Mg^{2+})$-ATPase activities as compared with the control group. These results indicated that, even in infarcted cardiac microsomes, $(Ca^{2+}-Mg^{2+})$-ATPase activity enhanced by EPA supplementation was unaffected, at least within the first 3 hours following coronary ligation.

We also demonstrated that there were no measurable differences in the inhibition of Na^+ pump function in both infarcted and noninfarcted areas between the EPA and control groups, indicating that a toxic dose of digitalis did not inhibit (Na^+-K^+)-ATPase pump activity in the presence of dietary EPA. These results further suggest that the $(Ca^{2+}-Mg^{2+})$-ATPase increased by EPA supplementation also plays an important role in preventing the intracellular Ca^{2+} overload enhanced by digitalis administration after coronary occlusion. Furthermore, the inhibition of intracellular Ca^{2+} overload during the early phase of infarction by increasing activities of $(Ca^{2+}-Mg^{2+})$-ATPase in cardiac microsomes also may have favorable effects on myocardial infarction by decreasing the incidence and severity of ventricular extrasystoles as well as by attenuating the progression of ischemic injury.

SUMMARY

We found that metabolites of AA, such as 5- or 12-HETEs, were increased in the infarcted area (IA). Thus, the effects of dietary supplementation with EPA of an n-3 unsaturated fatty acid on experimental myocardial infarction were examined in dogs. It was given as EPA ester (100 mg/kg body weight) for 8 weeks prior to coronary ligation for 3 days. In the results, the following was detected in the EPA group: (a) the ratio of EPA to AA in myocardial microsomal membrane increased significantly more than three times; (b) chemotactic response of neutrophils to leukotriene B was reduced; (c) the level of 12-HETE in infarcted myocardium was reduced; (d) ultimate size of infarcted myocardium was reduced; (e) infiltration of neutrophils in infarcted myocardium was less; and (f) contractile function of the infarcted ventricle was well preserved. The positive peak dp/dt in the EPA-treated group was 1408 ± 156 mmHg/sec^2, which was significantly higher than 933 ± 115 mmHg/sec^2 in controls. We conclude that dietary EPA attenuates ischemic myocardial damage, leading to prevention of postinfarcted heart failure.

Dietary supplementation with EPA significantly reduced the incidence and severity of arrhythmias during coronary artery occlusion. Immediately after coronary artery occlusion, all animals given a toxic dose of digitalis in the control group developed VT or Vf, whereas none of the animals in the EPA-supplemented group developed VT or Vf within 15 minutes of administration of digitalis. Irrespective of the presence of an infarcted area, the specific activity of the Ca^{2+}-pump enzyme, $(Ca^{2+}-Mg^{2+})$-ATPase, within the myocardial microsomal fraction of the EPA-supplemented group was significantly higher than in the control group.

These results indicated that EPA supplementation increases the $(Ca^{2+}-Mg^{2+})$-ATPase activity within myocardial membranes that is involved in Ca^{2+} metabolism in myocardial cells by increasing the ratio of EPA to AA within cellular membranes. These cellular alterations are likely to reduce the severity of ventricular arrhythmias by inhibiting the rapid accumulation of intracellular Ca^{2+} following ischemia.

REFERENCES

1. Prescott SM. The effect of eicosapentaenoic acid on leukotriene B production by human neutrophils. *J Biol Chem* 1984;259:7615–7621.
2. Curtis MJ, Macleod BA, Walker MJA. Models for the study of arrhythmias in myocardial ischaemia and infarction. *J Mol Cell Cardiol* 1987;9:339–419.
3. Minkes M, Stanford N, Chi MM-Y, et al. Cyclic adenosine 3'5'-monophosphate inhibits the availability of arachdonate to prostaglandin synthetase in human platelet suspensions. *J Clin Invest* 1977; 59:449–454.
4. Jones LR, Besch HR Jr. Isolation of cardiac sarcolemmal vesicles. *Methods Pharmacol* 1984;5:1–24.
5. Ozawa A, Nakamura E, Jimbo H, et al. Determination of higher fatty acids in various lipid fractions of human plasma, platelets and erythrocyte membrane using thin layer chromatography. *Bunseki Kagaku* 1982;32:174–177 (in Japanese, abstract in English).
6. Ozawa A, Takayanagi K, Fujita T, et al. Determination of long chain fatty acids in human total plasma lipids using gas-chromatography. *Bunseki Kagaku* 1983;31:87–91 (in Japanese, abstract in English).
7. Boyden S. The chemotactic effect of mixtures of antibody and antigen on polymorphonuclear leukocytes. *J Exp Med* 1962;115:453–466.
8. Fishbein MC, Meerbaum S, Rit J, et al. Early phase acute myocardial infarct size quantification: validation of triphenyl tetrazolium chloride tissue enzyme staining technique. *Am Heart J* 1981;101: 593–600.
9. Sanma H, Nakamura T. Effect of adriamycin and coenzyme Q10 on leukotriene C-like substance formation in the guinea pig heart. *Biochem Int* 1982;5:617–627.

10. Bradley PP, Priebat DA, Christensen R, Rothstein G. Measurement of cutaneous inflammation: estimation of neutrophil content with enzyme marker. *J Invest Dermatol* 1982;78:206–209.
11. Bednar M, Smith B, Pinto A, Mullane KM. Nafazatrom-induced salvage of ischemic myocardium in anesthetized dogs is mediated through inhibition of neutrophil function. *Circ Res* 1985;57:131–141.
12. Itoh K, Morimoto S, Shiraishi T, Taniguchi K, Onishi T, Kumahara Y. Increase of Ca^{2+}-Mg^{2+}-ATPase activity of renal basolateral membrane by parathyroid hormone via cyclic AMP-dependent membrane phosphorylation. *Biochem Biophys Res* 1988;150:263–270.
13. Pershadsingh H, McDaniel ML, Lacy PE, McDonald JM. Ca^{2+} activated ATPase and ATP-dependent calmodulin-stimulated Ca^{2+} transport in islet cell plasma membrane. *Nature* 1980;288:492–495.
14. Youngberg GE, Youngberg MV. Phosphorous metabolism: a system of blood phosphorus analysis. *J Lab Med* 1930;16:7501–7509.
15. Sottocasa GL, Kuylenstierna B, Ernster L, Bergstrand A. An electron-transport system associated with the outer membrane of liver mitochondria. A biochemical and morphological study. *J Cell Biol* 1967;32:415–438.

The Failing Heart, edited by N. S. Dhalla,
R. E. Beamish, N. Takeda, and M. Nagano.
Lippincott-Raven Publishers, Philadelphia © 1995.

6

Diastolic Dysfunction in Stunning: Its Prevention

Horacio E. Cingolani, *Susana M. Mosca, and †Abel E. Moreyra

*Cardiovascular Research Center, *Department of Physiology, La Plata School of
Medicine, La Plata, 1900 Argentina; †Department of Medicine, Division of Cardiology,
University of Medicine and Dentistry of New Jersey, Robert Wood Johnson Medical School,
New Brunswick, NJ 08903 United States*

In 1986, Murry et al. (1) provided the first evidence that repeated brief episodes of coronary artery occlusion limited infarct size caused by subsequent sustained ischemia. Paradoxically, then, myocardium that has been reversibly injured by ischemia is more tolerant of a subsequent episode of ischemia. This endogenous protection was called "ischemic preconditioning" (IP) and has been described in reference not only to infarct size, but also to arrhythmias (2) and stunning (3).

Stunning is defined as the prolonged but transient contractile dysfunction of viable myocardium after an ischemic period that did not result in irreversible damage. The protection from the systolic dysfunction of the stunning by IP is controversial and perhaps related to species differences (3–6). The diastolic dysfunction of the stunning and its prevention by IP and related maneuvers have been less studied.

In a model of global ischemia in rabbits, we describe the systolic and diastolic alterations of stunning and several interventions leading to its prevention.

METHODS

Rabbit hearts were perfused with Ringer's solution (118 mM NaCl; 2 mM $CaCl_2$; 5,9 mM KCl; 1,2 mM $MgSO_4$; 20 mM $NaHCO_3$; and 11.1 mM dextrose) by the nonrecirculating Langendorff technique. A latex balloon tied to the end of a polyethylene tube was passed into the left ventricle and connected to a pressure transducer. The balloon was filled with aqueous solution to a left ventricular end-diastolic pressure (LVEDP) of 8 to 14 mmHg. The coronary flow was maintained constant at 41 ± 1 ml/min. By subtracting LVEDP from the peak systolic pressure, the left ventricular developed pressure (LVDP) was obtained. Coronary perfusion pressure (CPP), left ventricular (LV) pressure, and its first derivative of LV (dP/dt) were obtained. Maximal velocity of increase of LV pressure ($+dP/dt_{max}$) was measured. The isovolumic relaxation was evaluated through the time constant of relaxation τ(7). The LVEDP at constant volume was used as an index of ventricular diastolic stiffness (8).

After the preparation was stabilized, myocardial stunning was induced in ten hearts by a 15-min period of global ischemia, followed by 30 min of reperfusion. Since Cohen et al. (3) found that only one 5-min occlusion cycle was enough to induce IP, in eight hearts, one period of 5 min of global ischemia before the longer ischemic period of 15 min was used for IP. In six hearts, adenosine (800 μg/min) was infused for 5 min, followed by 5 min of reperfusion without drug to mimic the effect of IP. In five hearts, dipyridamole (4 μg/min), infused for 5 min, was used to mimic the effect of IP. Eight hearts of rabbits pretreated orally with nicardipine (20 mg/d) for 1 month were isolated and compared with control hearts without any treatment with the same protocol. Nitroprusside (25 μg/min) infused during 5 minutes was injected into the coronary line at the end of the reperfusion period in four hearts in order to bring CPP to control values.

RESULTS

Figure 1 shows pooled data for LV pressure during and after global ischemia in the rabbit heart. Electron microscopic studies revealed that after the end of the ischemic period of 15 min all hearts exhibited predominantly normal ultrastructure, without evidence of irreversible injury (Fig. 2). In spite of this, a systolic dysfunction can be detected using either LVDP or $+dP/dt_{max}$ as the index of contractility (Fig. 1A,B). After the ischemic period LVDP was about 100 mmHg and at the end of reperfusion period, it stabilized at about 50% of control values.

Figure 1C,D shows the diastolic alterations detected by us in this model. The time constant of LV pressure fall, τ(Fig. 1C), from control values of 48 ± 4 msec peaked after 5 min of the onset of reperfusion, but gradually normalized at the end of the reperfusion period. In Fig. 1D, LVEDP increased monotonically from control values of 13 ± 1 mmHg to values of 41 ± 6 mmHg at the end of the reperfusion period.

The time dissociation between velocity of relaxation and diastolic chamber stiffness (LVEDP at constant volume) argues against incomplete relaxation as the cause of the increase in LVEDP. Because CPP (Fig. 1D) also increased monotonically during the reperfusion period, the possibility of an increase in LVEDP induced by the increase in CPP ("garden hose" effect) was considered. Because the normalization of CPP by the vasodilator nitroprusside did not normalize the altered diastolic stiffness, we can rule out this mechanism as the cause of the increased LVEDP. The increase in diastolic stiffness was probably increasing the coronary resistance through changes in the extravascular support.

Figures 3A (LVDP) and Fig. 3B ($+dP/dt_{max}$) on page 71 show how IP protects the heart from the systolic alterations of stunning. Figure 3C shows the attenuation

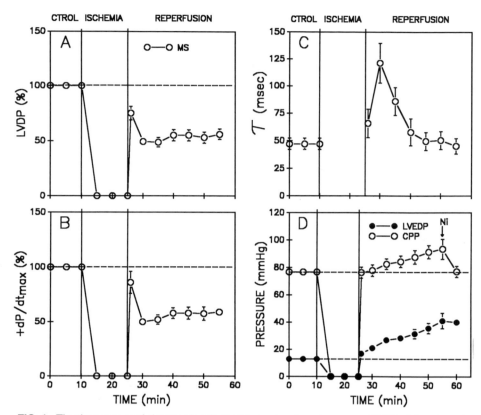

FIG. 1. The time course of changes in left ventricular developed pressure (LVDP) (**A**) and maximal rate of rise of LV pressure ($+dP/dt_{max}$) (**B**), both expressed as percentage of preischemic values. The time constant of relaxation τ, left ventricular end-diastolic pressure (LVEDP), and coronary perfusion pressure (CPP) are shown in panels **C** and **D**.

of the transitory prolongation of τ, and Fig. 3D shows the attenuation of the increase in LVEDP at constant diastolic volume (i.e., diastolic chamber stiffness).

Figures 4A (LVDP) and Fig. 4B ($+dP/dt_{max}$) on page 72 show the protection from the systolic alterations of stunning induced by adenosine infusion during a 5-min period. Figure 4C shows the attenuation of the transitory prolongation of τ, and Fig. 4D shows the attenuation of the increase in diastolic stiffness achieved by the drug.

Figures 5A (LVDP) and Fig. 5B ($+dP/dt_{max}$) on page 73 show the protection from the systolic alterations of stunning induced by the dipyridamole infusion during a 5-min period. Figures 5C (τ) and Fig. 5D (LVEDP) show the attenuation of diastolic alterations of stunning induced by the infusion of dipyridamole. Both the transitory impairment in relaxation and the increase in LVEDP detected in reperfusion were attenuated by this pharmacological intervention. This finding is in agree-

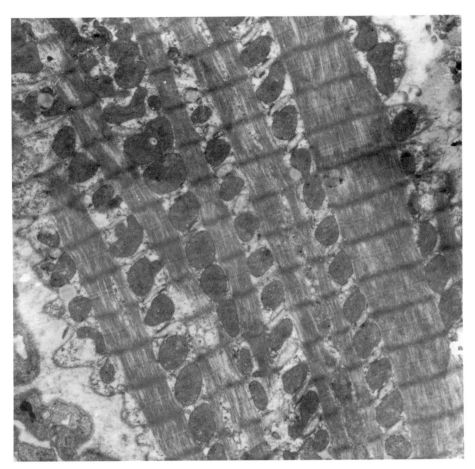

FIG. 2. Electron micrograph from the posterior wall of the left ventricle of the heart subject to 15 min of ischemia and 30 min of reperfusion. Aspect of contractile system and the mitochondria is essentially normal. Note the integrity of the sarcolemma. ×5300.

ment with the protection reported by the infusion of both adenosine deaminase inhibitor and a nucleoside transport blocker (9) and, in addition, answers a question raised by these authors: It is not necessary to block the release of adenosine to obtain the protection. The inhibition of both adenosine–deaminase activity and the entrance of adenosine to the cell bring protection.

Figures 6A (LVDP) and Fig. 6B (+ dP/dt$_{max}$) on page 74 show the protection from the systolic alterations of stunning by chronic pretreatment with nicardipine. Left ventricular developed pressure values of pretreated and control hearts were 89 ± 6 mmHg and 99 ± 3 mmHg, respectively. The + dP/dt$_{max}$ values in pretreated and control hearts were 1195 ± 82 mmHg/sec and 1289 ± 54 mmHg/sec, respec-

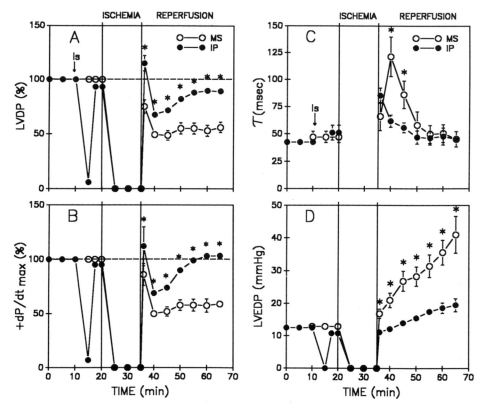

FIG. 3. The time course of changes in left ventricular developed pressure (LVDP) (**A**) and maximal rate of rise of LV pressure ($+dP/dt_{max}$) (**B**), both expressed as percentage of preischemic values. The time constant of relaxation τ and left ventricular end-diastolic pressure (LVEDP) in ischemic preconditioning (IP) are shown in (**C**) and (**D**). To facilitate the comparison, the parameters of the stunned group (MS) are depicted. Is, 5 min of ischemia; *, $p < 0.05$ with respect to the stunned group.

tively. In spite of the lack of negative inotropic effect induced by the pretreatment, an attenuation in the degree of stunning was detected with the chronic pretreatment with this calcium channel blocker. Figures 6C (τ) and Fig. 6D (LVEDP) show the attenuation of the diastolic alterations of stunning induced by this intervention.

DISCUSSION

In the model of global ischemia in the rabbit, the systolic dysfunction of stunning was accompanied by two diastolic alterations: (a) a transitory impairment in relaxation detected early in reperfusion and (b) a monotonic increase in LV chamber stiffness that persisted in spite of normalization of the relaxation rate. At the end of

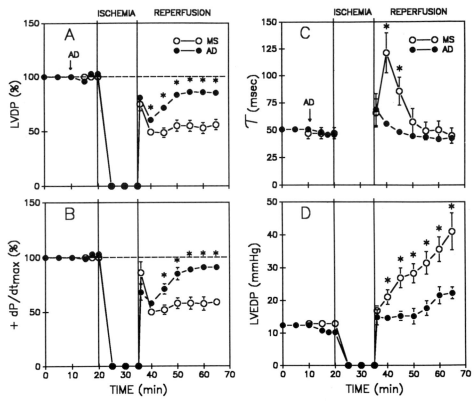

FIG. 4. The time course of changes in left ventricular developed pressure (LVDP) (**A**) and maximal rate of rise of LV pressure ($+dP/dt_{max}$) (**B**), both expressed as percentage of preischemic values. The time constant of relaxation τ and left ventricular end-diastolic pressure (LVEDP) in hearts perfused with adenosine (AD) are shown in (**C**) and (**D**). To facilitate the comparison, the parameters of the stunned group (MS) are depicted. AD, time of infusion of adenosine; *, p <0.05 with respect to the stunned group.

the reperfusion period, the velocity of relaxation does not differ significantly from control values, but LVEDP reaches its highest values. We could speculate that both diastolic alterations, the transitory impairment in relaxation and the increased diastolic stiffness, are the mechanical counterparts of two different cellular alterations: transitory Ca^{2+} overload and adenosine triphosphate (ATP) depletion, respectively. Our speculations are in agreement with previous investigations showing that increases in cytosolic Ca^{2+} are neither sufficient nor necessary for the inhibition of the ischemic contracture. Depletion of ATP, and not Ca^{2+} overload, seems to be the cause of the rise in diastolic stiffness due to the formation of rigor crossbridges (10).

Before discussing the prevention of these alterations by the different maneuvers assayed by us, we will discuss the possible mechanisms by which the diastolic alterations of the stunning take place (for review, see refs. 11,12).

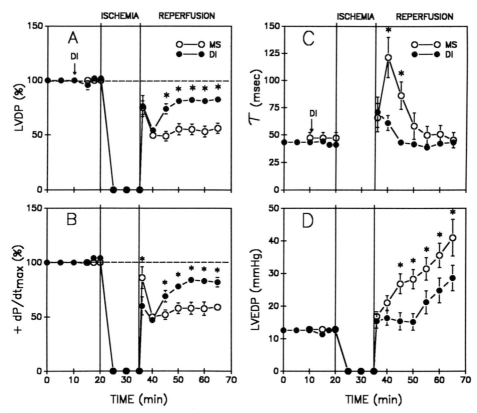

FIG. 5. The time course of changes in left ventricular developed pressure (LVDP) (**A**) and maximal rate of rise of LV pressure ($+dP/dt_{max}$) (**B**), both expressed as percentage of preischemic values. The time constant of relaxation τ and left ventricular end-diastolic pressure (LVEDP) in hearts perfused with dipyridamole (DI) are shown in (**C**) and (**D**). To facilitate the comparison, the parameters of the stunned group (MS) are depicted. DI, time of infusion of dipyridamole; *, p <0.05 with respect to the stunned group.

Two main mechanisms have been postulated to trigger myocardial stunning: calcium overload and free radical generation. These two mechanisms are not mutually exclusive, because free radical generation has been reported to induce calcium overload (13). An initial and transitory increase in cytosolic $[Ca^{2+}]_i$ acting on endogenous enzymes (i.e., Ca^{2+}-dependent proteases or lipases) (14) can induce the damage, including the decrease in myofilament sensitivity (11,15,16). Myocardial relaxation can become compromised when the calcium overload exceeds the functional capacity of the sarcoplasmic reticulum (SR) or the SR becomes leaky to Ca^{2+} after reperfusion. A later decline in cytosolic calcium would allow the sarcoplasmic reticulum to return to its normal functional capacity. The transient impairment of relaxation is compatible with previously proposed mechanisms of SR dysfunction during stunning (17,18).

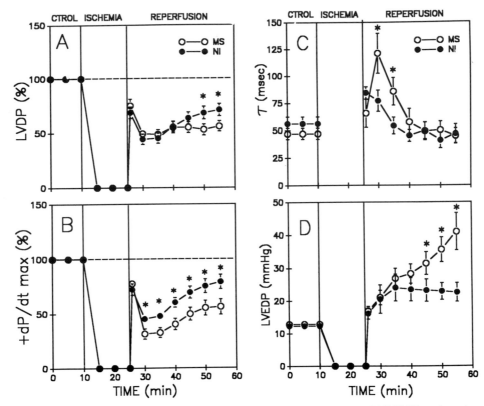

FIG. 6. The time course of changes in left ventricular developed pressure (LVDP) (**A**) and maximal rate of rise of LV pressure ($+dP/dt_{max}$) (**B**), both expressed as percentage of preischemic values. The time constant of relaxation τ and left ventricular end-diastolic pressure (LVEDP) in hearts pretreated with nicardipine (NI) are shown in (**C**) and (**D**). To facilitate the comparison, the parameters of the stunned group (MS) are depicted. *, $p < 0.05$ with respect to the stunned group.

We attenuated or prevented the systolic and diastolic alterations of stunning by the following interventions: ischemic preconditioning, adenosine and dipyridamole infusion, and chronic pretreatment of rabbits with the calcium channel blocker, nicardipine. A widely accepted theory to explain the protection induced by IP is the adenosine hypothesis (19,20). The protection seems to be mediated by ischemia inducing adenosine release and subsequent activation of A_1 adenosine receptors. A_1 receptors are coupled to G proteins, which will carry signal transduction (21).

One proposed mechanism to explain the protection brought about by adenosine involved the opening of K_{ATP}-dependent channels (22,23). This mechanism, by inducing hyperpolarization, would decrease the calcium influx through the L channels. If the hypothesis that the Ca^{2+} channel is the main pathway for Ca^{2+} entry during reperfusion is valid, the inhibition of Ca^{2+} influx by calcium antagonists during reperfusion should prevent Ca^{2+} overload. Most investigators, however, have failed to demonstrate a reduction of Ca^{2+} overload when Ca^{2+} antagonists were infused at the time of reperfusion (24–26). When these compounds were given prior to the ischemic period, Ca^{2+} accumulation during reperfusion was reduced (24–28). The calcium channels seem to be inactive after reoxygenation (24–26,29,30), however, and the pretreatment with Ca^{2+} antagonists can induce protection by mechanisms other than direct blockade of the channel. One of these mechanisms is that Ca^{2+} antagonists can delay the depletion of high-energy stores by reduction of myocardial contractility (26,31). This possibility was ruled out in our experiments in which the chronic pretreatment of rabbits with nicardipine was not inducing a detectable decrease in the contractile state. Actually, a higher, although not statistically significant, contractility was detected when hearts from pretreated rabbits were compared with nontreated animals before ischemia. One important question to be addressed is why the chronic pretreatment with this dihydropyridine did not induce a decrease in contractility in the chronically pretreated rabbits. Two possibilities should be considered: (a) The pharmacological action of these compounds is no longer present after isolation. This is an unlikely possibility because in in vitro pieces of myocardium, the persistence of the blockade seems to be longer (32). (b) Chronic pretreatment induced an up-regulation of the calcium channels that can perhaps offset a decrease in calcium influx. Implicit in these possibilities is the statement that chronic pretreatment with these compounds is not inducing calcium blockade in the heart and therefore probably not inducing protection through this mechanism. Several actions of the calcium channel blockers, other than direct calcium blockade, are listed in Table 1.

We do not know of any study showing up-regulation of calcium channels after chronic treatment with nicardipine. With the chronic pretreatment with the dihydropyridine nifedipine, however, we recently showed an up-regulation of the Ca^{2+} channels in the rabbit (33), in agreement with previous reports in avian hearts (34). This finding argues against a protection of calcium channel blockers by a direct calcium influx blockade.

TABLE 1. *Calcium antagonists: Mechanisms other than direct blockade of cardiac Ca^{2+} influx*

Protection of mitochondrial function (27)
Prevention of decrease in Na^+ pump activity (35)
Action on Na^+ channel (36–38)
Antiperoxidative mechanism (39)
Anti α_1 effect (40)
Decrease in Noradrenaline release (41)
Delay of depletion of ATP by the decrease in contractility (26,31)

Numbers within parentheses indicate references from which data were sourced.

SUMMARY

Using the model of global ischemia in rabbits, we described the systolic and diastolic alterations of stunning. Electron microscopic studies revealed that after the end of the ischemic period, all of the hearts exhibited predominantly normal ultrastructure without evidence of irreversible injury. In spite of this, systolic and diastolic dysfunction was detected using LVDP, LVEDP, $+dP/dt_{max}$, and the time constant of pressure fall, τ. τ increased at about 5 min after the onset of reperfusion, but gradually normalized at the end of the reperfusion period. The diastolic stiffness, however, increased monotonically through all of the reperfusion period. The time dissociation between velocity of relaxation and diastolic chamber stiffness (LVEDP at constant volume) argues against incomplete relaxation as the cause of the increase in LVEDP.

The systolic and diastolic alterations were prevented by preconditioning, adenosine or dipyridamole infusion prior to the ischemic period, and chronic pretreatment of rabbits with nicardipine.

ACKNOWLEDGMENT

We wish to thank Martin Carriquiriborde for his valuable technical assistance.

REFERENCES

1. Murry CE, Jennings R, Reimer KA. Preconditioning with ischemia: a delay of lethal cell injury in ischemic myocardium. *Circulation* 1986;74:1124–1136.
2. Shiki K, Hearse DJ. Preconditioning of ischemic myocardium: reperfusion-induced arrhythmias. *Am J Physiol* 1987;253:H1470–H1476.
3. Cohen MV, Liu GS, Downey JM. Preconditioning causes improved wall motion as well as smaller infarcts after transient coronary occlusion in rabbits. *Circulation* 1991;84:341–349.
4. Ovize M, Przylklenk K, Hale SL, Kloner R. Preconditioning does not attenuate myocardial stunning. *Circulation* 1992;85:2247–2255.
5. Miyamae M, Fujiwara H, Kida M, et al. Preconditioning improves energy metabolism during reperfusion but does not attenuate myocardial stunning in porcine hearts. *Circulation* 1993;88:223–234.
6. Asimakis G, Inners-McBride K, Medellin G, Conti V. Ischemic preconditioning attenuates acidosis and postischemic dysfunction in isolated rat hearts. *Am J Physiol* 1992;263:887–894.
7. Mosca SM, Gelpi RJ, Cingolani HE. Dissociation between myocardial relaxation and diastolic stiffness in the stunned heart: its prevention by ischemic preconditioning. *J Mol Cell Biochem* 1993; 129:171–178.
8. Mirsky I. Assessment of diastolic function: suggested methods and future considerations. *Circulation* 1984;64:836–841.
9. Zughaib ME, Abd-Elfattah AS, Jeroudi MO, et al. Augmentation of endogenous adenosine attenuates myocardial "stunning" independently of coronary flow or hemodynamic effects. *Circulation* 1993;88:2359–2369.
10. Koretsune Y, Marban E. Mechanism of ischemic contracture in ferret hearts: relative roles of $[Ca^{2+}]_i$ elevation and ATP depletion. *Am J Physiol* 1990;258(*Heart Circ Physiol* 27):H9–H19.
11. Kusuoka H, Marban E. Cellular mechanisms of myocardial stunning. *Annu Rev Physiol* 1992;54: 243–256.
12. Tani M. Mechanisms of Ca^{2+} overload in reperfused ischemic myocardium. *Annu Rev Physiol* 1990;52:543–559.

13. Correti M, Koretsune Y, Kusuoka H, Chacko VP, Zweier J, Marban E. Glycolitic inhibition and calcium overload as consequences of exogenously generated free radicals in rabbit hearts. *J Clin Invest* 1991;88:1014–1025.
14. Matsumura Y, Kusuoka H, Inoue M, Hori M, Kamada T. Protective effect of the protease inhibitor leupeptin against myocardial stunning. *J Cardiovasc Pharmacol* 1993;22:135–142.
15. Kusuoka H, Porterfield JK, Weisman HF, Weisfeldt ML, Marban E. Pathophysiology and pathogenesis of stunned myocardium: depressed Ca^{2+} activation of contraction as a consequence of reperfusion-induced cellular calcium overload in ferret hearts. *J Clin Invest* 1987;79:950–961.
16. Carrozza JP, Bentivegna LA, Williams ChP, Kuntz RE, Grossman W, Morgan JP. Decreased myofilament responsiveness in myocardial stunning follows transient calcium overload during ischemia and reperfusion. *Circ Res* 1992;71:1334–1340.
17. Davis M, Lebolt W, Feher J. Reversibility of the effects of normothermic global ischemia on the ryanodine-sensitive and ryanodine-insensitive calcium uptake of cardiac sarcoplasmic reticulum. *Circ Res* 1992;70:163–171.
18. Krause SM. Myocardial stunning opens the Ca^{2+} release channel in cardiac sarcoplasmic reticulum. *Circulation* 1989;80:II-601(abst).
19. Liu GS, Thornton J, Van Winkle DM, Stanley AWH, Olsson RA, Downey JM. Protection against infarction afforded by preconditioning is mediated by A_1 adenosine receptors in rabbit heart. *Circulation* 1991;84:350–356.
20. Thornton JD, Liu GS, Olsson RA, Downey JM. Intravenous pretreatment with A_1-selective adenosine analogues protects the heart against infarction. *Circulation* 1992;85:659–665.
21. Thornton JD, Liu GS, Downey J. Pretreatment with pertussis toxin blocks the protective effects of preconditioning evidence for a G-protein mechanism. *J Mol Cell Cardiol* 1993;25(3):311–320.
22. Auchampach JA, Gross GJ. Adenosine A_1 receptors, K_{ATP} channels, and ischemic preconditioning in dogs. *Am J Physiol* 1993;264:H1327–H1336.
23. Yao Z, Gross GP. Effects of the K_{ATP} channel opener bimakalim on coronary blood flow, monophasic action potential duration, and infarct size in dogs. *Circulation* 1994;89:1769–1775.
24. Bourdillon PD, Poole-Wilson PA. The effects of verapamil, quiescence, and cardioplegia on calcium exchange and mechanical function in ischemic rabbit myocardium. *Circ Res* 1982;50:360–368.
25. Lefer AM, Polansky EW, Bianchi CP, Narayan S. Influence of verapamil on cellular integrity and electrolyte concentrations of ischemic myocardial tissue in the cat. *Basic Res Cardiol* 1979;74:555–567.
26. Watts JA, Koch CD, LaNoue K. Effects of calcium antagonism on energy metabolism: Ca^{2+} and heart function after ischemia. *Am J Physiol* 1980;238:H909–H916.
27. Nayler WG, Ferrari R, Williams A. Protective effect of pretreatment with verapamil, nifedipine and propranolol on mitochondrial function in the ischemic and reperfused myocardium. *Am J Cardiol* 1980;46:242–248.
28. Poole-Wilson PA, Harding DP, Bourdillon PDV, Tones MA. Calcium out of control. *J Mol Cell Cardiol* 1984;16:175–187.
29. Linden J, Brooker J. Properties of cardiac contractions in zero sodium solutions: intracellular free calcium controls slow channel conductance. *J Mol Cell Cardiol* 1980;12:457–478.
30. Murphy JG, Smith TW, Marsh JD. Mechanisms of reoxygenation-induced calcium overload in cultured chick embryo heart cells. *Am J Physiol* 1988;254:H1133–H1141.
31. Lange R, Ingwall J, Hale SL, et al. Preservation of high-energy phosphates by verapamil in reperfused myocardium. *Circulation* 1984;70:734–741.
32. Le Grand B, Hatem S, Deroubaix E, Couetil JP, Coraboeuf E. Calcium current depression in isolated human atrial myocytes after cessation of chronic treatment with calcium antagonists. *Circ Res* 1991;69: 292–299.
33. Chiappe de Cingolani GE, Mosca SM, Vila Petroff M, Cingolani HE. Chronic administration of nifedipine induces up regulation of dihydropyridine receptors in rabbit heart. *Am J Physiol* 1994; 267:H1222–H1226.
34. Chapados RA, Gruver EJ, Ingwall JS, Marsh JD, Gwathmey JK. Chronic administration of cardiovascular drugs: altered energetics and transmembrane signaling. *Am J Physiol* 1992;263(*Heart Circ Physiol* 32):H1576–H1586.
35. Daly MJ, Elz JS, Nayler WG. The effects of verapamil on ischemia-induced changes to the sarcolemma. *J Mol Cell Cardiol* 1985;17:667–674.
36. Grima M, Freyss-Beguin M, Millanvoye Van Brussel E, Decker N, Schwartz J. Effects of various

antianginal drugs on sodium influx in rat brain synaptosomes and in rat heart muscle cells in culture. *Eur J Pharmacol* 1987;138:1–8.

37. Yatani A, Brown AM. The calcium channel blocker nitrendipine blocks sodium channels in neonatal rat cardiac myocites. *Circ Res* 1985;57:868–875.
38. Yatani A, Kunze DL, Brown AM. Effects of dihydropyrydine calcium channel modulators on cardiac sodium channels. *Am J Physiol* 1988;254:H140–H147.
39. Tong Mak I, Weglicki WB. Comparative antioxidant activities of propranolol, nifedipine, verapamil, and diltiazem against sarcolemmal membrane lipid peroxidation. *Circ Res* 1990;66:1449–1452.
40. Karliner JS, Motulsky HJ, Dunlap J, Brown JH, Insel PA. Verapamil competitively inhibits α1-adrenergic and mauscarinic but not β-adrenergic receptors in rat myocardium. *J Cardiovasc Pharmacol* 1982;4:515–520.
41. Nayler WG, Papagiotopoulos S, Elz JS, Daly MJ. Inhibitory effect of calcium antagonists on the depletion of cardiac norepinephrine during post ischemic reperfusion. *J Cardiovasc Pharmacol* 1985;7:581–587.

The Failing Heart, edited by N. S. Dhalla,
R. E. Beamish, N. Takeda, and M. Nagano.
Lippincott-Raven Publishers, Philadelphia © 1995.

7

Diastolic Dysfunction: Pathophysiology and Treatment Options

E. Douglas Wigle

Department of Medicine, Division of Cardiology, The University of Toronto, The Toronto Hospital–General Division, Toronto, Ontario, M5G 2C4 Canada

Traditionally, congestive heart failure has been attributed usually to left ventricular systolic dysfunction. In the past decade or so, however, it has become increasingly recognized that diastolic dysfunction is an important cause of heart failure. This fact, plus an enhanced understanding of the pathophysiology of diastolic dysfunction (1–3), has resulted in an increased interest in diastolic abnormalities as a cause of heart failure.

PATHOPHYSIOLOGY

In describing the pathophysiology of diastolic dysfunction, we will use hypertrophic cardiomyopathy (HCM) as a model because just about everything that can affect diastolic function adversely is present in HCM (4–7) (Figs. 1–4). Where appropriate, attention will be drawn to the manner in which other forms of heart disease are similarly affected. As was the case with most types of heart disease, diastolic dysfunction in HCM was originally attributed to decreased compliance (increased chamber stiffness) (8,9). With improved understanding of diastole (1–3), however, and the availability of a number of clinical measures of diastolic function, it is now realized that impaired relaxation is the dominant type of diastolic dysfunction that is encountered in HCM (4–7).

Prior to discussing the pathophysiology of diastolic dysfunction in HCM, it is important to draw attention to several features of this condition:

1. The hypertrophy in HCM is almost always asymmetrical (Fig. 1), and the extent of hypertrophy varies from being massive (Fig. 1) to being very localized and mild (4–10).

2. Myocardial fiber disarray and variable amounts of loose intercellular connective tissue and/or myocardial fibrosis are characteristic features of the microscopic picture in HCM (10) (Fig. 2).

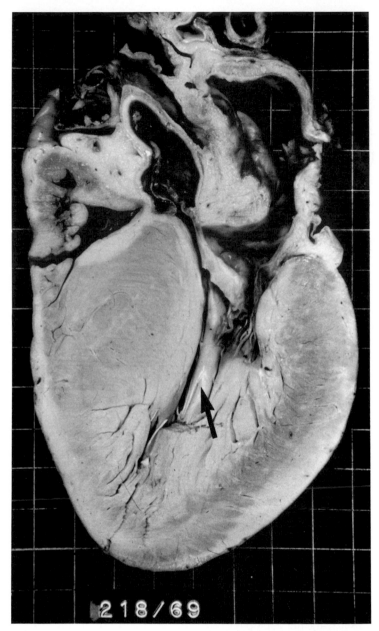

FIG. 1. Ventricular septal hypertrophy. Longitudinal section of the heart from a 32-year-old woman with subaortic obstructive HCM, who died suddenly while on propranolol therapy. Hemodynamic investigation had confirmed the presence of subaortic obstruction, as well as mitral regurgitation that was due partially to an abnormal mitral valve (insertion of an anomalous papillary muscle [*arrow*] onto the ventricular surface of the anterior mitral leaflet). Note the asymmetric hypertrophy with a grossly thickened ventricular septum and a narrowed outflow tract between the upper septum and the anterior mitral leaflet, which is very thickened and fibrosed from repeated mitral leaflet-septal contact. The increased myocardial mass and stiffness (due to interstitial fibrosis) and decreased chamber volume would all act to increase chamber stiffness (decrease compliance). The asymmetry (nonuniformity) of hypertrophy and the subaortic obstruction (contraction load) would act to impair relaxation. From Wigle et al. (4), with permission.

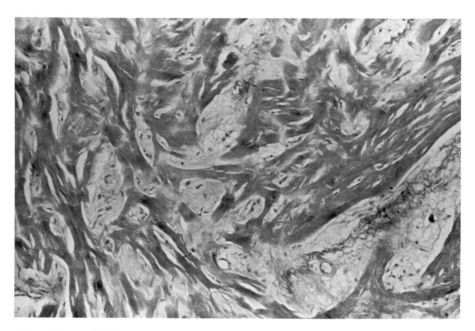

FIG. 2. Myocardial fiber disarray. Microscopic section taken from the ventricular septum of the 28-year-old patient with HCM, who died while jogging. This section shows a typical area of myocardial fiber disarray with the fibers running in all different directions. The muscle cells are short and plump, and the nuclei are large and hyperchromatic. Note the extensive amount of loose intercellular connective tissue that may become transformed into diffuse myocardial fibrosis late in the disease. × 100. From Wigle et al. (4), with permission.

3. The obstruction to left ventricular outflow is an important part of the clinical spectrum of HCM (4–9) and may adversely affect diastolic filling (4–7) (Fig. 3). Pharmacological (11) or surgical relief (12) of the outflow obstruction in HCM results in improved relaxation and a lowering of left ventricular end-diastolic (LVEDP) and left atrial pressures.

The principle determinants of diastolic function are listed in Table 1. The following is a description of how these factors are altered in HCM.

Chamber Stiffness

Chamber stiffness is a measure of the rate of change of pressure with respect to volume (dp/dv) during diastole in the left or right ventricle and is the inverse of compliance (dv/dp) (13). Chamber stiffness is directly related to myocardial mass and stiffness and inversely related to chamber volume. In HCM, all three determinants of chamber stiffness are altered in a way that increases chamber stiffness; that is, there is an increase in myocardial mass due to the hypertrophy, an increase in

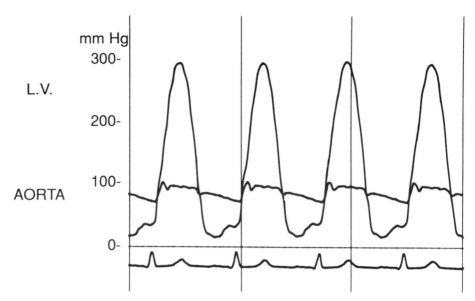

FIG. 3. Subaortic obstructive HCM. Simultaneous left ventricular (LV) and aortic pressures from a 19-year-old patient with severe, subaortic obstructive HCM. Note how early in systole the pressure gradient begins in the presence of severe obstruction, which acts as a contraction load to delay the onset and impair relaxation. Slow relaxation is suggested by the declining LV pressure in the first half of diastole at a time when the LV is filling (which should cause the pressure to rise) and also by the elevated LVEDP.

myocardial stiffness due to fibrosis, and a decrease in ventricular volume, related to the amount of hypertrophy present (4–7) (Figs. 1, 2, and 4). This increased chamber stiffness results in an increased ventricular diastolic pressure with respect to volume (increased dp/dv); that is, the diastolic pressure volume curve is shifted upward and to the left (13). Left ventricular hypertrophy due to systemic hypertension or aortic stenosis would also increase chamber stiffness in a similar fashion.

Active Relaxation

Brutsaert and colleagues have defined three basic factors that affect diastolic relaxation: load, inactivation, and nonuniformity of load and inactivation in space and time (1–3) (Fig. 4). Thus, "relaxation is governed by the continuous interplay of the sensitivity of the contractile system to the prevailing relaxation load, dissipating relaxation (inactivation), and to the temporal and regional (spatial) nonuniform distribution of load and inactivation" (2).

TABLE 1. *Determinants of diastolic function*

Chamber stiffness
Active relaxation
   Loads that affect relaxation
      Contraction load
      Relaxation loads
         Late systolic load
         End-systolic deformation load
         Coronary filling load
         Ventricular filling load
   Inactivation
   Nonuniformity of load and inactivation
Pericardial constraint and ventricular interaction
Extent of hypertrophy

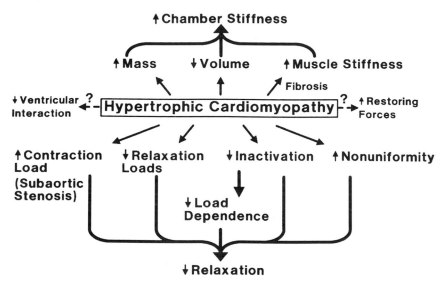

FIG. 4. Diastolic dysfunction in HCM. In HCM, there is increased chamber stiffness (dp/dv) (or decreased compliance [dv/dp]) as a result of the increased mass of muscle and the resulting decreased ventricular volume, as well as the increased muscle stiffness due to myocardial fibrosis. Thus, all three factors that affect the stiffness or compliance of the ventricle, are altered in a way that ventricular diastolic filling would be hindered by this mechanism. Left ventricular relaxation is impaired in HCM because of changes in loading conditions, decreased inactivation, and increased nonuniformity. The subaortic stenosis in obstructive HCM would represent a contraction load on the ventricle, which would delay and impair relaxation. The loads that aid in relaxation (coronary filling and ventricular filling loads) are reduced in HCM because of the degree of hypertrophy and other reasons. High myoplasmic calcium would result in decreased inactivation, which would directly impair relaxation, but would also indirectly impair it through reducing the load dependence of the relaxation process. Finally, there is a great deal of nonuniformity in HCM, which would also impair relaxation. Thus, all three factors that control relaxation—load, inactivation and nonuniformity—are altered in a way that relaxation would be impaired in HCM. The degree of impaired relaxation may be lessened by increased restoring forces. Ventricular interaction would be decreased because of the ventricular septal hypertrophy. From Wigle et al. (4), with permission.

Loads That Affect Relaxation

There are basically five loads that may affect diastolic relaxation in humans (1–3) (Table 1, Fig. 5). An increase in one, the contraction load, may impair relaxation, whereas an increase in any of the four relaxation loads enhances relaxation. A brief description of each of these loads as they would pertain in HCM follows (4–7).

In HCM the subaortic obstruction would have an affect similar to a load clamp applied during the first half of systole (1); that is, it would act as a contraction load and would act to delay the onset of relaxation and may slow the rate of relaxation. Pharmacological or surgical abolition of the subaortic obstruction improves active relaxation and often results in a lowering of left ventricular end-diastolic pressure (LVEDP) (11,12). The elevated left ventricular systolic pressure in hypertension and valvular aortic stenosis would similarly act as a contraction load to delay and impair relaxation in those conditions.

There are four loads that act to improve relaxation (relaxation loads) (1–3) (Table

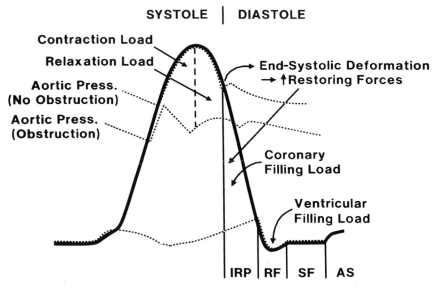

FIG. 5. Hemodynamic loads affecting ventricular relaxation in HCM. Diagram of left atrial, ventricular, and aortic pressures (with and without obstruction to outflow) together with the various loads that may affect diastolic relaxation in HCM. A contraction load (the subaortic obstruction) applied in the first half of systole would delay the onset and slow the rate of relaxation. The relaxation load that could be applied in the last half of systole is not felt to be important in HCM. The coronary filling load during the isovolumic relaxation period (IRP) and the ventricular filling load (during rapid filling [RF]) are both reduced in HCM as a result of the extent of hypertrophy and other factors. Exaggerated end-systolic deformation, due to extensive hypertrophy, could result in increased internal and external restoring forces, which would act during the IRP to improve relaxation, off-setting other factors acting to impair relaxation. SF, slow filling; AS, atrial systole. From Wigle et al. (4), with permission.

1, Fig. 5). There is no evidence that a late systolic relaxation load has any effect on left ventricular relaxation in humans. The generation of increased internal and external restoring forces could play an important role in the relaxation of the ventricle in HCM when the amount of hypertrophy present may result in greater than normal end-systolic deformation (4–7). These increased restoring forces could explain the apparent paradox of a normal LVEDP in the presence of extreme hypertrophy (4). These restoring forces could also be important in the left ventricular hypertrophy of systemic hypertension and aortic stenosis.

The filling of the coronary arterial tree during isovolumic relaxation represents a third load that may augment diastolic relaxation by applying an intramural load to the already relaxing muscle (1–3) (Table 1, Fig. 5). This "coronary kick" could be considerably blunted by a number of factors in HCM, including a reduced coronary perfusion pressure, small vessel disease with decreased coronary vasodilator capacity (14), septal perforator artery compression, and myocardial bridging (4–7). Impaired relaxation during the isovolumic relaxation period would also reduce the coronary filling load during this period (4–7), and the hypertrophy itself would reduce the impact of the coronary filling load. Consideration of all of these factors would suggest that the coronary filling load is reduced in HCM (4–7), as it would be in other forms of left ventricular hypertrophy. Coronary stenoses in coronary artery disease would reduce the coronary filling load in a nonuniform manner and result in nonuniform ischemia, and thus would impair relaxation by all three principle mechanisms.

The fourth relaxation load on the left ventricle in diastole is due to ventricular filling after mitral valve opening. The degree of ventricular filling is determined by the tension in the left ventricular wall, as indicated by the La Place relationship ($T = P \times r/2\ h$) (Fig. 5, Table 1) (1–3). Some authors prefer to think of this load as the left atrial–left ventricular pressure gradient in early diastole. In healthy subjects, although the filling pressure (P) is low, the rapid decrease in wall thickness (h) and the increase in left ventricular radius (r) result in an increased tension (T) or load on the left ventricular wall and ensure rapid diastolic filling (1–3). In HCM, however, wall thickness is increased, the rate of thinning of the wall is reduced, and the radius is reduced (15); all of these factors would decrease the wall tension or load that normally aids relaxation (2). These effects would, to some extent, be counteracted by the elevated left atrial (filling) pressure, which would increase the load on the left ventricular wall, and promote relaxation (4). Appropriately, this elevation of filling pressure is greatest in those patients with HCM, who have the greatest abnormalities in diastolic filling. These elevated filling pressures would partially compensate for, but not overcome, the effects of increased wall thickness and diminished radius, which act to diminish the hemodynamic ventricular filling load during rapid ventricular filling in HCM (4). Left ventricular hypertrophy from other causes would also result in a diminished ventricular filling load.

Thus, the contraction load in obstructive HCM, and a reduction in the principle relaxation loads (5) (coronary and ventricular filling loads), are believed to be important considerations in explaining impaired relaxation in HCM (2–7). Increased restoring forces may be important in some circumstances in HCM and would act to limit the impairment of relaxation caused by other factors. It is important to recall that ventricular relaxation is normally load dependent (1–3).

Inactivation

Inactivation is the second major factor affecting relaxation of the left ventricle (1–3); the term refers specifically to the deactivation of the force-generating sites, the actin–myosin crossbridges, in the myocardium. This deactivation process is generally attributed to the reuptake of myoplasmic calcium by the sarcoplasmic reticulum, which is an energy-dependent process, and to the extrusion of calcium to the extracellular space. With unchanging loads on the left ventricle, the rate of inactivation of contractile process is a principle determinant of the rate of myocardial relaxation (1–3). Inactivation is retarded by a high myoplasmic calcium, which may be primary in HCM (16,17) and/or due to myocardial ischemia. Inactivation not only impairs relaxation directly, but also diminishes the load dependency of relaxation (double-edged sword effect of decreased inactivation) (1–3). This latter effect would be particularly important in HCM where the principle relaxation loads are decreased (4–7). These considerations would also apply in other forms of left ventricular hypertrophy. In coronary artery disease, diminished inactivation due to myocardial ischemia would play an important role in causing impaired relaxation.

Nonuniformity of Load and Inactivation

The third major factor affecting diastolic relaxation is the nonuniform temporal and regional distribution of load and inactivation (1–3). Physiologic nonuniformity is believed to be present in the normal heart. Ample evidence suggests that pathologic nonuniformity is an important feature in cardiac hypertrophy, particularly in HCM. The essence of both the gross and microscopic pathologies in HCM is asymmetry and nonuniformity (4–7) (Figs. 1, 2). There is evidence to suggest that contraction and relaxation loading in HCM are nonuniform in distribution, and the same is undoubtedly true of the inactivation process (6,7). For example, because of septal perforator artery compression, the coronary filling load would be less in the septum than elsewhere in the left ventricle (4–7). Similarly, the asymmetrical nature of the hypertrophy would result in a nonuniform application of the ventricular filling load. Inactivation would also be nonuniform in HCM in that myoplasmic calcium would be higher in areas of myocardial fiber disarray (16,17) and there is evidence that myocardial ischemia is nonuniform in HCM, tending to occur in the areas of greatest hypertrophy.

In addition, incoordinate and/or asynchronous systolic and diastolic wall motion abnormalities have been reported in HCM and have been associated with impaired global left ventricular relaxation (18,19). It has been reported that drug-induced or disease-induced regional wall motion asynchrony in humans and animals results in global left ventricular relaxation abnormalities that are virtually identical to those seen in HCM (20). Studies by Bonow and colleagues have indicated that improvement in global left ventricular relaxation in HCM after the administration of verapamil is associated with a decrease in the asynchrony of contraction and relaxation (18). All of these observations suggest that regional nonuniformity of load and inactivation of space and time may play a major role in determining global left ventricular relaxation abnormalities in HCM.

Figure 6 demonstrates the interplay that exists between diminished and nonuniform loading, the occurrence of myocardial ischemia with impaired inactivation, and their impact on relaxation in HCM (4). This vicious cycle of diminished load, myocardial ischemia, and impaired relaxation in HCM would equally apply to coronary artery disease (Fig. 6).

In summary, there is evidence that abnormalities of left ventricular relaxation in HCM are due to a combination of altered load, impaired inactivation, and increased nonuniformity of load and inactivation of space and time. Thus, all three factors

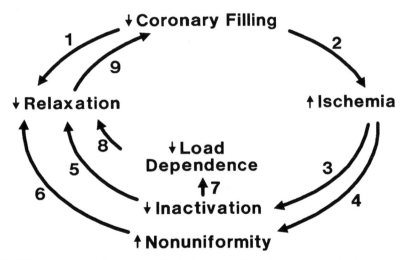

FIG. 6. Vicious cycle relating myocardial ischemia and impaired relaxation in HCM. There are many causes for impaired coronary filling and myocardial ischemia in HCM, including small vessel disease, septal perforator artery compression, myocardial bridges, decreased vasodilator capacity, and reduced capillary–myocardial fiber ratio. Decreased coronary filling during the isovolumic relaxation period will impair relaxation by the decreased load (*1*), as well as by producing myocardial ischemia (*2*), which in turn decreases inactivation (*3*) and increases nonuniformity (*4*), both of which act to slow the rate of relaxation (*5, 6*). Decreased inactivation decreases load dependency (*7*), which would further impair relaxation (*8*). Finally, impaired relaxation itself would reduce coronary filling (*9*) during the isovolumic relaxation period, and this would complete the vicious cycle by further reducing the coronary filling (relaxation) load (*1*) and producing more myocardial ischemia (*2*). A similar vicious cycle would exist in coronary artery disease where a coronary stenosis would reduce the coronary filling load, thereby impairing relaxation (*1*) and would also produce myocardial ischemia (*2*). From Wigle et al. (*4*), with permission.

involved in the triple control of relaxation are significantly altered in HCM (1–7) (Fig. 4).

Clinical Measures of Diastolic Function

Many different invasive and noninvasive techniques have been used to study diastolic dysfunction in humans. Thus, echocardiography (15,21,22), echophono-cardiography (23), Doppler (24–27), nuclear (28,29), and micromanometric (20, 27) techniques have been used to characterize the abnormalities during isovolumic relaxation, rapid filling, and atrial systolic filling. The noninvasive techniques suffer from the lack of knowing the hemodynamic loading conditions, particularly the ventricular filling load, but methods are now available to overcome at least some of these problems (27). Figure 7 demonstrates the pattern of ventricular filling when relaxation is impaired and in the presence of a restrictive filling pattern. In essence, impaired relaxation results in a decrease in the rate and volume of ventricular filling during the rapid filling phase, with a compensatory increase in atrial systolic filling, which results in a loud and often palpable fourth heart sound on clinical examination (6,7,28). In contrast, a restrictive filling pattern has an increased rate and volume of ventricular filling during the rapid filling period that is due to high left atrial pressure (increased ventricular filling load) (27). As a result, atrial systolic filling is often diminished.

Atrial Fibrillation

Atrial fibrillation in HCM is almost always related to an increase in left atrial size, as it is in most types of heart disease (4–7). This increase in left atrial size is seen most commonly in subaortic obstructive HCM (30), but also occurs in the presence of diastolic dysfunction (6,7). The onset of atrial fibrillation in the presence of impaired relaxation often results in dramatic hemodynamic deterioration (Fig. 8), because the rapid rate does not allow time for left ventricular relaxation to occur, and atrial systole, the most important compensatory mechanism for impaired relaxation, is lost (4–7).

TREATMENT OPTIONS

The treatment of diastolic dysfunction varies according to the type of heart disease; thus we will discuss treatment options for each of several common types of heart disease in which diastolic dysfunction is an important factor. Most therapy for diastolic dysfunction is directed at improving left ventricular relaxation, but where appropriate, mention will be made when therapy also affects chamber stiffness.

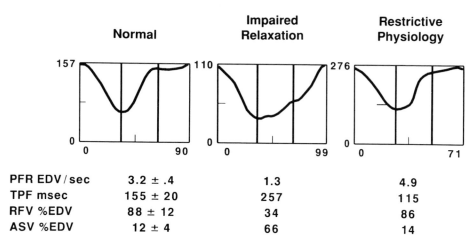

	Normal	Impaired Relaxation	Restrictive Physiology
PFR EDV/sec	3.2 ± .4	1.3	4.9
TPF msec	155 ± 20	257	115
RFV %EDV	88 ± 12	34	86
ASV %EDV	12 ± 4	66	14

FIG. 7. Two types of diastolic dysfunction in HCM. Nuclear diastolic function (time/activity) curves in a healthy subject (*left*) and in two patients with HCM, one with impaired relaxation and the other with a restrictive filling pattern. Impaired relaxation results in a reduced peak filling rate (PFR) and a prolonged time to peak filling (TPF) as well as reduced rapid filling volume (RFV) and, in compensation, an increased atrial systolic volume (ASV). The increased ASV accounts for these patients having a loud and often palpable fourth heart sound and the fact that if these patients go into atrial fibrillation, they may become profoundly symptomatic because of the loss of atrial systole, with the rapid rate not allowing time for ventricular relaxation (see Fig. 8). A restrictive filling pattern often develops in the later stages of diastolic dysfunction when the left atrial pressure is elevated. This increased ventricular filling load results in an increased PFR, a shortened TPF, a normal or increased RFV, and a normal or decreased ASV. The increased RFV accounts for these patients often having a loud third heart sound, and the normal or decreased ASV accounts for the fact that atrial fibrillation does not have profound hemodynamic consequences for these patients. Adapted from Wigle and Wilansky (6), with permission.

Hypertrophic Cardiomyopathy

Impaired relaxation in nonobstructive HCM is best managed with calcium antagonists (31,32), which have the potential to improve the coronary filling load, improve inactivation by decreasing myoplasmic calcium and relieving ischemia (33), and by reducing the degree of nonuniformity (18). Verapamil (28,29), and to a lesser extent nifedipine (34) and diltiazem, have been shown to improve left ventricular relaxation by one or more of these mechanisms, but calcium antagonists also have the potential to impair relaxation by their negative inotropic effect (29).

The treatment of subaortic obstructive HCM is directed at relieving the outflow obstruction by medical, pacemaker, or surgical means. Although the negative inotropic effect of verapamil usually decreases the gradient in obstructive HCM, the vasodilating action of this drug has the potential to worsen the obstruction unpredictably, leading to cardiogenic shock, pulmonary edema, and death (35). It is for this reason that we do not use calcium antagonists in the therapy of obstructive

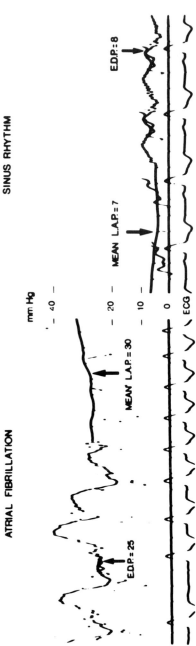

FIG. 8. Hemodynamic effects of atrial fibrillation in HCM. Left atrial and left ventricular end-diastolic pressures in a patient with subaortic obstructive HCM in sinus rhythm (*right*) and atrial fibrillation (*left*), demonstrating a dramatic rise in mean left atrial pressure from 7 to 30 mmHg with the onset of atrial fibrillation. Such a dramatic pressure rise, with the onset of this arrhythmia, would be expected in a patient with impaired relaxation because (a) the rapid rate would not allow time for relaxation and (b) the loss of atrial systole would deprive the patient of the most important compensatory mechanism for impaired ventricular filling during early diastole. From Wigle et al. (4), with permission.

HCM (4). We have used the type 1A antiarrhythmic drug disopyramide for its negative inotropic properties, and this has been demonstrated to decrease the gradient and the LVEDP (4,36,37) as well as improve left ventricular relaxation because of the decreased contraction load (the subaortic obstruction) (11). Dual chamber pacing reduces the pressure gradient in obstructive HCM and lowers LVEDP (38–40), but has been shown to impair left ventricular relaxation acutely, presumably because of the pacing induction of increased nonuniformity and the shortened atrioventricular interval (41). Myectomy surgery reduces or abolishes the gradient and the concomitant mitral regurgitation (4,5,12,42,43) in obstructive HCM, and also reduces the LVEDP (12). The latter may reflect improved relaxation due to abolition of the contraction load (the subaortic stenosis) (4), as well as relieve myocardial ischemia.

Hypertension

Left ventricular relaxation would be improved in hypertension by pharmacological reduction in the left ventricular systolic pressure (the contraction load) and by relief of ischemia that may accompany left ventricular hypertrophy. Resolution of the left ventricular hypertrophy would result in increased relaxation as well as a reduction in chamber stiffness (improved compliance).

Aortic Stenosis

Aortic valve replacement surgery would improve left ventricular relaxation by removing the contraction load (the stenotic valve) and by decreasing the degree of left ventricular hypertrophy in time, which would also improve relaxation as well as decrease chamber stiffness.

Coronary Artery Disease

Medical management of coronary artery disease would act to reduce the nonuniform ischemia, which would improve inactivation and restore load dependency as well as decrease nonuniformity, which together would improve left ventricular relaxation. In addition to these effects, angioplasty or bypass surgery would also increase the coronary filling load and reduce its nonuniformity, both of which would act to further improve left ventricular relaxation. Successful bypass surgery or angioplasty would reverse the vicious cycle of reduced coronary filling, myocardial ischemia, and impaired relaxation depicted in Fig. 6.

Miscellaneous

Restrictive Filling Defect

Patients with various types of heart disease may develop a restrictive type of filling defect that is basically related to an elevated atrial pressure (increased ventricular filling load) (27) (Fig. 7). These patients often will develop left and right heart failure and require diuretic therapy, which will lower atrial pressure and relieve pulmonary and systemic congestion. If the diuretic therapy is excessive, ventricular filling will suffer and cardiac output will decrease.

Atrial Fibrillation

Patients with impaired left ventricular relaxation develop increased left atrial size, which renders them liable to atrial fibrillation. Everything humanly possible should be done to attempt to maintain sinus rhythm because of the importance of atrial systole to these people (7) (Figs. 7, 8). This includes pharmacological and electrical cardioversion, anticoagulant therapy, and the use of amiodarone to maintain sinus rhythm when lesser antiarrhythmic agents fail.

Digitalis Glycosides

Digitalis glycosides are usually felt to be contraindicated in the presence of impaired relaxation in that they would act to increase myoplasmic calcium, which would impair inactivation and relaxation.

Transplantation

Cardiac transplantation is usually performed for end-stage systolic heart failure. It is also indicated in refractory cases of diastolic heart failure.

SUMMARY

Diastolic dysfunction is most commonly the result of impaired relaxation, but also may relate to an increase in passive chamber stiffness (decreased compliance). We have reviewed the triple control of relaxation by load, inactivation, and nonuniformity of load inactivation in space and time, indicating how these factors are altered in HCM as well as in hypertension, aortic stenosis, and coronary artery disease. The mechanisms by which medical and/or surgical therapy may improve relaxation and/or decrease chamber stiffness (improve compliance) have been discussed. In the late stages of diastolic dysfunction, a restrictive filling pattern may emerge, which is a difficult problem in management. Diastolic dysfunction and its management is now recognized to be an important aspect in the management of many cases of congestive heart failure.

REFERENCES

1. Brutsaert DL, Housmans PR, Goethais MA. Dual control of relaxation. Its role in the ventricular function in the mammalian heart. *Circ Res* 1980;47:637–652.
2. Brutsaert DL, Rademakers FE, Sys SU. Triple control of relaxation: implications in cardiac disease. *Circulation* 1984;69:190–196.
3. Brutsaert DL, Sys SU, Gillebert TC. Diastolic failure: pathophysiology and therapeutic implications. *J Am Coll Cardiol* 1993;22:318–325.
4. Wigle ED, Sasson Z, Henderson MA, et al. Hypertrophic cardiomyopathy. The importance of the site and the extent of hypertrophy. A review. *Prog Cardiovasc Dis* 1985;28:1–83.
5. Wigle ED. Hypertrophic cardiomyopathy: a 1987 viewpoint [Editorial]. *Circulation* 1987;75:311–322.
6. Wigle ED, Wilansky S. Diastolic dysfunction in hypertrophic cardiomyopathy. *Heart Failure* 1987; 3:82–93.
7. Wigle ED. Diastolic dysfunction in hypertrophic cardiomyopathy. In: Gaasch WH, Le Winter M, eds. *Left ventricular diastolic dysfunction and heart failure.* Philadelphia: Lea and Febiger; 1994;373–389.
8. Braunwald E, Morrow AG, Cornell WP, Aygen MM, Hilbish TF. Idiopathic hypertrophic subaortic stenosis. *Am J Med* 1960;29:924–945.
9. Wigle ED, Heimbecker RO, Gunton RW. Idiopathic ventricular septal hypertrophy causing muscular subaortic stenosis. *Circulation* 1962;26:325–340.
10. Teare RD. Asymmetrical hypertrophy of the heart in young adults. *Br Heart J* 1958;20:1–8.
11. Matsubara H, Nakatani S, Nagata S, Ishikura F, Beppu S, Miyatake K. Salutary effect of disopyramide on diastolic function in hypertrophic obstructive cardiomyopathy. *Circulation* 1993;88: I-135(abst).
12. Wigle ED, Chrysohou A, Bigelow W. Results of ventriculomyotomy in muscular subaortic stenosis. *Am J Cardiol* 1963;11:572–586.
13. Gaasch WH, Levine HJ, Quinones MA, Alexander JK. Left ventricular compliance: mechanisms and clinical implications. *Am J Cardiol* 1976;38:645–653.
14. Cannon RO, Rosing DR, Maron BJ, et al. Myocardial ischemia in patients with hypertrophic cardiomyopathy: contribution of inadequate vasodilator reserve and elevated left ventricular filling pressures. *Circulation* 1985;71:234–243.
15. Hanrath P, Mathey DG, Siegert R, Bleifeld W. Left ventricular relaxation and filling pattern in different forms of left ventricular hypertrophy. An echocardiographic study. *Am J Cardiol* 1980;45: 15–23.
16. Morgan MP, Morgan KG. Intracellular calcium levels during contraction and relaxation of mammalian cardiac vascular smooth muscle as detected with aequorin. *Am J Med* 1984;77:33–46.
17. Gwathmey JK, Warren SE, Briggs GM, et al. Diastolic dysfunction in hypertrophic cardiomyopathy. Effect on active force generation during systole. *J Clin Invest* 1991;87:1023–1031.
18. Bonow RO, Vitale DF, Maron BJ, Bacharach SL, Frederick TM, Green MV. Regional left ventricular asynchrony and impaired global ventricular filling in hypertrophic cardiomyopathy: effect of verapamil. *J Am Coll Cardiol* 1987;9:1108–1116.
19. Inoue T, Morooka S, Hayashi T, et al. Global and regional abnormalities of left ventricular diastolic filling in hypertrophic cardiomyopathy. *Clin Cardiol* 1991;14:573–577.
20. Pagani M, Pizzinelli P, Gussoni M, Craig WE, Pasipoularides A, Murgo JP. Diastolic abnormalities of hypertrophic cardiomyopathy reproduced by asynchrony of the left ventricle in conscious dogs. *J Am Coll Cardiol* 1983;1:641(abst).
21. Sanderson JE, Traill TA, St John Sutton MG, Brown DG, Gibson DG, Goodwin JF. Left ventricular relaxation and filling in hypertrophic cardiomyopathy. An echocardiographic study. *Br Heart J* 1978;40:596–601.
22. St. John Sutton MG, Tajik AJ, Gibson DG, Brown DG, Seward JB, Giuliani ER. Echocardiographic assessment of left ventricular filling and septal and posterior wall dynamics in idiopathic hypertrophic subaortic stenosis. *Circulation* 1978;57:512–520.

23. Hanrath P, Mathey DG, Kremer P, Sonntage F, Bleifeld W. Effect of verapamil on left ventricular isovolumic relaxation time and regional left ventricular filling in hypertrophic cardiomyopathy. *Am J Cardiol* 1980;45:1258–1264.

24. Yock PG, Hatle L, Popp RL. Patterns and timing of Doppler-detected intracavity and aortic flow in hypertrophic cardiomyopathy. *J Am Coll Cardiol* 1986;8:1047–1058.

25. Rakowski H, Sasson Z, Wigle ED. Echocardiographic and Doppler assessment of hypertrophic cardiomyopathy. *J Am Soc Echo* 1988;1:31–47.

26. Maron BJ, Spirito P, Greene KJ, Wesley YE, Bonow RO, Arce J. Noninvasive assessment of left ventricular diastolic function by pulsed Doppler echocardiography in patients with hypertrophic cardiomyopoathy. *J Am Coll Cardiol* 1987;10:733–742.

27. Appleton C, Hatle LK, Popp RL. Relation of transmitral flow velocity patterns to left ventricular diastolic function: new insights from a combined hemodynamic and Doppler echocardiographic study. *J Am Coll Cardiol* 1988;12:426–440.

28. Bonow RO, Frederick RM, Bacharach SL, et al. Atrial systole and left ventricular filling in hypertrophic cardiomyopathy: effect of verapamil. *Am J Cardiol* 1983;51:1386–1391.

29. Bonow RO, Ostrow HG, Rosing DR, et al. Effects of verapamil on left ventricular systolic and diastolic function in patients with hypertrophic cardiomyopathy: pressure volume analysis with a nonimaging scintillation probe. *Circulation* 1983;68:1062–1073.

30. Gilbert BW, Pollick C, Adelman AG, Wigle ED. Hypertrophic cardiomyopathy: subclassification by M-mode echocardiography. *Am J Cardiol* 1980;45:861–872.

31. Kaltenbach M, Hopf R, Kober G, Bussman WD, Keller M, Petersen Y. Treatment of hypertrophic obstructive cardiomyopathy with verapamil. *Br Heart J* 1979;42:35–42.

32. Rosing DR, Condit JR, Maron BJ, et al. Verapamil therapy: a new approach to the pharmacologic treatment of hypertrophic cardiomyopathy. III. Effects of long-term administration. *Am J Cardiol* 1981;48:545–553.

33. Dilsizian V, Bonow RO, Epstein SE, Fananapazir L. Myocardial ischemia detected by thallium scintigraphy is frequently related to cardiac arrest and syncope in young patients with hypertrophic cardiomyopathy. *J Am Coll Cardiol* 1993;22:796–804.

34. Lorell BH, Paulus WJ, Grossman W, Wynne J, Cohn PF. Modification of abnormal left ventricular diastolic properties by nifedipine in patients with hypertrophic cardiomyopathy. *Circulation* 1982;65:499–507.

35. Epstein SE, Rosing DR. Verapamil: its potential for causing serious complication in patients with hypertrophic cardiomyopathy. *Circulation* 1981;64:437–441.

36. Pollick C. Muscular subaortic stenosis. Hemodynamic and clinical improvement after disopyramide. *N Engl J Med* 1982;307:997–999.

37. Kimball BP, Bui S, Wigle ED. Acute dose-response effects of intravenous disopyramide in hypertrophic obstructive cardiomyopathy. *Am Heart J* 1993;125:1691–1697.

38. Duck HJ, Hutschemeiter W, Paneau H, Trenchkmann H. Atrioventricular stimulation with reduced AV delay time as a therapeutic principle in hypertrophic obstructive cardiomyopathy. *Z Gesamte Inn Med* 1984;39:437–447.

39. Fananapazir L, Cannon RO, Tripodi D, Panza JA. Impact of dual-chamber permanent pacing in patients with obstructive hypertrophic cardiomyopathy with symptoms refractory to verapamil and B-adrenergic blocker therapy. *Circulation* 1992;85:2149–2161.

40. Jeanrenaud X, Goy JJ, Kappenberger L. Effects of dual-chamber pacing in hypertrophic obstructive cardiomyopathy. *Lancet* 1992;339:1318–1323.

41. Symanski JD, Nishimura RA, Hayes DL, Tajik AJ. The effects of dual-chamber pacing on systolic and diastolic function in patients with hypertrophic cardiomyopathy: an acute Doppler/catheterization hemodynamic study. *Circulation* 1994;90:I-655(abst).

42. Wigle ED, Adelman AG, Felderhof CH. Medical and surgical treatment of cardiomyopathies. *Circ Res* 1974;35[Suppl II]:II-196–II-207.

43. Williams WG, Wigle ED, Rakowski H, Smallhorn J, LeBlanc J, Trusler GA. Results of surgery for idiopathic hypertrophic obstructive cardiomyopathy. *Circulation* 1987;76[Suppl V]:V-104–V-108.

The Failing Heart, edited by N. S. Dhalla,
R. E. Beamish, N. Takeda, and M. Nagano.
Lippincott-Raven Publishers, Philadelphia © 1995.

8

Cytoplasmic Calcium and Diastolic Dysfunction: Cardiac Hypertrophy and Failure

Kathleen A. Mansour and *James P. Morgan

*Department of Medicine (Cardiology), Emory University, Atlanta, Georgia 30322
United States; and *Department of Medicine, Cardiovascular Division,
Harvard Medical School, Beth Israel Hospital, Boston, Massachusetts 02215 United States*

Calcium ions play an integral part in regulating excitation–contraction coupling as well as in contractile performance in cardiac muscle. The release and re-uptake of intracellular calcium are necessary to maintain normal contraction and relaxation patterns in the mammalian heart. Consequently, abnormal modulation of intracellular calcium has been proposed as a major mechanism contributing to the systolic as well as diastolic dysfunction in cardiac hypertrophy and failure (1–3). Notably, these changes at the cellular level must be considered in the context of the overall function in an intact mammalian system, including the relationship and interdependence with peripheral and neurohumoral adaptive responses.

CALCIUM MODULATION

The central role of calcium in modulating excitation–contraction coupling in the mammalian heart is shown in Fig. 1 (1,4). The four major cellular sites for regulation of excitation–contraction coupling are the sarcolemma, sarcoplasmic reticulum, myofilaments, and regulatory complex. Intracellular calcium availability is regulated primarily by the sarcolemma and sarcoplasmic reticulum, which functionally correspond with the action potential and calcium transient, respectively. Calcium responsiveness is regulated predominantly by the myofilaments, actin and myosin, as well as by the regulatory troponin–tropomyosin complex, which functionally corresponds with the calcium sensitivity and maximum calcium-activated force (F_{max}) of fibers made permeable to calcium.

Depolarization initiates excitation–contraction coupling by allowing calcium to enter the myoplasm through voltage-dependent calcium channels in the sarcolemma. This calcium causes the release of a much larger quantity of activator cal-

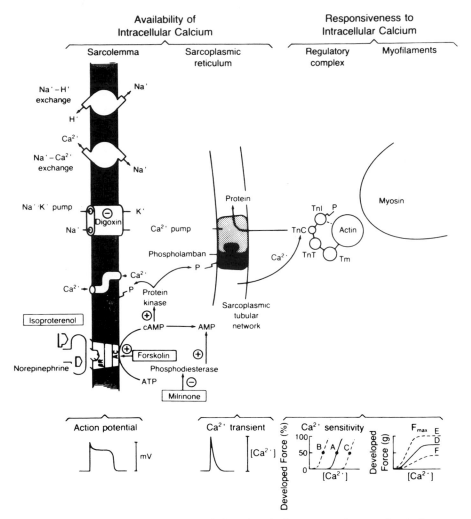

FIG. 1. Four major cellular sites for regulation of excitation–contraction coupling in the mammalian heart: sarcolemma, sarcoplasmic reticulum, regulatory complex, and myofilaments. Cardiac contractility may be altered by changing either the availability of intracellular calcium for activation or the responsiveness of the myofilaments to intracellular calcium. Calcium availability is regulated predominantly by sites in the sarcolemma and sarcoplasmic reticulum that can be functionally monitored by means of the action potential and calcium transient, respectively. Responsiveness to intracellular calcium is regulated predominantly by the troponin–tropomyosin complex, attached to actin, and the myofilaments, actin and myosin. These components can be functionally assessed by the calcium sensitivity and maximal calcium-activated force (F_{max}) of fibers rendered hyperpermeable to calcium. The Ca^{2+} transient is the depolarization-induced release and decrease in the intracellular calcium concentration ($[Ca^{2+}]$); Ca^{2+} sensitivity is the relation between the intracellular calcium concentration and cardiac activation, expressed as a percentage of peak developed force. Curves A and D are baseline values of the sensitivity of myofilaments to calcium and F_{max}, respectively. Ca^{2+} sensitivity and F_{max} can change independently of each other. Curves B and E show enhancement, and curves C and F depression, of sensitivity and F_{max}, respectively, TnI, troponin I; TnC, troponin C; TnT, troponin T; Tm, tropomyosin; βR, beta-adrenergic receptor; AD, adenylate cyclase; cAMP, cyclic AMP; P, phosphorylation. From Morgan (1).

cium from intracellular stores in the sarcoplasmic reticulum. The newly released calcium interacts with troponin C, an inhibitory regulatory complex on the myofilaments, causing a change in conformation, allowing actin and myosin to interact, crossbridges to form, and cardiac contraction to occur. Relaxation results from the dissociation of calcium from the contractile apparatus and its resequestration by the energy-dependent calcium ATPase pump of the sarcoplasmic reticulum (3,5,6). The heart maintains a 10,000-fold concentration gradient for calcium across the cell membrane through the synchronous function of each of these steps outlined in Fig. 1. These mechanisms regulating excitation–contraction coupling can be viewed schematically, as first observed by Blinks and Endoh (5), as (a) calcium-dependent "upstream" events (i.e., the events proximal to the interaction of calcium with troponin C), (b) events involving changes in the affinity of troponin C for calcium, and (c) "downstream" events (i.e., events occurring distal to the site of calcium and troponin C interaction).

Intracellular calcium homeostasis is maintained by sarcolemmal processes, including extrusion of calcium into the extracellular space, a sodium–calcium exchanger (Fig. 1) and an energy-dependent calcium pump (not shown). Initial membrane depolarization is associated with the entry of sodium into cells, which is eventually extruded by the sodium/potassium ATPase pump or by the sodium–calcium exchanger, which operates on the basis of concentration gradients. The sodium–hydrogen exchanger also has important regulatory actions, particularly in pathophysiologic conditions, such as ischemia. It is important to realize that dysfunction at any of these numerous sites outlined in Fig. 1 can result in abnormal intracellular calcium concentrations with subsequent disruption of excitation–contraction coupling, and consequently, contractile dysfunction and failure (6).

Cyclic AMP, generated by the action of adenylate cyclase on ATP, is another integral second messenger in the heart with a particularly important role in excitation–contraction coupling. Cyclic AMP activates a series of protein kinases that phosphorylate various sites within the cell, as shown in Figs. 1 and 2 (7,8). The various regions in which phosphorylation occurs include the region of the voltage-dependent calcium channels of the sarcolemma (which when phosphorylated increase the influx of calcium during depolarization), phosphorylation of the sarcoplasmic reticulum (a calcium regulatory unit, which when phosphorylated enhances calcium resequestration by the sarcoplasmic reticulum during diastole), and troponin I in the regulatory complex of the myofilaments (which decreases the affinity of troponin C for calcium when phosphorylated, thereby enhancing dissociation of calcium from this binding site). Phosphorylation of the sarcolemma increases systolic contraction and force generation by increasing calcium availability, whereas phosphorylation effects on the sarcoplasmic reticulum and troponin I enhance diastolic relaxation. The resulting net effect of an increase in cyclic AMP depends on the balance between the phosphorylation sites and is influenced by species differences as well as acute or chronic pathophysiologic disease states (1,3,4,7,9). In vivo, this process is initiated by the activation of beta-adrenergic receptors. Other potential second messengers that may play a part in the regulation of excitation–

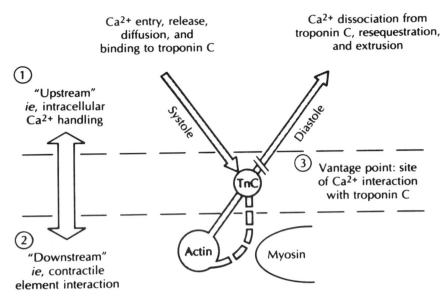

FIG. 2. Three major mechanisms (*1,2,3*) regulating the contractile state. Dashed line connecting TnC to actin depicts inhibitory action of troponin–tropomyosin complex on actin–myosin interaction. This inhibition is removed and crossbridges allowed to attach when Ca^{2+} binds to TnC. TnC, troponin C. From Apstein and Morgan (8).

contraction coupling include inositol triphosphate and diacylglycerol, but their ultimate roles have yet to be confirmed (2).

ABNORMAL REGULATION OF INTRACELLULAR CALCIUM

Abnormal intracellular calcium handling is a major cause of both systolic and diastolic dysfunction. Models of acute cardiac failure involve alteration in excitation–contraction coupling as the predominant cause of dysfunction, while chronic cardiac failure appears to include extracellular factors involving myocyte and connective tissue content in addition to abnormalities in excitation–contraction coupling. Hypertrophic cardiomyopathy is a unique state with signs and symptoms of diastolic dysfunction, which is due primarily to alteration in intracellular calcium handling in the hypertrophied cells (1–3,6,10).

A summary of the alterations in calcium regulation in various models of acute, subacute, and chronic heart failure, as well as hypertrophic cardiomyopathy, is shown in Tables 1 and 2 (6,9). Interestingly, the ability of the cardiac muscle to generate systolic tension is depressed under most experimental conditions. This decrease in systolic function does not always correlate with decreased availability of activator calcium, however. For example, in the model of acute systolic dysfunction produced by the drug butanedione monoxime (BDM), there is depressed systolic force generation with preserved intracellular calcium levels, suggesting an uncoup-

TABLE 1. *Experimental models of subacute, acute, and chronic heart failure and diastolic failure with hyperdynamic systolic function*

Models	Species	Preparation	Primary mechanism
Acute heart failure			
Drugs			
$\downarrow [Ca^{2+}]_o$	Ferret	SS/PM/WH	Upstream
Ca^{2+} channel blockers	Cat, ferret, human	PM	Upstream
Digitalis toxicity	Ferret	PM/WH	Upstream
Local anesthetics	Cat, ferret, human	PM	Upstream
Ryanodine	Cat, ferret, rabbit, human	PM/WH	Upstream
BDM	Ferret, human	PM	Downstream, TnC
Acidosis	Ferret	PM/WH	Upstream
Hypoxia	Ferret	PM	Downstream, TnC
Ischemia	Ferret	WH	Downstream, TnC
Bradycardia	Cat, ferret, human	PM/WH	Upstream
Subacute heart failure			
Postischemic stunning	Ferret	WH	Downstream, TnC
Chronic heart failure			
RV pressure overload	Ferret	PM	Extracellular
LV pressure overload	Ferret	WH	Upstream
Hypothyroidism	Ferret	PM	Upstream
Hypertrophic CMY	Hamster	PM	Upstream
Hypertensive CMY	Rat	PM	Extracellular
End-stage dilated CMY	Human	PM	Upstream
End-stage hypertrophic CMY	Human	PM	Upstream
Pacing-induced CMY	Dog	PM	Upstream
Hereditary dilated CMY	Hamster	WH	Upstream
Diastolic failure with hyper-dynamic systolic function			
Hypertrophic CMY	Human	PM	Upstream

Table from Perreault et al. (9); mechanisms adapted from Blinks and Endoh (5).
$\downarrow [Ca^{2+}]_o$, decreased extracellular calcium concentration; BDM, butanedione monoxime; RV, right ventricular; LV, left ventricular; CMY, cardiomyopathy; SS, single cell; PM, papillary muscle, trabeculae carneae; WH, whole heart; TnC, troponin C.

ling of calcium from contraction produced by a decrease in myofilament calcium responsiveness (6,11,12). In addition, in the ferret model of right ventricular pressure-overload hypertrophy with chronic failure, there is depressed systolic force generation, but the intracellular calcium levels are normal. The major abnormality resulting in impaired systolic function in this model appears to be an alteration in connective tissue content in the cardiac interstitium (13). Thus, the decrease in systolic force generation in the majority of these models correlates with decreased myofilament calcium responsiveness in acute heart failure and correlates with interstitial changes in chronic heart failure (9). In contrast, several other models including Syrian hamsters with end-stage dilated cardiomyopathy (14,15), diabetic rats (16), and rats after myocardial infarction (17) have demonstrated excellent correlation between systolic dysfunction and the decreased availability of activator calcium in cardiac muscle.

Although there appears to be a variable relation between systolic force generation

TABLE 2. *Relation of changes in intracellular calcium modulation and isometric contraction in hypertrophy and failure*

	Peak systolic level		End-diastolic level		Duration		Myofilament Ca²⁺ responsiveness	Morphologic and interstitial changes	References
	Cont. force	$[Ca^{2+}]_i$	Cont. force	$[Ca^{2+}]_i$	Cont. force	$[Ca^{2+}]_i$			
Acute heart failure									
Drugs									
↓$[Ca^{2+}]_o$	→↑	→↑	↕	↕	↕	↕	↕	0	12–14
Ca²⁺ channel blockers	→↑→	→↑↔→	↕	↕	↕	↕	↕↔→	0	15
Digitalis toxicity	→↑→	→↑↔→	↕	↕	↕	↕	↕↔→	0	16
Local anesthetics	→↑	→↑	↕←↑	↕←↑	↕↔→↑←	↕↔→↑←	→↑→↔→	0	17,18
Ryanodine	→↑	↕	↕	↕	→↔↑←	→↔↑←	→↔→↔→	0	12
BDM	→↑↔	↕	↕	↕↔←↑	↕→↑←	↕→↑←	→↔→↔	0	4
Acidosis	→→	↕	↕←↑	↕←↑	↕↑←	↕↑←	↑→	0	4
Hypoxia	→↔	↕↔←↑	↕	↕←←↑	↕↔↑←	↕↔↑←	↔→↑	0	8,19
Ischemia	→↔	↕↔←↑	↕	↕←←↑	↕↔↑←	↕↔↑←	↔→↑	0	8,20
Bradycardia	→→	↕	↕	↕	↕↑←	↕↑←	↕	0	21,22
Subacute heart failure									
Postischemic stunning	↓	↕←↑	↕	↕	↕↑←	↕↑←	→↑	0	23
Chronic heart failure									
RV pressure overload	→→→	↕←↑	↕	↕	←↑←	←↑←	↕	+	24
LV pressure overload	→→→	↕←↑	↕	↕	←↑←	←↑←	↕	+	25
Hypothyroidism	→→→	→→↔	↕	↕	←←←	←←←	↕	0	26
Hypertrophic CMY	→→→	→→↔	↕	↕→↔	←←←	←←←	↕	+	27
Hypertensive CMY	→→→	→→↔	↕→↔	↕→↔	←←←	←←←	↕	+	28,29
End-stage dilated CMY	↓↕	↕↕	↕↕←	↕↕←	←←←	←←←	→→↑	+	30–32
End-stage hypertrophic CMY	↓↕	→→→	↕←↑	↕←↑	←←←	←←←	→→↔	+	30–34
Pacing-induced CMY	→→→	→↑	↕	↕	←←←	←←←	↕	0	35
Hereditary dilated CMY	→→→	→↓	↕	↕	←←←	←←←	↕	+	36
Diastolic failure with hyperdynamic systolic function									
Hypertrophic CMY	↔↑	↔↑	↔↑	↔↑	↑↑	↑↑	↕	+	12

Data derived from models in Table 1 (from Perreault et al. [9]).
Cont. force, contractile force; $[Ca^{2+}]_i$, intracellular calcium concentration; $[Ca^{2+}]_o$, extracellular calcium concentration; BDM, butanedione monoxime; RV, right ventricular; LV, left ventricular; CMY, cardiomyopathy; ↔, no change; ↑, increase; ↓, decrease; 0, not a factor or minor factor; +, major factor.

and intracellular calcium, diastolic relaxation abnormalities appear to have a high positive correlation with end-diastolic calcium levels. Prolongation of relaxation was demonstrated in most of the models studied and correlated well with prolongation of the intracellular calcium transients as measured with the calcium indicator aequorin (9,18). Interestingly, in hypoxia, the increase in end-diastolic calcium levels are associated with increased end-diastolic tension (Fig. 3A), whereas in ischemia, there are marked increases in systolic and diastolic calcium concentrations associated with a marked decrease in force production (Fig. 3B), suggesting uncoupling of the calcium from the force generation (19–25).

Hypertrophic cardiomyopathy is notable for the normal or hyperdynamic systolic function associated with diastolic contractile abnormalities. At rapid heart rates there is incomplete relaxation between contractions, producing elevated end-diastolic calcium and tension (fusion phenomenon). Pretreatment of the myopathic muscle with relaxing agents (e.g., forskolin or isoproterenol), which increase cyclic AMP and increase sequestration of calcium by the sarcoplasmic reticulum, prevented the fusion. Conversely, if agents that increase intracellular calcium (e.g., digitalis) or prolong the calcium transient or twitch were given, the fusion was enhanced (1,10,26). Further evidence of altered intracellular calcium homeostasis was demonstrated by the exacerbation of contractile abnormalities of the hypertrophied muscles when exposed to increased extracellular calcium concentrations. It appears that the degree of hypertrophy directly correlates with abnormalities in excitation–contraction coupling, suggesting that the abnormality in calcium handling may reflect the degree of myocyte hypertrophy that is present rather than the heart failure per se (10,27).

HUMAN HEART FAILURE

Human heart failure occurs as a result of systolic dysfunction, diastolic dysfunction, or a combination of both and as such is a difficult area for experimental work (see Meuse et al. [28] for a review of contemporary studies). On the basis of numerous studies using human heart muscle loaded with the calcium indicator aequorin (29), however, there appear to be three "signatures" of heart failure in isolated human myocardium, as shown in Fig. 4 (9,27,30). These three hallmarks of human heart failure are (a) reversed force–frequency relation, (b) two components of intracellular calcium transient, and (c) decreased responsiveness to drugs that act by increasing cyclic AMP concentrations (9,30–32). The result of the reversal of force–frequency relation is that the myopathic human muscle generates less systolic force at higher pacing rates. Abnormal calcium modulation at the sarcoplasmic reticulum and sarcolemma cause the two-component calcium signal from the indicator aequorin (Fig. 5) (9). The decreased responsiveness to drugs that increase cyclic AMP appears to reflect deficient production of this nucleotide by the myopathic heart (1). One explanation for this depressed cyclic AMP production is an increase in the proportion of inhibitory to stimulatory G proteins that regulate adenylate

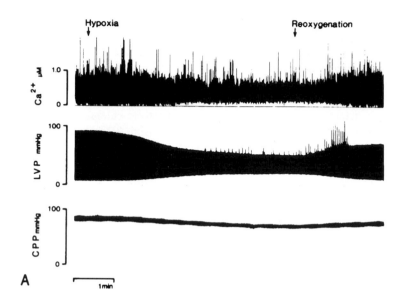

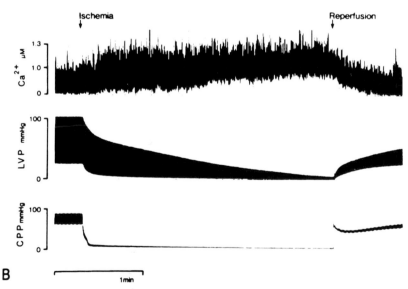

FIG. 3. Recordings from isolated buffer-perfused ferret heart at 30°C, and paced at 125 to 130 beats per minute. Simultaneous recording of $[Ca^{2+}]_i$ transients (*top*), isovolumic LV pressures (LVP) (*middle*), and coronary perfusion pressures (*bottom*) during 5 min of hypoxia followed by reoxygenation (**A**) or 3 min of global ischemia followed by reperfusion (**B**). Note that $[Ca^{2+}]_i$ and LVP correlate in hypoxia but appear to be uncoupled in ischemia. CPP, coronary perfusion pressure. From Perreault et al. (9).

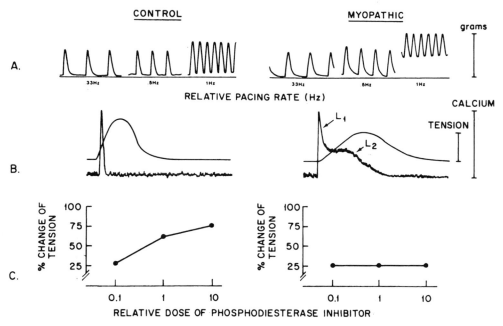

FIG. 4. Tracings showing signatures of heart failure in isolated human myocardium. **(A)** Reversal of force–frequency relation from positive to negative staircase going from lower to higher pacing frequencies. **(B)** Prolonged $[Ca^{2+}]_i$ transient and twitch; two components, L_1 and L_2, in $[Ca^{2+}]_i$ transient. **(C)** Markedly diminished response to phosphodiesterase inhibitors like milrinone. From Perreault et al. (9).

cyclase activity (30,31), and this inhibitory to stimulatory G protein ratio may depend on the etiology of the heart failure (33–35).

In addition to excitation–contraction coupling, myofilament responsiveness to calcium has an important role in regulating cardiac contractile performance (2). The degree of activation of the myofilaments is related directly to the binding of calcium to troponin C, but the degree of activation can be altered by numerous pathophysiologic states and pharmacologic agents, as shown in Fig. 6 (8). For example, alkalosis increases the responsiveness of myofilaments to calcium, whereas acidosis and the accumulation of inorganic phosphate decrease myofilament responsiveness. Interestingly, studies from 1991 have demonstrated that some endogenous substances such as alpha agonists, opioid agonists, and endothelin may produce intracellular alkalosis resulting in increased force production (i.e., inotropic activity), but with delayed relaxation due to enhanced myofilament calcium responsiveness (36–40). Of note, a study using the inotropic agent DPI 201-106 demonstrated a significant increase in calcium sensitivity of human cardiac muscle from patients with end-stage failure, yet had no effect on calcium sensitivity in normal heart muscle, thus suggesting that pharmacologic agents such as DPI 201-106 may produce differential effects on myofibrillar calcium sensitivity in normal and diseased

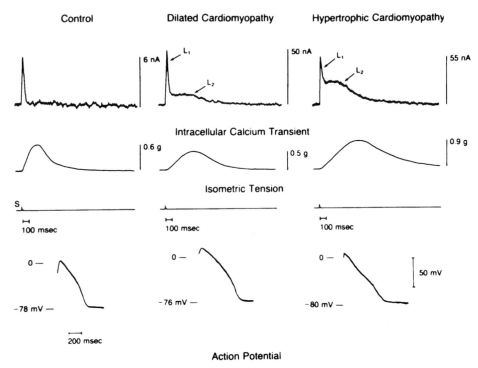

FIG. 5. Recordings representing, from top to bottom, aequorin light tracing (i.e., $[Ca^{2+}]_i$), isometric tension, stimulus(s) artifact, and action potentials from control and myopathic human trabeculae carneae, maintained in vitro. Light expressed in nanoamperes (nA) of anode current; tension in grams (g), action potentials in millivolts (mV). L_1, L_2, two components in $[Ca^{2+}]_i$ transient. From Perreault et al. (9).

cardiac states (41). Studies of myopathic myocardium, however, have demonstrated that a change in myosin isoforms must be present for a substantial change in calcium responsiveness of the ventricular muscle (6,29) and that pressure overload appears to play a major role in the cardiac myosin isoform shift (42,43) and may be an adaptive mechanism to the increased pressure overload (44). Additionally, alterations in myofibrils have been demonstrated in human heart failure. One study compared the myofibrillar ATPase activity from normal human ventricular muscle with that from patients with end-stage heart failure (45). Significantly lower amounts of myofibrillar protein were found in heart failure muscle regardless of severity of disease, in contrast to normal heart muscle, suggesting that the decrease in ventricular myofibrillar protein content may relate to progression of heart failure and to the development of subsequent diastolic dysfunction.

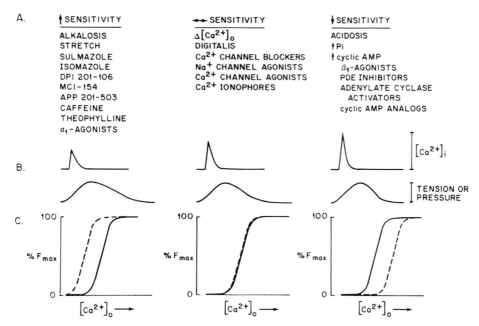

FIG. 6. Effects of interventions on the Ca^{2+} sensitivity of the contractile apparatus. (**A**) Summaries of the effects of interventions on myofilament calcium sensitivity. (**B**) The effects of equiinotropic concentrations of the agonists listed in A on the intracellular calcium transient. Note that drugs that decrease myofilament calcium sensitivity increase the amplitude of the calcium transient relative to drugs that do not change myofilament calcium sensitivity. (**C**) The effects of these agents on the force versus pCa relationship of skinned or hyperpermeabilized fibers. The interventions that increase myofilament sensitivity to calcium have the potential to cause or exacerbate diastolic dysfunction; conversely, agents that decrease myofilament sensitivity to calcium have a potential lusitropic effect. From Apstein and Morgan (8).

SUMMARY

Intracellular calcium homeostasis is an integral part of the maintenance of excitation–contraction coupling and contractile cardiac performance, both systolic and diastolic. Abnormalities in the regulation of intracellular calcium appear to be compensatory initially in cardiac hypertrophy, but these changes may contribute ultimately to subsequent failure (1). The challenge is not only to "fine-tune" the intracellular calcium regulatory system so as to optimize systolic function while minimizing diastolic dysfunction, but also to determine the causes of transition to heart failure itself.

REFERENCES

1. Morgan JP. Abnormal intracellular modulation of calcium as a major cause of cardiac contractile dysfunction. *N Engl J Med* 1991;325:625–632.
2. Rasmussen H. The calcium messenger system. *N Engl J Med* 1986;314:1094–1101, 1164–1170.

3. Katz AM. Cardiomyopathy of overload: a major determinant of prognosis in congestive heart failure. *N Engl J Med* 1990;322:100–110.

4. Feldman MD, Copelas L, Gwathmey JK, et al. Deficient production of cyclic AMP: pharmacologic evidence of an important cause of contractile dysfunction in patients with end-stage heart failure. *Circulation* 1987;75(2):331–339.

5. Blinks JR, Endoh M. Modification of myofibrillar responsiveness to Ca^{++} as an inotropic mechanism. *Circulation* 1986;73[Suppl III]:III85–III98.

6. Perreault CL, Meuse AJ, Bentivegna LA, Morgan JP. Abnormal intracellular calcium handling in acute and chronic heart failure: role in systolic and diastolic dysfunction. *Eur Heart J* 1990;11[Suppl C]:8–21.

7. Katz AM. Cyclic adenosine monophosphate effects on the myocardium: a man who blows hot and cold with one breath. *J Am Coll Cardiol* 1983;2:143–149.

8. Apstein CS, Morgan JP. Cellular mechanisms underlying left ventricular diastolic dysfunction. In: Gaasch WH, LeWinter MM, eds. *Left ventricular diastolic dysfunction and heart failure*. Philadelphia: Lea & Febiger; 1994:3–24.

9. Perreault CL, Williams CP, Morgan JP. Cytoplasmic calcium modulation and systolic versus diastolic dysfunction in myocardial hypertrophy and failure. *Circulation* 1993;87[Suppl VII]:VII31–VII37.

10. Gwathmey JK, Warren SE, Briggs GM, et al. Diastolic dysfunction in hypertrophic cardiomyopathy: effect on active force generation during systole. *J Clin Invest* 1991;87:1023–1031.

11. Blanchard EM, Alpert NR, Allen DG, Smith GL. The effect of 2,3-butanedione monoxime on the initial heat-tension integral relation and aequorin light output from ferret papillary muscles. *Biophys J* 1988;53:605a.

12. Ohkusa T, Gwathmey JK. The effects of 2,3-butanedione monoxime on twitch force and steady state force relationship in ferret papillary muscle. *Biophys J* 1989;55;100a.

13. Gwathmey JK, Morgan JP. Altered calcium handling in experimental pressure-overload hypertrophy in the ferret. *Circ Res* 1985;57:836–843.

14. Bentivegna LA, Ablin LW, Kihara Y, Morgan JP. Altered calcium handling in left ventricular pressure-overload hypertrophy as detected with aequorin in the isolated, perfused ferret heart. *Circ Res* 1991;69:1538–1545.

15. Wikman-Coffelt J, Stefenelli T, Wu ST, Parmley WW, Jasmin G. $[Ca^{2+}]_i$ transients in the cardiomyopathic hamster heart. *Circ Res* 1991;68:45–51.

16. Maher KA, Litwin SE, Perreault CL, Bentivegna LA, Shannon RP. Abnormalities in excitation-contraction coupling in diabetic cardiomyopathic rats. *Circulation* 1991;84[Suppl II]:II446.

17. Litwin SE, Morgan JP. Intracellular Ca^{2+} handling and beta-adrenergic responsiveness in surviving myocardium from rats with large infarctions. *Circulation* 1991;84[Suppl II]:II10.

18. Morgan JP, Morgan KG. Calcium and cardiovascular function: intracellular calcium levels during contraction and relaxation of mammalian cardiac and vascular smooth muscle as detected with aequorin. *Am J Med* 1984;77(5A):33–46.

19. Kihara Y, Gwathmey JK, Grossman W, Morgan JP. Mechanisms of positive inotropic effects and delayed relaxation produced by DPI 201-106 in mammalian working myocardium: effects on intracellular calcium handling. *Br J Pharmacol* 1989;96:927–939.

20. Levine MJ, Harada K, Meuse A, et al. Excitation-contraction coupling during ischemia in the blood perfused dog heart. *Biochem Biophys Res Commun* 1991;179:502.

21. MacKinnon R, Gwathmey JK, Morgan JP. Differential effects of reoxygenation on intracellular calcium and isometric tension. *Pflugers Arch* 1987;409:448–453.

22. Marban E, Kitakaze M, Kusuoka H, Porterfield JK, Yue DT, Chacko VP. Intracellular free calcium concentration measured with 19F NMR spectroscopy in intact ferret hearts. *Proc Natl Acad Sci USA* 1987;84:6005–6009.

23. Mohabir R, Lee HC, Kurz RW, Clusin WT. Effects of ischemia and hypercarbic acidosis on myocyte calcium transients, contraction and pH_i in perfused rabbit hearts. *Circ Res* 1991;69:1525–1537.

24. Kihara Y, Grossman W, Morgan JP. Direct measurement of changes in intracellular calcium transients during hypoxia, ischemia, and reperfusion of the intact mammalian heart. *Circ Res* 1989;65:1029–1044.

25. Carrozza JP, Bentivegna LA, Williams CP, Kuntz RE, Grossman W, Morgan JP. Decreased myofilament responsiveness in myocardial stunning follows transient calcium overload during ischemia and reperfusion. *Circ Res* 1992;71:1334–1340.

26. Li Q, Biagi B, Starling R, Hohl C, Altshuld R, Stokes B. Characteristics of calcium transients and electrophysiology in human ventricular myocytes. *Biophys J* 1989;55[Suppl]:488a.

27. Gwathmey JK, Copelas L, MacKinnon R, et al. Abnormal intracellular calcium handling in myocardium from patients with end-stage heart failure. *Circ Res* 1987;61:70–76.

28. Meuse AJ, Perreault CL, Morgan JP. Pathophysiology of cardiac hypertrophy and failure of human working myocardium: abnormalities in calcium handling. In: Hasenfuss G, Holusbarsch CH, Just H, Alpert NR, eds. *Cellular and molecular alterations in the failing human heart*. Darmstadt: Steinkopff Verlag; 1992:223–233.

29. Morgan JP, Erny RE, Allen PD, Grossman W, Gwathmey JK. Abnormal intracellular calcium handling, a major cause of systolic and diastolic dysfunction in ventricular myocardium from patients with heart failure. *Circulation* 1990;81[Suppl III]:III21–III32.

30. Feldman MD, Copelas L, Gwathmey JK, et al. Deficient production of cyclic AMP: pharmacologic evidence of an important cause of contractile dysfunction in patients with end-stage heart failure. *Circulation* 1987;75(2):331–339.

31. Feldman AM, Cates AE, Veazey WB, et al. Increase of the 40,000-mol wt pertussis toxin substrate (G protein) in the failing human heart. *J Clin Invest* 1988;82:189–197.

32. Phillips PJ, Gwathmey JK, Feldman MD, Schoen FJ, Grossman W, Morgan JP. Post-extrasystolic potentiation and the force-frequency relationship: differential augmentation of myocardial contractility in working myocardium from patients with end-stage heart failure. *J Mol Cell Cardiol* 1990;22:99–110.

33. Bohm M, Gierschik P, Jakobs KH, et al. Increase in $G_{i\ alpha}$ in human hearts with dilated but not ischemic cardiomyopathy. *Circulation* 1990;82:1249.

34. Neumann J, Scholz H, Doring V, Schmitz W, von Meyerinck L, Kolmar P. Increase in myocardial G_i-proteins in heart failure. *Lancet* 1988;2(8617):936–937.

35. Fleming JW, Wisler PL, Watanabe AM. Surgical transduction by G proteins in cardiac tissues. *Circulation* 1992;85(2):420–433.

36. Lompre AM, Lambert F, Lakatta EG, Schwartz K. Expression of sarcoplasmic reticulum Ca^{2+}-ATPase and calsequestrin genes in rat heart during ontogenic development and aging. *Circ Res* 1991;69:1380–1388.

37. Ventura C, Capogrossi MC, Spurgeon HA, Lakatta EG. Kappa-opioid peptide receptor stimulation increases cytosolic pH and myofilament responsiveness to Ca^{2+} in cardiac myocytes. *Am J Physiol* 1991;261:H1671–H1674.

38. Movsesian MA, Leveille C, Krall J, Colyer J, Wang JH, Campbell KP. Identification and characterization of proteins in sarcoplasmic reticulum from normal and failing human left ventricles. *J Mol Cell Cardiol* 1990;22:1477–1485.

39. Kramer BK, Smith TW, Kelly RA. Endothelin and increased contractility in adult rat ventricular myocytes. Role of intracellular alkalosis induced by activation of the protein kinase C-dependent Na^+-H^+ exchanger. *Circ Res* 1991;68:269–279.

40. Kelly RA, Eid H, Kramer BK, et al. Endothelin enhances the contractile responsiveness of adult rat ventricular myocytes to calcium by a pertussis toxin-sensitive pathway. *J Clin Invest* 1991;86:1164–1171.

41. Hauar RJ, Gwathmey JK, Briggs GM, Morgan JP. Differential effect of DPI 201-106 on the sensitivity of the myofilaments to Ca^{2+} in intact and skinned trabeculae from control and myopathic human hearts. *J Clin Invest* 1988;82:1578–1584.

42. Tsuchimochi H, Sugi M, Kuro-o M, et al. Isozymic changes in myosin of human atrial myocardium induced by overload. Immunohistochemical study using monoclonal antibodies. *J Clin Invest* 1984;74:662–665.

43. Kawana M, Kimata S, Taira A, et al. Isozymic changes in myosin human myocardium induced by pressures overload. *Circulation* 1986;74:II82.

44. Yazaki Y, Tsuchimochi H, Komuro I, Kurabayashi U, Takaku F. Molecular and biological aspects of cardiac hypertrophy. In: Toshima H, Maron BJ, eds. *Hypertrophic cardiomyopathy*. Tokyo: University of Tokyo Press; 1988:97–111.

45. Pagani ED, Alousi AA, Grant AM, Older TM, Dziuban SW Jr, Allen PD. Changes in myofibrillar content and Mg-ATPase activity in ventricular tissues from patients with heart failure caused by coronary artery disease, cardiomyopathy or mitral valve insufficiency. *Circ Res* 1988;63:380–385.

The Failing Heart, edited by N. S. Dhalla,
R. E. Beamish, N. Takeda, and M. Nagano.
Lippincott-Raven Publishers, Philadelphia © 1995.

9

Molecular Signaling in Cardiac Myofilaments

R. John Solaro

*Department of Physiology and Biophysics, University of Illinois at Chicago,
College of Medicine, Chicago, Illinois 60612-7342 United States*

Detailed understanding of the molecular processes by which regulatory proteins signal the myofilaments to turn on and turn off has taken on a new importance. There are compelling data indicating that length dependence of myofilament response to Ca^{2+} forms the basis of Starling's Law (1–3). Thus, length dependence of myofilament activation appears to be an important determinant of the shape of the relation between end systolic volume and end-systolic pressure. There is also substantial evidence that adrenergic stimulation of the heart is associated with phosphorylation of the myofilaments by, for example, protein kinase A, protein kinase C, and also myosin light chain (Ca^{2+}-calmodulin-dependent) protein kinase, to name the most well studied (4,5). Importantly, covalent modulation of the myofilament proteins via these kinases affects their activity and their control by Ca^{2+} (4,5).

Alterations in the response of the myofilaments to Ca^{2+} also occur during conditions associated with depressed cardiac function. One example is during acidosis, in which it has been shown that force-generating capabilities of heart muscle are considerably depressed under conditions in which the amplitude of Ca^{2+}-transient during the twitch is, in fact, increased (6). Similar effects occur during the depression in cardiac function associated with hypoxia and accumulation of adenosine diphosphate (ADP) or inorganic phosphate (Pi), the products of adenosine triphosphate (ATP) hydrolysis, and breakdown of creatine phosphate (1,7). There are also potential long-term changes in structure/function relations of the myofilaments associated with breakdown of myofilament proteins (8) or altered gene expression (9–11) that may affect the myofilament response to Ca^{2+}. Strong ties between altered gene expression and heart failure are the identification of mutations in the myosin-heavy chain gene that form the molecular basis of familial hypertrophic cardiomyopathy (10). More recent evidence also ties missense mutations in TnT and in tropomyosin (Tm) to this same syndrome, which is emerging as a "sarcomeric" disease (11). Reexpression of a fetal isoform of TnT has also been correlated with the well-known depression in maximum myofibrillar ATPase activity in various forms of heart failure (9).

The complexity of myofilament regulation suggests a rich array of possible mechanisms by which myofilament response to Ca^{2+} might be manipulated pharmacologically. Recent evidence indicates that pharmacological manipulation of the response of the myofilaments to Ca^{2+} may alter the energy requirements for pumping function of the heart. The inotropic agent Acardi (pimobendan; UDCG 115BS) increases Ca^{2+} binding to troponin C (TnC) in myofilaments and is also an inhibitor of cAMP phosphodiesterase (type III) (12). The introduction of Acardi into clinical use in heart failure in Japan shows early promise, but must await more extensive clinical experience and trials of this so-called Ca-sensitizer. Convincing evidence that such agents may affect cardiac energetics in humans comes from recent studies showing that the compound MCI-154 (13) reduces myocardial oxygen consumption in diseased human hearts. The proposed mechanism is that the altered response of the myofilaments to Ca^{2+} has reduced the cost of nonmechanical work (13).

CHEMOMECHANICAL COUPLING AND SWITCHING ON OF THIN FILAMENTS BY Ca^{2+}

Likely control steps in the actin–myosin reaction have been revealed by considering the kinetics of the crossbridge reaction with actin and the relation between hydrolysis of ATP and myofilament force and shortening (7,14–16). Crossbridges appear to be in one of the following three states with regard to their interaction with actin: (a) a blocked state, in which binding to the thin filament is blocked by Tn-Tm; (b) a weak binding state, in which crossbridges react with the thin filament in a rapid "on-off steady state" but do not generate force; and (c) a strong binding state that generates force and, as will be discussed, cooperatively turns on the thin filament. In the complete absence of Tn-Tm it is apparent that the thin filament is fully reactive. When Tn and Tm are present on the thin filament, the transition from the blocked or weakly bound state to a strong binding state is triggered by Ca^{2+}. The step in the reaction sequence most likely controlled by Ca^{2+}, according to the Millar and Homsher (7) model, is a slow step involving isomerization of a weak binding state, actin-myosin-ADP-Pi (7,14,15) to a strong, force-generating state. Accordingly, during diastole, in which Ca^{2+} is limiting, weakly bound or blocked crossbridges accumulate and myofilaments are in a resting condition.

SWITCHING THE THIN FILAMENT ON THROUGH Ca-TnC

There is ample evidence that the reaction of Ca^{2+} with TnC triggers transition of crossbridges to force generating states (1,2,17). A currently unresolved issue is just what is regulated when Ca^{2+} binds to TnC. One possibility is that Ca^{2+} acts as a switch and promotes the transition from the weak to the strong state in an "all-or-none" fashion (18). In this case, Tm acts to enhance the affinity of crossbridges for actin, and relative activation of the myofilaments by Ca^{2+} (e.g., at the 50% level) would involve 50% of the crossbridges "recruited" to the strong state. An opposite view is that Ca^{2+} increases the rate of transition from the weak to the strong state in a "graded" fashion (19). In this case, 50% relative activation of the myofilaments could involve all of the crossbridges in an activated state, but with the forward rate of transition between weak and strong states at some submaximal level (19). A choice between these possibilities is difficult in that the conclusions from particular experiments are dependent on the methods used and may be model-dependent (7). In any case, the actions of Tm are difficult to explain by a pure steric effect and are more readily explained by allosteric effects on actin structure. A model restricted to the idea that simple movement of Tm or Tn permits binding of myosin heads is probably too simple, and some allosteric effects on actin structure seem likely.

Whether all-or-none or graded in terms of activation of the thin filament, there is an emerging picture of how the reaction of Ca^{2+} with TnC is transduced to affect the reactivity of actin (1,17). Figure 1 illustrates the molecular processes that are believed to occur in triggering the actin–myosin crossbridge reaction and shows the thin filament in on and off states. The off state is associated with low cytosolic Ca^{2+}; there are weak interactions between TnC and TnI and possibly between TnC

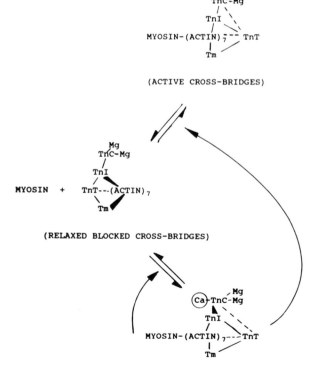

FIG. 1. Modes of activation of cardiac myofilaments by calcium and by strong crossbridges. This figure demonstrates that thin filaments are turned on by calcium through TnC and by the binding of the crossbridge.

and TnT; TnI binds to actin strongly (17). The off state also may be characterized by a poorly understood interaction of TnI with TnT, and a potential interaction of TnT with actin (20). These interactions, which are transmitted to Tm through TnT, hold Tm in a conformational state or location that alters actin activity such that the actin–crossbridge reaction is impeded. The strong interaction of TnI with actin in relaxing conditions also is likely to inhibit the reaction of crossbridges and has been speculated to produce the blocked state (21). As depicted in Fig. 1, these inhibitory reactions are reversed when Ca^{2+} binds to TnC and result in an activation of myofilament activity. A key reaction central to the release from inhibition is the tight binding of TnC with TnI upon Ca^{2+}-binding to the regulatory site of TnC (22). The topology of the interactions are presently being sorted out (23). An interesting feature of the cardiac variant of TnI (cTnI) is an amino terminal (N domain) extension of some 32 amino acids. This stretch of amino acids contains serines that are substrates for protein kinase A (4,5). Using NMR and selective isotope labeling, Krudy et al. have shown that the interaction of TnI with TnC is antiparallel; that is, the N domain of cTnC is opposite the C domain of cTnI (23). Moreover, Bremel et al. (24) have also shown that removal of the N domain of cTnI has no effect of Ca^{2+} activation of myofibrillar ATPase activity or its inhibition by acidic pH. Our hypothesis is that the unique N domain of cTnI is important only when it is phosphorylated. Phosphorylation of amino acids (Ser 23/24) in the unique N domain and just downstream (Ser 43/45) affect the Ca^{2+}-sensitivity and maximum actomyosin ATPase rate. This latter finding (Noland et al., unpublished data) indicates that the state of TnI may affect the ability of the thin filament to turn on even in saturating levels of Ca^{2+}.

SWITCHING THE THIN FILAMENT ON THROUGH STRONG CROSSBRIDGES

It is now clear that in striated muscle, myosin not only is a molecular motor but also is involved in activation of the thin filament. This action of myosin heads was first demonstrated clearly in vitro in the studies of Bremel et al. (24), who showed that rigor crossbridges could, in the presence of Tm or Tn-Tm, cooperatively turn on the thin filament as determined from measurement of acto-S-1 or acto-HMM ATPase activity, even in the absence of Ca^{2+}. That binding of S-1 affects further binding of S-1 was also shown by the experiments of Lehrer and Ishii (25), who probed the number of active Tm units using a fluorescent tag reporting the on configuration. These experiments showed that turning on of the thin filament is largely dependent on S-1 binding and is relatively weakly affected by Ca^{2+} binding to Tn. The cooperative turning on of the thin filament lies in two mechanisms. One is the fact that Tm covers seven actins so that with binding of S-1, seven actins are activated. The other is that the cooperative binding of S-1 requires end-to-end interactions between adjacent Tm molecules. Thus, near-neighbor interactions involving functional units consisting of actin:Tm:Tn in a 7:1:1 ratio are also involved.

CONCLUSION

Based on the current perception of myofilament activation, we can address the following question: What do we believe happens in the transition from the diastolic (relaxed) to the systolic (active) state? Release of Ca^{2+} into the myofilament space results in Ca^{2+} binding to a single regulatory site on TnC; Ca^{2+} acts at some distance from the S-1 binding site on actin (i.e., allosterically) to trigger contraction through a series of protein–protein interactions involving TnI, TnT, and Tm. The trigger may involve two types of processes: a release from a blocked state and an increase in the rate constants for transition from the weak to the strong binding state. Tropomyosin or TnI (and potentially TnT) are moved from a blocking position in a few functional units by strong crossbridges; near-neighbor crossbridges promote further activation of the thin filament and thus activation spreads and more functional units are engaged in the contraction. Thus, a particular contractile state may be perceived as a balance between the allosteric activation of the myofilaments by Ca^{2+} and the cooperative activation of the myofilaments by crossbridges. The force that is generated is a function of the distribution of crossbridge states and force generated by each state.

SUMMARY

Altered response of the myofilaments to Ca^{2+} is causal in heart failure associated with certain cardiac myopathies and diverse pathology arising, for example, from acidosis and ischemia. Importantly, the response of cardiac myofilaments to Ca^{2+} also may be manipulated pharmacologically. This chapter considers a current perception of the molecular interactions regulating myofilament activity in heart cells. Control of the actin–myosin reaction is not only through Ca^{2+} binding to TnC, but also through steric, cooperative, and allosteric processes involving all of the main myofilament proteins—actin, myosin, Tm, TnC, TnT, and TnI. The process is modulated by covalent and noncovalent mechanisms.

ACKNOWLEDGMENT

The author is supported by research grants NIH RO1-HL22231 and R01 HL49934.

REFERENCES

1. Solaro RJ, Pan BS. Control and modulation of contractile activity of cardiac myofilaments. In: Sperelakis N, ed. *Physiology and pathophysiology of the heart*. Boston: Kluwer Academic; 1988: 291–293.
2. Moss RL. Ca^{2+} regulation of mechanical properties of striated muscle: mechanistic studies using extraction and replacement of regulatory proteins. *Circ Res* 1992;70:865–884.

3. Allen DG, Kentish JC. The cellular basis of the length-tension relation in cardiac muscle. *J Mol Cell Cardiol* 1985;17:821–840.
4. Solaro RJ. Protein phosphorylation and the cardiac myofilaments. In: Solaro RJ, ed. *Protein phosphorylation in heart*. Boca Raton, FL: CRC Press; 1986:129–156.
5. Solaro RJ. Modulation of activation of cardiac myofilaments by beta-adrenergic agonists. In: Lee JA, Allen DG, eds. *Modulation of cardiac calcium sensitivity*. Oxford: Oxford University Press; 1993:161–177.
6. Solaro RJ, Lee J, Kentish J, Allen DA. Differences in the response of adult and neonatal heart muscle to acidosis. *Circ Res* 1988;63:779–787.
7. Millar N, Homsher E. The effect of phosphate and Ca on force generation in glycerinated rabbit skeletal muscle fibers. *J Biol Chem* 1990;265:20234–20240.
8. Westfall MV, Solaro RJ. Alterations in myofibrillar function and protein profiles following global ischemia in rat hearts. *Circ Res* 1992;70:302–313.
9. Anderson PAW, Malouf NN, Oakeley A, Pagani ED, Allen PD. Troponin T isoform expression in humans: a comparison among normal and failing adult heart, fetal heart, and adult and fetal skeletal muscle. *Circ Res* 1991;60:1226–1233.
10. Tanigawa G, Jarcho JA, Kass S, et al. A molecular basis for familial hypertrophic cardiomyopathy: an α/β cardiac myosin heavy chain hybrid gene. *Cell* 1990;622:991–998.
11. Thierfelder L, Watkins H, MacRae C, et al. Alpha-tropomyosin and cardiac troponin T mutations cause familial hypertrophic cardiomyopathy: a disease of the sarcomere. *Cell* 1994;77:701–712.
12. Fujino K, Sperelakis N, Solaro RJ. Sensitization of dog and guinea pig cardiac myofilaments to Ca^{2+}-activation and inotropic effect of pimobendan: comparison with milrinone. *Circ Res* 1988;63:911–922.
13. Mori M, Takeuchi M, Takaoka H, et al. New Ca^{2+} sensitizer, MCI-154, reduces myocardial oxygen consumption for non-mechanical work in diseased human hearts. *Circulation* 1994;I217.
14. Kawai M, Saeki Y, Zhao Y. Crossbridge scheme and the kinetic constants of elementary steps deduced from chemically skinned papillary and trabecular muscles of the ferret. *Circ Res* 1993;73:35–50.
15. Walker JW, Lu Z, Moss RL. Effects of Ca^{2+} on the kinetics of phosphate release in skeletal muscle. *J Biol Chem* 1992;267:2459–2466.
16. Lehrer S. The regulatory switch of the muscle thin filament: Ca^{2+} or myosin heads? *J Muscle Res Cell Motil* 1994;15:232–236.
17. Zot AS, Potter JD. Structural aspects of troponin-tropomyosin regulation of skeletal muscle contraction. *Annu Rev Biophys Chem* 1987;16:535–559.
18. Kress M, Huxley HE, Faruqi AR, Hendrix J. Structural changes during activation of frog muscle studied by time resolved X-ray diffraction. *J Mol Biol* 1986;188:325–342.
19. Brenner B. Changes in calcium sensitivity at the cross-bridge level. In: Lee JA, Allen DG, eds. *Modulation of cardiac calcium sensitivity*. Oxford: Oxford University Press; 1993:197–214.
20. Heeley DH, Smillie LB. Interaction of rabbit skeletal muscle troponin T and F-actin at physiological ionic strength. *Biochemistry* 1988;27:8227–8231.
21. Geeves MA, Lehrer SS. Dynamics of the muscle thin filament regulatory switch: the size of the cooperative unit. *Biophys J* 1994;67:273–282.
22. Krudy G, Kleerkoper Q, Guo X, Howarth JW, Solaro RJ, Rosevear PR. NMR studies delineating spatial relationships within the cardiac troponin I-troponin C complex. *J Biol Chem* 1994;269:23731–23735.
23. Guo X, Wattanapermpool J, Palmiter KA, Murphy AM, Solaro RJ. Mutagenesis of cardiac troponin I: role of the unique NH_2-terminal peptide in myofilament activation. *J Biol Chem* 1994;269:15210–15216.
24. Bremel R, Murray J, Weber A. Manifestations of cooperative behavior in the regulated actin filament during actin-activated ATP hydrolysis in the presence of calcium. *Cold Spring Harbor Symp Quant Biol* 1973;37:267–275.
25. Lehrer S, Ishii Y. Fluorescence properties of acrylodan-labeled tropomyosin and tropomyosin-actin: evidence for myosin subfragment 1 induced changes in geometry between tropomyosin and actin. *Biochemistry* 1988;27:5899–5906.

The Failing Heart, edited by N. S. Dhalla,
R. E. Beamish, N. Takeda, and M. Nagano.
Lippincott-Raven Publishers, Philadelphia © 1995.

10

Skeletal Muscle Metabolic Alterations in Heart Failure

Roberto Ferrari, *Claudio Ceconi, †Federica de Giuli,
†Evasio Pasini, †Palmira Bernocchi, ‡Cristina Opasich, and
†Amerigo Giordano

*Universita' degli Studi di Brescia, 25123 Brescia, Italy; *Spedali Civili, 25123
Brescia, Italy; †Fondazione Clinica del Lavoro, Centro di Fisiopatologia Cardiovascolare
"S. Maugeri," 25064 Gussago, Brescia, Italy; and ‡Fondazione Clinica del Lavoro,
Centro di Montescano, Montescano, 27040 Pavia, Italy*

Exertional intolerance is a major clinical problem in patients with chronic heart failure, and it is associated with both muscle fatigue and dyspnea (1). Usually, these symptoms are alleviated by diuretics, digitalis, and vasodilator therapy, with the majority of patients experiencing complete resolution of symptoms at rest. Many of them, however, continue to complain of exertional symptoms, despite optimal diuresis and medical therapy (2,3). It follows that their daily life is severely limited, and during maximal exercise testing, they must terminate the exercise early because of leg fatigue.

Exertional fatigue in heart failure has been attributed traditionally to skeletal muscle under perfusion. It has been shown that leg blood flow responses to bicycle exercise in patients with heart failure are significantly lower than that of normal subjects (4). Patients who exhibit improved exercise capacity after therapy with angiotensin-converting enzyme inhibitors also exhibit improved leg blood flow (5).

BLOOD FLOW IN SKELETAL MUSCLE

The reduced capacity of patients with heart failure to increase flow proportionally to the working skeletal muscle might depend on a reduction in cardiac output coupled to an impaired arteriolar vasodilation, as evidenced by a failure of leg vascular resistance to decrease normally during exercise (6,7). It has been suggested that sodium retention impairs arteriolar vasodilation by compressing the capillary bed (8). Removal of excess fluid and sodium retention, however, does not normalize arterial vasodilation (9). The abnormal increase of noradrenaline and angiotensin II induced by exercise in patients with heart failure could also impair vasodilation, although blocking these systems does not necessarily improve blood flow (10,11). Other proposed possibilities include an abnormality of vascular endothelium, leading to a reduced production of vasodilating factor (12); a vascular remodeling due to increased angiotensin II (13); and an impaired release of vasodilators metabolites by the skeletal muscle (1). Whatever the cause, muscle underperfusion results in an intramuscular lactic acidosis, which, in turn, produces muscular fatigue.

Recent observations from our (14,15) and other laboratories (16) have shown that there is a subset of patients with heart failure who show a normal increase of skeletal muscle blood flow during exercise but who develop exertional fatigue and abnormal lactic acidosis. This suggests that abnormalities other than underperfusion of the working skeletal muscle might contribute to exertional fatigue. This concept is reinforced by several other findings. The increase in cardiac output caused by vasodilators, even when associated with enhanced oxygen transport to skeletal muscle, is not associated with increased exercise capacity and peak oxygen consumption in patients with chronic heart failure (14). When oxygen delivery to type I and IIA muscle fibers that depend on oxidative muscle is enhanced, oxygen utilization is not augmented, at least not acutely (15). Numerous experimental and human studies have shown that exercise training induces major adaptations in skeletal muscle and improves exertional fatigue, independently of skeletal muscle perfusion (16,17).

INTRINSIC ABNORMALITIES OF SKELETAL MUSCLE IN HEART FAILURE

The observations described above have prompted the hypothesis that in chronic heart failure there are intrinsic abnormalities of skeletal muscle that prevent acute improvement in peak VO_2 and lead to excessive accumulation of lactate (1,18). Three types of observations support this concept: (a) Skeletal muscle biopsy studies have provided evidence of intrinsic skeletal muscle abnormalities; (b) anthropometric and magnetic resonance imaging studies have demonstrated skeletal muscle atrophy in the majority of the patients; and (c) metabolic studies have shown abnormal responses to exercise in patients with heart failure unrelated to muscle underperfusion. All of these changes could impair muscle performance and contribute to exertional fatigue.

FINDINGS FROM SKELETAL MUSCLE BIOPSIES

To determine if an abnormality of skeletal muscle could be demonstrated in patients with heart failure, several authors have taken skeletal muscle biopsies from a heterogenous group of patients with heart failure. These demonstrated a variety of different and, in part, conflicting abnormalities (19–24).

Histological examination of skeletal muscle revealed a variable extent of atrophy, increased interstitial cellular space, and an increase in type IIB fibers (20–22).

From the biochemical point of view, Lipkin et al. (20) noted a variety of abnormalities but no specific pattern of changes. The activity of citrate synthase, an oxidative enzyme, was normal in six patients but decreased in three. An increase in acid phosphatase was observed in six patients. In the gastrocnemius muscle of patients with heart failure, Mancini et al. (21) found a decrease in β-hydroxyacyl–CoA activity, a mitochondrial-based enzyme involved in fatty acid metabolism. Citrate synthase, however, was normal, suggesting normal oxidative enzyme levels. Phosphofructokinase levels were also normal, suggesting maintenance of enzymes involved in glycolysis. In biopsies from the vastus lateralis of patients with heart failure, Drexler and colleagues (25) noted a decrease in volume and surface density of mitochondrial cristae and inner boundary membranes. In addition, they discovered an increase in triadic junction cisternae, which are involved in intracellular and extracellular calcium release. Based on these data, the authors suggest that muscular fatigue in heart failure may be, in part at least, related to reduced oxidative capacity of skeletal muscle, possibly caused by Ca^{2+} overloading.

FINDINGS FROM ANTHROPOMETRIC MEASUREMENTS

The detection of type II fiber atrophy, consistently found in skeletal muscle biopsy studies, suggested the possibility of skeletal muscle atrophy in patients with heart failure. A reduction of muscle mass diminishes the maximum strength of the muscle group and may cause changes of gas exchange on exercise similar to those seen in heart failure. Because the smaller-mass muscle is undertaking a similar work load, the biochemical changes in the muscle will be different from normal. If atrophy is selective for particular fiber types, the use of specific substrates will be altered, and there may also be alterations of the mechanical efficiency of the muscle (26).

To determine if such generalized muscle atrophy is present in patients with heart failure, Mancini et al. (27) performed anthropometric measurements in 62 patients with heart failure and compared calf muscle volume (assessed with magnetic resonance imaging) of patients with heart failure to control subjects.

With these technologies, skeletal muscle atrophy was noted in more than 50% of patients. Interestingly, anthropometric measurements failed to detect reduction in fat stores in the majority of the patients. This suggests that muscle atrophy is not accompanied by a generalized loss of total body weight and fat stores.

FINDINGS FROM METABOLICAL STUDIES

The first metabolic studies have been conducted using phosphorus-31 nuclear magnetic resonance (NMR), a technology that permits the noninvasive monitoring of phosphocreatine, inorganic di-adenosine [DI-(ADP)] and tri-adenosine [TRI-(ATP)] phosphates, as well as pH in working muscle. A series of studies examined the metabolic behavior of both forearm and calf muscles in patients with heart failure. The data obtained show a more pronounced increase in the organic phosphate/phosphocreatine ratio and a more pronounced decrease in muscle pH than in normal subjects performing a comparable work load (28–30). In addition, patients with heart failure showed a delayed time constant of recovery for phosphocreatine resynthesis after exercise (31). This NMR spectroscopy analysis of the recovery period after exercise has the advantage, compared with classical NMR spectroscopy, to focus only on metabolic changes taking place during exercise, independently of the muscle volume (31). Interestingly, the time constant of recovery correlates better with the work slope than with the muscle volume, thus suggesting that intrinsic and metabolic alterations rather than muscle atrophy are at the basis of reduced exercise tolerance in heart failure. Furthermore, these observations fit with previous findings in patients with chronic heart failure, showing that the extent of intrinsic and ultrastructural alterations of skeletal muscle is related to exercise capacity (32).

All of these metabolic abnormalities are not due simply to skeletal muscle ischemia because they also occur in the presence of a normal forearm blood flow (30). In other studies, the arterial-venous femoral difference has been measured at rest and during exercise. By using this technique, we could demonstrate that in patients with heart failure, the uptake of free fatty acid (FFA) is impaired both at rest and during exercise (14,15). In addition, we and others have shown that the skeletal muscle metabolism in heart failure is abnormally dependent on anaerobic glycolysis, resulting in excessive accumulation and release of lactic acid (16). These biochemical changes could not be explained by impaired blood flow or reduced oxygen delivery alone. One metabolic change that would explain these observations is a decrease in glucose and FFA oxidation relative to glycolysis. Such an imbalance would accelerate tissue acidosis during exercise.

Support for metabolic changes in chronic heart failure also comes from studies using the pyruvate dehydrogenase complex stimulator, dichloroacetate (DCA). Wilson et al. gave 35 mg/kg of DCA intravenously to 18 male patients with chronic heart failure before exercise in a double-blind cross-over trial. No adverse effects were observed. In this acute intravenous study, a significant improvement in serum lactate levels during exercise was noted, but exercise time did not change (33). Wargovich et al. studied the effects of DCA on cardiac hemodynamic and coronary blood flow during cardiac catheterization and found beneficial acute hemodynamic effects (34). Bersin et al. compared the effects of intravenous DCA (50 mg/kg) with clinically optimized doses of dobutamine in seven patients with severe heart failure and found that DCA significantly improved myocardial mechanical efficiency (35).

POTENTIAL MECHANISM OF SKELETAL MUSCLE CHANGES IN HEART FAILURE

It is clear, on the basis of the observations described above, that multiple factors can contribute to exercise intolerance in patients with heart failure. At the present time, the most important factors are likely to be skeletal muscle underperfusion and deconditioning.

The cause of underperfusion or of an increased resistance in the vessel supplying the limbs is unknown. The effect seems to be related neither to structural changes in the arterioles and endothelial cells nor to activation of the sympathetic or the renin–angiotensin systems. Clear abnormality of endothelial cell function has not yet been shown in humans. Another possibility is that the response of receptors and of ion channels involved in the control of vascular resistance is abnormal. Interestingly, after heart transplantation, the forearm resistance does not return to normal for at least 4 weeks (36). This strongly suggests that the changes are not directly linked to central hemodynamics.

Deconditioning is likely to occur because patients with heart failure, partly following the physician's advice, restrict their own physical activity or are hospitalized and subjected to long periods of bed rest. Deconditioning, in turn, produces muscle atrophy and reduction in mitochondrial-based enzymes. Consistent with this concept, bicycle training in patients with heart failure has been shown to improve exercise tolerance by peripheral mechanisms, such as delaying the onset of anaerobic metabolism (37). Training induces improvement of peripheral muscle metabolism and function appears to be independent of systemic adaptations.

Although these observations suggest that the alterations of skeletal muscle in chronic heart failure are a result of deconditioning, other potential factors should not be ignored. A decreased caloric and protein intake may be a major contributor to skeletal muscle atrophy, at least in certain subsets of patients, such as those with alcoholic cardiomyopathy. Other factors may include increased oxygen-free radical activity (38), increased sympathetic tone, elevated cortisol levels (39), or monocyte activation with increased plasma levels of tumor necrosis factor (40).

We are only beginning to realize the complexity of the peripheral alteration in heart failure. Further studies should provide important information on the role of cytokine, endothelial dysfunction, and neuroendocrine activation. From the clinical point of view, the available information suggests that more attention should be focused on detecting and eventually correcting skeletal muscle changes. If deconditioning and/or malnutrition are diagnosed, appropriate interventions should be instituted. Restriction of physical activity should be substituted by an appropriate exercise program.

SUMMARY

The factors that limit exercise capacity in patients with chronic heart failure are poorly understood. Recent evidence suggests that the major mechanism is not related to central hemodynamics but to a combination of muscle underperfusion and muscle deconditioning. Several abnormalities have been demonstrated in skeletal muscle of patients with heart failure, including reduced FFA uptake and abnormal lactic acid production during exercise, reduced levels of mitochondrial-based enzymes, higher percentage of type I and IIA fibers, and muscle atrophy. These abnormalities seem to be due, at least in part, to deconditioning and to exercise-induced ischemia, although other factors such as malnutrition, increased tissue necrosis factor, elevated cortisol levels, and endothelial dysfunction cannot, at the present time, be ruled out.

ACKNOWLEDGMENTS

This work has been supported by the National Research Council (CNR) target project, "Prevention and Control Disease Factors," n. 9100156 pf 41, and by the CNR target project, "Biotechnology and Bioinstrumentation." We thank Miss Roberta Bonetti for secretarial help.

REFERENCES

1. Wilson JR, Mancini DM. Factors contributing to the exercise limitation of heart failure. *J Am Coll Cardiol* 1993;22:93A–98A.
2. Wilson JR, Ferraro N. Exercise intolerance in patients with chronic left heart failure: relationship to oxygen transport and ventilatory abnormalities. *Am J Cardiol* 1983;51:1358–1363.
3. Weber KT, Kinasewitz GT, Janicki JS, Fishman AP. Oxygen utilization and ventilation during exercise in patients with chronic cardiac failure. *Circulation* 1982;65:1213–1223.
4. Wilson JR, Martin JL, Schwartz D, Ferraro N. Exercise intolerance in patients with chronic heart failure: role of impaired skeletal muscle nutritive flow. *Circulation* 1984;69:1079–1087.
5. Drexler H, Banhardt U, Meinertz T, Wollschlager H, Lehmann M, Just H. Contrasting peripheral short-term and long-term effect of converting enzyme inhibition in patients with congestive heart failure. *Circulation* 1989;79:491–502.
6. Sullivan MJ, Knight JD, Higginbotham MB, Cobb FR. Relation between central and peripheral hemodynamics during exercise in patients with chronic heart failure. *Circulation* 1989;80:769–781.
7. LeJemtel TH, Maskin CS, Lucido D, Chadwick BJ. Failure to augment maximal limb blood flow in response to one-leg versus two-leg exercise in patients with severe heart failure. *Circulation* 1989;80:769–781.
8. Zelis R, Flaim SF. Alterations in vasomotor tone in congestive heart failure. *Prog Cardiovasc Dis* 1982;24:437–459.
9. Sinoway L, Minotti J, Musch T, et al. Enhanced metabolic vasodilation secondary to diuretic therapy in decompensated congestive heart failure secondary to coronary artery disease. *Am J Cardiol* 1987;60:107–111.
10. Wilson JR, Ferraro N, Wiener DH. Effect of the sympathetic nervous system on limb circulation and metabolism during exercise in heart failure. *Circulation* 1985;72:72–81.
11. Wilson JR, Ferraro N. Effect of the renin-angiotensin system on limb circulation and metabolism during exercise in heart failure. *J Am Coll Cardiol* 1985;6:556–563.
12. Katz SD, Schwarz M, Yuen J, LeJemtel TH. Impaired acetylcholine-mediated vasodilation in patients with congestive heart failure. Role of endothelium-derived vasodilating and vasoconstricting factors. *Circulation* 1993;88:55–61.
13. Dzau VJ. Role of endothelium-derived vasoactive substances in the regulation of vascular tone via structural remodeling of blood vessels. In: Ryan US, Rubanyi GM, eds. *Endothelial regulation of vascular tone*. New York: Marcel Dekker; 1992:331–339.
14. Ferrari R, Bernocchi P, Boraso A, Visioli O. Insufficienza cardiaca congestizia dal muscolo cardiaco al muscolo scheletrico. *Cardiologia* 1993;38:45–50.
15. de Giuli F, Cargnoni A, Pasini E, et al. Effect of propionyl-l-carnitine (PLC) on skeletal muscle metabolism in patients with chronic heart failure (CHF). *Can J Cardiol* 1994;10:74(abst).
16. Wilson JR, Mancini DM, Dunkman WB. Exertional fatigue due to skeletal muscle dysfunction in patients with heart failure. *Circulation* 1993;87:470–475.
17. Barlow CW, Qayyum MS, Davey PP, Conway J, Paterson DJ, Robbins PA. Effect of physical

training on exercise induced hyperkalemia in chronic heart failure: relation with ventilation and catecholamines. *Circulation* 1994;89:1144–1152.

18. Drexler H. Skeletal muscle failure in heart failure. *Circulation* 1992;85:1621–1623.
19. Drexler H, Riede U, Schafer H. Reduced oxidative capacity of skeletal muscle in patients with severe heart failure. *Circulation* 1987;76[Suppl IV]:IV-178(abst).
20. Lipkin DP, Jones DA, Round JM, Poole-Wilson PA. Abnormalities of skeletal muscle in patients with chronic heart failure. *Int J Cardiol* 1988;18:187–195.
21. Mancini DM, Coyle E, Coggan A, et al. Contribution of intrinsic skeletal muscle changes to 31P-NMR skeletal muscle metabolic abnormalities in patients with chronic heart failure. *Circulation* 1989;80:1338–1346.
22. Sullivan MJ, Green HJ, Cobb FR. Skeletal muscle biochemistry and histology in ambulatory patients with long-term heart failure. *Circulation* 1990;81:518–527.
23. Dunnigan A, Staley NA, Smith SA, et al. Cardiac and skeletal muscle abnormalities in cardiomyopathy: comparison of patients with ventricular tachycardia or congestive heart failure. *J Am Coll Cardiol* 1987;10:608–618.
24. Caforio ALP, Rossi B, Risalti R, et al. Type 1 fiber abnormalities in skeletal muscle of patients with hypertrophic and dilated cardiomyopathy: evidence of subclinical myogenic myopathy. *J Am Coll Cardiol* 1989;14:1464–1473.
25. Drexler H, Reide U, Munzel T, Konig H, Funke E, Just H. Alterations of skeletal muscle in chronic heart failure. *Circulation* 1992;85:1751–1759.
26. Poole-Wilson PA, Buller NP, Lindsay DC. Blood flow and skeletal muscle in patients with heart failure. *Chest* 1992;101:330S–332S.
27. Mancini DM, Walter G, Reichek N, et al. Contribution of skeletal muscle atrophy to exercise intolerance and altered muscle metabolism in heart failure. *Circulation* 1992;85:1364–1373.
28. Wilson JR, Fink L, Maris J, et al. Evaluation of skeletal muscle energy metabolism in patients with heart failure using gated phosphorus-31 nuclear magnetic resonance. *Circulation* 1985;71:57–62.
29. Mancini DM, Ferraro N, Tuchler M, Chance B, Wilson JR. Detection of abnormal calf muscle metabolism in patients with heart failure using phosphorus-31 nuclear magnetic resonance. *Am J Cardiol* 1988;62:1234–1240.
30. Wiener DH, Fink LI, Maris J, Jones RA, Chance B, Wilson JR. Abnormal skeletal muscle bioenergetics during exercise in heart failure: role of reduced muscle blood flow. *Circulation* 1986;73:1127–1136.
31. Mancini DM, Walter G, Reichek N, et al. Contribution of skeletal muscle atrophy to exercise intolerance and altered muscle metabolism in heart failure. *Circulation* 1992;85:1364–1373.
32. Drexler H, Riede U, Hiroi M, Munzel T, Holubarsch C, Meinertz T. Ultrastructural analysis of skeletal muscle in chronic heart failure: relation to exercise capacity and indices of left ventricular dysfunction. *Circulation* 1988;78[Suppl II]:II-107(abst).
33. Wilson JR, Mancini DM, Ferraro N, Egler J. Effect of dichloroacetate on the exercise performance of patients with heart failure. *J Am Coll Cardiol* 1988;12:1464–1469.
34. Wargovich TJ, MacDonald RG, Hill JA, Feldman RL, Stacpoole PW, Pepine CJ. Myocardial metabolic and hemodynamic effects of dichloroacetate in coronary artery disease. *Am J Cardiol* 1988;61:65–70.
35. Bersin R, Kwasman M, Wolfe C, et al. Improved hemodynamic function in congestive heart failure with the metabolic agent sodium dichloroacetate (DCA). *J Am Coll Cardiol* 1990;15[Suppl A]:157A (abst).
36. Sinoway LI, Minotti JR, Davis D, et al. Delayed reversal of impaired vasodilation in congestive heart failure after heart transplantation. *Am J Cardiol* 1988;61:1076–1079.
37. Sullivan MJ, Higginbotham MB, Cobb FR. Exercise training in patients with severe left ventricular dysfunction: hemodynamic and metabolic effects. *Circulation* 1988;78:506–515.
38. Belch JJF, Bridges AB, Scott N, Chopra M. Oxygen free radicals and congestive heart failure. *Br Heart J* 1991;65:245–248.
39. Holloszy JO, Coyle EF. Adaptations of skeletal muscle to endurance exercise and their metabolic consequences. *J Appl Physiol* 1984;56:831–838.
40. Levine B, Kalman J, Mayer LM, Fillit H, Packer M. Elevated circulating levels of tumor necrosis factor in severe chronic heart failure. *N Engl J Med* 1990;323:236–241.

The Failing Heart, edited by N. S. Dhalla,
R. E. Beamish, N. Takeda, and M. Nagano.
Lippincott-Raven Publishers, Philadelphia © 1995.

11

Respiratory Sleep Disorders in Patients with Chronic Heart Failure

Carlo Sacco, Alberto Braghiroli, *Amerigo Giordano, and
Claudio F. Donner

*Division of Pulmonary Disease, "Clinica del Lavoro" Foundation,
Medical Center of Rehabilitation, I-28010 Veruno, Italy; and *Fondazione Clinica del
Lavoro, Centro di Montescano, 25064 Gussago, Bresia, Italy*

It is well known that subjects with chronic heart failure (CHF) and low ejection fraction (EF) are often prone to respiratory sleep disorders (RSDs) (1). Central sleep apnea is the most common breathing disorder in patients with CHF, but is also found in a heterogeneous group of patients with different disorders (2). Central sleep apnea is characterized by the complete cessation of airflow at the nose and mouth, with no evidence of thoracoabdominal movements for at least 10 seconds. As mentioned, central sleep apnea is often associated with a variety of clinical disorders and can be classified according to the different pathogenetic mechanisms causing its occurrence.

An abnormal regulation of the respiratory response to chemoreceptor stimuli results in central apneas and hypopneas during sleep and hypoventilation during wakefulness (1). This form of disordered breathing is secondary to various neuromuscular conditions such as muscular dystrophy, Guillain-Barré syndrome, myasthenia gravis, diaphragmatic paralysis, and thoracoskeletal deformities. Other causes can be related to structural lesions of the brainstem such as trauma, tumor, and infection (3). Primary alveolar hypoventilation is the condition in which the cause cannot be identified during sleep or wakefulness. Moreover, idiopathic central sleep apnea may be present in normal subjects during the transition from wakefulness to sleep until sleep becomes more stable (1,4,5).

Transitory fluctuations in the central respiratory drive without clear alterations of the control system seem to play a potentially key role in determining central apneas in patients suffering from severe CHF. During sleep, in patients with low EF, central apneas can assume a regular, cyclic respiratory pattern: the so-called periodic breathing (PB) or Cheyne-Stokes respiration (CSR). Periodic breathing is sometimes present in normal subjects (6), and its occurrence increases with age, especially in obese subjects (7). It is often associated with exposure to high altitude

(8), neurological disease (intracerebral hemorrhage, brain tumors, and encephalitis) (3), Ondine's syndrome (9), and is found in premature infants (rarely in full-term infants), possibly representing a risk factor for sudden infant death (10,11).

PATHOPHYSIOLOGY OF CHEYNE-STOKES RESPIRATION

For several days his breathing was irregular; it would entirely cease for a quarter of a minute, then it would become perceptible, though very low, then by degrees it became heaving and quick, and then it would gradually cease again. This revolution of his breathing occupied a minute during which there were about thirty acts of respiration.

This is the first description by J. Cheyne, in 1818, of a peculiar respiratory pattern (12).

CSR, which may be regarded as an exaggerated form of PB, is characterized by a cyclic crescendo–decrescendo pattern of ventilation alternating with apnea or hypopnea. This seems to be the consequence of instability in the respiratory control system. The apneas are usually central, but obstructive and mixed apneas and hypopneas are often observed. Oxygen saturation has characteristic rises and falls that follow the cyclic trend of the ventilatory pattern (13).

Under normal conditions, breathing is regulated by two different integrated systems: the chemical (metabolic) system, which acts to maintain blood gas homeostasis and acid-base balance, and the behavioral respiratory control system that during wakefulness can stimulate respiration independently of the chemical control (1,14). The metabolic (automatic) control system consists of two different types of chemoreceptors which sense the levels of O_2 and CO_2 content in blood and transmit the information to the respiratory areas in the brain. The peripheral chemoreceptors consist of the carotid bodies and similar structures which sense O_2 levels and, partially, CO_2 levels. The central chemoreceptors are not encased in a single structure, but are probably placed just under the ventral surface of the medulla and contain a tissue sensitive to CO_2 (15,16).

Animal experiments have led to the claim that the extracellular $[H^+]$ could be of prime importance as the final stimulus of these chemoreceptors; however, there is a lack of in vivo evidence that cerebro spinal fluid $[H^+]$ is the actual stimulus (17).

The behavioral control system located in the cerebral cortex controls acts such as speaking, swallowing, talking, and eating, which need changes in ventilation that override the automatic control. The final regulation of respiratory and upper airways muscles is controlled by bulbo pontine neurons which integrate the afferences from the peripheral receptors, each controlling a single function (14,15).

The homeostatic control of arterial blood gases tension is achieved through a negative feedback system based on a peripheral controller (the chemoreceptors located in the medulla and carotid bodies) which senses fluctuations in blood gas tension and acts mainly by changing the level of ventilation. The mechanoreceptors in the thorax and the stretch receptors in the lung act by regulating the pattern of breathing (1,13–16).

During wakefulness, the metabolic and behavioral systems interact to determine the level and pattern of breathing. During sleep, however, the behavioral control system becomes quiescent, and breathing depends on the metabolic system. At sleep onset, there are repeated transitions between wakefulness and sleep stages 1 and 2. These transitions induce significant changes in ventilation depending on the decrease in tidal volume and breathing frequency, with changes in the ventilatory response to chemical stimuli often determining a small increase in $PaCO_2$ and a small drop in oxygen content. On the contrary, slow-wave sleep (stages 3 and 4) is characterized by a stable pattern of breathing that is thought to be controlled almost exclusively by automatic mechanisms, while during REM sleep the behavioral control system may again assume a functional role in the control of ventilation (13,15).

As mentioned at the beginning of the chapter, CSR is frequently found in patients with CHF and low EF and seems to be related to an instability in the respiratory control system. One of the factors involved in the instability of the respiratory control system is thought to be the prolonged circulation time causing delays in the recognition of changes in arterial blood gas tensions from the lungs to the chemoreceptors (1,13–15,18). This is the result of both low cardiac output and dilatation of the ventricles. Simplifying, it is possible to think that a stimulus is able to increase ventilation and decrease $PaCO_2$ to the apnea threshold. Ventilation is restored when the central sensor detects a $PaCO_2$ above this critical threshold, but this feedback signal is delayed because of the delayed circulation time. Hence, while in the lung there is a decrease in $PaCO_2$ level in response to increased ventilation, $PaCO_2$ rises to the level of the chemoreceptor causing a further but improper increase in ventilation and a progressive hypocapnia. On the contrary, PaO_2 shows an opposite trend. During ventilation, PaO_2 is lowest when $PaCO_2$ is highest at the chemoreceptors; but during the apneic phase, PaO_2 increases the gain of the CO_2 chemoreceptor (15).

Many factors overimpose to this relatively simple mechanism:

1. The reduction of the venous return and the delayed circulation time lead to a reduction of O_2 reserves.
2. Subjects suffering from CHF present a metabolic alkalosis induced by hyperaldosteronism and diuretic therapy. For this reason these patients are hypocapnic and therefore closer to the apnea threshold.
3. Pulmonary sub-edema stimulates the mechanoreceptors, causing hyperventilation, as described at high altitude (8).
4. Baroreceptors have an important role in the control of breathing and may often present changes induced by drugs, hypertension, or alterations of the autonomous nervous system function (19).

Generally, the triggering factor is identified in a hyperventilation that is usually caused by an arousal during the night. While the patient is sleeping, different stimuli or even the regular alternating of sleep stages can waken the subject, causing an increase in ventilation which reduces $PaCO_2$ below the critical level necessary to precipitate an apnea. As a result, CSR appears and in some cases can last all night.

This happens in patients whose $PaCO_2$ is below the normal value and remains near the apneic threshold during sleep (13,15).

CLINICAL FEATURES

Cheyne-Stokes respiration can occur in normal subjects at sleep onset. In this case, the apnea threshold is not reached, but PB is induced by a regular cyclic pattern of hyperventilation and hypoventilation phases with slight oxygen desaturations. In such instances CSR has no effect on sleep quality, and subjects are usually asymptomatic. On the contrary, most patients with CHF and CSR present important alterations of sleep architecture. In 1989 Hanly et al. (20) determined the prevalence and distribution of CSR during sleep in ten male patients with stable heart failure and left ventricular ejection fraction <35%. He found that all of the patients had CSR during sleep, total sleep time was reduced, and CSR was predominant in sleep stages 1 and 2, determining deep desaturations in most patients. Slow-wave sleep was markedly reduced, with a high frequency of sleep stage changes and arousals. Most of these arousals were found during light sleep and followed the onset of breathing. These results also reflect our findings (21).

Despite normal arterial oxygenation when awake, patients with CSR and reduced EF can develop severe hypoxemia during sleep. Periodic hypoxemia may have long-term consequences on the cardiovascular system of these patients, compromising cardiac function, one of the major determinants of the clinical outcome. Systemic blood pressure monitoring shows an increment during the hyperventilation phase (20).

In the morning, patients with CSR present symptoms similar to those of patients suffering from obstructive sleep apnea (OSA). They complain of excessive daytime sleepiness, asthenia, and sometimes morning headache. These subjects may present with impaired memory and daytime performances. Their mood may be depressed or tense (13).

TREATMENTS

The treatment of these patients should be aimed at reducing CSR and consolidating sleep and consequently the cardiovascular sequelae. Another important aim is to improve daytime function and the quality of life in these patients. The improvement in cardiac function should be considered the first therapeutic approach, as it is the *conditio sine qua non* of CSR. As cardiac function improves, CSR disappears, as shown in patients who undergo heart transplantation (22). In some patients, however, CSR persists albeit they are clinically stable and under the best possible pharmachological treatment. In such cases, it seems that there are no anthropometric or clinical features able to discriminate subjects at risk of CSR. To date, the main therapeutic approaches aim to reduce the symptoms or to act at the level of one of the factors that perpetuate the CSR. For this reason, hypnotics have been used to reduce arousals during sleep. The inhalation of O_2 or CO_2 at low concentration or nasal continuous positive airway pressure (CPAP) has been found to modify the ventilatory drive and improve the baseline hemodynamics of these patients.

Nasal Continuous Positive Airway Pressure

Mechanical ventilation can improve patients with overt CHF (23), and the contemporary association of nasal CPAP with oxygen has proved to be effective in the treatment of severe cardiogenic pulmonary edema (24). Nasal CPAP is effective in CHF patients suffering from both OSA and CSR: The application of a positive intrathoracic pressure reduces left ventricular afterload and, as a result, increases cardiac output (25). In these patients, who may be only snorers (26) or present all the characteristics of OSA (27), nasal CPAP reduces upper airways resistances, achieving a definite improvement in the EF and often the disappearance of CSR.

Bradley et al. (28) studied the acute hemodynamic effects of CPAP in patients with CHF. Patients were divided into two groups based on their baseline pulmonary capillary wedge pressure (PCWP). The authors found that the application of nasal CPAP at 5 cm H_2O increased both cardiac index and stroke volume index in the group with high PCWP, but there was a deterioration in hemodynamics in the low-PCWP group. In conclusion, the study failed to identify the precise mechanisms involved. It is likely that this was due to the great interindividual variability of their subjects, who could not be identified as responders or nonresponders according to predictive clinical parameters or hemodynamic values.

Data on chronic administration of CPAP are less encouraging. Studies by Buckle et al. (29) and Davies et al. (30) clearly show that in CHF patients with CSR without upper airways obstruction, nasal CPAP treatment showed no benefits on sleeping respiration, sleep quality, daytime symptoms, or left ventricular function. Most of these patients did not tolerate nasal CPAP therapy, and in some cases it was detrimental.

Oxygen Therapy

It is well known that the administration of oxygen is effective in the treatment of CSR, for instance, in subjects exposed to high altitude (8) or in premature infants (31). Reduced oxygen stores and hypoxemia play an important role in the pathogenesis of CSR in patients with CHF (32). Consequently, oxygen supply would correct hypoxemia and reduce CSR. Hanly et al. (33) studied the effects of supplemental oxygen on CSR in nine patients with severe, stable CHF and concluded that oxygen therapy reduces CSR, corrects nocturnal hypoxemia, and consolidates sleep, improving the clinical status of these patients.

To date, there have been no control studies on the effectiveness of long-term oxygen therapy on CSR, but preliminary data do show that 6 months of oxygen therapy significantly decreases PB, improves the quality of sleep, and reduces oxyhemoglobin desaturations in these patients at high cardiovascular risk (21). In conclusion, further studies are needed to investigate the relationship between sleep breathing disorders and cardiovascular disease and, consequently, to adopt a correct and individual therapeutical approach.

SUMMARY

Nocturnal CSR, which is characterized by a cyclic crescendo–decrescendo pattern of ventilation alternating with apnea or hypopnea, seems to be a widespread feature in patients with CHF and low EF. Under normal conditions, breathing is regulated by the metabolic and behavioral control systems. During sleep, the behavioral control system becomes quiescent, and breathing depends on the metabolic system. The automatic regulation of the respiratory drive in patients with CHF seems to be influenced by a prolonged circulation time between the carotid body and the lung, conditioning a distortion of the feedback regulation. This is the result of both low cardiac output and dilatation of the ventricles. Furthermore, a reduction of body stores of oxygen and an altered apneic threshold induced by the respiratory alkalosis is usually reported in these patients. Patients with CHF present important alterations of sleep quality and sleep architecture. Apneas induce nocturnal oxyhemoglobin desaturations, despite normal oxygenation while awake. Periodic hypoxemia compromises cardiac function, one of the major determinants of the clinical outcome. In the morning, patients with CSR present symptoms that are similar to those of patients suffering from OSA.

The treatment of these patients should be focused on reducing CSR, improving cardiac function, consolidating sleep, and improving the patients' quality of life. To date, the main therapeutic approaches aim to reduce symptoms or to act at the level of one of the factors that perpetuate the CSR. For this reason, hypnotics have been used to reduce arousals during sleep. Nasal CPAP is effective in patients suffering from both OSA and CSR, while data on the chronic administration of CPAP are less encouraging and in some cases nasal CPAP therapy is detrimental. On the contrary, there are encouraging data on the effectiveness of long-term oxygen therapy on CSR.

REFERENCES

1. Cistulli PA, Sullivan CE. Pathophysiology of sleep apnea. In: Saunders NA, Sullivan CE, eds. *Sleep and breathing*. 2nd ed. New York: Marcel Dekker; 1994:157–190.
2. Dowell AR, Buckley CE III, Cohen R, Whalen RE, Sieker HO. Cheyne-Stokes respiration. *Arch Intern Med* 1971;127:712–726.
3. Brown H, Plum F. The neurologic basis of Cheyne-Stokes respiration. *Am J Med* 1961;30:849–860.
4. Chapman KR, Bruce E, Gothe B, Cherniack NS. Possible mechanisms of periodic breathing during sleep. *J Appl Physiol* 1988;64:1000–1008.
5. Bradley TD, Phillipson EA. Central sleep apnea. *Clin Chest Med* 1992;13:493–505.
6. Phillipson EA. Control of breathing during sleep. *Am Rev Respir Dis* 1978;118:909–939.
7. Cherniack NS. Sleep apnea and its causes. *J Clin Invest* 1984;73:1501–1506.

8. Weil JV, Kryger MH, Scoggin CH. Sleep and breathing at high altitude. In: Guilleminault C, Dement WC, eds. *Sleep apnea syndromes*. New York: Alan R. Liss; 1978:119–136.
9. Mellins RB, Balfour HH Jr, Turino GM, Winters RW. Failure of automatic control of ventilation (Ondine's curse). *Medicine* 1970;49:487–504.
10. Rigatto H, Brady JP. Periodic breathing and apnea in the preterm infants. I. Evidence for hypoventilation possibly due to central respiratory depression. *Pediatrics* 1972;50:202–218.
11. Nugent ST, Finley JP. Spectral analysis of periodic and normal breathing in infants. *IEEE Trans Biomed Eng* 1983;10:672–675.
12. Cheyne JA. A case of apoplexy in which the fleshy part of the heart was converted into fat. *Dublin Hosp Rep* 1818;2:216–223.
13. Bradley TD. Breathing during sleep in cardiac disease. In: Saunders NA, Sullivan CE, eds. *Sleep and breathing*. 2nd ed. New York: Marcel Dekker; 1994:787–821.
14. Cherniack NS, Longobardo GS. Abnormalities in respiratory rhythm. In: Cherniach NS, Widdicombe JG, eds. *Handbook of physiology*. Vol. II: *Control of breathing*, Pt 2. Bethesda: American Physiological Society; 1986:729–749.
15. Cherniack NS, Longobardo GS. Periodic breathing during sleep. In: Saunders NA, Sullivan CE, eds. *Sleep and breathing*. 2nd ed. New York: Marcel Dekker; 1994:787–821.
16. Bradley G. Control of ventilation. In: Scadding JG, Cumming G, eds. *Scientific foundations of respiratory medicine*. London: Heinemann Medical; 1981:162–172.
17. Loeschcke HH. Respiratory physiology. In: Widdicombe JG, ed. *MTB international review of science*. Physiology Series 1, Vol 2. Baltimore: University Park Press; 1974:167–196.
18. Khoo MCK. Periodic breathing. In: Crystal RG, West JB, eds. *The lung: scientific foundations*. New York: Raven Press; 1991:1419–1431.
19. Coleridge HM, Coleridge JCG, Jordan D. Integration of ventilatory and cardiovascular control system. In: Crystal RG, West JB, eds. *The lung: scientific foundations*. New York: Raven Press; 1991: 1405–1418.
20. Hanly PJ, Millar TW, Steljes DG, Baert R, Frais MA, Kryger MK. Respiration and abnormal sleep in patients with congestive heart failure. *Chest* 1989;96:480–488.
21. Braghiroli A, De Vito F, Sacco C, et al. Six months oxygen therapy in patients with congestive heart failure: preliminary results. *Am Rev Respir Dis* 1992;145:A446.
22. Dark DS, Pingleton SK, Kerby GR, et al. Breathing pattern abnormalities and arterial oxygen desaturation during sleep in the congestive heart failure syndrome. *Chest* 1987;91:833–836.
23. Luce JM. The cardiovascular effects of mechanical ventilation and positive end-expiratory pressure. *JAMA* 1984;252:807–811.
24. Bernsten AD, Holt AW, Vedig AE, Skowronski GA, Baggoley CJ. Treatment of severe cardiogenic pulmonary edema with continuous positive airway pressure delivered by face mask. *N Engl J Med* 1991;325:1825–1830.
25. Buda AJ, Pinsky MR, Ingels NB, Daughters GT, Stinson EB, Alderman EL. Effects of intrathoracic pressure on left ventricular performance. *N Engl J Med* 1979;301:453–459.
26. Takasaki Y, Orr D, Popkin J, Rutherford R, Liu P, Bradley TD. Effect of continuous positive airway pressure on sleep apnea in congestive heart failure. *Am Rev Respir Dis* 1989;140:1578–1584.
27. Malone S, Liu PP, Holloway R, Rutherford R, Xie A, Bradley TD. Obstructive sleep apnoea in patients with dilated cardiomyopathy: effects of continuous positive airway pressure. *Lancet* 1991; 338:1480–1484.
28. Bradley TD, Holloway RH, McLaughlin PR, Ross BL, Walters J, Liu PP. Cardiac output response to continuous positive airway pressure in congestive heart failure. *Am Rev Respir Dis* 1992;145: 377–382.
29. Buckle P, Millar T, Kryger M. The effect of short-term nasal CPAP on Cheyne-Stokes respiration in congestive heart failure. *Chest* 1992;102:31–35.
30. Davies RJO, Harrington KJ, Ormerod OJM, Stradling JR. Nasal continuous positive airway pressure in chronic heart failure with sleep-disordered breathing. *Am Rev Respir Dis* 1993;147:630–634.
31. Weintraub Z, Alvaro R, Kwiatkowski K, Cates D, Rigatto H. Effects of inhaled oxygen (up to 40%) on periodic breathing and apnea in preterm infants. *J Appl Physiol* 1992;72:116–120.
32. Moshenifar Z, Amin D, Jasper AC, Shah PK, Koerner SK. Dependence of oxygen consumption on oxygen delivery in patients with chronic congestive heart failure. *Chest* 1987;92:447–450.
33. Hanly PJ, Millar TW, Steljes DG, Baert R, Frais MA, Kryger MH. The effect of oxygen on respiration and sleep in patients with congestive heart failure. *Ann Intern Med* 1989;111:777–782.

The Failing Heart, edited by N. S. Dhalla,
R. E. Beamish, N. Takeda, and M. Nagano.
Lippincott-Raven Publishers, Philadelphia © 1995.

12

Cardiac Contractile Failure and Ultrastructural Abnormalities during the Development of Diabetic Cardiomyopathy

Leonard S. Golfman, *Nobuakira Takeda, Robert E. Beamish, and
Naranjan S. Dhalla

*Division of Cardiovascular Sciences, Faculty of Medicine, University of Manitoba,
St. Boniface General Hospital Research Centre, Winnipeg, Manitoba R2H 2A6 Canada;
and *Department of Internal Medicine, Aoto Hospital, Jikei University, Tokyo 125, Japan*

It is becoming clear that the term *diabetic cardiomyopathy* is loosely used in clinical circles to describe cardiac dysfunction in patients with chronic diabetes. It occurs not only because of insufficient coronary perfusion of the myocardium associated with occlusive coronary atherosclerosis but also because of a unique cardiomyopathy which is expressed in the form of hemodynamic and contractile abnormalities as well as structural derangement. In many instances, the etiology of diabetic cardiomyopathy is unknown (1); however, it is emphasized that numerous clinical reports have confirmed that human diabetics appear particularly susceptible to heart failure, a leading cause of death in these patients. Factors that appear largely to account for the increased incidence of cardiovascular dysfunction in chronic diabetes include atherosclerosis of the coronary arteries, microangiopathy, and autonomic neuropathy. It has also become apparent, however, that these factors are not always responsible for the cardiac dysfunction associated with diabetes. For example, a significant number of diabetic patients who do not develop atherosclerosis, microangiopathy, and autonomic neuropathy still suffer from cardiomegaly, left ventricular dysfunction, and clinically overt congestive heart failure (2). These observations suggest that a specific cardiac muscle disease may occur during diabetes, and this disease (diabetic cardiomyopathy) is possibly a consequence of a direct effect of insulin deficiency on myocardial cell function. The diagnosis of diabetic cardiomyopathy is to be considered in those patients in whom coronary artery disease, alcoholism, hypertensive cardiovascular disease, and other etiological factors producing myocardial dysfunction have been contraindicated. Evidence to support an impairment of performance due to a lesion of cardiac muscle itself comes from postmortem findings, abnormalities in contractile function in absence of major vessel disease, and ultrastructural derangement of cardiac tissue. Accordingly, it is intended to examine the involvement of myocardial ultrastructural changes, microvascular changes, and impairment of contractile function, which are manifested in diabetic cardiomyopathy.

MYOCARDIAL ULTRASTRUCTURAL CHANGES IN DIABETES

Several types of cells having unique and specialized functions are responsible for the structure and performance of the heart. Cardiomyocytes, smooth muscle, endothelial, fibroblasts, and other nonmuscle cells represent just a few of the various cell types found in the heart. The cardiac muscle cells are the primary functional component of the myocardium and determine the force generation of the heart. It is for this reason that cardiomyocytes have attracted the most attention in studies on diabetic cardiomyopathy. Although these contractile cells are not predominant in the heart in number, cardiomyocytes compose some 80% to 85% of the volume of the heart (3,4) and account for more than half of its weight (5).

Various techniques are available for examining the structure of the myocardium; these include morphological methods, freeze-fracture cytochemical methods, and vadioiodination techniques (6–10). One of the most informative methods employs the electron microscope for examining the structure of the myocardial cell (6–10). This method has allowed investigators to examine the myocyte's organelles in extreme detail; the principle organelles that have been targeted in various studies of diabetic animals include the contractile proteins, mitochondria, sarcoplasmic reticulum, the transverse tubular system, sarcolemma, and the nucleus. Because each organelle, by virtue of its unique function, contributes to the maintenance of the myocardial cell in a constant functional state, a lesion in any of these subcellular organelles may result in a compromised condition, and thus ultimately in a functional defect. The use of electron microscopic and morphometric techniques has revealed that the myofibrils and the mitochondria account for nearly 50% and 33% to 43% of the rat's total cell volume of its myocytes, respectively, with much smaller volumes occupied by other subcellular structures (transverse tubular system, 1%; sarcoplasmic reticulum, 2%; nucleus, 5%; sarcolemma, very low; lysosomes, very low) (5–11).

A number of studies have observed derangement in the contractile proteins in the hearts of diabetic animals. These alterations have been described as loss of contractile proteins (11–14), degeneration of myofibrils (15–17), lysis of myofibrils (17–19), derangements in the Z-band region (16,17,20), disorganization of myofibrils (12,13,17), and contraction of sarcomeres (13–16). These findings have been reported in spontaneous diabetes (11,18,19) and in chemically induced (alloxan or streptozotocin) diabetes in rats and rabbits (12–16,18–20). The implications of these ultrastructural alterations are that cardiac performance in diabetes may be depressed severely by an inefficiency or inability of the myofibrillar proteins to generate contractile force development.

The membranous systems in the heart, when examined under the electron microscope, also appear to be abnormal during diabetes. The sarcoplasmic reticular system shows signs of disruption in the spontaneously diabetic KK mouse heart (17). In drug-induced diabetes in animals, many investigators have reported swollen sarcoplasmic reticular tubules (14,18,19,21), mild edema immediately adjacent to the sarcoplasmic reticulum (22), and loss of sarcoplasmic reticulum (12,13). In addition, the membrane that envelopes the cell is also disturbed by the diabetic condition. It was observed that portions of the sarcolemmal membrane had lifted away from the myocardial cell surface; there were also considerable blebbing and vacuolization immediately adjacent to that area (23). Because similar changes have been noticed in experimental models of cardiac dysfunction due to intracellular Ca^{2+} overload (24), it is possible that the observed alterations in the diabetic heart may be a consequence of the occurrence of intracellular Ca^{2+} overload. These sarcolemmal changes may be involved in increased permeability characteristics of the heart observed during diabetes (25). In addition, local thickening of the cardiac sarcolemma during diabetes has also been reported (11,19). In studies with alloxan diabetic rats (12,13), complete loss of transverse tubules has also been observed. Furthermore, cell-to-cell contact has been observed by a number of investigators to be altered in the hearts of diabetic animals. In drug-induced diabetic animals (12–15,19,26) the intercalated disc region is visibly separated and widened along the fascial adherents (12,13), with maintenance of both desmosomes and gap junctions (12,13,19). This may disturb intercellular communication and may partially explain, at least from an ultrastructural standpoint, the enhanced arrhythmogenic capacity of the diabetic heart (27).

Mitochondrial abnormalities are the most common ultrastructural disturbance reported in the heart during diabetes. Mitochondrial swelling is frequently observed (15–17,19–22,26,28); however, one study observed mitochondrial shrinkage (11), but Thompson (13) reported that mitochondrial size and architecture were rarely altered in alloxan-induced diabetic rats. On the other hand, generalized mitochondrial disruption (11,14) is evident in the form of vacuolization of the mitochondria (29), clearing of the matrix (15,29), separated cristae (16,19), and lysis of both inner and outer mitochondrial membranes (29). This damage could be the result of increased lysosomal activity in hearts from diabetic animals. An incorporation of lysosomal membranes into the mitochondrial matrix has been observed (15). An increase in the number of electron-dense particles in the mitochondria has also been reported (11,22); this may reflect an accumulation of Ca^{2+} ions. Other structural alterations have also become evident from electron microscopic examination of the diabetic animal heart. Lysosomes have been shown to increase in number in myocardium from diabetic animals (14,15,29). The lysosomes were reported to be found more frequently near large amounts of glycogen and lipid droplets in the cell (29). Alterations in the nuclei of myocardial cells during diabetes have also been noticed. Condensation of nuclear chromatin (15) and the presence in the nuclei of perichromatin granules with a bright "halo" (19) have been described. Seager and co-workers (15) reported a folding of the nuclear membranes. An abnormal increase in perivascular space around the nucleus has also been observed (14). Giacomelli and Wiener (11) have reported degenerative nerve endings in the diabetic heart.

CHANGES IN METABOLIC SUBSTRATES IN DIABETIC MYOCARDIUM

Evidence from electron microscopic studies indicates that there are changes occurring with respect to the storage of metabolic substrates in the myocardial cell from diabetic animals; these changes corroborate similar findings by traditional biochemical methods. Several studies have observed an increased number of lipid droplets in myocardial cells from diabetic animals (11–16,19,21,22). These lipid droplets have been seen to be situated in close proximity to the Z-line (14,30) in both chemically induced and spontaneous models of diabetes. Another common observation in the diabetic myocardium is an increase in electron-dense glycogen particles (14,19,29,31). Again using the electron microscope, this finding correlates well with biochemical evidence of an increase in myocardial glycogen content during diabetes (32).

The extracellular space in the heart contains a matrix of polyanionic, protein–mucopolysaccharide sites (33); collagen is the primary protein in the extracellular matrix. Collagen fibrils may run in very close apposition to the membrane surface in smooth-muscle cells and myocardial cells and, in some cases, may even become embedded in the membrane wall (33). Collagen is an important extracellular structure and is thought to maintain myocardial function by a number of mechanisms. Due to its viscoelastic properties, collagen fibrils may transmit and distribute force generation during muscular contraction (34). Collagen may also influence muscle function through an interaction with Ca^{2+} ions as it may serve as an extracellular Ca^{2+} binding site (33) or alter the diffusion of extracellular Ca^{2+} into muscle cells (35). In disease states such as experimental hypertension and hypertrophy, increases in collagen synthesis by smooth-muscle cells have been demonstrated (36). Some controversy regarding the status of collagen in hearts of diabetic animals still exists, however. Where some investigators report evidence in favor of an increase in collagen content of the heart in diabetes (13,18,20,37–39), others have found no change (17,31). It has been suggested that the nature of the diabetic condition may represent an important factor in the accumulation of collagen in the heart during diabetes (40). Particularly, moderate and chronic models of diabetes appear to exhibit a consistently higher myocardial collagen content (20,37,38). It is the contention of many investigators that an increase in collagen content inhibits myocardial distensibility and alters cardiac performance.

FACTORS INFLUENCING THE DEVELOPMENT OF ULTRASTRUCTURAL CHANGES IN THE HEART DURING DIABETES

Although it is becoming clear that insulin-dependent diabetes produces a progressive pattern of ultrastructural changes in the myocardium of different diabetic animal models, it should be stated that ultrastructural derangement in the myocardium does not always accompany diabetes mellitus. For example, reports of diabetic effects on myocyte ultrastructure range from no effect (38) to myocytolysis and contraction bands (14). In this regard, several factors have been identified in the diabetic state that may affect the development of ultrastructural abnormalities in the heart. These include the duration and severity of diabetes, the type of diabetes, and the presence of other accompanying diseases. Modification of any of these factors will result in dramatic changes in the expression of structural damage to the heart during diabetes mellitus.

One of the most closely examined factors that influences the progression of ultrastructural damage in the heart is the length of time that the animal is exposed to diabetes. In short-term diabetes, ultrastructural changes in the heart are minimal. Electron microscopic examination of sections of the myocardium in rats 2 to 4 days after the induction of a diabetic state by alloxan injection revealed no alterations in the structure of cellular organelles (30). Only an increase in lipid droplets was observed so soon after alloxan injection (31). In the drug-induced diabetic rat model, it is difficult to ascertain precisely when significant ultrastructural derangement can be documented. As early as 7 days after the induction of diabetes, mitochondrial swelling and dilation of sarcoplasmic reticular tubules have been reported (21); however, others have reported no changes in myocardial ultrastructure as late as 6 weeks after injection of streptozotocin (14). Tarach (19), however, reported increases in cardiac lipid and glycogen deposition as well as swelling of the fascial adherents of the intercalated disk in 6-week alloxan-diabetic rats. Thompson (13) observed loss of myofibrils, disorganization of remaining myofibrils, disruption of banding pattern, loss of sarcoplasmic reticular elements and transverse tubules, and separation at the intercalated discs along the fascial adherents in 6-week alloxan-diabetic rats. Some investigators have found gross ultrastructural alterations at 8 weeks (15), 12 weeks, and 24 weeks (13,14) after the induction of the diabetic state with both streptozotocin and alloxan. Thus, although the duration of the diabetes does influence myocardial ultrastructure, the presence of abnormalities represents a gradual and very subtle progression. The changes may be so subtle that conventional electron microscopic techniques may not detect them. This view is supported by the observation that functional depression of the heart preceded the manifestation of ultrastructural abnormalities in the heart (14).

In the spontaneously diabetic mouse (C57BL/KsJ dbt/dbt), Giacomelli and Weiner (11) documented the ultrastructural alterations of the heart as a function of the age of the animal. As early as 5 weeks of age, myocardial cells exhibited mitochondrial changes, disruption of sarcomeres, and focal thickening of the sarcolemma; severe damage was present in the hearts of 6- to 7-month-old diabetic mice. In contrast, little evidence of damage to the arterial vessels and capillaries was present at 5 weeks of age in diabetic animals (11). At 12 weeks of age, some alterations were observed in endothelial and smooth-muscle cells; these included dense mitochondria, focal areas of lysis, and increased amounts of endoplasmic reticulum and Golgi bodies. By 24 and 28 weeks of age, diabetic mouse heart exhibited an increase in collagen content, destruction of capillary lumen, mitochondrial loss, and thickened basal lamina of arteries (11). The most significant finding was the difference in the time course of the appearance of ultrastructural defects in the myocardial cell, as opposed to alterations in the arterial vessels and capillaries. The observation that changes in myocardial cells preceded those in the vasculature (11,13,15) represents important evidence that diabetes is attended by a primary cardiomyopathic condition.

Not every investigator has observed ultrastructural derangement in hearts from diabetic animals (37,38,41). Part of the reason for this discrepancy may involve the severity of the diabetic state. One group (37,38) has consistently used an alloxan-induced model of diabetes in dogs which does not exhibit resting hyperglycemia but does show abnormal glucose tolerance. They found little or no evidence of changes in the ultrastructure of cellular organelles in the hearts of these animals. In addition, no changes in the vasculature were noted. Alterations in myocardial composition (an increase in collagen content and lipid droplets) were the only unusual features associated with this type of diabetes. The severity of the diabetes may represent a plausible explanation for the presence or absence of ultrastructural changes in the heart during diabetes (40). The degree of severity of insulin-dependent diabetes was examined in a time-course study of alloxan-diabetic rats (12). Even with the same degree of hyperglycemia, glycosuria, polydipsia, and polyuria, moderately diabetic animals did not develop the degenerative ultrastructural changes seen in myocardium from more severely diabetic rats. These include decreased cardiocyte size, loss and disorganization of myofibrils, and loss of sarcoplasmic reticulum and transverse tubules.

The hypothesis that the severity of diabetes may represent a plausible explanation for the presence or absence of ultrastructural changes in the heart during diabetes was given further indirect support by studies that have examined myocardial ultrastructure by electron microscopy in insulin-treated diabetic animals. Daily insulin administration to diabetic animals reversed all myocardial ultrastructural defects, which were associated with short-term diabetes (21). This was also true for the most part in diabetes of longer duration. Some mitochondrial abnormalities and vascular resistance to a normalization in ultrastructure in response to insulin treatment were observed, however (22). These studies stress the increased difficulty in normalizing vascular ultrastructural alterations with insulin as opposed to changes in cardiac muscle cells.

The presence of other diseases in diabetic animals or patients has also been shown to augment cardiac ultrastructural damage. The hypertensive diabetic animal is one such example. A far greater incidence and severity of ultrastructural abnormalities were observed in diabetic animals that were also hypertensive (41). Disorganization of sarcomeres, increased numbers of mitochondria, and alterations in the intercalated disc region in the myocardial cell from hypertensive diabetic rats were reported (41). A thickened pericapillary basal lamina and an increase in endothelial pinocytotic vesicles in myocardial capillaries were also found. All of these changes were less severe in the hypertensive rat or in the diabetic rat in comparison with those observed in the hypertensive diabetic rat hearts (41). Similar findings were reported using the light microscope on myocardial sections obtained from hypertensive diabetic rats (42) and diabetic patients with hypertension (43). Considering the reported prevalence of hypertension in the diabetic population (44), the presence of cardiac ultrastructural alterations in the diabetic community may be more widespread than originally assumed.

From the foregoing discussion it is evident that ultrastructural changes in the heart are dependent on the duration, severity, and type of diabetes present. Alterations in myocardial ultrastructure can occur in the absence of arterial or capillary changes, whereas increase in the number of lipid droplets appears to be one of the earliest abnormalities detected in the diabetic cardiac muscle cell. Sarcomere disorganization, myofibrillar loss, and mitochondrial swelling and clearing are among the more common ultrastructural lesions reported. Less frequently observed but still notable are nuclear abnormalities and T-tubule and sarcoplasmic reticulum swelling. Sarcolemmal alterations and separation of the intercalated disc region have also been reported. Vascular defects, when observed, usually appear in the form of thickened arterial or capillary basal lamina. Micropinocytotic activity associated with the capillary wall has also been reported. These lesions are aggravated by the presence of hypertension in the diabetic subject. A relationship of these ultrastructural abnormalities in the heart during diabetes to cardiac functional depression has been challenged by others; however, the presence of such damage does provide clear, undeniable evidence that the heart is undergoing a process of pathological regression.

CONTRIBUTION OF SMALL VESSEL DISEASE IN DIABETIC CARDIOMYOPATHY

The crucial function of the cardiocyte, and subsequently the function of the heart, is critically dependent on proper support by the other components of the heart. In particular, the cardiocyte is dependent on the ability of the microvasculature to supply metabolic substrates and hormonal factors, remove metabolic wastes, and regulate both the ionic and osmotic environment of the tissue. Abnormalities in the capillaries and arterioles take the form of local constrictions of the vessel, abnormal vascular flow patterns, aneurysms, vessel permeability changes, and alterations in reactivity to various stimuli. These injuries may lead to reperfusion damage in the myocardium and have been implicated by many as a primary cause of cardiac contractile dysfunction and failure. The possibility that this complication may be a contributing factor in heart dysfunction during diabetes has received much attention and has led to much controversy.

Several studies have reported no atherosclerotic plaque formation in the myocardial arteries of diabetic animals (15,17,45). In addition, no structural changes in smooth-muscle or endothelial cells in the small arteries, arterioles, or capillaries of the heart during diabetes (8 weeks, streptozotocin-diabetic rats) were evident (15). Furthermore, no basement membrane thickening has been observed in hearts from diabetic KK mice (17). These results, however, are in conflict with several other animal studies that document a thickening of small arteries and the basal lamina of capillaries in the heart during diabetes (13,18,19,31,46). A thickened densa in the presence of a loss of the lamina lucida has been observed in myocardial capillary walls during diabetes (46). Pinocytotic activity in the capillary walls has also been reported (13,20,46), with increased number and size of micropinocytotic vesicles (13,46). The explanation for the controversy in findings in the vasculature of the heart during diabetes in experimental animals may be related to the duration and severity of diabetes. It is also of interest that insulin administration to chronically STZ-diabetic rats did not prevent capillary basement membrane thickening in the myocardium (46). On the other hand, insulin administration to chronically alloxan-diabetic rats (13) reversed the diabetic-induced capillary abnormalities. The endothelium was smooth and of normal thickness, and the micropinocytotic vesicles were of normal size and distribution (13).

In the past, the role of small vessels in the pathogenesis of the diabetic heart in humans has been questioned by some investigators. Resnecov (47) considered the increased incidence of heart failure among diabetic patients to be probably caused by microangiopathy. The rarity of small vessel disease in nondiabetic patients with cardiomyopathy was also stressed. Regan et al. (48) examined ten uncomplicated diabetics and found significant luminal narrowing of extramural or intramural coronary arteries in one patient. All had accumulation of periodic acid-Schiff (PAS) material in the left ventricular interstitium, interstitial fibrosis, and hypertrophy. Factor et al. (49) noted microaneurysms of myocardial capillaries. Thickening of the basement membrane (basal lamina) was reported by Silver et al. (50) in postmortem samples and by Fischer et al. (51) in tissues removed during bypass surgery. Shirley et al. (52) included 12 patients with diabetes mellitus in a group of 139 patients with primary myocardial disease. Based on biopsy findings, autopsies were performed in two diabetic patients, and there was no small vessel involvement. Ledet (53) reported no significant changes in capillaries of postmortem human myocardium of young juvenile diabetics. Negative results in reporting small vessel disease may be due to technical difficulties or to the imperfection of the technique. Biopsy techniques may miss focal changes of the myocardium (54). For example, in the studies by Zoneraich and Silverman (55), four paraffin blocks from seven areas were taken; each block was sectioned at 6 μm and four sections were stained. They found small vessel disease alone in 50% of the 36 diabetics.

The causes and importance of capillary basement thickening as a result of diabetes have been discussed extensively elsewhere (56,57). It has been suggested that this thickening occurs independently of the lowered insulin levels and is perhaps due to hyperglycemia and/or other metabolic and hormonal imbalances. This might explain why insulin treatment failed to prevent changes in streptozotocin-diabetic rats, as reported by McGrath and McNeill (46); it does not, however, explain the contrary findings by Thompson (13) with alloxan-diabetic rats. Many investigators have suggested that the increased microvascular permeability to macromolecules, such as plasma proteins, plays an important role in the pathogenesis of diabetic complications in several organs (58). There are numerous reports of increased microvascular permeability to macromolecules in diabetic patients and experimental diabetic animals. Although the mechanism remains to be elucidated, it has been suggested (46) that the observed increase in the number of micropinocytotic vesicles may explain the increased vascular permeability reported in diabetes and may thus influence cardiac dysfunction.

Most of the evidence supporting involvement of the microvasculature in the depression of cardiac performance during diabetes is still, unfortunately, largely conjectural. Many past studies have reported abnormalities in heart function or electrocardiographic recordings from diabetic patients and, after observing no evidence of coronary stenosis or ischemic heart disease, have concluded the cause of this dysfunction to be microvascular in origin (59–62). No direct evidence, however, supports such a conclusion in these studies.

The existence of focal changes in microvessels are not sufficient to account for the diffuse myocardial degeneration with interstitial fibrosis, which is a pathomorphological feature of diabetic cardiomyopathy (63). Furthermore, the presence of functional microangiopathy (increased microvascular permeability) in the diabetic myocardium was not identified until 1993 when Yamaji et al. (63) provided evidence for increased capillary permeability in the diabetic rat myocardium. By using an in situ perfusion method, which is the most direct way of investigating microvascular permeability to macromolecules, it was reported that capillary permeability to albumin was markedly increased in the diabetic rat myocardium because of enhanced vesicular transport. It was hypothesized that this may play an important role in the pathogenesis of diabetic cardiomyopathy. The increased capillary permeability in diabetic rat myocardium shown in this study was a remarkable functional change seen in almost all capillaries. This observation, seen diffusely in diabetic myocardium, was considered to be much more significant than focal structural abnormalities of microvessels.

It has been suggested that abnormally increased extravasation of plasma constituents such as albumin may cause myocardial edema (increased interstitial matrix), which would be followed by interstitial fibrosis during a long period of disease (64). Both interstitial edema and fibrosis, which are frequent histopathological features of diabetic myocardium (13,65–67), may contribute to the development of diastolic dysfunction through increased ventricular stiffness. Several investigators have suggested the significance of advanced glycosylated end product in the pathogenesis of vascular complications (68). Advanced glycosylation end products accumulated on vessel-wall proteins and collagen may decrease protein removal, increase new protein deposition, and stimulate cellular proliferation in the interstitium by forming cross-links with extravascular plasma proteins (68). Such studies have provided evidence that one of the principal pathophysiological features of diabetic complications is the morphological and functional alterations of microvessels, called "diabetic microangiopathy." Morphological microangiopathy of both the relatively large intramyocardial vessels as well as arterioles and capillaries has been identified in diabetic myocardium of experimental animals and human diabetic patients. The exact relationship of microangiopathy to the pathogenesis of diabetic cardiomyopathy remains controversial, however. It has been suggested recently that microangiopathy, in association with the formation of advanced glycosylation end products, may play an important role in the pathogenesis of diabetic cardiomyopathy in a manner similar to that for retinopathy or nephropathy (1).

HEART FUNCTION DURING DIABETES

As a pump, the heart of a diabetic patient is in a compromised condition. Several techniques have been employed to evaluate cardiac function in both humans and experimental diabetic animals. Noninvasive methods, including electrocardiography, phonocardiography, graphic recording of carotid pulsation, echocardiography, and radionuclide perfusion, have been used individually, or in some cases in combination, in order to measure the performance of the heart. These methods are carried out in a clinical setting with little compromise or discomfort to the patient; however, interpretation of the data is difficult, and conclusions from such studies are often limited. The use of invasive techniques extends the quantity and quality of information that must be obtained regarding force generation by the cardiac muscle. Cardiac catheterization, heart–lung preparations, isolated hearts, ventricular wall strips, interventricular septal preparations, and isolated papillary muscles represent only a few of the methods and models whereby cardiac contractile force generation may be directly monitored in an invasive manner. Because of their invasive natures, their use is restricted, by ethical considerations, to animal studies. These data, unfortunately, also have limited value, in this case with respect to the direct application of these animal results to heart function in humans. Nonetheless, in the past two decades, a number of both invasive and noninvasive studies have been conducted in human diabetics and experimental animals to more clearly define the alterations of cardiac physiology and to evaluate pump performance in diabetes and diabetic cardiomyopathy. In this section, different aspects of cardiac performance are discussed, including (a) human diabetic studies, (b) animal studies, and (c) methods to normalize cardiac function in diabetes.

Human Diabetic Studies

Results from analyses of cardiac performance during diabetes have been reported by various investigators. Resting heart rate was similar in control and diabetic subjects (69,70) or higher in diabetics (71,72). Manipulation of external variables unmasked significant differences in heart rate. For example, the ingestion of small quantities of alcohol did not alter heart rate in control subjects, but stimulated heart rate in diabetics (69). Ambulatory monitoring of heart function for a 24-hour period revealed higher diurnal heart rates in diabetic men (73). This was especially true for those patients suspected of autonomic neuropathy. Under intense exercise stress, Abenavoli and co-workers (74) found that diabetic subjects without evidence of clinical heart disease had lower maximal heart rates than control subjects. Blood pressure measurements were shown to be dependent on the presence of atherosclerotic complications in the arterial system during diabetes; hypertension in the diabetic population has been reported (75). In relatively asymptomatic diabetic men, systolic blood pressure tended to be higher in those patients with autonomic neuropathy but lower in diabetics considered to have peripheral neuropathy (73). Diastolic blood pressure changes may correlate with pathological alterations. Shapiro and colleagues (76) discovered that the posterior wall of the heart was thicker in diabetic patients if the diastolic blood pressure was between 100 and 125 mmHg than if it was less than 100 mmHg. Cardiac hypertrophy has been considered an indicator of clinical heart disease and part of the pathology of diabetic cardiomyopathy (77,78).

The majority of investigations on cardiac function in diabetic patients has used systolic time intervals as a measure of cardiac performance. The measurements are accomplished by simultaneous recording of the electrocardiogram, phonocardiogram, and carotid pulse tracing. The critical parameters within the systolic time interval are the pre-ejection period (PEP), left ventricular ejection time (LVET), the PEP/LVET ratio, the conduction time, and the isovolumic contraction time or isovolumic relaxation time. Cardiac dysfunction has been associated with increases in PEP, PEP/LVET ratio, and isovolumic contraction time, whereas stimulated cardiac performance was associated with decrease in these systolic time interval measurements (79,80). It is important to note, however, that systolic time intervals have a limited value in individuals in whom the carotid pulse wave was difficult to record, or when septal defects or vascular disease were present (79). The application of systolic time interval measurements to cardiac performance in diabetes has revealed significant defects in almost all of the values. Systolic time intervals (81), especially the ratio of PEP/LVET has been shown to correlate with invasively determined parameters of contractile performance, such as ejection fraction (82). Several independent investigators have reported an increase in PEP (69,76,79,82,83), an increase in the PEP/LVET ratio (28,69,76,79,82–84), a prolonged isovolumic contraction time (79), an increase in conduction time (79), and a prolonged isovolumic relaxation time (76,84). This was observed in both insulin-dependent diabetics and non–insulin-dependent diabetic patients; one study, however, noted more pronounced defects in the former (76). Although one group found no correlation between the duration of diabetes and changes in systolic time interval (79), another found that in diabetic patients under 20 years of age there was a significant correlation between these indices (84). Alterations in systolic time intervals in diabetic patients have also been correlated with glycosylated hemoglobin levels (82) and blood glucose levels (85). Uusitupa and co-workers (86) found that when blood glucose concentrations were better controlled, PEP and PEP/LVET ratio declined and LVET increased toward control values. On closer examination of their data, they found that only those diabetic patients whose fasting blood glucose concentrations had improved ≥3 mmol/l demonstrated significant changes in systolic time interval. Thus, these studies would support a close relationship between cardiac dysfunction, as evidenced by abnormal systolic time intervals, and the diabetic condition (especially hyperglycemia).

Doppler echocardiography has been utilized increasingly to assess systolic and diastolic function of the left ventricle in a variety of conditions (87). Pulsed Doppler ultrasound examination of mitral inflow velocities affords a simple and reproducible method for evaluating diastolic and systolic variables that correlate with radionuclide and invasive techniques (88–90). Doppler echocardiography is independent of factors that alter ventricular geometry and can be employed easily. Ventricular diameters are calculated from the echocardiograms during systole and diastole to determine the ejection fraction, which is an indicator of cardiac pump fraction. A larger than normal ejection fraction represents an augmentation in contractile function of the heart, whereas a decrease in the myocardial ejection fraction has been considered to be an indicator of heart disease. Zoneraich and colleagues (83) could find no evidence of any defects in left ventricular function in a group of diabetics using echocardiography, even though systolic time intervals demonstrated significant dysfunction. Only in a selected subgroup of diabetic patients did significant left ventricular dysfunction become evident by echocardiography (83). Notwithstanding these findings, several investigations using echocardiography have revealed defects in cardiac pump performance in diabetes. The percentage of myocardial fractional shortening was lower in diabetics than nondiabetics (74,91,92). The ejection fraction was also subnormal in diabetic patients (91,92). The end-systolic left ventricular volume was greater in diabetics (92). The left ventricular wall movement and mitral valve opening had less of a temporal relationship than usual (61). In fact, mitral valve opening was often delayed in diabetic subjects and, in some patients, the outward left ventricular wall movement was recorded prior to the opening of the mitral valve (61). The latter finding is consistent with ischemic heart disease, and in view of the patency of large vessels, it may be interpreted as indicating small vessel disease (61); other observations support this conclusion (91). Echocardiograms from diabetic patients in other studies, however, were suggestive of left ventricular hypertrophy (93) and altered compliance, possibly due to an accumulation of interstitial glycoproteins (93,94).

Radionuclide angiography has also been employed to assess cardiac performance in control and diabetic patients. The majority of investigations using radionuclide angiography has observed no difference in the resting left ventricular ejection fraction between control and diabetic patients (94–97). Manipulation of several external variables, however, revealed significant defects in cardiac performance in diabetic patients. If blood glucose levels rose, the mean ejection fraction at rest rose significantly higher than in the normoglycemic period (94). The explanation of this effect is unknown. If diabetic patients were exercised, significant depression in the ejection fraction was observed in comparison to control patients (95,96). This was observed frequently enough in one study (95) to allow investigators to conclude that as many as one-third of their diabetic patients exhibited subclinical left ventricular dysfunction. Another investigation unmasked cardiac dysfunction in diabetics only when stress-tested by cold stimulation (98). The mechanism responsible for this effect was unclear, although autonomic complications may represent one possible factor (98). Abenavoli and colleagues (74) observed a decrease in percentage of myocardial fractional shortening in diabetic patients. In all of the studies, macrovascular disease was eliminated as a factor involved in the cardiac dysfunction.

The presence of a defect in left ventricular contractile function during diabetes is supported by other investigators who have used other measurement techniques, including catheterization and contrast ventriculography. Myocardial dysfunction during diabetes is evidenced by a decrease in ejection fraction (99,100), an increase in left ventricular end-diastolic pressure (28,65,99,100), an increase in end-diastolic volume (28,65,100), a decrease in cardiac index (100), mean systolic ejection rate (100) and stroke volume (28,65), and an increase in the left ventricular end-diastolic pressure to volume ratio (65). Increasing the afterload of the heart in diabetics resulted in higher filling pressures without altering the stroke volume (65). Large vessel complications were not considered to contribute to these indices of cardiac dysfunction in these studies. Instead, small vessel disease (99,100) and alterations in ventricular compliance due to the accumulation of collagen (28,65) have been suggested to account for the depressed cardiac performance during diabetes.

In the preceding discussion, impairment of the left ventricular systolic and diastolic functions has been detected frequently with type I diabetes and has been related to specific diabetic complications and the duration of disease. Overall, there are few reports on early changes in left ventricular function in asymptomatic cardiac diabetic patients. Some have stated that diastolic function is more commonly impaired than systolic function and that diastolic dysfunction may be the primary abnormality in patients with diabetes (87,101). In a recent study, Raev (70) found that myocardial damage in cardiac asymptomatic type I diabetic patients affects diastolic function before systolic function. To minimize the influence of factors other than diabetes on left ventricular function, this study excluded heart failure and/or arterial hypertension, coronary artery disease, other cardiac and noncardiac diseases, above-average physical activity, and the use of drugs (with the exception of regular doses of insulin). A high prevalence of diastolic dysfunction (impaired active and passive properties of the left ventricle) with preserved systolic function in young cardiac asymptomatic type I diabetic patients was observed. The results showed further that diastolic dysfunction was twice as common as systolic dysfunction (27% vs. 12%). Of the diabetic patients with systolic dysfunction, 83% had impaired diastolic function, whereas only 30% of diabetic patients with diastolic dysfunction had systolic dysfunction. On the other hand, only 3 of 157 diabetic patients (1.9%) had systolic dysfunction with preserved diastolic function. Furthermore, diastolic dysfunction, represented by the interval from minimal left ventricular dimension to mitral valve opening, was seen in diabetic patients approximately 8 years after onset of diabetes and systolic dysfunction, represented by fractional shortening, after about 18 years. In addition, diastolic dysfunction, represented by isovolumic relaxation time, was found in the presence of mild complications, while systolic dysfunction, represented by fractional shortening, was found only in the presence of more severe complications.

In many other disorders, such as congestive heart failure (102), hypertension (103), and coronary artery disease (104), systolic abnormalities have been preceded by diastolic dysfunction. Diastolic dysfunction with intact systolic function in patients with diabetes has been reported previously by many authors (76,105–108). Thus, these findings also confirm those of Raev (70) that the abnormalities of diastolic function may therefore be an earlier sign of diabetic heart muscle disease than impaired systolic function. In terms of clinical implications, the results of Raev's study (70) indicate that the cardiopathic process in patients with diabetes affects diastolic function before systolic function and show that an isolated examination of the systolic function in diabetic patients is not sensitive enough for the early discovery of left ventricular dysfunction. Intentional assessment of diastolic function in patients with diabetes is advisable (70) for the early detection of left ventricular dysfunction before appearance of the clinical symptoms and for follow-up of any deterioration of cardiac status. Thus, the detection of diastolic abnormalities may be a useful indicator for the prognosis of cardiovascular mortality in diabetic subjects. A 3-year follow-up study comparing groups of diabetic patients with normal diastolic function with those with diastolic dysfunction revealed that the former group had survival rates close to those predicated, but 31% of patients with diastolic dysfunction, even those who were asymptomatic, developed heart failure, and 19% died (109).

Animal Studies

The use of animals for studying changes in cardiac contractility is particularly advantageous because of the number of parameters that can be more critically and accurately measured. In vitro heart preparations, such as atrial preparations, isolated hearts, working hearts, papillary muscle preparations,'and in vivo hemodynamic studies, have been performed with diabetic animals. These experimental studies have been necessary in order to obtain a better understanding of the pathophysiology of diabetic cardiomyopathy, which is characterized by a decrease in both systolic and diastolic function. This decrease in heart function can occur in diabetes mellitus independent of the presence of any other risk factors associated with cardiovascular disease (110). Detailed experiments have shown the presence of a cardiomyopathy in both chemically (alloxan or streptozotocin) and spontaneously diabetic rats similar to that observed in diabetic patients.

Many of the studies from several independent laboratories have reported alterations in cardiac performance in diabetic animals. With all but one exception (37), the investigators have shown that the heart is in a depressed functional state during diabetes. The most extensive studies, which were carried out in the mid-1970s (37) and early 1980s (111,112), still remain landmark investigations. Many parameters have been monitored to assess cardiac performance in animals during diabetes. In general, the findings with diabetic animal hearts, which demonstrate a significant depression in contractile performance of the cardiac muscle, correspond to those obtained with human diabetics. These can be subdivided into tension (force) generation and relaxation. Generally, all indices of force generation in the hearts of diabetic animals were subnormal. The ability to generate a peak amount of force or pressure was depressed. In addition, the rate of force or pressure development was slower (113–127). These defects were translated into functional depressions in hemodynamic parameters such as aortic output, stroke volume, cardiac work, and cardiac output (37,111,114,116,118,119,128). In addition, other affected indices of force generation in hearts from diabetic animals include augmentation of time to peak tension, time to peak shortening, and time to peak shortening velocity (112). Alterations in end-diastolic volume have been reported (37,111); probably depending on the severity and duration of diabetes, however, the direction of the change and its relationship to pressure development were found to be variable (37,111). The change in the ability of the heart to relax during diabetes can be even more dramatic than the change in force generation (112). The presence of diabetes appears to slow the rate of relaxation and prolongs the amount of time it takes to dissipate tension. Changes in tension generation and relaxation in papillary muscles from diabetic and control animals were demonstrated in a study by Fein and colleagues (112). When one considers various indices of relaxation affected in hearts from diabetic animals, studies have overwhelmingly shown attenuation of peak velocity of relaxation ($-dP/dt$ as well as $-dT/dt$) and augmentation of such parameters as time to peak relaxation velocity, time for peak tension to fall by 50%, and time to peak rate of tension fall (111–113,115,121,122).

As stated earlier, one factor that influences cardiac performance during diabetes is duration of diabetes. Miller (114) observed a depression in systolic pressure development, cardiac output, and aortic output of the isolated perfused working heart from diabetic rats as early as 3 days after the induction of diabetes with an injection of alloxan. This impairment in cardiac performance could be normalized by including insulin in the perfusate or elevating perfusate glucose concentrations substantially. Thus, it was concluded that the defect in cardiac function was due to an inability of the acutely diabetic rat heart to use glucose (114). This, however, was not found to be the case in the chronically diabetic animal. The defects in cardiac performance in rats made diabetic for several weeks have been shown to be corrected to some extent (111,118,119) by altering glucose delivery to the heart, but these hearts still exhibited significant functional depression in contrast to controls (111–113). Thus, the defect in cardiac performance observed in chronically diabetic rats may not be due primarily to an inability to utilize perfusate glucose. Instead, intrinsic defects in the cardiac excitation–contraction coupling process have been suggested as the cause of the functional impairment (121,129,130). Various studies have shown that 1 month of diabetes is necessary before contractile deficiencies can be observed in hearts from chemically induced diabetic rats (112,113). In other studies the duration of diabetes is required to be 2½ to 3 months before cardiac dysfunction is apparent in the chemically induced diabetic rabbit (39,131). Data from various laboratories support the contention that the type of diabetes present does not affect the appearance of cardiac dysfunction. Insulin-dependent diabetes of a spontaneous (132,133) or chemically induced nature produces structural and/or functional changes in the heart. Cardiac dysfunction in a chemically induced model of non-insulin diabetes has been reported (118); the characteristics of this diabetic model (fasting euglycemia in the presence of glucose intolerance), however, may instead reflect an insulin-deficient state of lesser severity rather than a true non–insulin-dependent diabetes mellitus.

The severity of diabetes mellitus may also represent an important factor in determining the expression of cardiac disease. Most studies of chemically induced diabetes have employed rather large dosages of alloxan or streptozotocin (≥ 50 mg/kg body weight) to produce highly elevated fasting blood glucose levels (>400 mg%) (111–114,120). The contractile dysfunction associated with this condition has been significant as well. In contrast, Regan and co-investigators (37) have used low doses of alloxan (20 mg/kg body weight) on multiple occasions (three times at monthly intervals) in dogs to produce a mild diabetic condition. Fasting blood sugar levels were normal, but glucose intolerance was observed in addition to lower end-diastolic volume in diabetic dogs and double the increase in end-diastolic pressure in ventricles from diabetic dogs in response to volume expansion tests (37). These findings are in opposition to those of Penpargkul and co-workers (111), who used a more severe model of diabetes in rats. The conflict in results is important because of their implications regarding the mechanism responsible for the functional defects in the heart. Regan and colleagues (37) concluded that the cardiac dysfunction is caused by a reduced compliancy of the ventricular wall, whereas Penpargkul and co-workers (111) concluded that their results are consistent with a contractile defect rather than a compliancy factor. Further examination of the factors responsible for the conflicting results is warranted; such a difference in results, however, is further complicated by the possibility that species difference also may have influenced the findings. This is more directly supported by a study by Fein et al. (112,120), who found important differences in the time dependency of the appearance of some mechanical alterations in the heart. Alterations in myocardial glycoprotein composition have been observed in chemically induced diabetic rabbits (39) and dogs (37) but not consistently in rats (41,133). Again, these discrepancies have important implications with respect to the mechanisms responsible for the cardiomyopathy in diabetes.

Alterations in the performance of hearts from diabetic animals are unmasked by various interventions. The response of the heart to increasing Ca^{2+} concentrations in the perfusate shows a difference between control and diabetic animals (116,134). In the study by Bielefeld et al. (116), both left ventricle pressure development and aortic output were depressed at low but not higher calcium concentrations in diabetic preparations in contrast to control preparations. Supraphysiological Ca^{2+} concentrations again revealed a depression in cardiac function (116); these results have suggested that the myocardium cannot regulate intracellular Ca^{2+} concentrations. Variations have also been reported for the response of cardiac preparations from diabetic animals to glycosidic stimulation (124,134). Perfusion of papillary muscles with varying concentrations of ouabain resulted in a greater rise in resting tension and a larger fall in developed tension in diabetic preparations as compared with control preparations; this resulted in contractures at a ouabain concentration of 0.1 mM (124). Changes in inotropic response of the heart to other agonists have also been observed. β-adrenoceptor agonist, isoproterenol, was shown to be far more potent in stimulating inotropy in cardiac muscles from control rats as opposed to diabetic rats (76).

Myocardial dysfunction has been observed in newborn children of diabetic mothers (135). In this regard, an interesting investigation by Nakanishi and colleagues (136) dealt with myocardial excitation–contraction coupling in the fetal hearts from diabetic rabbits. Diabetes was induced by alloxan injection in pregnant diabetic rabbits by day 14 of gestation, and the fetal heart was removed 14 days later for mechanical analysis. These investigators discovered no difference in force generation between control and diabetic preparations in the presence of 1.5 mM Ca^{2+}; at higher perfusate Ca^{2+} concentrations, however, the inotropic effect was more pronounced, and the toxic effect was significantly less in the fetal heart preparations from the diabetic mother as opposed to the nondiabetic mother (136). These changes in myocardial Ca^{2+} regulation appeared to be due to alterations in Ca^{2+} movements across the sarcolemmal membrane and not due to changes in the accumulation of Ca^{2+} by intracellular membrane systems (136). Similar defects in myocardial regulation of Ca^{2+} flux at the sarcolemmal membrane level have been described in diabetes in adult animals (137).

Methods to Normalize Cardiac Function in Diabetics

The presence of significant abnormalities in cardiac performance during diabetes is thought to be related to epidemiological and autopsy findings of an increased frequency of cardiac lesions and cardiac failure in the diabetic population. This has led researchers to investigate methods of treating the cardiac dysfunction and pose such questions as the following: (a) Can the depression in heart function during diabetes be normalized? (b) What kinds of therapy can most effectively treat heart disease in the diabetic patient? The most direct approach to the problem, and the one most frequently employed, has been to examine whether correction of the hyperglycemic condition of animals results in a normalization of cardiac function. Insulin administration to diabetic animals has been the obvious method of choice in most investigations; however, other means of achieving normal glycemic status have been used to determine its effect on heart performance. Because of the presence of concomitant alterations in hormones other than insulin in the diabetic state, the normalization of such hormonal balance in the presence of diabetes has also been examined with regard to its effect on myocardial performance. Because of ethical considerations, the withdrawal and administration of diabetic therapy has been studied only in animal models. Accordingly, the effects of insulin therapy on diabetic cardiomyopathy were studied by Fein and colleagues (138). At 5 to 8 weeks after inducing diabetes in rats by streptozotocin injection, insulin was administered to the animals by daily subcutaneous injection for 4 weeks. This treatment normalized plasma glucose concentration and corrected the changes in body and heart weight associated with the diabetic condition (138). Furthermore, isometric contractile defects evident in papillary muscles from diabetic rats were corrected by the insulin treatment (138). Because addition of insulin to the muscle bath of diabetic preparations did not correct the contractile deficiencies (138), it was concluded that the normalization was a result of insulin therapy.

Duration of insulin treatment is an important factor in normalizing muscle function of diabetic rats. This, however, is not correlated with blood glucose levels, which are almost immediately corrected by insulin administration (138). In left ventricular papillary muscle functional studies of insulin-treated diabetic rats, a gradual reversal of the prolongation of time to peak tension was observed (138). Insulin treatment for 10 days was sufficient to partially reverse this contractile defect. A full 4 weeks of insulin administration to diabetic rats normalized these contractile defects. The dosage of insulin was also found to be important regarding the ability of insulin therapy to reverse cardiac dysfunction. At 7 to 8 weeks after the induction of diabetes in rats by streptozotocin injection, animals were given daily subcutaneous injections of insulin for a further 6 weeks (139). Papillary muscles were dissected from control or diabetic rats, which were given doses of insulin varying from 0 to 2.5 U/d; the results demonstrated a graded recovery in muscle function, depending on the dose of insulin (139).

Several other factors are important concerning the effects of insulin therapy on cardiac performance in diabetic animals. The studies just discussed used a duration of diabetes of about 2 to 3 months (138,139). Insulin therapy also partially or totally reversed the alterations in cardiac function associated with long-term diabetes (5 to 6 months) in rats (38); this was not the case, however, in mildly diabetic dogs. The myocardial abnormalities observed in dogs maintained in a diabetic state for 1 year could not be reversed by insulin administration (38); these findings may be qualified by longer durations of insulin treatment. The cardiac dysfunction that can be reversed by insulin treatment can also be prevented by insulin treatment. If, instead of administering insulin to diabetic animals that already exhibit cardiac abnormalities, insulin is given immediately after inducing diabetes, the appearance of cardiac dysfunction is prevented (140). Thus insulin therapy of diabetic animals may yield some information regarding the factors that contribute to the cardiac performance defects. On the basis of results obtained by varying the insulin dose in diabetic animals (139,140) or administering insulin to control animals (141), it has been suggested that insulin deficiency rather than hyperglycemia may be a more important factor in cardiac dysfunction during diabetes. It is known that insulin can exert an inotropic effect in the heart that is independent of its effects on substrate supply (142). Furthermore, insulin has been shown to alter ion interactions with several myocardial subcellular organelles (129). The topic of the role of insulin deficiency versus hyperglycemia in diabetic cardiomyopathy, however, requires further investigation before firm conclusions can be reached.

Therapy other than insulin has been given to rats in an effort to reverse or prevent depression in cardiac performance. Various methods of restoring euglycemia to insulin-deficient diabetic animals have been utilized by different laboratories. Hungarian investigators (143) compared the effects of insulin therapy and sulfonylurea therapy on the myocardium in diabetic dogs. After injection with the diabetic agent, alloxan, animals were treated with insulin, carbutamide, or glibenclamide for 3 months. Insulin was injected subcutaneously and the sulfonylurea drugs were given orally to the animals at meal time. After the treatments, there was a significant improvement in myocardial performance, ventricular compliancy, and accumulation of connective tissue in hearts from the diabetic dogs (143), but no difference was observed among the three agents with respect to myocardial recovery from the diabetes-related performance defects. Carbutamide treatment caused a significant elevation in arterial blood pressure in the diabetic dogs (143). Because sulfonylurea drugs can improve cardiac performance by simply including the drug in the perfusion medium and stimulating energy metabolism (119), its mechanisms of action are thought to involve both pancreatic and myocardial sites of action (119,144).

Another method used to prevent the decline in cardiac performance during diabetes was vanadate treatment. Vanadate is the oxidized form of the trace element vanadium; it has an insulin-like action in the cell (145). Vanadate, when included in the drinking water of diabetic rats, restored plasma glucose levels to control without influencing plasma insulin concentrations (146,147). Left ventricular developed pressure, $+dP/dt$ and $-dP/dt$, were significantly depressed in the diabetic animals. After vanadate treatment, these functional parameters were normalized. Unfortunately, side effects of vanadate may limit its clinical usefulness, at least in the near future. Because cardiac dysfunction recovered without any improvement in plasma insulin concentrations, but with a dramatic improvement in blood sugar levels, this would support a role for hyperglycemia and not hypoinsulinemia in diabetes-induced cardiac disease. The validity of this contention, however, is complicated and seriously threatened by the knowledge that the molecular mode of action of vanadate is very much like that of insulin (145).

Circulating thyroid hormone concentrations are depressed in both diabetic rats (115,148,149) and humans (150). Hypothyroid animals demonstrate a depression in cardiac pump function (151); these abnormalities in cardiac performance in the hypothyroid state are similar to those exhibited by the diabetic animal. It is possible, therefore, that the cardiac dysfunction present in diabetics may be due to accompanying thyroid hormone deficiency. Several investigators have examined this possibility by administering thyroid hormone to diabetic animals. Normalization of circulating thyroid hormone levels did not restore cardiac performance (148), nor did it bring the activity of several subcellular organelles, which are associated with force generation in the heart, back to control values (115,149). Administration of pharmacological doses of thyroid hormone was found to normalize contractile protein enzymatic activity (149); the results, however, do not support a role for depressed circulating thyroid concentrations in diabetic cardiomyopathy. This view was further strengthened by evidence of depressed cardiac function in animal species that maintained normal circulating thyroid hormone levels during diabetes (39,132).

Dichloroacetate (DCA), a pyruvate dehydrogenase activator, is a pharmacological agent that is effective in increasing myocardial glucose oxidation in normal and diabetic rat hearts perfused with glucose and insulin (152,153). Nicholl and co-workers (154) indicated that even in the presence of elevated levels of fatty acids, DCA dramatically stimulated glucose oxidation in chronically diabetic rat hearts. In this study, it was demonstrated that diabetic hearts perfused with palmitate plus DCA showed marked improvement in function. Heart rate and the heart rate–peak systolic pressure product in spontaneously beating hearts, as well as left ventricular diastolic pressure and $+dP/dt$ in paced hearts, were all restored to control heart values. Etomoxir, which is also considered to promote glucose oxidation by inhibiting fatty-acid oxidation as well as lowering plasma free fatty acids, has been shown to prevent a depression in sarcoplasmic reticular Ca^{2+}-ATPase as well as redistribution of myosin isozymes in the diabetic heart (155). In fact, lowering the plasma free fatty acids in diabetic animals by hydralazine was found to prevent impairment in cardiac contractile function of the diabetic heart (156). Whether the beneficial effects of the lipid-lowering agents in diabetic animals is due to a decrease in lipid oxidation or their ability to promote glucose oxidation cannot be stated with certainty; it seems, however, that a therapy of diabetic patients with a combination of lipid-lowering agents and insulin could prove useful.

MECHANISMS OF CARDIAC DYSFUNCTION IN CHRONIC DIABETES

From the foregoing discussion, it is evident that heart dysfunction in chronic diabetes is due primarily to insulin deficiency; the exact stimulus for contractile failure in this condition, however, is poorly understood. Extensive work by using streptozotocin-induced and alloxan-induced diabetes in rats has revealed that contractile abnormalities in diabetic hearts may be due to Ca^{2+}-handling abnormalities in the cell as well as remodeling of myofibrils (115,137,139,149,157–165). In this regard, sarcolemmal (SL) Na^{+}-Ca^{2+} exchange and Ca^{2+}-pump activities, as well as sarcoplasmic reticulum (SR) Ca^{2+}-pump activities, are impaired in diabetic rat heart; these explain the Ca^{2+}-handling defects. Furthermore, myofibrillar Ca^{2+}-stimulated ATPase activity in diabetic rat heart is decreased markedly. The subcellular changes in SR Ca^{2+}-transport and myofibrillar ATPase activities in addition to heart dysfunction were partially prevented on treating the diabetic rats with a Ca^{2+} antagonist, verapamil (122,166).

It can be seen from data in Table 1 that treatment of streptozotocin-induced diabetic rats with verapamil did not affect the body weight loss, increased heart/body weight ratio, plasma glucose, or plasma insulin levels. The depressed level of cardiac adenosine triphosphate (ATP) or adenosine triphosphate/adenosine diphosphate (ATP/ADP) ratio and elevated levels of ADP or adenosine monophosphate (AMP), were, however, normalized by treatment of diabetic animals with verapamil. Furthermore, hemodynamic assessment of animals revealed that heart dysfunction in diabetic animals was prevented by verapamil treatment, but the increased QRS complex was not affected (Table 2). Verapamil treatment also prevented the devel-

TABLE 1. *General characteristics as well as myocardial high-energy stores of control, diabetic, and verapamil-treated diabetic rats*

	Control	Diabetic	Verapamil-treated diabetic
Body wt (g)	462 ± 7	270 ± 16[a]	305 ± 10
Heart/body wt (mg/g)	2.25 ± 0.06	2.74 ± 0.07[a]	2.65 ± 0.09
Plasma glucose (mg/dl)	155 ± 16	473 ± 20[a]	460 ± 16
Plasma insulin (mU/dl)	3.1 ± 0.25	0.9 ± 0.10[a]	0.9 ± 0.10
ATP (μmol/g)	4.95 ± 0.15	3.72 ± 0.10[a]	4.45 ± 0.19[b]
ADP (μmol/g)	1.47 ± 0.04	1.85 ± 0.11[a]	1.56 ± 0.12[b]
AMP (μmol/g)	0.44 ± 0.01	0.90 ± 0.01[a]	0.65 ± 0.04[b]
ATP/ADP ratio	3.20 ± 0.15	2.10 ± 0.14[a]	3.21 ± 0.57[b]

Data from Afzal et al. (122).
[a]p <0.05 (diabetic vs. control).
[b]p <0.05 (treated vs. untreated diabetic).
Each value is a mean ± SE of 6 to 12 experiments. Diabetes in rats was induced by streptozotocin (65 mg/kg; i.v.). One group of 4-week diabetic animals was treated with verapamil (8 mg/kg in two doses; subcutaneously) for 4 weeks; this treatment was started 1 day after inducing diabetes.
ATP, adenosine triphosphate; ADP, adenosine diphosphate; AMP, adenosine monophosphate.

opment of ultrastructural defects in diabetic heart (122). These results indicate that Ca^{2+}-handling abnormalities play an important role in the genesis of heart dysfunction in chronic diabetes.

To establish whether the changes observed in cardiac subcellular organelles are limited to the rat model of diabetes, the alloxan-induced diabetes in rabbits was employed to study changes in the heart. Table 3 shows the general characteristics of the control and diabetic rabbits. Body weights and heart weights were significantly depressed in diabetic rabbits, compared with control rabbits, 12 weeks after alloxan

TABLE 2. *Hemodynamic, electrocardiographic, and cardiac contractile changes in control, diabetic, and verapamil-treated diabetic rats*

	Control	Diabetic	Verapamil-treated diabetic
LVSP (mmHg)	151 ± 2	123 ± 3[a]	142 ± 7[b]
LVDP (mmHg)	3 ± 2	19 ± 1[a]	6 ± 2[b]
HR (beats/min)	357 ± 6	283 ± 7[a]	321 ± 9[b]
TME (mmHg/min)	53,138 ± 1,172	34,628 ± 992[a]	45,339 ± 1,471[b]
PR interval (ms)	10 ± 0.26	9.1 ± 0.20	9.6 ± 0.18
QRS amplitude (mm)	9.9 ± 0.26	16.1 ± 0.5[a]	17.3 ± 0.74
+ dP/dt (mmHg/s)	6,137 ± 176	4,332 ± 226[a]	7,220 ± 158[b]
− dP/dt (mmHg/s)	5,415 ± 158	3,610 ± 173[a]	5,776 ± 154[b]

Data from Afzal et al. (122).
[a]p <0.05 (diabetic vs. control).
[b]p <0.05 (treated vs. untreated diabetic).
Each value is a mean ± SE of 8 to 12 experiments.
LVSP, left ventricular systolic pressure; LVDP, left ventricular diastolic pressure; HR, heart rate; TME, total mechanical energy (HR × LVSP).

TABLE 3. *General characteristics of control and diabetic rabbits*

	Control	Diabetic
Body weight (kg)	4.50 ± 0.25	3.10 ± 0.15^a
Heart weight (g)	6.53 ± 0.51	3.60 ± 0.62^a
Plasma glucose (mg/dl)	133.5 ± 11.3	457.9 ± 40.6^a
Plasma insulin (mU/l)	20.3 ± 2.1	15.1 ± 1.0^a
Plasma cholesterol (mmol/dl)	2.06 ± 0.25	4.81 ± 0.35^a

[a]Significantly different form control; $p < 0.05$.

Values are means $\pm$ SE of 5 to 6 animals for each experimental group. Diabetes was induced by injecting alloxan (125 mg/kg; i.v.); sham control received buffered vehicle. Animals were used 12 weeks later.

administration. A marked increase in plasma glucose and cholesterol levels was seen in experimental rabbits, whereas plasma insulin levels were decreased. Table 4 shows that myofibrillar Ca^{2+}-stimulated ATPase was significantly depressed (32%) in diabetic rabbits compared with controls; myofibrillar Mg^{2+}-stimulated ATPase, however, was unaffected. In diabetic rabbits, both Ca^{2+}-stimulated and Mg^{2+}-stimulated SR ATPase activity was reduced in comparison with control rabbits. Table 5 reveals that the SL Na^+-dependent Ca^{2+} exchange activity was severely depressed (41%) in the diabetic rabbits compared with the control; neither the SL Na^+-K^+-ATPase activity nor the Ca^{2+} pump indices (Ca^{2+}-stimulated ATPase and ATP-dependent Ca^{2+} uptake) were affected.

It should be pointed out that the diabetic (hyperglycemic-glycosuric) rabbit, as a model of human diabetes, has been produced by reduction in pancreatic mass and injury to pancreatic beta cells (167). Since the first report of hyperglycemia induced by alloxan in the rabbit, a variety of dosages and methods of administration have been utilized by several investigators to achieve a permanent state of diabetes in the rabbit (168). These investigators (168) report that there is extreme variability in individual rabbit susceptibility to the diabetogenic effects of alloxan. In a study presented here (Table 3), a single dose of 125 mg/kg alloxan in the rabbits resulted

TABLE 4. *Influence of diabetes on myofibrillar and sarcoplasmic reticulum ATPase activity in rabbit hearts*

	Control	Diabetic
Myofibrillar ATPase activity (μmol Pi/mg/hr)		
Mg^{2+}-stimulated	1.80 ± 0.13	1.59 ± 0.18
Ca^{2+}-stimulated	8.18 ± 0.23	5.60 ± 0.46^a
Sarcoplasmic reticulum ATPase activity (μmol Pi/mg/5 min)		
Mg^{2+}-stimulated	6.6 ± 0.2	4.2 ± 0.3^a
Ca^{2+}-stimulated	0.81 ± 0.07	0.54 ± 0.05^a

[a]Significantly different from control; $p < 0.05$.

Values are means $\pm$ SE of 4 to 7 experiments. Diabetes was induced with alloxan (125 mg/kg; i.v.). Both myofibrils and SR were isolated from the control and diabetic hearts (12 weeks), and their activities determined.

TABLE 5. *Influence of diabetes on rabbit heart sarcolemmal enzymes*

	Control	Diabetic
Na^+-dependent Ca^{2+} uptake (nmol Ca^{2+}/mg/2 sec)	3.50 ± 0.56	$2.05 \pm 0.50^*$
Na^+-K^+ ATPase (μmol Pi/mg/hr)	9.8 ± 1.0	7.8 ± 0.93
ATP-dependent Ca^{2+} uptake (nmol Ca^{2+}/mg/5 min)	12.1 ± 2.0	9.9 ± 1.85
Ca^{2+}-stimulated ATPase (μm Ca^{2+}) (μmol Pi/mg/hr)	6.95 ± 1.0	5.45 ± 0.8
Mg^{2+}-stimulated ATPase (μmol Pi/mg/hr)	125 ± 10.5	131 ± 15.2

[a]Significantly different from control; $p < 0.05$.
Values are means $\pm$ SE of 4 to 6 experiments. Diabetes was induced by alloxan (125 mg/kg; i.v.), and the hearts were used 12 weeks later. The sarcolemmal vesicles were isolated and their Ca^{2+} uptake, and enzyme activities were determined.

in a stable, long-term diabetic state characterized by elevated plasma cholesterol and glucose levels and reduced plasma insulin levels. Our study is in agreement with others (16,39,120,131,169,170) with respect to changes in body weights and heart weights, as well as plasma alterations of glucose, insulin, and cholesterol. Bhimji et al. (39) reported that hyperglycemia alone did not significantly affect body weight of the diabetic animals. Hyperglycemia in the presence of hyperlipidemia, however, significantly decreased not only the body weight, but also the heart and left ventricular weights of diabetic animals. Bhimji et al. (16) also reported significant myocardial morphological damage in alloxan-induced diabetic rabbits. They observed myofibrillar disarrangement, mitochondrial damage, increased lipid droplets and glycogen granules, and dilated SR that contained varying degrees of electron-dense material. All of these ultrastructural alterations were quite evident by 10 weeks after alloxan administration.

Our results of depressed myofibrillar Ca^{2+}-stimulated ATPase and SR Ca^{2+}- and Mg^{2+}-stimulated ATPase are consistent with previously described hemodynamic correlates reported for this study with alloxan-diabetic rats and is in agreement with the study by Bhimji et al. (39) using alloxan-diabetic rabbits. They reported that hemodynamic parameters in anesthetized rabbits, such as left ventricular pressure, + dP/dt, and heart rate, were significantly depressed in diabetic rabbits at 10 weeks. In addition, in agreement with our study, depressions in SR-ATPase activity were observed, whereas sarcolemmal Na^+-K^+ ATPase was unchanged. Bhimji et al. (39), however, reported significant depression in myofibrillar Mg^{2+}-ATPase activity, whereas we did not observe any significant change; no reason at this time can be advanced for this observation.

In the study by Pollack et al. (170), no statistically significant difference was reported in actin-activated Mg^{2+}-ATPase activity. It is thought that small differences between experimental animals and heterogenous control groups might be missed at the low level of activities of this enzyme. Ca^{2+}-stimulated ATPase activity of the myofibrils was significantly depressed in the Pollack et al. study (170). Although we did not examine V_1, V_2, and V_3 composition in our rabbits, Pollack et al. reported significant elevations (90% to 95% V_3) in the percentage of V_3 in diabetic rabbit heart at 1, 3, and 6 months after alloxan administration. Our reported biochemical studies in myofibrils, SR, and depression in the Na^+-Ca^{2+} exchange not only are in agreement with the observed in vivo hemodynamic changes reported by Bhimji et al. (39), but also are in accord with the papillary muscle experiments conducted by Fein et al. (120) in the alloxan model of diabetes. In that study, they demonstrated marked differences in myocardial mechanics between chronically diabetic rabbits and normoglycemic controls. These changes included prolonged time to peak tension and one-half relaxation isometric contraction as well as prolonged time to peak shortening and diminished shortening velocity in isotonic contraction. Although the rate of contraction was slowed, duration of contraction was increased so that developed tension and peak shortening were generally unaltered in comparison with controls. The results of our studies with diabetic rabbits illustrate a common depression in myofibrillar Ca^{2+} ATPase and in SR-Ca^{2+} ATPase in diabetic rabbits as was found in diabetic rats. While we examined only subcellular activities at approximately 10 to 12 weeks, it is unclear in the rabbit (as we reported with the rat) which of the subcellular organelles displays the earliest biochemical defect. The exact molecular mechanism(s) responsible for the regulation of the Na^+-Ca^{2+} exchanger in normal rats and rabbits as well as in pathological states, such as diabetes, is not known. Because the activity of the Na^+-Ca^{2+} exchanger was depressed in both diabetic rats and rabbits, unlike the Ca^{2+} pump, it is thus possible that the Na^+-Ca^{2+} exchanger activity is the most sensitive Ca^{2+} transport protein to either hypoinsulinemic, hyperglycemic, or hyperlipidemic (or any combination of these) manifestations of the diabetic state.

It is also of note that thyroid hormone levels of the diabetic rabbits in the previously mentioned studies (39,170), unlike diabetic rats, were not significantly altered with respect to their age-matched controls. Thus, because thyroid hormone status has been shown to be important for myocardial function and cardiac subcellular enzymatic activities, and because this difference between rats and rabbits with respect to thyroid status in diabetes may not be important for Na^+-Ca^{2+} exchange activity in diabetic rabbit heart sarcolemma, future studies should examine Na^+-Ca^{2+} exchange regulation in more detail. In addition, other determinants of Ca^{2+} transport (i.e., Ca^{2+} channels) in relation to the Na^+-Ca^{2+} exchanger need further study. At this time, an explanation for lack of depression in the Ca^{2+} and Na^+ pump in the diabetic rabbit heart sarcolemma awaits further study. Taken together, however, our studies suggest a lack of Ca^{2+} handling (either Ca^{2+} overload/impairment in Ca^{2+} handling) in both the alloxan diabetic rat and rabbit.

SUMMARY

Although chronic diabetes has been shown to result in cardiomyopathy and contractile failure, the relationship between ultrastructural abnormalities and heart dysfunction is poorly understood. The cardiomyopathy in diabetes may or may not be associated with atherosclerosis, microangiopathy, or neuropathy. It is becoming evident that diabetic cardiomyopathy may be a consequence of Ca^{2+}-handling defects and subsequent occurrence of intracellular Ca^{2+} overload in the myocardial cell. By employing streptozotocin-induced and alloxan-induced diabetes in rats, various subcellular organelles, such as myofibrils SR and SL, have been shown to change their functions. These alterations do not seem to be limited to the rat model of diabetes, because Ca^{2+}-stimulated ATPase activities of myofibrils and SR as well as SL Na^+-Ca^{2+}-exchange activity in the heart were also found to be depressed in alloxan-induced diabetes in rabbits. It appears that the reduced ability of the diabetic heart to generate contractile force is due to depressed myofibrillar Ca^{2+}-stimulated ATPase activity, whereas the impaired ability of the diabetic heart to relax is due to a defect in SR Ca^{2+}-pump activity. Although cardiac defects in diabetes are due to insulin deficiency or ineffectiveness, the exact stimulus for heart dysfunction is far from understood. Recent work from our laboratory has suggested that promoting the oxidation of glucose or lowering the plasma lipids and their oxidation in the myocardium is beneficial in preventing diabetes-induced cardiac defects. Accordingly, it is proposed that therapy with lipid-lowering agents or verapamil in combination with insulin may prove useful in patients with uncontrolled diabetes.

ACKNOWLEDGMENTS

The work reported in this chapter was supported by grants from the Canadian Diabetes Association and the Racing Automobile Memorial Foundation, Tokyo.

REFERENCES

1. Pierce GN, Beamish RE, Dhalla NS. Dysfunction of the cardiovascular system during diabetes. In: *Heart dysfunction in diabetes*. Boca Raton, FL: CRC Press; 1988:51–71.
2. Rodrigues B, McNeill JH. The diabetic heart: metabolic causes for the development of a cardiomyopathy. *Cardiovasc Res* 1992;26:913–922.
3. Weiner J, Giacomelli F, Loud AV, Anversa P. Morphometry of cardiac hypertrophy induced by experimental renal hypertension. *Am J Cardiol* 1979;44:919–925.
4. Page E, McAllister LP. Quantitative electron-microscopic description of heart muscle cells: application to normal, hypertrophied and thyroxin-stimulated hearts. *Am J Cardiol* 1973;31:172–181.
5. Opie LH, ed. *The heart: physiology and metabolism*. 2nd ed. New York: Raven Press, 1989.
6. Singal PK, Dhalla NS. Morphological methods for studying heart membranes. In: Dhalla NS, ed. *Methods in studying cardiac membranes*. Vol. 2. Boca Raton, FL: CRC Press; 1984:3–16.
7. Severs NJ. Freeze-fracture cytochemical methods for studying the distribution of cholesterol in heart membranes. In: Dhalla NS, ed. *Methods in studying cardiac membranes*. Vol. 2. Boca Raton, FL: CRC Press; 1984:27–44.
8. Panagia V, Pierce GN, Michiel D, Dhalla NS. Methods for studying biochemical structure of heart membrane. In: Dhalla NS, ed. *Methods in studying cardiac membranes*. Vol. 2. Boca Raton, FL: CRC Press; 1984:45–58.
9. Benenson A, Mercel M, Heller M, Pinson A. Radioiodination techniques for localization of lipids and proteolipids in membranes: application to heart cells in cultures. In: Dhalla NS, ed. *Methods in studying cardiac membranes*. Vol. 2. Boca Raton, FL: CRC Press; 1984:59–82.
10. Frank JS. Application of freeze-fracture technique for studying heart cell membranes. In: Dhalla

NS, ed. *Methods in studying cardiac membranes.* Vol. 2. Boca Raton, FL: CRC Press; 1984:17–26.

11. Giacomelli F, Wiener J. Primary myocardial disease in the diabetic mouse: an ultrastructural study. *Lab Invest* 1979;40:460–473.
12. Thompson EW, Baker JC, Kamoss SA, Anderson WH. The severity of diabetes is a major determinant of myocardial damage in the rat. *Proc Soc Exp Biol Med* 1991;196:230–233.
13. Thompson EW. Structural manifestations of diabetic cardiomyopathy in the rat and its reversal by insulin treatment. *Am J Anat* 1988;182:270–282.
14. Jackson CV, McGrath GM, Tahiliani AG, Vadlamudi RVSV, McNeill JH. A functional and ultrastructural analysis of experimental diabetic rat myocardium: manifestation of a cardiomyopathy. *Diabetes* 1985;34:876–883.
15. Seager MJ, Singal PK, Orchard R, Pierce GN, Dhalla NS. Cardiac cell damage: a primary myocardial disease in streptozotocin-induced chronic diabetes. *Br J Exp Pathol* 1984;65:613–623.
16. Bhimji S, Godin DV, McNeill JH. Myocardial ultrastructural changes in alloxan-induced diabetes in rabbits. *Acta Anat* 1986;125:195–200.
17. Saito K, Nishi S, Kashima T, Tanaka H. Histologic and ultrastructural studies on the myocardium in spontaneously diabetic KK mice: a new animal model of cardiomyopathy. *Am J Cardiol* 1984;53:320–323.
18. Onishi S, Nunotani H, Fushimi H, Tochino Y. A pathomorphological study on the diabetogenic drug-induced heart disease in the rat. *J Mol Cell Cardiol* 1981;13[Suppl 2]:34.
19. Tarach JS. Histomorphological and ultrastructural studies of a rat myocardium in experimental conditions. *Z Mikrosk Anat Forsch* 1976;90:1145–1157.
20. Koltai MZ, Balogh I, Wagner M, Pogatsa G. Diabetic myocardial alterations in ultrastructure and function. *Exp Pathol* 1984;25:215–221.
21. Renila A, Akerblom HK. Ultrastructure of heart muscle in short-term diabetic rats: influence of insulin treatment. *Diabetologia* 1984;27:397–402.
22. McGrath GM, McNeill JH. Cardiac ultrastructural changes in streptozotocin-induced diabetic rats: effects of insulin treatment. *Can J Cardiol* 1986;2:164–169.
23. Pierce GN, Beamish RE, Dhalla NS. Ultrastructural abnormalities of the heart during diabetes. In: *Heart dysfunction in diabetes.* Boca Raton, FL: CRC Press; 1988:137–150.
24. Singal PK, Matsukubo MP, Dhalla NS. Calcium-related changes in the ultrastructure of mammalian myocardium. *Br J Exp Pathol* 1979;60:96–106.
25. Kuo TH, Moore KH, Giacomelli F, Weiner J. Defective oxidative metabolism of heart mitochondria from genetically diabetic mice. *Diabetes* 1983;32:781–787.
26. Senevirante BIB. Diabetic cardiomyopathy: the preclinical phase. *Br Med J* 1977;1:1444–1445.
27. Bakh S, Arena J, Lee W, et al. Arrhythmia susceptibility and myocardial composition in diabetes: influence of physical conditioning. *J Clin Invest* 1986;77:382–395.
28. Regan TJ, Ahmed SS, Levinson GE, et al. Cardiomyopathy and regional scar in diabetes mellitus. *Trans Assoc Am Phys* 1975;88:217–223.
29. Lebkova NP, Bondarenko MF, Kolesova OE, Azaryan GP. Ultrastructural manifestation of early metabolic disturbances in the myocardium of dogs with alloxan diabetes. *Bull Exp Biol Med (USSR)* 1980;89:684–687.
30. Orth DN, Morgan HE. The effect of insulin, alloxan, diabetes and anoxia on the ultrastruture of the rat heart. *J Cell Biol* 1962;15:509–523.
31. Fischer VW, Leskiw ML, Barner HB. Myocardial structure and capillary basal laminar thickness in experimentally diabetic rats. *Exp Mol Pathol* 1981;35:244–256.
32. Chen V, Ianuzzo CD, Fonz BC, Spitzer JJ. The effects of acute and chronic diabetes on myocardial metabolism in rats. *Diabetes* 1984;33:1078–1084.
33. Frank JS, Langer GA. The myocardial interstitium: its structure and its role in ionic exchange. *J Cell Biol* 1974;60:586–601.
34. Borg TK, Johnson LD, Lill PH. Specific attachment of collagen to cardiac myocytes: in vivo and in vitro. *Dev Biol* 1983;97:417–423.
35. Daniel EE, Grover AK, Kwan CY. Calcium. In: Stephens NL, ed. *Biochemistry of smooth muscle.* Vol. 3. Boca Raton, FL: CRC Press; 1983:1.
36. Leung DYM, Glagov S, Mathews MB. A new in vitro system for studying cell response to mechanical stimulation. *Exp Cell Res* 1977;109:285–298.
37. Regan TJ, Ettinger PO, Kahn MI, et al. Altered myocardial function and metabolism in chronic diabetes mellitus without ischemia in dogs. *Circ Res* 1974;35:222–237.

38. Regan TJ, Wu CF, Yeh CK, Oldewurtel HA, Haider B. Myocardial composition and function in diabetes: the effects of chronic insulin use. *Circ Res* 1981;49:1268–1277.
39. Bhimji S, Godin DV, McNeill JH. Biochemical and functional changes in hearts from rabbits with diabetes. *Diabetologia* 1985;28:452–457.
40. Regan TJ. Congestive heart failure in the diabetic. *Annu Rev Med* 1983;34:161–168.
41. Factor SM, Minase T, Bhan R, Wolinsky H, Sonnenblick EH. Hypertensive diabetic cardiomyopathy in the rat: ultrastructural features. *Virchows Arch* 1983;398:305–317.
42. Factor SM, Bhan R, Minase T, Wolinsky H, Sonnenblick EH. Hypertensive-diabetic cardiomyopathy in the rat: an experimental model of human disease. *Am J Pathol* 1981;102:219–228.
43. Factor SM, Minase T, Sonnenblick EH. Clinical and morphological features of human hypertensive-diabetic cardiomyopathy. *Am Heart J* 1980;74:446–458.
44. Christlieb AR. Diabetes and hypertensive vascular disease. *Am J Cardiol* 1973;32:592–606.
45. Fluckiger W, Perrin IV, Rossi GL. Morphometric studies on retinal microangiopathy and myocardiopathy in hypertensive rats (SHR) with induced diabetes. *Virchows Arch [B]* 1984;47:79–85.
46. McGrath GM, McNeill JH. Cardiac ultrastructural changes in streptozotocin-induced diabetic rats: effects of insulin treatment. *Can J Cardiol* 1986;2:164–169.
47. Resnecov L. Endocrine disease and the cardiovascular system in cardiology. In: Chatterjee K, Cheitlim MD, Karliner J, Parmley WW, Rapaport E, Scheiman M, eds. *Cardiology*. Philadelphia: JB Lippincott; 1991:1382–1384.
48. Regan TS, Haider B, Lyons MM. Altered ventricular function and metabolism in diabetes mellitus. In: Zoneraich S, ed. *Diabetes and the heart*. Springfield, IL: Charles C. Thomas; 1978:133.
49. Factor SM, Okun EM, Minase T. Capillary microaneurysms in the human diabetic heart. *N Engl J Med* 1980;302:384–388.
50. Silver MD, Huckell VS, Lorber M. Basement membranes of small cardiac vessels in patients with diabetes and myxoedema: preliminary observations. *Pathology* 1977;9:213–220.
51. Fischer VW, Barner HB, Leskiw L. Capillary basal laminar thickness in diabetic human myocardium. *Diabetes* 1979;28:713–719.
52. Shirley EK, Proudfit WL, Hawk WA. Primary myocardial disease. Correlation with clinical findings, angiography and biopsy diagnosis: follow-up of 139 patients. *Am Heart J* 1980;99:198–207.
53. Ledet T. Diabetic cardiomyopathy: quantitative histological studies of the heart from young juvenile diabetics. *Acta Pathol Microbiol Scand* 1976;84:421–428.
54. Zoneraich S, Mollura JL. Diabetes and the heart: state of the art in the 1990s. *Can J Cardiol* 1993;9:293–299.
55. Zoneraich S, Silverman G. Myocardial small vessel disease in diabetic patients. In: Zoneraich S, ed. *Diabetes and the heart*. Springfield, IL: Charles C. Thomas; 1978:3–18.
56. Williamson JR, Kilo C. Capillary basement membranes in diabetes. *Diabetes* 1983;32:96–100.
57. Tilton RG, Hoffman PL, Kilo C, Williamson JR. Pericyte degeneration and basement membrane thickening in skeletal muscle capillaries of human diabetics. *Diabetes* 1981;30:326–334.
58. Viberti GC. Increased capillary permeability in diabetes mellitus and its relationship to microvascular angiopathy. *Am J Med* 1983;75:81–84.
59. Kannel WB, Hjortland M, Castelli WP. Role of diabetes in congestive heart failure: the Framingham study. *Am J Cardiol* 1974;34:29–34.
60. Rubler S, Dlugash J, Yuceoglu YZ, Kumral T, Branwood AW, Grishman A. New type of cardiomyopathy associated with diabetic glomerulosis. *Am J Cardiol* 1972;30:595–602.
61. Sanderson JE, Brown DJ, Rivellese A, Kohner E. Diabetic cardiomyopathy. An echocardiography study of young diabetics. *Br Med J* 1978;1:404–407.
62. Shah S. Cardiomyopathy in diabetes mellitus. *Angiology* 1980;31:502–504.
63. Yamaji T, Fukuhara T, Kinoshita M. Increased capillary permeability to albumin in diabetic rat myocardium. *Circ Res* 1993;72:947–957.
64. Lane GA, Allen SJ. Left ventricular myocardial edema: lymph flow, interstitial fibrosis, and cardiac function. *Circ Res* 1991;68:1713–1721.
65. Regan TJ, Lyons MM, Ahmed SS, et al. Evidence for cardiomyopathy in familial diabetes mellitus. *J Clin Invest* 1977;60:885–899.
66. Fein FS, Sonnenblick EH. Diabetic cardiomyopathy. *Prog Cardiovasc Dis* 1985;27:255–270.
67. van Hoeven KH, Factor SM. A comparison of the pathological spectrum of hypertensive, diabetic and hypertensive-diabetic heart disease. *Circulation* 1990;82:848–855.
68. Brownlee M, Cerami A, Vlassara H. Advanced glycosylation end products in tissue and the biochemical basis of diabetic complications. *N Engl J Med* 1988;318:1315–1321.

69. Rubler S, Sajadi MRM, Araoye MA, Holford MD. Noninvasive estimation of myocardial performance in patients with diabetes. *Diabetes* 1978;27:127–134.
70. Raev DC. Which left ventricular function is impaired earlier in the evolution of diabetic cardiomyopathy? An echocardiographic study of young type I diabetic patients. *Diabetes Care* 1994;17: 633–639.
71. Flugelman MY, Kanter Y, Abinaer EG, Lewis BS, Barzilai D. Electrocardiographic patterns in diabetics without clinical ischemic heart disease. *Isr Med Sci* 1983;19:252–258.
72. Airaksinen KEJ. Electrocardiogram of young diabetic subjects. *Ann Clin Res* 1985;17:135–140.
73. Rubler S, Chuy DA, Bruzzone CL. Blood pressure and heart rate responses during 24-hour ambulatory monitoring and exercise in men with diabetes mellitus. *Am J Cardiol* 1985;55:801–806.
74. Abenavoli T, Rubler S, Fisher VJ, Axelrod H, Zuckerman KP. Exercise testing with myocardial scintigraphy in asymptomatic diabetic males. *Circulation* 1981;63:54–64.
75. Goldenberg S, Alex M, Blumenthal HT. Sequelae of arteriosclerosis of the aorta and coronary arteries. *Diabetes* 1958;7:98–108.
76. Shapiro LM, Howat AP, Calter MM. Left ventricular function in diabetes mellitus. I. Methodology and prevalence and spectrum of abnormalities. *Br Heart J* 1981;45:122–128.
77. Olsen EGJ. The pathology of cardiomyopathies: a critical analysis. *Am Heart J* 1979;98:385–394.
78. Fein FS. Diabetic cardiomyopathy. *Diabetes Care* 1990;13:1169–1179.
79. Ahmed SS, Levinson GE, Schwartz CJ, Ettinger PO. Systolic time intervals as measure of the contractile state of the left ventricular myocardium in man. *Circulation* 1970;46:559–565.
80. Garrard CL, Weissler AM, Dodge HT. The relationship of alterations in systolic time intervals to ejection fraction in patients with cardiac disease. *Circulation* 1970;42:455–462.
81. Weissler AM, Harris WS, Schoenfeld CD. Bedside techniques for the evaluation of ventricular function in man. *Am J Cardiol* 1969;23:577–583.
82. Jermendy G, Koltai MZ, Kammerer L, et al. Myocardial systolic alterations of insulin-dependent diabetics in rest. *Acta Cardiol* 1984;39:185–192.
83. Zoneraich S, Zoneraich O, Rhee JJ. Left ventricular performance in diabetic patients without clinical heart disease: evaluation by systolic time intervals and echocardiography. *Chest* 1977;72:748–751.
84. Shapiro LM, Leatherdale BA, Mackinnon J, Fletcher RF. Left ventricular function in diabetes mellitus. II. Relation between clinical features and left ventricular function. *Br Heart J* 1981;45: 129–132.
85. Shapiro LM, Leatherdale BA, Coyne ME, Fletcher RF, Mackinnon J. Prospective study of heart disease in untreated maturity onset diabetics. *Br Heart J* 1980;44:342–348.
86. Uusitupa M, Siitonen O, Aro A, Korhonen T, Pyorala K. Effect of correction of hyperglycemia on left ventricular function in non–insulin-dependent (type 2) diabetics. *Acta Med Scand* 1983;213: 363–368.
87. Zarich SW, Arbuckle BE, Cohen LR, Roberts M, Nesto RW. Diastolic abnormalities in young asymptomatic diabetic patients assessed by pulsed Doppler echocardiography. *J Am Coll Cardiol* 1988;12:114–120.
88. Rokey R, Kuo LC, Zoghbi WA, Limacher MC, Quinones MM. Determination of left ventricular diastolic filling with pulsed Doppler echocardiography: comparison with cineangiography. *Circulation* 1985;71:543–550.
89. Friedman BJ, Brinkovic N, Miles H, Shih WJ, Mazzoleni A, DeMaria AN. Assessment of left ventricular diastolic function: comparison of Doppler echocardiography and gated blood pool scintigraphy. *J Am Coll Cardiol* 1986;8:1348–1354.
90. Spirito P, Marion BJ, Bonow RO. Noninvasive assessment of left ventricular diastolic function: comparative analysis of Doppler echocardiography and radionuclide angiographic techniques. *J Am Coll Cardiol* 1986;7:518–526.
91. Nagano M, Dhalla NS, eds. *The diabetic heart*. New York: Raven Press, 1991.
92. Friedman NE, Levitsky LL, Vitullo DA, Lacina SJ, Chiemmongkoltip P. Echocardiographic evidence for impaired myocardial performance in children with type I diabetes mellitus. *Am J Med* 1982;73:846–850.
93. Gregor P, Widimsky P, Rostlapil J, Cervenka V, Visek V. Echocardiographic picture in diabetes mellitus. *Jpn Heart J* 1984;25:969–974.
94. Goldweit RS, Borer JS, Jovanovic LG, et al. Relation of hemoglobin A1 and blood to cardiac function in diabetes mellitus. *Am J Cardiol* 1985;56:642–650.
95. Mildenberger RR, Bar-Shlomo B, Druck MN, et al. Clinically unrecognized ventricular dysfunction in young diabetic patients. *J Am Coll Cardiol* 1984;4:234–238.

96. Vered Z, Battler A, Segal P, et al. Exercise-induced left ventricular dysfunction in young men with asymptomatic diabetes mellitus (diabetic cardiomyopathy). *Am J Cardiol* 1984;54:633–637.

97. Nicod P, Lewis SE, Corbett JC, et al. Increased incidence and clinical correlation of persistently abnormal technetium pyrophosphate myocardial scintigrams following acute myocardial infarction in patients with diabetes mellitus. *Am Heart J* 1982;103:822–829.

98. Harrower ADB, McFarlane G, Parekh P, Young K, Railton R. Cardiac function during stress testing in long-standing insulin-dependent diabetics. *Acta Diabetol Lat* 1983;20:179–183.

99. D'Elia JA, Weinrauch LA, Healy RW, Libertino RW, Bradley RF, Leland OS. Myocardial dysfunction without coronary artery disease in diabetic renal failure. *Am J Cardiol* 1979;43:193–199.

100. Hamby RI, Zoneraich S, Sherman L. Diabetic cardiomyopathy. *JAMA* 1974;229:1749–1754.

101. Ruddy TD, Shumak SL, Liu PP, et al. The relationship of cardiac diastolic dysfunction to concurrent hormonal and metabolic status in type I diabetes mellitus. *J Clin Endocrinol Metab* 1988;66: 113–118.

102. Soufer RA, Wohlgelanter DH, Vita NH. Intact systolic left ventricular function in clinical congestive heart failure. *Am J Cardiol* 1985;55:1032–1036.

103. Fouad-Tarazi FM. Ventricular diastolic function of the heart in systemic hypertension. *Am J Cardiol* 1990;65:85G–88G.

104. Aroesty JM, McKay RG, Heller GV, Royal HD, Als AV, Grossman W. Simultaneous assessment of left ventricular systolic and diastolic dysfunction during pacing-induced ischemia. *Circulation* 1985;71:889–900.

105. Airaksinen J, Ikaheimo M, Kaila J, Linnaluoto M, Takkunen J. Impaired left ventricular filling in young female diabetics. *Acta Med Scand* 1984;216:509–516.

106. Uusitupa M, Mustonen J, Laasko M, et al. Impairment of diastolic function in middle-aged type I (insulin-dependent) and type II (non–insulin-dependent) diabetic patients free of cardiovascular disease. *Diabetologia* 1988;31:783–791.

107. Raev D. Evolution of cardiac changes in young insulin-dependent (type I) diabetic patients: one more piece of the puzzle of diabetic cardiomyopathy. *Clin Cardiol* 1993;16:784–790.

108. Attali JR, Sachs RN, Valensi P, et al. Asymptomatic diabetic cardiomyopathy: a noninvasive study. *Diabetes Res Clin Pract* 1988;4:183–190.

109. Shapiro LM. Diabetes-induced heart muscle disease and left ventricular dysfunction. *Pract Cardiol* 1985;11:79–91.

110. Kannel WB, McGee DL. Diabetes and cardiovascular disease. *JAMA* 1979;241:2035–2038.

111. Penpargkul S, Schaible T, Yipintsoi T, Scheuer J. The effect of diabetes on performance and metabolism of rat hearts. *Circ Res* 1980;47:911–921.

112. Fein FS, Kornstein LB, Strobeck JE, Capasso JM, Sonnenblick EH. Altered myocardial mechanics in diabetic rats. *Circ Res* 1980;47:922–933.

113. Vadlamudi RVSV, Rodgers RL, McNeill JH. The effect of chronic alloxan- and streptozotocin-induced diabetes on isolated rat heart performance. *Can J Physiol Pharmacol* 1982;60:902–911.

114. Miller TB. Cardiac performance of isolated perfused hearts from alloxan diabetic rats. *Am J Physiol* 1979;236:H808–H812.

115. Ganguly PK, Pierce GN, Dhalla KS, Dhalla NS. Defective sarcoplasmic reticulum calcium transport in diabetic cardiomyopathy. *Am J Physiol* 1983;244:E528–E535.

116. Bielefeld DR, Pace CS, Boshell BR. Altered sensitivity of chronic diabetic rat heart to calcium. *Am J Physiol* 1983;245:E560–E567.

117. Ramanadham S, Tenner TE. Alterations in cardiac performance in experimentally-induced diabetes. *Pharmacology* 1983;27:130–136.

118. Schaffer SW, Tan BH, Wilson GL. Development of a cardiomyopathy in a model of non–insulin-dependent diabetes. *Am J Physiol* 1985;248:H179–H185.

119. Tan BH, Wilson GL, Schaffer SW. Effect of tolbutamide on myocardial metabolism and mechanical performance of the diabetic rat. *Diabetes* 1984;33:1138–1145.

120. Fein FS, Miller-Green B, Sonnenblick EH. Altered myocardial mechanics in diabetic rabbits. *Am J Physiol* 1985;248:H729–H736.

121. Heyliger CE, Pierce GN, Singal PK, Beamish RE, Dhalla NS. Cardiac alpha- and beta-adrenergic receptor alterations in diabetic cardiomyopathy. *Basic Res Cardiol* 1982;77:610–618.

122. Afzal N, Ganguly PK, Dhalla KS, Pierce GN, Singal PK, Dhalla NS. Beneficial effects of verapamil in diabetic cardiomyopathy. *Diabetes* 1988;37:936–942.

123. Haider B, Ahmed SS, Moschos CB, Oldewurtel HA, Regan TJ. Myocardial function and coronary blood flow response to acute ischemia in chronic canine diabetes. *Circ Res* 1977;40:577–583.

124. Ku DD, Sellers BM. Effects of streptozotocin diabetes and insulin treatment on myocardial sodium pump and contractility of the rat heart. *J Pharmacol Exp Ther* 1982;222:395–400.
125. Ingebretsen CG, Moreau P, Hawelu-Johnson C, Ingebretsen WR. Performance of diabetic rat hearts: effects of anoxia and increased work. *Am J Physiol* 1980;239:H614–H620.
126. Strobek JE, Factor SM, Bhan A, et al. Hereditary and acquired cardiomyopathies in experimental animals: mechanical, biochemical and structural features. *Ann NY Acad Sci* 1979;317:59–88.
127. Tahliani AG, Vadlamudi RVSV, McNeill JH. Prevention and reversal of altered myocardial function in diabetic rats by insulin treatment. *Can J Physiol Pharmacol* 1983;61:516–523.
128. Doursout M-F, Kashimoto S, Chelly JE. Cardiac function in the diabetic concious rat. In: Nagano M, Dhalla NS, eds. *The diabetic heart*. New York: Raven Press; 1991:11–19.
129. Dhalla NS, Pierce GN, Innes IR, Beamish RE. Pathogenesis of cardiac dysfunction in diabetes mellitus. *Can J Cardiol* 1985;1:263–281.
130. Pierce GN, Dhalla NS. The association of membrane alterations with heart dysfunction during experimental diabetes mellitus. In: Dhalla NS, Singal PK, Beamish RE, eds. *Pathophysiology of heart disease*. Boston: Martinus Nijhoff; 1987:177.
131. Bhimji S, Godin DV, McNeill JH. Coronary artery ligation and reperfusion in rabbits made diabetic with alloxan. *J Endocrinol* 1987;112:43–49.
132. Malhotra A, Mordes JP, McDermot L, Schaible TF. Abnormal cardiac biochemistry in spontaneously diabetic Bio-Breeding/Worcester rat. *Am J Physiol* 1985;249:H1051–H1055.
133. Spiro MJ, Kumar BRR, Crowley TJ. Myocardial glycoproteins in diabetes: type VI collagen is a major PAS-reactive extracellular matrix protein. *J Mol Cell Cardiol* 1992;24:397–410.
134. Fein FS, Aronson RS, Nordin C, Miller-Green B, Sonnenblick EH. Altered myocardial response to ouabain in diabetic rats: mechanics and electrophysiology. *J Mol Cell Cardiol* 1983;15:769–776.
135. Gutgesell HP, Speer ME, Rosenberg HS. Characterization of the cardiomyopathy in infants of diabetic mothers. *Circulation* 1980;61:441–450.
136. Nakanishi T, Matsuoka S, Uemura S, et al. Myocardial excitation-contraction coupling in the fetus of alloxan-diabetic rabbit. *Pediatr Res* 1984;18:1344–1350.
137. Pierce GN, Kutryk MJB, Dhalla NS. Alterations in calcium binding and composition of the cardiac sarcolemmal membrane in chronic diabetes. *Proc Natl Acad Sci USA* 1983;80:5412–5416.
138. Fein FS, Strobeck JE, Malhotra A, Scheuer J, Sonnenblick EH. Reversibility of diabetic cardiomyopathy with insulin in rats. *Circ Res* 1981;49:1251–1261.
139. Fein FS, Malhotra A, Miller-Green B, Scheuer J, Sonnenblick EH. Diabetic cardiomyopathy in rats: mechanical and biochemical response to different insulin doses. *Am J Physiol* 1984;247:H817–H823.
140. Rubinstein M, Schaible TF, Malhotra A, Scheuer J. Effects of graded insulin therapy on cardiac function in diabetic rats. *Am J Physiol* 1984;246:H453–H458.
141. Schaible TF, Malhotra A, Bauman WA, Scheuer J. Left ventricular function after chronic insulin treatment in diabetic and normal rats. *J Mol Cell Cardiol* 1983;15:445–458.
142. Lucchesi BR, Medina M, Kniffen FJ. The positive inotropic action of insulin in the canine heart. *Eur J Pharmacol* 1972;18:107–115.
143. Pogatsa G, Bihari-Varga M, Szinay G. Effect of diabetes therapy on the myocardium in experimental diabetes. *Acta Diabetol Lat* 1979;16:129–138.
144. Kramer JH, Lampson WG, Schaffer SW. Effect of tolbutamide on myocardial energy metabolism. *Am J Physiol* 1983;245:H313–H319.
145. Tamura S, Brown TA, Whipple JH, et al. A novel mechanism for the insulin-like effect of vanadate on glycogen synthase in rat adipocytes. *J Biol Chem* 1984;259:6650–6658.
146. Heyliger CE, Tahiliani AG, McNeill JH. Effect of vanadate on elevated blood glucose and depressed cardiac performance of diabetic rats. *Science* 1985;227:1474–1477.
147. Yuen VG, Orvig C, Thompson KH, McNeill JH. Improvement in cardiac dysfunction in streptozotocin-induced diabetic rats following chronic oral administration of bis(maltolato) oxovanadium (IV). *Can J Physiol Pharmacol* 1993;71:270–276.
148. Tahiliani AG, McNeill JH. Lack of effect of thyroid hormone on diabetic rat heart function and biochemistry. *Can J Physiol Pharmacol* 1984;62:617–621.
149. Dillmann WH. Influence of thyroid hormone administration on myosin ATPase activity and myosin isoenzyme distribution in the heart of diabetic rats. *Metabolism* 1982;31:199–204.
150. Saunders J, Hall SEH, Sonksen PH. Thyroid hormones in insulin requiring diabetes before and after treatment. *Diabetologia* 1978;15:29–35.

151. Hall R, Scanbon MF. Hypothyroidism: clinical features and complications. *Clin Endocrinol Metab* 1979;8:29–34.
152. McAllister A, Allison SP, Randle PJ. Effects of dichloroacetate on the metabolism of glucose, pyruvate, acetate, 3-hydroxybutyrate and palmitate in rat diaphragm and heart muscle in vitro and on extraction of glucose, lactate, pyruvate and free fatty acids by dog heart in vivo. *Biochem J* 1973;13:1067–1081.
153. Stacpoole PW. Review of the pharmacologic and therapeutic effects of diisopropyl-ammonium dichloroacetate (DIPA). *J Clin Pharmacol* 1969;9:282–291.
154. Nicholl TA, Lopaschuk GD, McNeill JH. Effects of free fatty acids and dichloroacetate on isolating working diabetic rat heart. *Am J Physiol* 1991;261:H1053–H1059.
155. Rupp H, Elimban V, Dhalla NS. Modification of myosin isozymes and SR Ca^{2+}-pump ATPase of the diabetic rat heart by lipid-lowering interventions. *Mol Cell Biochem* 1994;132:69–80.
156. Rodrigues B, Goyal RK, McNeill JH. Effects of hydralazine on streptozotocin-induced diabetic rats: prevention of hyperlipidemia and improvement in cardiac function. *J Pharmacol Exp Ther* 1986;237:292–299.
157. Pierce GN, Dhalla NS. Mechanisms of the defect in cardiac myofibrillar function during diabetes. *Am J Physiol* 1985;248:E170–E175.
158. Penpargkul S, Fein F, Sonnenblick EH, Scheuer J. Depressed sarcoplasmic reticular function for diabetic rats. *J Mol Cell Cardiol* 1981;13:303–309.
159. Lopaschuk GD, Katz S, McNeill JH. The effect of alloxan- and streptozotocin-induced diabetes on calcium transport in rat cardiac sarcoplasmic reticulum. The possible involvement of long chain acyl-carnitines. *Can J Physiol Pharmacol* 1983;61:439–448.
160. Lopaschuk GD, Tahiliani AG, Vadlamudi RVSV, Katz S, McNeill JH. Cardiac sarcoplasmic reticulum function in insulin- or carnitine-treated diabetic rats. *Am J Physiol* 1984;245:H969–H976.
161. Heyliger CE, Prakash A, McNeill JH. Alterations in cardiac sarcolemmal Ca^{2+} pump activity during diabetes mellitus. *Am J Physiol* 1987;252:H540–H544.
162. Makino N, Dhalla KS, Elimban V, Dhalla NS. Sarcolemmal Ca^{2+} transport in streptozotocin-induced diabetic cardiomyopathy in rats. *Am J Physiol* 1987;253:E202–E207.
163. Pierce GN, Ramjiawan B, Dhalla NS, Ferrari R. Na^+-H^+ exchange in cardiac sarcolemmal vesicles isolated from diabetic rats. *Am J Physiol* 1990;258:H255–H261.
164. Malhotra A, Penpargkul S, Fein FS, Sonnenblick EH, Scheuer J. The effect of streptozotocin-induced diabetes in rats on cardiac contractile proteins. *Circ Res* 1981;49:1243–1250.
165. Pierce GN, Dhalla NS. Cardiac myofibrillar ATPase activity in diabetic rats. *J Mol Cell Cardiol* 1981;13:1063–1069.
166. Afzal N, Pierce GN, Elimban V, Beamish RE, Dhalla NS. Influence of verapamil on some subcellular defects in diabetic cardiomyopathy. *Am J Physiol* 1989;256:E453–E458.
167. Bailey CC, Bailey OT, Leech RS. Alloxan diabetes with diabetic complications. *N Engl J Med* 1944;230:533–536.
168. Zhao Z-H, Watschinger B, Brown CD, Beyer MM, Friedman EA. Variations of susceptiblity to alloxan induced diabetes in the rabbit. *Horm Metab Res* 1987;19:534–537.
169. Fein FS, Miller-Green B, Zola B, Sonnenblick EH. Reversibility of diabetic cardiomyopathy with insulin in rabbits. *Am J Physiol* 1986;250;H108–H113.
170. Pollack PS, Malhotra A, Fein FS, Scheuer J. Effects of diabetes on cardiac contractile proteins in rabbits and reversal with insulin. *Am J Physiol* 1986;251:H448–H454.

The Failing Heart, edited by N. S. Dhalla,
R. E. Beamish, N. Takeda, and M. Nagano.
Lippincott-Raven Publishers, Philadelphia © 1995.

13

Structural Remodeling of the Myocardium in Ischemic and Hypertensive Heart Disease

Karl T. Weber, Yao Sun, *Anna Ratajska,
†Jack P.M. Cleutjens, and Suresh C. Tyagi

*Department of Medicine, Division of Cardiology, University of Missouri Health Sciences Center,
Columbia, Missouri 65212 United States; *Department of Anatomy, University of Iowa,
Iowa City, Iowa 52242 United States; and †Department of Pathology, Cardiovascular
Research Center Maastricht, University of Limburg, Maastricht, 6200 MD The Netherlands*

The fact that heart failure is a major health problem of ever-increasing proportions is recognized worldwide. Major etiologic factors responsible for ventricular diastolic and/or systolic dysfunction that eventuate in symptomatic heart failure include ischemic heart disease (IHD), with previous myocardial infarction (MI), and hypertensive heart disease (HHD) (1). A progressive downhill clinical course, punctuated by recurrent episodes of symptomatic failure that often require hospitalization, is characteristic and shortens survival (2). Insights into the progressive nature of heart failure are urgently needed.

What contributes to the progressive nature of heart failure? Answers will likely be multifactorial. From our perspective, they include the heart and renin-angiotensin-aldosterone system (RAAS) and sympathetic nervous system (SNS). Survival, for example, is inversely correlated with the degree of circulating neurohormonal activation (3,4). Moreover, circulating effector hormones of the RAAS and SNS promote a remodeling of myocardial microscopic structure that ultimately impairs its diastolic and systolic ventricular function (5,6). Emerging experimental evidence further implicates locally generated peptides, including angiotensin II (AngII), as contributory to the remodeling process (7–9). Herein, we consider the progressive structural remodeling of the myocardium that appears in IHD and HHD and the role of hormonal factors that contribute to the remodeling of myocyte and nonmyocyte compartments of the myocardium. These include (a) chronic, inappropriate (relative to dietary sodium intake and intravascular volume) elevations in *circulating* AngII and aldosterone (ALDO), as well as catecholamines; and (b) *locally generated* AngII, endothelins, bradykinin (BK), and prostaglandins. It is our overall hypothesis that the ongoing structural remodeling of the myocardium is a major determinant of the progressive nature of heart failure.

STRUCTURAL REMODELING IN ISCHEMIC HEART DISEASE

Cardiac myocyte necrosis follows a critical reduction in nutrient coronary blood flow. Individual myocytes or an entire population of myocytes contained within a segment of myocardium can be affected, depending on the extent to which coronary flow has been compromised. Impending cell death is heralded by a hyperpermeable plasmalemma membrane (10) that permits large macromolecules to gain entry into injured myocytes. In the rat, immunofluorescent labeling of myocytes with an antibody to plasma fibronectin or the contractile protein myosin has been used as a sensitive, early marker of myocyte necrosis following coronary artery ligation (11) or subsequent to the administration of a catecholamine (12) or AngII (13,14). Following myocyte necrosis, a complex wound-healing response appears and includes exudative, inflammatory, and subsequent fibrogenic phases.

Healing following Myocardial Infarction

Infarct Site

Chemical mediators of inflammation (e.g., BK and prostaglandins) and cytokines (e.g., platelet-derived growth factor and interleukins) orchestrate exudative and inflammatory phases that prevail during days 1 to 4 post-MI. Polymorphonuclear leukocytes and subsequently macrophages are the predominant inflammatory cells involved in this stage of tissue repair. The involvement of fibroblasts and fibroblast-like cells (or myofibroblasts) follows; their transcription and synthesis of fibrillar types I and III collagens account for the appearance of scar tissue at the site of necrosis. Morphologic evidence of scarring is first evident by day 7 (15–17). A progressive rise in tissue collagen concentration, expressed biochemically by its hydroxyproline concentration (18) or morphometrically as its collagen volume fraction (17), follows over the course of 6 to 8 weeks. Type I collagen ultimately predominates (19) and accounts for this reparative fibrosis that restores the structural integrity of infarcted tissue. During weeks 6 to 8, scar tissue undergoes its own transformation, including retraction and thinning (18).

Collagen degradation is also an early component of tissue repair. Matrix metalloproteinases (MMP) reside in the myocardium in a latent or inactive form (20,21). Cellular production of MMP-1 is not needed to initiate collagen degradation. Once activated, MMP-1 (or interstitial collagenase) will degrade fibrillar collagen into characteristic one- and three-quarter fragments; MMP-2 and MMP-9 are gelatinases that degrade these smaller fragments. A transient increase in collagenase activity appears in the infarcted left ventricle on day 2, peaks at day 7, and declines thereafter, together with a concomitant increase and contribution in collagenolytic activity of gelatinases (22). This collagenase activity comes from the latent pool because an increase in collagenase (MMP-1) mRNA expression does not appear until day 7 in the infarcted ventricle. Changes in MMP-1 activity or mRNA expression are not observed at sites remote to the infarct. Tissue inhibitors (TIMPs) neutralize collagenolytic activity. Transcription of TIMP mRNA occurs at 6 hours in the infarcted ventricle, peaks on day 2, and slowly declines thereafter (22). No change in TIMP mRNA expression is observed at remote sites. Fibroblast-like cells are responsible for the transcription of MMP-1 and TIMP mRNAs.

Hence, at the site of infarction, posttranslational activation of latent collagenase (MMP-1) plays a dominant role in tissue repair. Transcription of collagenase mRNA occurs when latent extracellular MMP-1 is reduced through the activation of the latent pool of collagenase and gelatinases. In turn, TIMP mRNA synthesis is regulated by the activation of MMPs. The balance between collagenase activation and TIMP inhibition therefore determines collagenolysis in infarcted tissue. Fibroblasts and/or fibroblast-like cells, and their synthesis and degradation of collagen, are essential to fibrogenesis and subsequent remodeling of fibrous tissue.

These various events, which occur at the tissue level, could influence ventricular chamber architecture and geometry. Within several days after MI, a slippage of cardiac myocytes has been observed in association with ventricular dilatation (23). This architectural remodeling of the myocardium is temporally coincident with the activation of collagenase that appears postinfarction (22). Fibrillar collagen degradation has been proposed as the anatomic requisite for myocyte slippage (24). Left ventricular (LV) chamber dilatation is progressive over the course of 6 weeks (18) and is associated with a thinning of the ventricular wall; scar thinning is also evident at 6 weeks.

Remote Sites

Following a loss of myocytes to MI, remaining cells will hypertrophy as their loading conditions are increased. This occurs in the infarcted left ventricle (25), particularly involving cells that border on the site of necrosis (26). Right ventricular myocytes may hypertrophy as well (25), provided there is increased pulmonary venous pressure.

Fibrous tissue not only appears at the site of MI, but at remote sites as well (Fig. 1). In the interventricular septum this includes endocardial fibrosis (17,27); in the right ventricle and septum, microscopic scars and perivascular/interstitial fibrosis are found (16,17,28). Fibrosis of the visceral pericardium involving the infarcted ventricle may also appear (17).

Chronic Ischemic Heart Disease

Remodeling of the failing, explanted human myocardium, due to previous MI, has been studied extensively by Beltrami et al. (29). In these hearts obtained from patients with advanced, chronic symptomatic heart failure due to IHD, and in whom activation of the RAAS would be expected (3,30), there was evidence of both LV and right ventricular hypertrophy. Evidence of hypertrophy was present by tissue

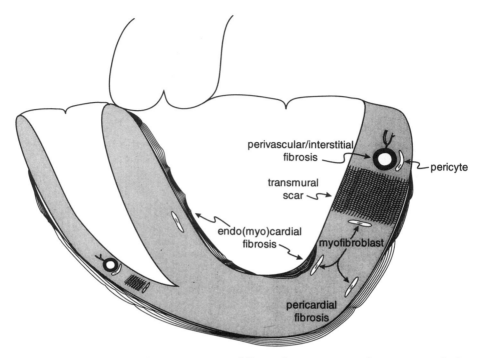

FIG. 1. Composite view of multiple patterns of fibrous tissue responses that can appear in the myocardium of both ventricles either postinfarction or in hypertensive heart disease. Cells thought to be involved are also represented.

weight, aggregate myocyte mass, and myocyte cell volume per nucleus (29). Myocyte loss was responsible for the difference in the extent of hypertrophy assessed at the organ, tissue, and cellular levels. In explanted human hearts, specific changes in cardiac myocyte geometry have been observed in association with their growth, or hypertrophy (29,31). This consists primarily of an increase in myocyte length (vis-à-vis cell diameter). Such lengthening of myocytes, together with a reduction in the number of myocytes per ventricular wall thickness, is consistent with myocyte slippage. In both ventricles, fibrosis was evident as segmental and microscopic scarring and as a perivascular/interstitial fibrosis. This collective remodeling process accounted for an increase in LV chamber volume and reduction in mass to volume ratio.

The mechanisms responsible for the architectural and geometric remodeling of the myocardium and ventricular chamber in IHD are not fully understood. Collagenolytic activity in the dilated failing human heart due to previous MI has been examined and compared with normal human cardiac tissue (32). Tissue homogenates were prepared from normal tissue and from infarcted and noninfarcted tissue collected from the endo- and epimyocardium of the infarcted LV and noninvolved right ventricle at the time of cardiac transplantation. Sodium dodecyl sulfate poly-acrylamide gel electrophoresis (SDS-PAGE) was used to determine total protein concentration, while collagenolytic activity was measured by zymography. After normalization for total protein concentration, collagenolytic activity in normal tissue was found to be 3% and could be activated to 80% to 90% by trypsin or plasmin, indicating that collagenase is normally inactive. By contrast, in endo- and epimyocardium of infarcted tissue, collagenolytic activity was increased significantly. This was also the case in noninfarcted tissue, but to a lesser extent. Thus, collagenase activity was increased in both infarcted and noninfarcted tissue in the dilated heart with advanced failure requiring transplantation. Similar findings have been observed in endomyocardial biopsies obtained from patients with idiopathic (dilated) cardiomyopathy (33).

HORMONAL REGULATION OF POSTINFARCT REMODELING

Circulating Angiotensin II and Aldosterone

Circulating effector hormones of the RAAS are generally not increased in humans following acute MI (34). In the rat, plasma renin activity and plasma levels of AngII and/or ALDO are neither increased during the first 4 weeks following coronary artery ligation (35–37) nor at 12 weeks postinfarction. It therefore is not likely that circulating AngII or ALDO adversely contribute to the ongoing structural remodeling seen in the right and left ventricles soon after MI. In chronic IHD with symptomatic heart failure, on the other hand, the circulating RAAS is activated (30).

Tissue Hormones

Infarct Site

Scars, a site of high collagen turnover postinfarction, are associated with high-density angiotensin-converting enzyme (ACE) binding (in vitro autoradiography). Angiotensin-converting enzyme binding density, in fact, is increased markedly in scar tissue that appears at sites of cardiac myocyte necrosis, irrespective of the etiologic basis of cell loss. This, for example, includes the macroscopic scarring that follows coronary artery ligation (17,38,39), the endomyocardial fibrosis that appears following isoproterenol-induced necrosis (40), and the microscopic scarring associated with chronic AngII or ALDO administration (41). The density of ACE binding postinfarction or with AngII or ALDO infusion increases in parallel with the progressive accumulation of fibrillar collagen at these sites (17,41). At the site of infarction, ACE-producing cells have been identified by ACE monoclonal antibody (42) and found to include fibroblast-like cells, macrophages, and endothelial cells in new blood vessels.

Remote Sites

Fibrosis that appears remote to infarction and involving the right ventricle and interventricular septum or within the visceral pericardium are other sites of high-density ACE binding (16,17,28). In the right ventricle, this is expressed as a perivascular fibrosis and microscopic scars, while in the septum, an endocardial fibrosis appears. At these remote sites, immunohistochemistry identified ACE in fibroblast-like cells, which were also labeled with anti-alpha smooth-muscle actin antibody. We therefore consider that these cells are likely myofibroblasts (43). In situ hybridization further identified that each of these ACE-producing myofibroblasts express the transcript for type I collagen (17).

The anatomic coincidence between ACE binding in normal and pathologic expressions of connective tissue formation is evident. High-density ACE binding is a marker of active collagen turnover. ACE-producing myofibroblasts express type I collagen mRNA. Stroma and its mesenchymal cells therefore appear to form a metabolic entity whose purpose may be to regulate local collagen turnover via the elaboration of peptide hormones (40). Accordingly, these cells are able to govern the connective tissue composition of the heart postinfarction. If stroma and its constituent cells elaborate peptide hormones involved in regulating myofibroblast collagen turnover at the site of or remote to MI, precursors, proteases, and products must be identified (Fig. 2). Indeed, the majority of Ang peptides are generated locally (44).

Angiotensin Peptides

Angiotensinogen is the only known precursor for Ang peptides. It therefore is obligatory to tissue Ang generation and requires demonstration of angiotensinogen synthesis (44). On exposure to renin, the isolated crystalloid-perfused rat heart generates AngI and AngII (45). The generation of these Ang peptides could be blocked by renin and ACE inhibitors, respectively. Dexamethasone induces angiotensinogen mRNA expression and angiotensinogen release into coronary venous effluent. Cells responsible for the release of precursor are uncertain. In the adult rat heart and aorta, in situ hybridization localized mRNA expression of angiotensinogen within fibroblasts and brown adipocytes (46,47). In the neonatal rat heart, this transcript is localized to atria and ventricles (ventricles more than atria) and within their cardiac myocytes and fibroblasts (48). Both AngI and AngII have been detected in these cells (49). Neonatal rat cardiac fibroblasts also contain the transcript for renin (48) and other serine and aspartyl proteases, such as cathepsin G and D, respectively (50,51). Thus the neonatal phenotype of cardiac fibroblast, which may resemble a phenotypically transformed form of myofibroblast involved in wound healing, would appear capable of generating AngII.

Local production of Ang peptides is likely influenced by tissue-specific mechanisms of regulation. These may include either intra- or extracellular pathways (9).

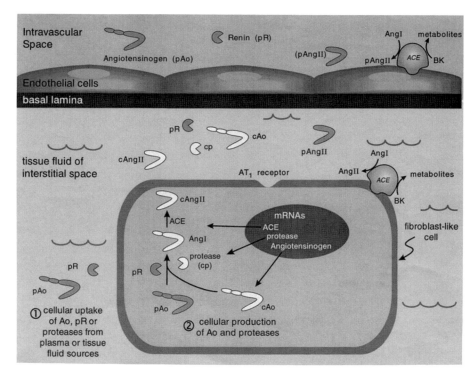

FIG. 2. A theoretical model of tissue antiotensin II–generating system that could be involved in the regulation of fibrous tissue formation in the heart. See text for details.

AngI and II may be generated intracellularly from cleavage of either locally synthesized angiotensinogen, angiotensinogen derived from plasma, or that which has been taken up by the cell from the interstitial space (see Fig. 2). Various proteases, likewise produced by the cell or procured from its environment, may be involved in the generation of these Ang peptides. They include cathepsin D, pepsin, and other aspartyl proteases that can generate AngI; and tonin, cathepsin G, trypsin, and other serine proteases that release AngII directly from angiotensinogen. Renin would not be obligatory to such a tissue Ang system.

The involvement of AngII in tissue repair and fibrogenesis that follows inflammation can be inferred from studies of healing that follow infarction. Local angiotensinogen production may lead to a significant increase in the concentration of this precursor in interstitial fluid. For any constant amount of protease in tissue fluid, the increase in angiotensinogen should be paralleled by an increase in Ang. On day 5 following coronary artery ligation, the expression of angiotensinogen mRNA was found to be increased in the rat left ventricle (52). This precedes the morphologic appearance of fibrillar collagen in the form of a scar (15–18,53,54). During the first 2 weeks postligation, AngII content of infarcted tissue has not been measured. It was found to be increased at 21 days and could be attenuated by delapril treatment initiated at the time of infarction (55). Plasma renin and AngII concentrations were not increased in this model. In tissue homogenates, evidence of increased mRNA expression and ACE activity have been observed at sites remote to MI (e.g., right ventricle) as long as 12 weeks after coronary ligation (36). Moreover, plasma renin and ACE activity were not increased while the increase in ACE mRNA expression and activity was organ-specific. This is in keeping with the concept of contained fibrous tissue formation within an injured organ (heart).

Bradykinin and Prostaglandins

Kinins and prostanoids are also endogenous hormones. Their role as chemical mediators of inflammation is well recognized. Bradykinin, prostaglandin I_2 (PGI$_2$), and prostaglandin E_2 (PGE$_2$) have each been detected in coronary sinus drainage. During myocardial ischemia or following infarction, BK in sinus effluent rises severalfold (56–59). A similar response is observed for the sinus concentration of AngII (59) and PGE$_2$ (60). Endothelial cells are able to elaborate BK and various prostanoids. Whether the early release of BK following infarction arises from the coronary vasculature and/or other cells is presently unknown. During the first several days after infarction, the release of PGE$_2$ is markedly increased by administration of BK, suggesting that inflammatory cells may be involved (60).

Various mesenchymal cells are also able to synthesize prostanoids. These include squamous epithelial cells of visceral and parietal pericardium, pleura and peritoneum (61–63), fibroblasts of various organs (64–66), and cultured mesothelial cells of pericardium (67). Whether these nonendothelial cells also release BK, a stimulus to prostaglandin synthesis (64) is yet uncertain. Both BK and PGE$_2$ alter cultured cardiac fibroblast collagen turnover (64,68,69). Fibroblast-like cells, isolated from the site of infarction 7 days after coronary ligation, demonstrate increased cyclooxygenase activity and increased prostanoid production, including PGE$_2$ (70). At 30 days after infarction, BK-induced release of PGE$_2$ from the heart is increased (60). Prostaglandin synthesis is increased in microsomes prepared from infarcted myocardium at 3 weeks and 3 months after coronary ligation. Thus, there is a persistence of PGE$_2$ production well beyond the inflammatory phase of tissue repair.

In Vivo Studies of Collagen Turnover

The elaboration of Ang peptides, BK, or PGE$_2$ by myofibroblasts has not yet been determined. Nonetheless, receptor–ligand binding is a requisite if locally generated peptides are to influence fibrogenesis. Normally, high-density AngII receptor binding in the heart is confined to its pacemaker and conduction tissue (71). Depending on the experimental model, autoradiographic localization of type I AngII and BK receptor binding is anatomically coincident with sites of myocardial fibrosis and ACE binding (72).

The role of AngII and BK in regulating fibrogenesis can be inferred from in vivo studies wherein pharmacologic agents that interfered with their elaboration or receptor binding were used. Six-week treatment with enalapril in 4-week-old rats retarded collagen formation in both the right and left ventricles, aorta, and superior mesenteric artery (73). A small dose of quinapril, which did not prevent hypertension in 4-week-old spontaneously hypertensive rats (SHR), was found to inhibit aortic ACE activity by 60% without reducing plasma ACE activity. The expected rise in aortic collagen volume fraction, observed in untreated SHRs at 30 weeks of age, was not seen in quinapril-treated animals (74).

Angiotensin-converting enzyme inhibitors reduce fibrous tissue formation following infarction. Perindopril, given 1 week after infarction, decreased the endomyocardial fibrosis that appeared in the nonnecrotic segment of left ventricle (27). Captopril treatment commenced at the time of coronary artery ligation prevented the expected proliferation of fibroblasts and fibrosis of the right ventricle and septum that appeared at 1 and 2 weeks following infarction (54). A type I AngII receptor antagonist, losartan, prevented fibrosis, but not fibroblast, proliferation at these remote sites (75). In the model of cardiac myocyte necrosis associated with chronic AngII administration (13,14), lisinopril attenuated microscopic scarring despite the presence of myocyte injury (76).

The evidence gathered to date, albeit indirect, implicates ACE as an integral component of an AngII-generating system found in connective tissue and which can be attributed to mesenchymal cells involved in fibrillar collagen formation under normal and pathologic conditions. Pharmacologic inhibition of fibrous tissue ACE or antagonism of type I AngII receptor attenuates fibrosis at various sites in the myocardium and arterial vasculature. The relative importance of AngII and BK in the paradigm of reciprocal regulation to collagen turnover (77) requires further study. In vitro studies, however, shed light on this topic.

In Vitro Studies of Collagen Turnover

Peptide hormones influence adult rat cardiac fibroblast collagen turnover. In serum-deprived cells, incubation with AngII increases net collagen production (78) by increased type I and III collagen synthesis (79,80). Moreover, AngII reduces collagenolytic activity of culture medium (79). The mitogenic potential of these cells was not altered by AngII (78,79), which contrasts to the growth response seen in neonatal cardiac fibroblasts (81,82). The presence of AngII receptors in adult and neonatal cardiac fibroblasts has been identified and found to be predominantly type I (78,83). Inhibitors of cardiac fibroblast collagen synthesis include BK and PGE_2, while these hormones stimulate collagenolytic activity (80). A dual effect of ACE inhibitors may prevent the appearance of myocardial fibrosis, either at or remote to the site of MI. These agents reduce local AngII concentration while augmenting local levels of BK and, indirectly, PGE_2. The relative importance of AngII has been considered by using a type I AngII receptor antagonist, as noted earlier. The contribution of BK and PGE_2 needs to be addressed by pharmacologic antagonism of type I and II BK receptors and cyclooxygenase inhibitors, respectively.

STRUCTURAL REMODELING IN HYPERTENSIVE HEART DISEASE

Hypertrophied Left Ventricle

In the absence of other responsible etiologic factors, an increase in LV mass, verified by postmortem LV weight or by echocardiographic derivation, is an essential first criterion to establish the diagnosis of HHD. In some patients, LV hypertrophy (LVH) may precede the appearance of resting hypertension. Right ventricular hypertrophy will accompany LVH when there is long-standing LV failure (84).

Left ventricular hypertrophy can be expressed as a proportionate thickening of the LV free wall and interventricular septum (85). This is the *concentric* pattern of LVH. It is the most common echocardiographic presentation of LVH in patients with HHD. Systolic ventricular function (i.e., ejection fraction and fractional shortening) is commonly preserved in these patients (86,87), while diastolic dysfunction (e.g., prolonged relaxation time and reduced rates of diastolic filling) may be present (88–91). Thirty percent of patients with symptomatic heart failure will have primary diastolic dysfunction with preserved ejection fraction. This is most often associated with HHD or coronary artery disease (92).

Less common is a disproportionate (relative to the posterior free wall) thickening of the interventricular septum (93–97). Septal thickness, however, does not reach values commonly attained in hypertrophic cardiomyopathy. An *eccentric* pattern of hypertrophy accompanies the appearance of systolic dysfunction with LV chamber enlargement. Here, wall thickness returns to or toward normal values. Nonetheless, myocardial mass remains increased unless there is considerable myocyte necrosis. It therefore is essential to not make the diagnosis of LVH solely on the basis of echocardiographic wall thickness. Instead, LV mass must be calculated (86,98).

Structural Remodeling

The growth of parenchyma, or muscle mass, must be balanced with proportionate growth of stroma, or collagen (99), if LVH is to be adaptive. In HHD, however, there is a structural remodeling of intramyocardial arteries and arterioles and their neighboring interstitial space by an abnormal accumulation of fibrous tissue. It is because of this remodeling that the proportion between parenchyma and stroma, or muscle mass to collagen mass, respectively, is distorted to create pathologic hypertrophy.

Cardiac myocytes of the left ventricle are enlarged in HHD. Expressed as an increase in myocyte cross-sectional area (not length), myocyte hypertrophy is due to the in-parallel addition of myofibrillar units (100). In long-standing hypertension, myocyte hyperplasia is also seen (101). Myocytes of the right ventricle remain normal in size until there exists a chronic pressure overload due to pulmonary venous hypertension; thereafter they, too, hypertrophy. Myocyte growth in either ventricle is closely related to ventricular loading (102–104) present at rest and during physical activity.

Coronary resistance vessels, like their counterparts in systemic arteries and arterioles (105–108), are remodeled in HHD. This includes a perivascular fibrosis of intramyocardial coronary arteries and arterioles, together with thickening of their media (109–117). This medial thickening is caused by hypertrophy and/or hyperplasia of vascular smooth-muscle cells. A structural realignment of these cells with enhanced accumulation of extracellular structural proteins (i.e., collagen and elastin) is also contributory (106,110,111). Other features of this vascular structural remodeling include intimal hyalinization and endothelial hyperplasia (106). Collectively, these changes in coronary resistance vessels serve to reduce their wall thickness to lumen ratio and adversely influence their capacity for vasodilatation (112, 118). Vascular remodeling of systemic and coronary resistance vessels may precede the appearance of hypertension (118) and indeed may be the cause of elevated arterial pressure and impaired vasodilator reserve. Hypertensive patients with LVH are at increased risk of myocardial ischemia (119). Responsible mechanisms may include the structural remodeling of coronary resistance vessels (120), prevailing coronary perfusion pressure (121), and coexistence of epicardial coronary artery disease.

Fibrosis is another well-recognized feature of the adverse structural remodeling found in the myocardium in HHD. Myocardial fibrosis has been observed in postmortem and endomyocardial biopsy tissues (116,117). The pathologic accumulation of collagen presents in several distinct morphologic patterns (see Fig. 1). A *perivascular fibrosis* of intramyocardial coronary arteries and arterioles appears from which fibrillar collagen extends outward for variable distances into the interstitial space, where it represents an *interstitial fibrosis*. This is a progressive process involving ever-increasing amounts of the interstitium (122). This *reactive* perivascular/interstitial fibrous tissue response is present throughout the free wall of the left ventricle and the interventricular septum (113) and involves the normotensive, nonhypertrophied right ventricular free wall as well (123). Individual muscle fibers of both ventricles become encircled by thickened collagen fibers, which impairs their ability to be stretched and to contract and ultimately leads to myocyte atrophy (124). The increase in collagen volume fraction, or interstitial fibrosis, found in biopsies taken from human HHD, has been correlated with abnormal diastolic function of the left ventricle (125,126). Distinct from this perivascular/interstitial fibrosis are discrete focal collections of fibrillar collagen that represent microscopic scars (a *reparative* fibrosis) that replace necrotic cardiac myocytes. These scars, often found in the endomyocardium, preserve the structural integrity of the myocardium associated with the loss of myocytes. Fibrosis may also present as an endocardial accumulation of collagen, where it is considered an *endocardial fibrosis*. These reactive and reparative forms of myocardial fibrosis are seen in essential hypertension (109–115). The perivascular fibrosis has also been found in systemic arterioles (e.g., pancreas and adrenal glands) in patients with autopsy-proven adrenal adenoma (127).

The normal concentration of fibrillar collagen in the myocardium is an important determinant of its stiffness (128). An increase in collagen concentration, representing a disproportionate growth of stroma relative to parenchyma and defined as myocardial fibrosis, is primarily expressed as type I collagen (19,129). Type I collagen has the tensile strength of steel (130). In experimental studies, a two- to threefold rise in collagen concentration is associated with an increase in diastolic stiffness, while resting systolic stiffness and ejection fraction are preserved (131–134). A further rise in collagen concentration (fourfold or more), particularly within the endomyocardium, raises diastolic stiffness even further and is now associated with the appearance of systolic dysfunction (134–137). This more advanced rise in myocardial collagen concentration is seen late in HHD and is related to the reactive fibrosis and to a reparative fibrosis that replaces lost cardiac myocytes, particularly within the endomyocardium. In patients with LVH and diastolic dysfunction, endomyocardial biopsy has demonstrated the presence of myocardial fibrosis (125,126). The importance of diastolic dysfunction as a cause of symptomatic heart failure and potential contributory mechanisms has recently been reviewed (138).

In preventing the rise in collagen concentration tissue in the rat heart, stiffness remains normal (139). Absence of fibrous tissue response in the hypertrophied ventricle does not raise diastolic stiffness (140,141), while the presence of fibrosis in the absence of LVH raises stiffness (142). The importance of fibrillar collagen to the mechanical behavior of the myocardium is further emphasized in studies where fibrosis was regressed from hearts with both established LVH and fibrosis. With or without a regression of LVH, regression of fibrosis served to normalize stiffness (143).

HORMONAL REGULATION OF REMODELING IN HYPERTENSIVE HEART DISEASE

Circulating Angiotensin II and Aldosterone

A reactive and a reparative fibrosis have each been observed in the myocardium in some but not all experimental models of HHD (144). The reactive perivascular/interstitial fibrosis appears after surgically induced unilateral renal ischemia, where plasma AngII and ALDO are each increased (132,133,145–147). The normotensive, nonhypertrophied right ventricle is also involved (146), implicating a role for these circulating hormones. In this connection, pre- and continued treatment with captopril in these animals could prevent this remodeling process (139). Evidence of enhanced collagen concentration in the nonhypertrophied left ventricle and hypertrophied right ventricle that followed pulmonary artery banding in cats (148), a model known to be associated with activation of the RAAS and the appearance of pleural effusions and ascites (149), further implicates these hormones. Bilateral renal ischemia, created by suprarenal abdominal aortic banding, is accompanied by an increase in myocardial collagen synthesis (150), which is prevented by digitoxin treatment (151). Expression of type I and III collagen mnRNAs, the major fibrillar collagens of the myocardium, is increased early after surgical induction of unilateral renal ischemia (152). This is followed by accumulation of type I collagen in perivascular and interstitial locations weeks later.

Pathologic fibrous tissue accumulation does not occur with the pressure overload hypertrophy induced by infrarenal aortic banding (146). It likewise does not appear with either the volume overload hypertrophy associated with uninephrectomy and a high-sodium diet (146), a compensated arteriovenous fistula (147,153), chronic anemia (154), atrial septal defect (140), or the hypertrophy induced by chronic thyroxine administration (154,155). In each of these circumstances, the RAAS is not activated.

A perivascular fibrosis of both ventricles and systemic arterioles has been observed in uninephrectomized rats on a high-sodium diet that received either d-ALDO (146,156) or deoxycorticosterone acetate for weeks (157). In these models of chronic mineralocorticoid excess, plasma renin activity and AngII are each suppressed. In rats receiving ALDO, pre- and continued treatment with an ALDO receptor antagonist, spironolactone, prevented both the perivascular fibrosis and scarring of the myocardium. This was true for both a small dose of spironolactone, which did not prevent hypertension or LVH, and a large dose, which achieved these endpoints (158). To further address the role of arterial pressure, captopril was used to prevent hypertension in rats receiving ALDO for 8 weeks; given the independent source of ALDO, captopril did not interfere with the effects of this hormone, and as a result, it did not prevent the reactive myocardial fibrosis. Finally, the administration of ALDO to uninephrectomized rats on a low-sodium diet was associated with a marked elevation in plasma ALDO, but not the reactive fibrosis. The results of the various in vivo studies suggest a clear association between chronic inappropriate (relative to sodium intake) elevations in circulating AngII and/or ALDO and the reactive fibrous tissue response. Fibrogenic mechanism(s) remain uncertain and may indeed be quite distinct for each hormone.

To further address the role of AngII and ALDO in promoting myocardial fibrosis, either hormone was administered by implanted minipump in a dose that initially did not elevate arterial pressure (41). Weber et al. (159) had suggested that the fibrogenic response to AngII administration was secondary to coronary vascular hyperpermeability. In rats receiving AngII, macromolecular permeability was monitored using an antibody to plasma fibronectin, while the temporal appearance of myocardial fibrosis was examined using the picrosirius red stain specific for fibrillar collagen (160). On day 1 of AngII infusion, intramyocardial coronary arterioles of both ventricles were morphologically intact and resembled untreated controls. On day 2, localized deposits of plasma fibronectin were evident within the media and adventitia of these vessels, with protrusions into the adjacent interstitial space. Immunolabeling of large intramural arteries or veins was not detected. A cellular response was also now evident within the adventitia of these vessels and appeared to involve fibroblasts and macrophages. On day 4, plasma fibronectin staining of the media and adventitia of arterioles was more extensive and widespread than that seen earlier, while its extension into the interstitial space was more advanced. On day 7 of AngII, the walls of intramyocardial coronary arterioles had become thicker with diffuse fibronectin labeling evident in the media, adventitia, and neighboring interstitial space. The increased cellularity of the adventitia was still evident in involved vessels on days 4 and 7. Although fibroblasts and macrophages were still apparent by day 7, no polymorphonuclear cells were found.

By days 10 and 14 of AngII infusion, a widespread involvement of intramyocardial coronary arterioles was evident, and plasma fibronectin labeling was present in the media and adventitia of these vessels. Again, larger intramural arteries and veins were not involved. The presence of an increased number of cells, presumably fibroblasts and macrophages, was still evident, while a perivascular fibrosis of arterioles, represented by an increased accumulation of fibrillar collagen, was evident in both ventricles on day 14. Each fibrous tissue response became more extensive over the course of 6 weeks AngII treatment.

Type I collagen mRNA–producing cells were seen only in the myocardium of AngII-infused animals. They appeared in both ventricles on days 4 and 7 of the infusion. Grains were abundant in these cells, which were located in the adventitia and perivascular space of many, but not all, coronary arterioles. Within the interstitial space there were also mRNA–synthesizing cells. Based on their morphologic features, which included an elongated fusiform shape with elongated nuclei and prominent nucleoli, these cells appeared to be fibroblasts or a fibroblast-like phenotype. These cells were not seen in control animals.

In uninephrectomized rats on a high-sodium diet receiving ALDO, reactive or reparative fibrosis was not evident until 4 weeks when it appeared in both ventricles, becoming more extensive at 6 weeks. Thus, while fibrosis was seen in both ventricles with each model, a combined elevation in circulating AngII and ALDO led to a more rapid appearance of the fibrous tissue response than the elevation in plasma ALDO alone. Mechanisms involved in promoting fibrogenesis require further investigation.

Chronic activation of the RAAS is also associated with cardiac myocyte necrosis and a subsequent reparative fibrosis. Even in the absence of hypertension, myocyte necrosis accompanies inappropriate elevations in plasma AngII (13,14). Anticardiac myosin or antifibronectin antibodies have been used to detect myocyte injury (13,14) seen in association with AngII administration. In AngII-infused animals, both ventricles were found to contain multifocal areas of cardiac myocyte injury on day 1. This was associated with scattered polymorphonuclear leukocytes and clusters of macrophages. On day 7, these areas of injured myocytes with wound healing contained fibroblasts. Microscopic scars were evident on day 14. To address the role of AngII-induced release of adrenal catecholamines or ALDO, animals receiving AngII either had preceding bilateral total adrenalectomy, bilateral adrenal medullectomy, or were given the ALDO receptor antagonist spironolactone. The same histologic pattern of necrosis and scarring was observed in animals receiving AngII together with spironolactone. In rats with total adrenalectomy who received AngII only, a few scattered foci of myocyte necrosis were seen, and scarring was not found on day 14. Attenuated myocyte injury not accompanied by microscopic scarring was also noted in animals with bilateral adrenal medullectomy. Thus, it would appear that AngII-induced release of adrenal medullary catecholamines lead to myocyte injury.

Myocyte necrosis and scarring is also evident after weeks of mineralocorticoid excess created by d-ALDO (156,161) or deoxycorticosterone acetate (157,162) in previously uninephrectomized rats receiving a high-sodium diet. Spironolactone and amiloride each have potassium-sparing effects albeit through different mechanisms of action. Each was found to prevent the appearance of microscopic scarring in the ventricles in rats treated with ALDO for 8 weeks (161,163). Dietary potassium chloride supplementation has a similar protective effect (162). Spironolactone, but not amiloride, on the other hand, prevents the perivascular fibrosis (158,161), indicating potassium loss is not responsible for this reactive fibrosis. Thus, myocardial potassium depletion in the setting of chronic mineralocorticoid excess contributes to myocyte necrosis and reparative fibrosis. This would explain the microscopic scarring of the myocardium reported in a patient with Bartter's syndrome (164) as well as in a weightlifter taking anabolic steroids (165) and where androgens create a chronic excess of deoxycorticosterone by 11β-hydroxylase inhibition (166).

Elevations in circulating catecholamines have a cytotoxic effect on the myocardium expressed as cardiac myocyte necrosis that often favors the endomyocardium of the left and right ventricles (12,15,167,168).

Tissue Hormones

In SHRs, a progressive accumulation of collagen has been observed in the myocardium with aging (132,169). This fibrosis involves intramural vessels as well as a replacement of lost myocytes (132,170). In SHRs, circulating levels of AngII and ALDO are not increased above the expected "normal range," but are abnormal given the presence of hypertension. Hormones generated within cardiovascular tissue, such as AngII, may be contributory to this remodeling process in SHRs (171). In treating nonhypertensive 4-week-old SHRs with hydralazine for 32 weeks, it was possible to prevent hypertension and LVH (142), but not the perivascular fibrosis of intramural coronary vessels which was evident at 32 weeks in treated animals as well as nontreated SHRs with LVH and hypertension. Enalapril introduced early in HHD was able to prevent the appearance of myocardial fibrosis (172). Importantly, this was associated with a reduction in the propensity for spontaneous and inducible ventricular arrhythmias.

Abnormalities in collagen turnover, where collagen synthesis exceeds its degradation, are likely responsible for promoting this fibrous tissue response in SHRs.

Sen et al. (173) observed an elevation in collagen synthesis in the myocardium of these animals at 4 weeks of age, before they had become hypertensive, as well as at 8 weeks when arterial pressure was elevated. Thereafter collagen synthesis was no different from Wistar Kyoto (WKY) controls until 24 weeks of age, when it again was increased. This again underscores the fact that hypertension per se does not contribute to this fibrous tissue response. Moreover, the perivascular fibrosis of systemic arterioles may herald the appearance of hypertension.

Collectively, these various studies indicate the following: (a) Ventricular hypertrophy, an increment in parenchymal mass based on cardiac myocyte growth, is primarily regulated by either ventricular pressure or volume loading; (b) perivascular fibrosis is associated with chronic inappropriate elevations in circulating effector hormones of the RAAS, not ventricular loading; (c) scarring, or reparative fibrosis, follows myocyte necrosis of diverse cause and is related to adrenal catecholamines released alone or in association with increased plasma AngII (13,14) and myocardial potassium depletion due to chronic mineralocorticoid excess (162); and (d) separate regulatory controls (174,175) determine whether hypertrophy involves a preservation or distortion in stromal structure and, accordingly, whether LVH will be adaptive or pathologic (5,137).

SUMMARY

Heart failure is a major health problem characterized by a relentless downhill clinical course. Major etiologic factors are IHD, with previous MI, and HHD. Factors that contribute to the progressive nature of heart failure are likely multifactorial, but certainly include an adverse remodeling of myocardial microscopic structure that ultimately impairs diastolic and systolic ventricular function. Emerging experimental evidence implicates AngII, ALDO, and catecholamines in this remodeling. The progressive structural remodeling of the myocardium in IH and HHD was reviewed and the role of hormonal factors examined.

ACKNOWLEDGMENTS

This work was supported in part by NIH grant RO1-HL-31701 and was conducted during Dr. Ratajska's tenure as a Fogarty International Research Fellow (1F05 TWO 4577-1) and Dr. Cleutjens' tenure with the Netherlands Organization for Scientific Research (NWO) (Grant S93.221.92) and Netherlands Heart Foundation (Grant 90.282).

REFERENCES

1. Kannel WB. Epidemiological aspects of heart failure. *Cardiol Clin* 1989;7:1–9.
2. Ho KKL, Anderson KM, Kannel WB, Grossman W, Levy D. Survival after the onset of congestive heart failure in Framingham Heart Study patients. *Circulation* 1993;88:107–115.

3. Swedberg K, Eneroth P, Kjekshus J, Wilhelmsen L. Hormones regulating cardiovascular function in patients with severe congestive heart failure and their relation to mortality. CONSENSUS Trial Study Group. *Circulation* 1990;82:1730–1736.
4. Cohn JN, Johnson G, Ziesche S, et al. A comparison of enalapril with hydralazine-isosorbide dinitrate in the treatment of chronic congestive heart failure. *N Engl J Med* 1991;325:303–310.
5. Weber KT, Brilla CG. Pathological hypertrophy and cardiac interstitium: fibrosis and renin-angiotensin-aldosterone system. *Circulation* 1991;83:1849–1865.
6. Weber KT, Brilla CG, Janicki JS. Myocardial fibrosis: functional significance and regulatory factors. *Cardiovasc Res* 1993;27:341–348.
7. Meggs LG, Coupet J, Huang H, et al. Regulation of angiotensin II receptors on ventricular myocytes after myocardial infarction in rats. *Circ Res* 1993;72:1149–1162.
8. Reiss K, Capasso JM, Huang H-E, Meggs LG, Li P, Anversa P. ANG II receptors, c-*myc*, and c-*jun* in myocytes after myocardial infarction and ventricular failure. *Am J Physiol* 1993;264: H760–H769.
9. Weber KT, Sun Y, Tyagi SC, Cleutjens JPM. Collagen network of the myocardium: function, structural remodeling and regulatory mechanisms. *J Mol Cell Cardiol* 1994;26:279–292.
10. Reimer KA, Jennings RB. Myocardial ischemia, hypoxia, and infarction. In: Fozzard HA, Haber E, Jennings RB, Katz AM, Morgan HE, eds. *The heart and cardiovascular system.* New York: Raven Press; 1986:1133–1201.
11. Nolan AC, Clark WA Jr, Karwoski T, Zak R. Patterns of cellular injury in myocardial ischemia determined by monoclonal antimyosin. *Proc Natl Acad Sci USA* 1983;80:6046–6050.
12. Benjamin IJ, Jalil JE, Tan LB, Cho K, Weber KT, Clark WA. Isoproterenol-induced myocardial fiborosis in relation to myocyte necrosis. *Circ Res* 1989;65:657–670.
13. Tan LB, Jalil JE, Pick R, Janicki JS, Weber KT. Cardiac myocyte necrosis induced by angiotensin II. *Circ Res* 1991;69:1185–1195.
14. Ratajska A, Campbell SE, Sun Y, Weber KT. Angiotensin II associated cardiac myocyte necrosis: role of adrenal catecholamines. *Cardiovasc Res* 1994;28:684–90.
15. Pick R, Jalil JE, Janicki JS, Weber KT. The fibrillar nature and structure of isoproterenol-induced myocardial fibrosis in the rat. *Am J Pathol* 1989;134:365–371.
16. van Krimpen C, Schoemaker RG, Cleutjens JPM, et al. Angiotensin I converting enzyme inhibitors and cardiac remodeling. *Basic Res Cardiol* 1991;86[Suppl 1]:149–155.
17. Sun Y, Cleutjens JPM, Diaz-Arias AA, Weber KT. Cardiac angiotensin converting enzyme and myocardial fibrosis in the rat. *Cardiovasc Res* 1994;28:1423–32.
18. Jugdutt BI, Amy RWM. Healing after myocardial infarction in the dog: changes in infarct hydroxyproline and topography. *J Am Coll Cardiol* 1986;7:91–102.
19. Bishop J, Greenbaum J, Gibson D, Yacoub M, Laurent GJ. Enhanced deposition of predominantly type I collagen in myocardial disease. *J Mol Cell Cardiol* 1990;22:1157–1165.
20. Tyagi SC, Matsubara L, Weber KT. Direct extraction and estimation of collagenase(s) activity by zymography in microquantities of rat myocardium and uterus. *Clin Biochem* 1993;26:191–198.
21. Tyagi SC, Ratajska A, Weber KT. Myocardial matrix metalloproteinase(s): localization and activation. *Mol Cell Biochem* 1993;126:49–59.
22. Cleutjens JP, Guarda E, Weber KT. Transcriptional and post-transcriptional regulation of interstitial collagenase after myocardial infarction in the rat heart. *Circulation* 1993;88[Suppl I]:I-380 (abst).
23. Olivetti G, Capasso JM, Sonnenblick EH, Anversa P. Side-to-side slippage of myocytes participates in ventricular wall remodeling acutely after myocardial infarction in rats. *Circ Res* 1990;67: 23–34.
24. Weber KT. Cardiac interstitium in health and disease: the fibrillar collagen network. *J Am Coll Cardiol* 1989;13:1637–1652.
25. Anversa P, Loud AV, Levicky V, Guideri G. Left ventricular failure induced by myocardial infarction. I. Myocyte hypertrophy. *Am J Physiol* 1985;248:H876–H882.
26. Olivetti G, Capasso JM, Meggs LG, Sonnenblick EH, Anversa P. Cellular basis of chronic ventricular remodeling after myocardial infarction in rats. *Circ Res* 1991;68:856–869.
27. Michel J-B, Lattion A-L, Salzmann J-L, et al. Hormonal and cardiac effects of converting enzyme inhibition in rat myocardial infarction. *Circ Res* 1988;62:641–650.
28. Volders PGA, Willems IEMG, Cleutjens JPM, Arends J-W, Havenith MG, Daemen MJAP. Interstitial collagen is increased in the non-infarcted human myocardium after myocardial infarction. *J Mol Cell Cardiol* 1993;25:1317–1323.

29. Beltrami CA, Finato N, Rocco M, et al. Structural basis of end-stage failure in ischemic cardio-myopathy in humans. *Circulation* 94;89:151–163.
30. Francis GS, Benedict C, Johnstone DE, et al. Comparison of neuroendocrine activation in patients with left ventricular dysfunction with and without congestive heart failure: a substudy of the Studies of Left Ventricular Dysfunction (SOLVD). *Circulation* 1990;82:1724–1729.
31. Gerdes AM, Kellerman SE, Moore JA, et al. Structural remodeling of cardiac myocytes in patients with ischemic cardiomyopathy. *Circulation* 1992;86:426–430.
32. Tyagi SC, Reddy HK, Voelker DJ, Tjahja IE, Weber KT. Myocardial collagenase in failing human heart. *Clin Res* 1993;41:681A(abst).
33. Reddy HK, Tyagi SC, Tjahja IE, Voelker DJ, Campbell SE, Weber KT. Activated myocardial collagenase in idiopathic dilated cardiomyopathy: a marker of dilatation and remodeling. *Clin Res* 1993;41:660A(abst).
34. Rouleau JL, de Champlain J, Klein M, et al. Activation of neurohormonal systems in postinfarc-tion left ventricular hypertrophy. *J Am Coll Cardiol* 1993;22:390–398.
35. Hodsman GP, Kohzuki M, Howes LG, Sumithran E, Tsunoda K, Johnston CI. Neurohumoral responses to chronic myocardial infarction in rats. *Circulation* 1988;78:376–381.
36. Hirsch AT, Talsness CE, Schunkert H, Paul M, Dzau VJ. Tissue-specific activation of cardiac angiotensin converting enzyme in experimental heart failure. *Circ Res* 1991;69:475–482.
37. Yamaguchi T, Ikekita M, Kizuki K, Moriva H. Distribution of angiotensin I converting enzyme in male reproductive systems of various vertebrates and properties of the genital enzymes. *Adv Exp Med Biol* 1989;247B:377–382.
38. Johnston CI, Mooser V, Sun Y, Fabris B. Changes in cardiac angiotensin converting enzyme after myocardial infarction and hypertrophy in rats. *Clin Exp Pharmacol Physiol* 1991;18:107–110.
39. Fabris B, Jackson B, Kohzuki M, Perich R, Johnston CI. Increased cardiac angiotensin-converting enzyme in rats with chronic heart failure. *Clin Exp Pharmacol Physiol* 1990;17:309–314.
40. Weber KT, Sun Y, Katwa LC, Cleutjens JPM. Connective tissue: a metabolic entity? *J Mol Cell Cardiol* 1995;27:107–20.
41. Sun Y, Ratajska A, Zhou G, Weber KT. Angiotensin converting enzyme and myocardial fibrosis in the rat receiving angiotensin II or aldosterone. *J Lab Clin Med* 1993;122:395–403.
42. Danilov SM, Faerman AI, Printseva OY, Martynov AV, Sakharov IY, Trakht IN. Immunohisto-chemical study of angiotensin-converting enzyme in human tissues using monoclonal antibodies. *Histochemistry* 1987;87:487–490.
43. Gabbiani G. The myofibroblast: a key cell for wound healing and fibrocontractive diseases. In: Deyl Z, Adam M, eds. *Connective tissue research: chemistry. biology, and physiology.* New York: Liss; 1981:183–194.
44. Campbell DJ. Circulating and tissue angiotensin systems. *J Clin Invest* 1987;79:1–6.
45. Lindpaintner K, Jin M, Niedermaier N, Wilhelm MJ, Ganten D. Cardiac angiotensin and its local activation in the isolated perfused beating heart. *Circ Res* 1990;67:564–573.
46. Campbell DJ, Habener JF. Cellular localization of angiotensinogen gene expression in brown adipose tissue and mesentery: quantification of messenger ribonucleic acid abundance using hy-bridization *in situ. Endocrinology* 1987;121:1616–1626.
47. Cassis LA, Lynch KR, Peach MJ. Localization of angiotensinogen messenger RNA in rat aorta. *Circ Res* 1988;62:1259–1262.
48. Dostal DE, Rothblum KN, Chernin MI, Cooper GR, Baker KM. Intracardiac detection of angio-tensinogen and renin: a localized renin-angiotensin system in neonatal rat heart. *Am J Physiol* 1992; 263:C838–C850.
49. Dostal DE, Rothblum KN, Conrad KM, Cooper GR, Baker KM. Detection of angiotensin I and II in cultured rat cardiac myocytes and fibroblasts. *Am J Physiol* 1992;263:C851–C863.
50. Klickstein LB, Kaempfer CE, Wintroub BU. The granulocyte-angiotensin system. Angiotensin I–converting activity of cathepsin G. *J Biol Chem* 1982;257:15042–15046.
51. Pearl LH, Taylor WR. A structural model for the retroviral proteases [Letter]. *Nature* 1987;329: 351–354.
52. Lindpaintner K, Lu W, Niedermajer J, et al. Selective activation of cardiac angiotensinogen gene expression in post-infarction ventricular remodeling in the rat. *J Mol Cell Cardiol* 1993;25:133–143.
53. Judd JT, Wexler BC. Prolyl hydroxylase and collagen metabolism after experimental myocardial infarction. *Am J Physiol* 1975;228:212–216.

54. van Krimpen C, Smits JFM, Cleutjens JPM, et al. DNA synthesis in the non-infarcted cardiac interstitium after left coronary artery ligation in the rat heart: effects of captopril. *J Mol Cell Cardiol* 1991;23:1245–1253.
55. Yamagishi H, Kim S, Nishikimi T, Takeuchi K, Takeda T. Contribution of cardiac renin-angiotensin system to ventricular remodelling in myocardial-infarcted rats. *J Mol Cell Cardiol* 1993; 25:1369–1380.
56. Baumgarten CR, Linz W, Kunkel G, Schölkens BA, Wiemer G. Ramaprilat increases bradykinin outflow from isolated hearts of rat. *Br J Pharmacol* 1993;108:293–295.
57. Kimura B, Sumners C, Phillips MI. Changes in skin angiotensin II receptors in rats during wound healing. *Biochem Biophys Res Commun* 1992;187:1083–1090.
58. Hashimoto K, Hirose M, Furukawa K, Hayakawa H, Kimura E. Changes in hemodynamics and bradykinin concentration in coronary sinus blood in experimental coronary artery occlusion. *Jpn Heart J* 1977;18:679–689.
59. Noda K, Sasaguri M, Ideishi M, Ikeda M, Arakawa K. Role of locally formed angiotensin II and bradykinin in the reduction of myocardial infarct size in dogs. *Cardiovasc Res* 1993;27:334–340.
60. Evers AS, Murphree S, Saffitz JE, Jakschik BA, Needleman P. Effects of endogenously produced leukotrienes, thromboxane, and prostaglandins on coronary vascular resistance in rabbit myocardial infarction. *J Clin Invest* 1985;75:992–999.
61. Herman AG, Claeys M, Moncada S, Vane JR. Biosynthesis of prostacyclin (PGI$_2$) and 12L-hydroxy-5,8,10,14-eicosatetraenoic acid (HETE) by pericardium, pleura, peritoneum and aorta of the rabbit. *Prostaglandins* 1979;18:439–452.
62. Dusting GJ, Nolan RD. Stimulation of prostacyclin release from the epicardium of anaesthetized dogs. *Br J Pharmacol* 1981;74:553–562.
63. Nolan RD, Dusting GJ, Jakubowski J, Martin TJ. The pericardium as a source of prostacyclin in the dog, ox and rat. *Prostaglandins* 1982;24:887–902.
64. Goldstein RH, Polgar P. The effect and interaction of bradykinin and prostaglandins on protein and collagen production by lung fibroblasts. *J Biol Chem* 1982;257:8630–8633.
65. Bareis DL, Manganiello VC, Hirata F, Vaughan M, Axelrod J. Bradykinin stimulates phospholipid methylation, calcium influx, prostaglandin formation, and cAMP accumulation in human fibroblasts. *Biochemistry* 1983;80:2514–2518.
66. Ahumada GG, Sobel BE, Needleman P. Synthesis of prostaglandins by cultured rat heart myocytes and cardiac mesenchymal cells. *J Mol Cell Cardiol* 1980;12:685–700.
67. Satoh K, Prescott SM. Culture of mesothelial cells from bovine pericardium and characterization of the arachidonate metabolism. *Biochim Biophys Acta* 1980;930:283–296.
68. Baum BJ, Moss J, Breul SD, Crystal RC. Association in normal human fibroblasts of elevated levels of adenosine 3′:5′-monophosphate with a selective decrease in collagen production. *J Biol Chem* 1978;253:3391–3394.
69. Zhou G, Tyagi SC, Weber KT. Bradykinin regulates collagen turnover in cardiac fibroblasts. *Clin Res* 1993;41:630A(abst).
70. Weber DR, Stroud ED, Prescott SM. Arachidonate metabolism in cultured fibroblasts derived from normal and infarcted canine heart. *Circ Res* 1989;65:671–683.
71. Allen AM, Yamada H, Mendelsohn FAO. In vitro autoradiographic localization of binding to angiotensin receptors in the rat heart. *Int J Cardiol* 1990;28:25–33.
72. Sun Y, Diaz-Arias AA, Weber KT. Angiotensin-converting enzyme, bradykinin and angiotensin II receptor binding in rat skin, tendon and heart valves: an in vitro quantitative autoradiographic study. *J Lab Clin Med* 1994;123:372–377.
73. Keeley FW, Elmoselhi A, Leenan FHH. Enalapril suppresses normal accumulation of elastin and collagen in cardiovascular tissues of growing rats. *Am J Physiol* 1992;262:H1013–H1021.
74. Albaladejo P, Bouaziz H, Duriez M, et al. Angiotensin converting enzyme inhibition prevents the increase in aortic collagen in rats. *Hypertension* 1994;23:74–82.
75. Smits JFM, van Krimpen C, Schoemaker RG, Cleutjens JPM, Daemen MJAP. Angiotensin II receptor blockade after myocardial infarction in rats: effects on hemodynamics, myocardial DNA synthesis, and interstitial collagen content. *J Cardiovasc Pharmacol* 1992;20:772–778.
76. Sun Y, Weber KT. Nonendothelial ACE and myocardial fibrosis in rats receiving angiotensin II: inhibition by lisinopril. *Am J Hypertens* 1993;6:4A(abst).
77. Weber KT. Hormones and fibrosis: a case for lost reciprocal regulation. *News Physiol Sci* 1994;9: 123–28.

78. Villarreal FJ, Kim NN, Ungab GD, Printz MP, Dillman WH. Identification of functional angiotensin II receptors on rat cardiac fibroblasts. *Circulation* 1993;88:2849–2861.
79. Brilla CG, Zhou G, Matsubara L, Weber KT. Collagen metabolism in cultured adult cardiac fibroblasts: response to angiotensin and aldosterone. *J Mol Cell Cardiol* 1994;26:809–20.
80. Zhou G, Brilla CG, Weber KT. Angiotensin II–mediated stimulation of collagen synthesis in cultured cardiac fibroblasts. *FASEB J* 1992;6:A1914(abst).
81. Schorb W, Booz GW, Dostal DE, Conrad KM, Chang KC, Baker KM. Angiotensin II is mitogenic in neonatal rat cardiac fibroblasts. *Circ Res* 1993;72:1245–1254.
82. Sadoshima J, Izumo S. Molecular characterization of angiotensin II–induced hypertrophy of cardiac myocytes and hyperplasia of cardiac fibroblasts. Critical role of the AT_1 receptor subtype. *Circ Res* 1993;73:413–423.
83. Katwa LC, Weber KT. Angiotensin type I and type II receptors in cultured adult rat cardiac fibroblasts. *J Mol Cell Cardiol* 1993;25[Suppl III]:S89(abst).
84. Jones RS. The weight of the heart and its chambers in hypertensive cardiovascular disease with and without failure. *Circulation* 1953;7:357–369.
85. Weber KT, Brilla CG, Janicki JS. Myocardial remodeling and pathologic hypertrophy. *Hosp Pract* 1991;26(Apr.):73–80.
86. Devereux RB, Savage DD, Drayer JIM, Laragh JH. Left ventricular hypertrophy and function in high, normal, and low-renin forms of essential hypertension. *Hypertension* 1982;4:524–531.
87. Devereux RB, Savage DD, Sachs I, Laragh JH. Relation of hemodynamic load to left ventricular hypertrophy and performance in hypertension. *Am J Cardiol* 1983;51:171–176.
88. Echeverria HH, Bilsker MS, Myerburg RJ, Kessler KM. Congestive heart failure: echocardiographic insights. *Am J Med* 1983;75:750–755.
89. Fouad FM, Slominski JM, Tarazi RF. Left ventricular diastolic function in hypertension: relation to left ventricular mass and systolic function. *J Am Coll Cardiol* 1984;3:1500–1506.
90. Cuocolo A, Sax FL, Brush JE, Maron BJ, Bacharach SL, Bonow RO. Left ventricular hypertrophy and impaired diastolic filling in essential hypertension. Diastolic mechanisms for systolic dysfunction during exercise. *Circulation* 1990;81:978–986.
91. Grossman E, Oren S, Messerli FH. Left ventricular filling and stress response pattern in essential hypertension. *Am J Med* 1991;91:502–506.
92. Kessler KM. Heart failure with normal systolic function: update of prevalence, differential diagnosis, prognosis, and therapy. *Arch Intern Med* 1988;148:2109–2111.
93. Dunn FG, Chandraratna P, deCarvalho JGR, Basta LL, Frohlich ED. Pathophysiologic assessment of hypertensive heart disease with echocardiography. *Am J Cardiol* 1977;39:789–795.
94. Maron BJ, Edwards JE, Epstein SE. Disproportionate ventricular septal thickening in patients with systemic hypertension. *Chest* 1978;73:466–470.
95. Safar ME, Lehner JP, Vincent MI, Plainfosse MT, Simon AC. Echocardiographic dimensions in borderline and sustained hypertension. *Am J Cardiol* 1979;44:930–935.
96. Cohen A, Hagan AD, Watkins J, et al. Clinical correlates in hypertensive patients with left ventricular hypertrophy diagnosed with echocardiography. *Am J Cardiol* 1981;47:335–341.
97. Yokota Y, Teng S-S, Emoto R, et al. Mechanism of development of asymmetric septal hypertrophy in patients with essential systemic hypertension. *Jpn Circ J* 1989;53:1173–1184.
98. Devereux RB, Reichek N. Echocardiographic determination of left ventricular mass in man: anatomic validation of the method. *Circulation* 1977;55:613–618.
99. Montfort I, Pérez-Tamayo R. The muscle collagen ratio in normal and hypertrophic human hearts. *Lab Invest* 1962;11:463–470.
100. Anversa P, Ricci R, Olivetti G. Quantitative structural analysis of the myocardium during physiologic growth and induced cardiac hypertrophy: a review. *J Am Coll Cardiol* 1986;7:1140–1149.
101. Anversa P, Palackal T, Sonnenblick EH, Olivetti G, Meggs LG, Capasso JM. Myocyte cell loss and myocyte cellular hyperplasia in the hypertrophied aging rat heart. *Circ Res* 1990;67:871–885.
102. Weber KT, Anversa P, Armstrong PW, et al. Remodeling and reparation of the cardiovascular system. *J Am Coll Cardiol* 1992;20:3–16.
103. Weber KT, Brilla CG, Cleland JGF, et al. Cardioreparation and the concept of modulating cardiovascular structure and function. *Blood Pressure* 1993;2:6–21.
104. Liebson PR, Grandits G, Prineas R, et al. Echocardiographic correlates of left ventricular structure among 844 mildly hypertensive men and women in the Treatment of Mild Hypertension Study (TOMHS). *Circulation* 1993;87:476–486.

105. Imbriglia JE. Pathology of hypertension as a generalized vascular disease. In: Moyer JH, ed. *Hypertension: the First Hahnemann Symposium on Hypertensive Disease*. Philadelphia: W.B. Saunders; 1959:3–8.
106. Moritz AR, Oldt MR. Arteriolar sclerosis in hypertensive and non-hypertensive individuals. *Am J Pathol* 1937;13:679–728.
107. Kernohan JW, Anderson EW, Keith NM. The arterioles in cases of hypertension. *Arch Intern Med* 1929;44:395–423.
108. Morlock CG. Arterioles of the pancreas, liver, gastrointestinal tract and spleen in hypertension. *Arch Intern Med* 1939;63:100–118.
109. Tanaka M, Fujiwara H, Onodera T, et al. Quantitative analysis of narrowing of intramyocardial small arteries in normal hearts, hypertensive hearts, and hearts with hypertrophic cardiomyopathy. *Circulation* 1987;75:1130–1139.
110. Mulvaney MJ. Contractile properties of resistance vessels related to cellular function. In: Lee RMKW, ed. *Blood vessel changes in hypertension: structure and function*. Vol. 1. Boca Raton, FL: CRC Press; 1989:1–24.
111. Ito H. Vascular connective tissue changes in hypertension. In: Lee RMKW, ed. *Blood vessel changes in hypertension: structure and function*. Vol. 1. Boca Raton, FL: CRC Press; 1989:99–122.
112. Strauer BE. Development of cardiac failure by coronary small vessel disease in hypertensive heart disease? *J Hypertens* 1991;9[Suppl 2]:S11–S21.
113. Pearlman ES, Weber KT, Janicki JS, Pietra G, Fishman AP. Muscle fiber orientation and connective tissue content in the hypertrophied human heart. *Lab Invest* 1982;46:158–164.
114. Huysman JAN, Vliegen HW, Van der Laarse A, Eulderink F. Changes in nonmyocyte tissue composition associated with pressure overload of hypertrophic human hearts. *Pathol Res Pract* 1989;184:577–581.
115. Anderson KR, St. John Sutton MG, Lie JT. Histopathological types of cardiac fibrosis in myocardial disease. *J Pathol* 1979;128:79–85.
116. Campbell SE, Weber KT, Motz W, Krayenbuehl HP. Myocardial fibrosis in hypertensive patients with cardiac hypertrophy: assessment using endomyocardial biopsy. *J Am Coll Cardiol* 1993;21 [Suppl A]:332A(abst).
117. Schwartzkopff B, Motz W, Vogt M, Strauer BE. Heart failure on the basis of hypertension. *Circulation* 1993;87[Suppl IV]:IV66–IV72.
118. Antony I, Nitenberg A, Foult J-M, Aptecar E. Coronary vasodilator reserve in untreated and treated hypertensive patients with and without left ventricular hypertrophy. *J Am Coll Cardiol* 1993;22:514–520.
119. Otterstad JE. Ischaemia and left ventriculary hypertrophy. *Eur Heart J* 1993;14[Suppl F]:2–6.
120. Scheler S, Motz W, Strauer BE. Transient myocardial ischaemia in hypertensives: missing link with left ventricular hypertrophy. *Eur Heart J* 1992;13[Suppl D]:62–65.
121. Mansour P, Bostrom PA, Mattiasson I, Lilja B, Berglund G. Low blood pressure levels and signs of myocardial ischaemia: importance of left ventricular hypertrophy. *J Human Hypertens* 1993;7: 13–18.
122. Silver MA, Pick R, Brilla CG, Jalil JE, Janicki JS, Weber KT. Reactive and reparative fibrosis in the hypertrophied rat left ventricle: two experimental models of myocardial fibrosis. *Cardiovasc Res* 1990;24:741–747.
123. Weber KT, Sun Y, Guarda E. Nonclassic actions of angiotensin II and aldosterone in nonclassic target tissue (the heart): relevance to hypertensive heart disease. In: Laragh JH, Brenner BM, eds. *Hypertension: pathophysiology, diagnosis, and management*. 2nd ed. v. 2. New York: Raven Press; 1995;2203–23.
124. Jalil JE, Janicki JS, Pick R, Abrahams C, Weber KT. Fibrosis-induced reduction of endomyocardium in the rat after isoproterenol treatment. *Circ Res* 1989;65:258–264.
125. Ohsato K, Shimizu M, Sugihara N, Konishi K, Takeda R. Histopathological factors related to diastolic function in myocardial hypertrophy. *Jpn Circ J* 1992;56:325–333.
126. Sugihara N, Genda A, Shimizu M, et al. Diastolic dysfunction and its relation to myocardial fibrosis in essential hypertension. *J Cardiol* 1988;18:353–361.
127. Campbell SE, Diaz-Arias AA, Weber KT. Fibrosis of the human heart and systemic organs in adrenal adenoma. *Blood Pressure* 1992;1:149–156.
128. Borg TK, Ranson WF, Moshlehy FA, Caulfield JB. Structural basis of ventricular stiffness. *Lab Invest* 1981;44:49–54.

129. Weber KT, Janicki JS, Shroff SG, Pick R, Chen RM, Bashey RI. Collagen remodeling of the pressure-overloaded, hypertrophied nonhuman primate myocardium. *Circ Res* 1988;62:757–765.
130. Burton AC. Relation of structure to function of the tissues of the wall of blood vessels. *Physiol Rev* 1954;34:619–642.
131. Averill DB, Ferrario CM, Tarazi RC, Sen S, Bajbus R. Cardiac performance in rats with renal hypertension. *Circ Res* 1976;38:280–288.
132. Thiedemann KU, Holubarsch C, Medugorac I, Jacob R. Connective tissue content and myocardial stiffness in pressure overload hypertrophy. A combined study of morphologic, morphometric, biochemical and mechanical parameters. *Basic Res Cardiol* 1983;78:140–155.
133. Doering CW, Jalil JE, Janicki JS, et al. Collagen network remodeling and diastolic stiffness of the rat left ventricle with pressure overload hypertrophy. *Cardiovasc Res* 1988;22:686–695.
134. Jalil JE, Doering CW, Janicki JS, Pick R, Shroff SG, Weber KT. Fibrillar collagen and myocardial stiffness in the intact hypertrophied rat left ventricle. *Circ Res* 1989;64:1041–1050.
135. Weber KT, Janicki JS, Pick R, Capasso J, Anversa P. Myocardial fibrosis and pathologic hypertrophy in the rat with renovascular hypertension. *Am J Cardiol* 1990;65:1G–7G.
136. Capasso JM, Palackal T, Olivetti G, Anversa P. Left ventricular failure induced by long term hypertension in rats. *Circ Res* 1990;66:1400–1412.
137. Bing OHL, Sen S, Conrad CH, Brooks WW. Myocardial function structure and collagen in the spontaneously hypertensive rat: progression from compensated hypertrophy to haemodynamic impairment. *Eur Heart J* 1984;5[Suppl F]:43–52.
138. Brutsaert DL, Sys SU, Gillebert TC. Diastolic failure: pathophysiology and therapeutic implications. *J Am Coll Cardiol* 1993;22:318–325.
139. Jalil JE, Janicki JS, Pick R, Weber KT. Coronary vascular remodeling and myocardial fibrosis in the rat with renovascular hypertension: response to captopril. *Am J Hypertens* 1991;4:51–55.
140. Marino TA, Kent RL, Uboh CE, Fernandez E, Thompson EW, Cooper G. Structural analysis of pressure versus volume overload hypertrophy of cat right ventricle. *Am J Physiol* 1985;18:H371–H379.
141. Tomanek RJ, Palmer PJ, Peiffer GL, Schreiber KL, Eastham CL, Marcus ML. Morphometry of canine coronary arteries, arterioles, and capillaries during hypertension and left ventricular hypertrophy. *Circ Res* 1986;58:38–46.
142. Narayan S, Janicki JS, Shroff SG, Pick R, Weber KT. Myocardial collagen and mechanics after preventing hypertrophy in hypertensive rats. *Am J Hypertens* 1989;2:675–682.
143. Brilla CG, Janicki JS, Weber KT. Cardioreparative effects of lisinopril in rats with genetic hypertension and left ventricular hypertrophy. *Circulation* 1991;83:1771–1779.
144. Weber KT, Brilla CG, Janicki JS. Structural remodeling of myocardial collagen in systemic hypertension: functional consequences and potential therapy. *Heart Failure* 1990;6:129–137.
145. Jalil JE, Doering CW, Janicki JS, Pick R, Clark WA, Weber KT. Structural vs. contractile protein remodeling and myocardial stiffness in hypertrophied rat left ventricle. *J Mol Cell Cardiol* 1988; 20:1179–1187.
146. Brilla CG, Pick R, Tan LB, Janicki JS, Weber KT. Remodeling of the rat right and left ventricle in experimental hypertension. *Circ Res* 1990;67:1355–1364.
147. Michel JB, Salzmann JL, Ossondo Nlom M, Bruneval P, Barres D, Camilleri JP. Morphometric analysis of collagen network and plasma perfused capillary bed in the myocardium of rats during evolution of cardiac hypertrophy. *Basic Res Cardiol* 1986;81:142–154.
148. Buccino RA, Harris E, Spann JF, Sonnenblick EH. Response of myocardial connective tissue to development of experimental hypertrophy. *Am J Physiol* 1969;216:425–428.
149. Davis JO, Howell DS, Southworth JL. Mechanisms of fluid and electrolyte retention in experimental preparations in dogs. III. Effect of adrenalectomy and subsequent desoxycorticosterone acetate administration on ascites formation. *Circ Res* 1953;1:260–270.
150. Lindy S, Turto H, Uitto J. Protocollagen proline hydroxylase activity in rat heart during experimental cardiac hypertrophy. *Circ Res* 1972;30:205–209.
151. Turto H. Collagen metabolism in experimental cardiac hypertrophy in the rat and effect of digitoxin treatment. *Cardiovasc Res* 1977;11:358–366.
152. Chapman D, Weber KT, Eghbali M. Regulation of fibrillar collagen types I and III and basement membrane type IV collagen gene expression in pressure overloaded rat myocardium. *Circ Res* 1990;67:787–794.
153. Weber KT, Pick R, Silver MA, et al. Fibrillar collagen and the remodeling of the dilated canine left ventricle. *Circulation* 1990;82:1387–1401.

154. Bartosova D, Chvapil M, Korecky B, et al. The growth of the muscular and collagenous parts of the rat heart in various forms of cardiomegaly. *J Physiol* 1969;200:285–295.
155. Holubarsch C, Holubarsch T, Jacob R, Medugorac I, Thiedemann K. Passive elastic properties of myocardium in different models and stages of hypertrophy: a study comparing mechanical, chemical and morphometric parameters. In: Alpert NR, ed. *Myocardial hypertrophy and failure.* New York: Raven Press; 1983:323–336. (Katz AM, ed; *Perspectives in cardiovascular research;* vol 7).
156. Hall CE, Hall O. Hypertension and hypersalimentation. I. Aldosterone hypertension. *Lab Invest* 1965;14:285–294.
157. Selye H. The general adaptation syndrome and the diseases of adaptation. *J Clin Endocrinol* 1946;6:117–230.
158. Brilla CG, Matsubara LS, Weber KT. Anti-aldosterone treatment and the prevention of myocardial fibrosis in primary and secondary hyperaldosteronism. *J Mol Cell Cardiol* 1993;25:563–575.
159. Weber KT, Brilla CG, Campbell SE, Guarda E, Zhou G, Sriram K. Myocardial fibrosis: role of angiotensin II and aldosterone. *Basic Res Cardiol* 1993;88[Suppl]:107–124.
160. Ratajska A, Campbell SE, Cleutjens JPM, Weber KT. Angiotensin II and structural remodeling of coronary vessels in rats. *J Lab Clin Med* 1994;124:408–15.
161. Brilla CG, Weber KT. Reactive and reparative myocardial fibrosis in arterial hypertension in the rat. *Cardiovasc Res* 1992;26:671–677.
162. Darrow DC, Miller HC. The production of cardiac lesions by repeated injections of desoxycorticosterone acetate. *J Clin Invest* 1942;21:601–611.
163. Campbell SE, Janicki JS, Matsubara BB, Weber KT. Myocardial fibrosis in the rat with mineralocorticoid excess: prevention of scarring by amiloride. *Am J Hypertens* 1993;6:487–495.
164. Potts JL, Dalakos TG, Streeten DHP, Jones D. Cardiomyopathy in an adult with Bartter's syndrome: hemodynamic, angiographic, and metabolic studies. *Am J Cardiol* 1977;40:995–999.
165. Campbell SE, Farb A, Weber KT. Pathologic remodeling of the myocardium in a weightlifter taking anabolic steroids. *Blood Pressure* 1993;2:213–216.
166. Fink CS, Gallant S, Brownie AC. Peripheral serum corticosteroid concentrations in relation to the rat adrenal cortical circadian rhythm in androgen-induced hypertension. *Hypertension* 1980;2:617–622.
167. Todd GL, Baroldi G, Pieper GM, Clayton FC, Eliot RS. Experimental catecholamine-induced myocardial necrosis. I. Morphology, quantification and regional distribution of acute contraction band lesions. *J Mol Cell Cardiol* 1985;17:317–338.
168. Todd GL, Baroldi G, Pieper GM, Clayton FC, Eliot RS. Experimental catecholamine-induced myocardial necrosis. II. Temporal development of isoproterenol-induced contraction band lesions correlated with ECG, hemodynamic and biochemical changes. *J Mol Cell Cardiol* 1985;17:647–656.
169. Pfeffer JM, Pfeffer MA, Fishbein MC, Froehlich ED. Cardiac function and morphology with aging in the spontaneously hypertensive rat. *Am J Physiol* 1979;6:H461–H468.
170. Brilla CG, Janicki JS, Weber KT. Impaired diastolic function and coronary reserve in genetic hypertension: role of interstitial fibrosis and medial thickening of intramyocardial coronary arteries. *Circ Res* 1991;69:107–115.
171. Asaad MM, Antonaccio MJ. Vascular wall renin in spontaneously hypertensive rats. Potential relevance to hypertension maintenance and antihypertensive effect of captopril. *Hypertension* 1982;4:487–493.
172. Pahor M, Bernabei R, Sgadari A, et al. Enalapril prevents cardiac fibrosis and arrhythmias in hypertensive rats. *Hypertension* 1991;18:148–157.
173. Sen S, Bumpus FM. Collagen synthesis in development and reversal of cardiac hypertrophy in spontaneously hypertensive rats. *Am J Cardiol* 1979;44:954–958.
174. Lund DD, Twietmeyer TA, Schmid PG, Tomanek RJ. Independent changes in cardiac muscle fibres and connective tissue in rats with spontaneous hypertension, aortic constriction and hypoxia. *Cardiovasc Res* 1979;13:39–44.
175. Kozlovskis PL, Fieber LA, Pruitt DK, et al. Myocardial changes during the progression of left ventricular pressure-overload by renal hypertension or aortic constriction: myosin, myosin ATPase and collagen. *J Mol Cell Cardiol* 1987;19:105–114.

The Failing Heart, edited by N. S. Dhalla,
R. E. Beamish, N. Takeda, and M. Nagano.
Lippincott-Raven Publishers, Philadelphia © 1995.

14

Structural Basis and Consequences of Ventricular Remodeling following Acute Myocardial Infarction

Edmund H. Sonnenblick, *Giorgio Olivetti, *Federico Quaini,
*Peng Li, and *Piero Anversa

*Department of Medicine, The Albert Einstein College of Medicine,
Bronx, New York 10461 United States; and *Department of Medicine,
New York Medical College, Valhalla, New York 10595 United States*

Aside from less common unexplained cardiomyopathies and unrelieved pressure and volume overloads, most cases of heart failure result from ischemic heart disease. The pathology of ischemic heart disease involves a substantial amount of the myocardium replaced by fibrous tissue with the remaining myocytes inadequate in number or capacity to maintain required cardiac pump function despite various adaptations, including reactive myocyte hypertrophy (1). Experimental acute myocardial infarction and its sequelae, as studied in the rat, provides the clearest model of this process (2–5). Following obstruction of a coronary artery, ischemia develops in the anatomical region supplied by the artery involved with survival of myocardium in the region at risk, determined by residual blood flow, whether from existing collaterals or reperfusion of the obstructed artery, with a time limitation for survival measured in a few hours. Although in humans and dogs, collateral blood flow may be substantial, resulting in significant survival of epicardial tissue, in the rat, which has served as a model for these events, there are no significant collaterals, and a well-defined transmural myocardial infarction ensues following ligation of a coronary artery (2). This has made the rat model of acute myocardial infarction particularly attractive for quantitative analysis of structured alterations that follow the acute event (2,4–7). Following ligation of the left anterior descending coronary artery in the rat, the ejection fraction falls as a direct function of an increasing size of the infarct (8). Pump function is maintained by an increase in the end-diastolic volume of the heart with myocyte elongation, largely due to expansion of the remaining well-perfused myocardium. In the perfused portion of the ventricle, increased force of contraction and enhanced shortening occurs (Frank–Starling Relation) and stroke volume is preserved. Depending on the size of the infarct, substantial changes in the pressure volume relations of the ventricle occur over a period of time (9–11). With small infarcts, elevations of left ventricular diastolic filling pressures are small, and with apparent shrinkage of the infarction scar, the pressure–volume curve of the left ventricle is unaltered or actually moves to the left (10,12). With larger infarctions, diastolic filling pressures are elevated, and a progressive rightward movement of the pressure volume curve occurs so that there is an increased diastolic volume for any given filling pressure (10).

Such increases in diastolic volumes and filling pressures create important consequences related to the ultimate development of clinical heart failure. Given the LaPlace Relation (12), major increases in tension occur in the ventricular wall as a function of increased diastolic filling pressure. In diastole, as will be discussed later, such augmented tensions may result in myocyte distortion and myocyte death, progressive ventricular dilation, and functional mitral insufficiency. A shift to the right in the equilibrium volume of the ventricle (Vo), the volume at zero filling pressure, may also alter diastolic recoil and thus reduce early ventricular filling, with a resultant rise in mean filling pressures.

Against this background, we have studied the structural alterations that occur in the ventricular wall, following induction of an acute myocardial infarction in the rat, using quantitative morphometry preceded by careful hemodynamic measurements and subsequent perfusion fixation of the heart under controlled conditions (6,7). This has permitted cross-correlations of physiologic measurements with ultrastructured changes following an acute myocardial infarction. Two days following proximal ligation of the left anterior descending coronary artery in the rat, where 40% of the animals do not survive, a large infarction of the anterior wall of the left ventricle occurs involving approximately 55% of the ventricular free wall of the ventricle (i.e., left ventricle less the septum) (6). In survivors, hemodynamic measurements showed a 30% decrease in left ventricular dp/dt with an eightfold increase in the left ventricular end-diastolic pressure (LVEDP). The ventricles were fixed at Vo and even at 2 days, a large increase in chamber volume (Vo) was observed, accompanied by an expected concomitant decrease in left ventricular wall thickness. This resulted in a 700% to 800% increase in the stress in the ventricular wall *in diastole*, as calculated from the Laplace Relation (6). In contrast, the ventricular wall stress in systole was increased by a trivial 10%. Thus, the increase in tension faced by the ventricle following a large infarction occurs in diastole, not in systole. At a structural level, certain natural consequences occur from this acute increase in diastolic ventricular wall stress. First, an increase in myocyte volume occurs, even by 2 days. This amounted to 22% in the free wall and 16% in the septum. The major part of this change is an increase in myocyte length of 12%, although a minor increase in width of 6.5% was observed. Of note, sarcomere length at Vo was unchanged, averaging 2.04 μm, a value consonant with measurements of sarcomere length in normal diastole in the dog (15). These changes in overall geometry of the ventricle are consistent with *eccentric hypertrophy*, as is observed primarily with a volume overload. Integrity of other cytoplasmic components, such as mitochondria and matrix, is well preserved with a lack of edema.

With an abrupt increase in diastolic wall stress, the sarcomeres and myocytes could not elongate adequately in this initial stage, and major alterations in the organizational structure of the wall were seen. Supporting this view is the increase in Vo with the same sarcomere length. The increase in Vo was accompanied by a 36% decrease in the number of myocytes remaining *across* the free wall of the ventricle, supporting the view that "myocyte slippage" (as we have termed this process) had occurred. Due to this decrease in myocytes across the ventricular wall, the stress for each myocyte is further augmented (6). This augmented stress is greatest in the endocardial layers of the ventricular wall. Augmented diastolic stress with myocyte slippage helps to create a vicious cycle for progressive ventricular dilatation following infarction.

The process of myocyte slippage, combined with reactive myocyte growth, composes the process of ventricular remodeling. For slippage to occur, it is probable that myocytes arranged in series would need to disengage or die. With this in mind, we have observed death of single myocytes (16), which could result directly from massive, acute overstretching of myocytes, that is, mechanical cell death (Sonnenblick et al., *submitted for publication*). Such a process would serve to further amplify the infarction itself and could add to progressive ventricular dilation. How this is mediated is currently being studied in our laboratory, but may produce substantial damage in what has usually been thought to be preserved tissue.

It is also of interest that when myocytes have been isolated from the surviving myocardium in the first few days (Sonnenblick et al., *submitted for publication*), as well as 1 week (17) after the infarction, mechanical performance is reduced relative to that observed in sham-operated animals. This decreased extent shortening and velocity of shortening is observed in myocytes isolated from well-perfused regions of the myocardium, well away from the infarcted region. This reduced contractility occurs before substantial cellular hypertrophy has evolved. The biochemical basis and course with time of these alterations have not been defined. Thus, there are important *qualitative* changes in surviving myocytes following infarction as well as a *quantitative* problem of myocyte loss, even in the surviving "normal" myocardium that remains.

To study ventricular remodeling once the infarcted region has healed, hearts have been studied 40 days after ligation of the left anterior descending coronary artery (7). Infarcts were segregated as small, involving 38% of the left ventricular free wall (or about 25% of the total left ventricle), and as large, involving about 60% of the left ventricular free wall (or 40% of the total left ventricle). Small infarcts resulted in minor hemodynamic changes, with LVEDP remaining normal, while large infarcts were associated with a marked increase in left ventricular filling pressures rising from 3 to 17 mmHg. Consequently, only a 6% increase in ventricular chamber diameter was found with small infarcts, but a substantial 27% increase was observed with large infarcts. The result of these changes in ventricular volume and wall thickness was to produce a 2.3-fold increase in calculated wall stress in small infarcts and a ninefold increase with large infarcts. With large infarcts, an 81% increase in the ventricular cavity was found, but unlike with a small infarct, the ratio of myocardial mass to volume actually decreased. The consequence was a 50% decrease in the mass/chamber ratio with large infarcts that did not occur with small infarcts. Thus, in small infarcts, the extent of reactive myocardial hypertrophy was adequate to offset increments in diastolic volume so that mass/volume ratios were preserved. In large infarcts, the extent of hypertrophy was less than the increase in volume such that mass/volume decreased. This defines *decompensated eccentric hypertrophy* in response to very large infarctions, which is an inadequate response to a volume overload.

In terms of structural changes, myocytes in the free wall increased in volume: 43% in small infarcts and 81% in large infarcts. The major part of this enlargement was in myocyte length rather than in width. Sarcomere length was not increased at Vo despite the fact that Vo was markedly increased. When myocyte slippage was studied in these healed large infarcts, an 11% decrease in myocytes across the wall was determined, although this was not observed with small infarcts. This degree of myocyte slippage is substantially less than that observed in acute studies at 2 days (6), as noted previously, which raises the possibility that reversal of myocyte slippage can occur as permitted by progressive myocyte elongation. The mechanism by which this can occur has yet to be defined.

As with the acute infarction, even after 40 days, the increase in diastolic left ventricular filling pressures and volumes resulted in persistent massive increments in diastolic wall tension, increasing from the epicardium to the endocardium. These observations are consistent with other studies that show a rightward shift of the left ventricular pressure–volume curve as a function of infarct size and time after infarction.

It has been generally assumed that following an acute myocardial infarction, the remaining, normally perfused myocardium would manifest normal contractile activity. Because the posterior papillary muscle is largely outside the ischemic region, we undertook to study this muscle in vitro, using methods previously employed. Unfortunately, contractile activity was very variable and generally substantially reduced in the first few days after infarction. Moreover, structural studies revealed significant amounts of damage in the muscles which vitiated quantitative analysis of contractile function. Accordingly, we have studied contractile behavior of isolated myocytes from the noninfarcted portions of the ventricular wall. One week after a large acute myocardial infarction, when severe left ventricular dysfunction was evident, a substantial depression of myocyte contractile function was present (17). This was characterized by a 40% decrease in extent of shortening and a 46% decrease in peak velocity of shortening. Such changes are associated with substantial myocyte elongation appropriate to the eccentric hypertrophy associated with large infarctions, as discussed previously. It is of interest that captopril administration partially prevented the structural alterations as well as the contractility depression (17). The mechanism by which contractile function is reduced is not clear. Current studies (Sonnenblick et al., *unpublished data*) would support the view that excessive diastolic stretch of the myocardium produces irreversible damage to myocytes.

Using the foregoing observations, we have concluded that a large myocardial infarction of the left ventricle imposes primarily a major volume load on the ventricle, the response to which is primarily myocyte lengthening (eccentric hypertrophy). Myocyte thickening with lateral growth takes place to a lesser degree because the excess load in systole is modest. Acute, large diastolic loads may produce mechanical death of myocytes with associated myocyte slippage and ventricular wall thinning (i.e., decompensated eccentric hypertrophy). Complex growth factors, including angiotensin II, contribute to these changes, and blockade of angiotensin II activation modifies these events. It is unclear why myocyte function in mechanically stretched but well-perfused regions of the ventricle is also reduced, but this qualitative deficit may add importantly to the quantitative deficit of losing myocytes.

SUMMARY

The studies cited above provide a structural basis for understanding some of the factors that produce the evolution of myocyte loss as illustrated by the progression of acute myocardial infarction to progressive ventricular dilatation and congestive failure. With substantial myocyte loss, the greatest load on the myocardium is in *diastole*. Acutely, myocyte stretch is accompanied by "myocyte slippage" and myocyte death in well-perfused myocardium. If reactive hypertrophy is inadequate, decompensated eccentric ventricular hypertrophy and failure ensues. Dysfunction is not only quantitative but qualitative, since contractile depression occurs in even the well-perfused remaining myocardium, perhaps also as a result of excessive diastolic stretch.

Such findings lend support to the view that after a large infarction filling pressures should be controlled, initially with nitrates (19) and subsequently with angiotensin-converting enzyme (ACE) inhibitors (20) in order to vitiate ventricular remodeling (21–23). This forms a logical basis for the promising studies of the use of ACE inhibitors in reduction of post-infarction mortality in man (24).

ACKNOWLEDGMENTS

This work was supported by grants HL38132, HL39902, HL40561, and HL37412 from the National Heart, Lung, and Blood Institute.

REFERENCES

1. Anversa P, Capasso J, Puntillo E, Sonnenblick EH, Olivetti G. Morphometric analysis of the infarcted heart. *Pathol Res Pract* 1989;185:544–550.
2. Anversa P, Loud AV, Levicky V, Guideri G. Left ventricular failure induced by myocardial infarction. I. Myocyte hypertrophy. *Am J Physiol* 1985;248 (*Heart Circ Physiol* 17):H876–H882.
3. Pfeffer MA, Pfeffer JM, Fishbein MC, et al. Myocardial infarct size and ventricular function in rats. *Circ Res* 1979;44:503–512.
4. Pfeffer MA and Pfeffer JM. Ventricular enlargement following a myocardial infarction. *J Cardiovasc Pharmacol* 1987;9[Suppl 2]:S18–S20.

5. Anversa P, Beghi C, Kikkawa Y, Olivetti G. Myocardial infarction in rats. Infarct size, myocyte hypertrophy, and capillary growth. *Circ Res* 1986;58:26–37.
6. Olivetti G, Capasso JM, Sonnenblick EH, Anversa P. Side-to-side slippage of myocytes participates in ventricular wall remodeling acutely after myocardial infarction in rats. *Circ Res* 1990;67:23–34.
7. Olivetti G, Capasso JM, Meggs LG, Sonnenblick EH, Anversa P. Cellular basis of chronic ventricular remodeling after myocardial infarction in rats. *Circ Res* 1991;68:856–869.
8. McKay RG, Pfeffer MA, Pasternak RC, et al. Left ventricular remodeling after myocardial infarction: a corollary to infarct expansion. *Circulation* 1986;74(4):693–702.
9. Pfeffer JM, Pfeffer MA, Braunwald E. Influence of chronic captopril therapy on infarcted left ventricle of the rat. *Circ Res* 1985;57:84–95.
10. Pfeffer JM, Pfeffer MA, Fletcher PJ, Braunwald E. Progressive ventricle remodeling in rat with myocardial infarction. *Am J Physiol* 1991;260(*Heart Circ Physiol* 29):H1401–H1414.
11. Pfeffer MA, Pfeffer JM, Lamas GA. Development and prevention of congestive heart failure following myocardial infarction. *Circulation* 1993;87 [Suppl IV]:IV-120–IV-125.
12. Gaudron P, Eilles C, Ertl G, Kochsiek K. Early remodelling of the left ventricle in patients with myocardial infarction. *Eur Heart J* 1990;11 [Suppl B]:139–146.
13. Sonnenblick EH, Strobeck JE, Capasso JM, Factor SM. Ventricular hypertrophy: models and methods. NIH workshop on hypertrophy, Sept. 21–22, 1981, Bethesda, Maryland. *Perspectives in cardiovasc res*. Vol 8, edited by Tarazi RC, Dunbar JB, pp. 13–20. New York: Raven Press; 1983.
14. Yellin EL, Sonnenblick EH, Frater RWM. Dynamic determinants of left ventricular filling. In Baan, Artzenius, Yellin, eds. *Cardiac dynamics*. The Hague: Martinus Nijhoff; 1980:158.
15. Ross J Jr, Sonnenblick EH, Taylor RR, Spotnitz HM, Covell JW. Diastolic geometry and sarcomere lengths in the chronically dilated canine left ventricle. *Circ Res* 1971;28:49–61.
16. Capasso JM, Li P, Anversa P. Non-ischemic myocardial damage induced by non-occlusive constriction of coronary artery in rats. *Am J Physiol* 1991;29:H651–H661.
17. Capasso JM, Anversa P. Mechanical performance of spared myocytes after myocardial infarction in rats: effects of captopril treatment. *Am J Physiol* 1992;263:H841–H849.
18. Meggs LG, Coupet J, Huang H, et al. Regulation of angiotensin II receptors on ventricular myocytes after myocardial infarction in rats. *Circ Res* 1993;72:1149–1162.
19. Bodh IJ, Warnica W. Intravenous nitroglycerin therapy to limit myocardial infarct size, expansion, and complications. Effect of timing, dosage, and infarct location. *Circulation* 1988;78:906–919.
20. Pfeffer MA, Braunwald E. Ventricular remodeling after myocardial infarction. *Circulation* 1990; 81:1161–1172.
21. Capasso JM, Li P, Zhang X, Anversa P. Heterogeneity of ventricular remodeling after acute myocardial infarction in rats. *Am J Physiol* 1992;262(*Heart Circ Physiol* 31):H486–H495.
22. Visser CA, Delemarre BJ, Peels K. Left ventricular remodeling following anterior wall myocardial infarction. *Am J Cardiac Imaging* 1992;6(2):127–133.
23. Weisman HF, Bush DE, Mannisi JA, Weisfeldt ML, Healy B. Cellular mechanisms of myocardial infarct expansion. *Circulation* 1988;78:186–201.
24. Pfeffer MA, Gervasio AL, Vaughan DE, Parisi AF, Braunwald E. Effect of captopril on progressive ventricular dilatation after anterior myocardial infarction. *N Engl J Med* 1988;319:80–86.

The Failing Heart, edited by N. S. Dhalla,
R. E. Beamish, N. Takeda, and M. Nagano.
Lippincott-Raven Publishers, Philadelphia © 1995.

15

Prevention and Reversal of Ventricular Remodeling: Experimental and Clinical Observations

Jay N. Cohn

Department of Medicine, Cardiovascular Division, University of Minnesota Medical School, Minneapolis, Minnesota 55455 United States

Patients with heart failure usually exhibit a reduction of left ventricular ejection fraction, which serves as a guide to the severity of left ventricular dysfunction. The magnitude of reduction of ejection fraction is a powerful predictor of mortality rate in this syndrome (1). Although a reduced ejection fraction is often assumed to reflect an impairment of myocardial contractility, the major contributor to this ejection fraction decrease now is known to be an increase in end-diastolic volume. This volume increase does not relate to an increase in sarcomere length, but actually results from a process that can be called *ventricular remodeling*. Consequently, the prognosis in patients with heart failure appears to be related directly to the left ventricular remodeling process.

EXPERIMENTAL VENTRICULAR REMODELING

An experimental canine model of left ventricular remodeling has been developed in the laboratory at the University of Minnesota Medical School to explore the mechanisms and potential therapeutic response. Localized left ventricular damage is produced by repetitive DC shock using a wire electrode advance retrograde into the left ventricle and a paddle placed on the left ventricular apex in the anesthetized dog (2). One 80-J shock per kilogram body weight produces a transmural scar averaging approximately 18% of the left ventricular myocardium and usually occupying the anteroapical portion of the left ventricle. After induction of this scar, a global left ventricular remodeling process is initiated that results 4 mo later in a dilated and hypertrophied left ventricle with global systolic dysfunction, as reflected by a reduced left ventricular ejection fraction. The syndrome produced by this single episode of localized myocardial damage is similar to the syndrome of asymptomatic left ventricular dysfunction observed in patients after an acute myocardial infarction. Plasma norepinephrine is elevated and left ventricular end-diastolic pressure is elevated. Most importantly, the syndrome appears to be progressive because the left ventricular ejection fraction continues to decline and the left ventricle continues to dilate during the first year after the damage is produced.

Several pharmacologic interventions have been tested in the early phase of remodeling. When instituted the day following induction of the left ventricular damage, converting-enzyme inhibitors (3) and nitrates (4) administered over a 3-month period of time completely inhibit the hypertrophy and dilatation. The mechanism of this favorable effect is not entirely clear because it may involve both a reduction of hemodynamic load and an effect on neurohormonal or local tissue hormonal activity. Nonetheless, these intervention data demonstrate that the process of remodeling does not require a continuing external stimulus and that the remodeling process can be pharmacologically inhibited.

CLINICAL REMODELING

In the Vasodilator Heart Failure Trial (V-HeFT), radionuclide left ventricular ejection fraction was monitored sequentially in a large number of patients with clinical heart failure. In V-HeFT I, a placebo group of 243 patients receiving only digoxin and diuretic exhibited a progressive decline over 5 years of follow-up in left ventricular ejection (5). Both enalapril and the combination of hydralazine and isosorbide dinitrate resulted in a sustained increase in left ventricular ejection fraction and prevention of the progressive decline (6) observed in the placebo group. These data support the animal research, indicating that even in clinical cardiac disease, the remodeling process is progressive and can be inhibited pharmacologically.

In V-HeFT, both interventions that inhibited progressive remodeling were associated with a reduction of mortality rate. Indeed, the magnitude of improvement in left ventricular ejection fraction in response to therapy was strikingly correlated with the benefit on survival (7). Consequently, these data support the concept that left ventricular remodeling is an unwanted progressive process in patients with heart failure and that therapeutic interventions effective in slowing or reversing this remodeling process should have a favorable effect on prognosis.

A clinical model more consistent with the canine model developed in our laboratory is the study of interventions introduced immediately after acute myocardial infarction. In both the Acute Infarction Ramipril Efficacy (AIRE) and Survival and Ventricular Enlargement (SAVE) studies, converting-enzyme inhibitors introduced early after acute myocardial infarction prevented or slowed progressive left ventricular remodeling and reduced mortality rate (8–10).

STRUCTURAL BASIS OF REMODELING

The precise structural basis of the remodeling process that results in dilation of the left ventricular chamber is unresolved. Protein synthesis resulting in sarcomeres being laid down in series with the existing sarcomere structure would lead to lengthening of the myofiber and an increase in chamber circumference (11). This myocyte hypertrophy process accounts for at least some of the increase in chamber volume in both clinical and experimental remodeling, because isolated myocytes in both human and animal experiments exhibit lengthening. Myocyte slippage and interstitial growth also may be factors in the remodeling process, but are more difficult to quantitate. The mechanism by which pharmacologic agents inhibit this remodeling process, or even reverse it, has not been established. Such information is critical for better definition of the syndrome and for the development of more selective interventions to affect it favorably.

SUMMARY

Mortality in patients with heart failure is related to pump failure or sudden electrical events. Both of these endpoints are directly correlated with the severity of left ventricular dilatation and thus the magnitude of left ventricular remodeling. Because it now appears that these structural alterations can respond to pharmacologic intervention, the opportunity to profoundly affect the development of heart failure and mortality from heart disease is now clearly before us.

REFERENCES

1. Cohn JN, Johnson GR, Shabetai R, et al., for the V-HeFT VA Cooperative Studies Group. Ejection fraction, peak exercise oxygen consumption, cardiothoracic ratio, ventricular arrhythmias and plasma norepinephrine as determinants of prognosis in heart failure. *Circulation* 1993;87:VI-5–VI-16.
2. Carlyle PF, Cohn JN. A non-surgical canine model of chronic left ventricular myocardial dysfunction. *Am J Physiol* 1983;244:H769–H774.
3. McDonald KM, Garr M, Carlyle PF, et al. Relative effects of α_1 adrenoceptor blockade, converting enzyme inhibitor therapy, and angiotensin II subtype 1 receptor blockade on ventricular remodeling in the dog. *Circulation* 1994;90:3034–3046.
4. McDonald KM, Francis GS, Matthews JH, Hunter D, Cohn JN. Long-term oral nitrate therapy prevents chronic ventricular remodeling in the dog. *J Am Coll Cardiol* 1993;21:514–522.
5. Cohn JN, Archibald DG, Ziesche S, et al. Effect of vasodilator therapy on mortality in chronic congestive heart failure. Results of a Veterans Administration Cooperative Study (V-HeFT). *N Engl J Med* 1986;314:1547–1552.
6. Cohn JN, Johnson G, Ziesche S, et al. A comparison of enalapril with hydralazine-isosorbide dinitrate in the treatment of chronic congestive heart failure. *N Engl J Med* 1991;325:303–310.
7. Cintron G, Johnson G, Francis G, Cobb F, Cohn JN, for the V-HeFT VA Cooperative Studies Group. Prognostic significance of serial changes in left ventricular ejection fraction in patients with congestive heart failure. *Circulation* 1993;87:VI-17–VI-23.
8. The Acute Infarction Ramipril Efficacy (AIRE) Study Investigators. Effect of ramipril on mortality and morbidity of survivors of acute myocardial infarction with clinical evidence of heart failure. *Lancet* 1993;342:821–828.

9. Pfeffer MA, Braunwald E, Moyé LA, et al., on behalf of the SAVE Investigators. The effect of captopril on mortality and morbidity in patients with left ventricular dysfunction following myocardial infarction: results of the survival and ventricular enlargement (SAVE) trial. *N Engl J Med* 1992; 327:669–677.
10. Sutton MSJ, Pfeffer MA, Plappert T, et al., for the SAVE Investigators. Quantitative two-dimensional echocardiographic measurements are major predictors of adverse cardiovascular events after acute myocardial infarction: the protective effects of captopril. *Circulation* 1994;89:68–75.
11. Anversa P, Ricci R, Olivetti G. Quantitative structural analysis of the myocardium during physiologic growth and induced cardiac hypertrophy: a review. *J Am Coll Cardiol* 1986;7:1140.

The Failing Heart, edited by N. S. Dhalla,
R. E. Beamish, N. Takeda, and M. Nagano.
Lippincott-Raven Publishers, Philadelphia © 1995.

16

Implications of Cardiomyocyte Remodeling in Heart Dysfunction

A. Martin Gerdes, *Scott E. Kellerman, and
†Douglas D. Schocken

*Department of Anatomy and Structural Biology, University of South Dakota
School of Medicine, Vermillion, South Dakota 57069 United States;
*Department of Pediatrics, Rainbow Babies and Childrens Hospital,
Cleveland, Ohio 44106 United States; and †Division of Cardiology,
Department of Internal Medicine, University of South Florida,
Tampa, Florida 33612 United States*

Ventricular dilation and an increase in the chamber radius:wall thickness ratio are common endpoints for congestive heart failure due to dilated cardiomyopathy (DCM) and ischemic cardiomyopathy (ICM) (1–3). Although the relative contributions of interstitial and myocyte remodeling to the dilation process are not clear, it is believed currently that slippage of cardiac myocytes past one another is largely responsible for the chamber dilation (4,5). Recent, isolated myocyte data from six patients with ischemic cardiomyopathy, however, suggest that increased myocyte lengthening alone (e.g., series addition of new sarcomere units) may account for chamber dilation in heart failure (6). Furthermore, the increased chamber radius:wall thickness ratio characteristic of this disease was reflected at the cellular level by an increase in myocyte length:width ratio. It is not known if similar changes in myocyte shape occur in other cardiac diseases that lead to chamber dilation and congestive heart failure.

In this study, changes in cardiac myocyte shape associated with DCM are reported for the first time. New data from patients with ICM are also included for comparison. Cellular dimensions were collected from myocytes isolated from freshly explanted hearts obtained through our cardiac transplantation program. Data from subjects with DCM and ICM were compared to similar data from five control subjects. Additionally, measures of left ventricular size and global left ventricular systolic function are included and compared with the isolated myocyte observations.

METHODS

Cell size data were collected in the following manner from controls (n = 5) and patients with failure due to dilated (n = 5) and ischemic (n = 5) cardiomyopathy. Transmural pieces of fresh tissue weighing approximately 25 g were rapidly excised from the left ventricular free wall (usually near the apex) and immediately placed into ice-cold cardioplegic solution for transportation to the research lab. The sampling site varied slightly because areas with obvious scarring were avoided. A coronary arterial branch was cannulated with P.E. 50 tubing for perfusion with media containing collagenase. If arterial branches were too small, an epicardial vein was cannulated for retrograde perfusion. Similar results were obtained with either arterial or venous perfusion. Distal, superficial branches were ligated to obtain improved perfusion of penetrating vessels. The cell isolation protocol, used previously to isolate myocytes from experimental animals, has been described in detail elsewhere (7). The cannulated vessel was perfused with calcium-free Joklik media containing 0.01 mM ethylene glycol bis (β-aminoethyl ether)-N,N,N^1,N^1-tetraacetic acid (EGTA) followed by Joklik media plus collagenase (Worthington Biochemical Company, Freehold, NJ; 200 U activity/ml). After approximately 20 to 30 minutes of collagenase perfusion, softened tissue was minced and poured through 250-μm nylon mesh to collect myocytes. Freshly isolated cardiac myocytes were fixed immediately in a manner that does not alter cell volume (8). The isolated cell suspensions were centrifuged through a Ficoll gradient to remove capillaries, blood cells, and other unwanted debris (7).

Cell volume was measured using a Coulter Channelyzer. The Coulter system determines cell volume by measuring the change in electrical resistance due to displacement of electrolyte as cells move through the aperture. The reliability of this method has been extensively documented (7). Values reported are the mean of three different sample sites within the perfused piece of tissue (sample sites were generally about 1 to 2 cm apart; approximately 12,000 cells were measured per sample site). Using a microscope, the maximum myocyte length parallel to the long axis was measured from 40 cells from each sample (120 cells per heart). Myocyte cross-sectional area was calculated from cell volume and length (cross-sectional area = volume/length). Therefore, calculations represent average values for myocyte cross-sectional area along the entire length of the cell. This method gives the same results as direct measurements obtained morphometrically from sectioned myocytes, if those measurements are corrected for all known sources of error and the sampling procedure provides a representative sample of cross-sectioned profiles (7). Myocyte diameter was also calculated from cross-sectional area using the formula for a circle (area = πr^2; diameter = 2r). Because there were no significant differences between sample sites within a given piece of perfused tissue, data were pooled.

Sarcomere length was measured using a Bioquant Meg IV image analysis system. Ten sarcomeres each were measured from 20 different myocytes from each heart. One-way ANOVA was used to compare individual data from the DCM, ICM, and control groups. When present, statistically significant differences were identified using Scheffe's test. Linear regression was used to compare changes in myocyte length to alterations in echocardiographically determined end-diastolic diameter and left ventricular ejection fraction determined by multigated radionuclide ventriculography (9).

RESULTS

Coronary artery disease was excluded as a potential cause of heart failure in all patients with DCM. Conversely, all hearts from patients with ICM had significant coronary artery disease. Left ventricular ejection fraction averaged 20% and 16% in patients with DCM and ICM, respectively (Table 1). Unsuitable donor hearts with widely patent coronary arteries, normal chamber volumes, and normal ejection fractions served as nonfailing controls.

Isolated cell preparations contained approximately 75% rod-shaped, structurally intact myocytes. Changes in left ventricular myocyte dimensions are shown in Table 2. There was a trend toward larger volumes, smaller widths, and smaller cross-sectional areas in isolated myocytes from patients with ICM and DCM, but the differences did not reach statistical significance. The shape of cardiac myocytes from patients with either DCM or ICM, however, significantly differed from controls. Although cell width was similar in all three groups, myocyte length was longer ($p<0.01$) and myocyte length:width ratio was substantially larger ($p< 0.01$) in patients with DCM and ICM. There were no significant differences in cellular dimensions between the DCM and ICM groups. Sarcomere length was similar in myocytes from each group.

Comparison of ventricular size and systolic function measurements to cellular dimensions disclosed several significant findings and trends. First, end-diastolic diameter was directly related to cell length ($p<0.05$) (Fig. 1). Second, when left ventricular ejection fraction was compared with cell length, a highly significant inverse relationship was seen ($p<0.001$) (Fig. 2). Clinical data from this study and the previous study (6) were pooled so that cellular and clinical changes could be correlated for the first time using linear regression analysis (Figs. 1 and 2). End-

TABLE 1. *Patient data*

Patient group	Age	Sex	BW (kg)	LVEF (%)
DCM (n = 5)				
Mean	38	4M, 1F	80	20
ICM (n = 5)				
Mean	51	5M	76	16
C (n = 5)				
Mean	43	1M, 4F	57	65

Data from patients with DCM, ICM, and unsuitable donors with patent coronary arteries and nonfailing, nondilated ventricles (C).
Body weight, BW; LVEF, left ventricular ejection fraction; M, male; F, female.

TABLE 2. *Isolated myocyte data*

Patient group	Cell volume (μm³)	Cell length (μm)	C.S. area (μm²)	Cell width (μm)	Cell L/W ratio	Sarcomere length (μm)
DCM (n = 5)						
Mean	48,670	194[a]	251	17.9	10.9[a]	2.04
± SE	3,417	6	14	0.5	0.4	0.01
% change from C	↑ 18	↑ 41	↓ 16	↓ 7	↑ 49	↑ 2
ICM (n = 5)						
Mean	53,190	194[a]	268	17.9	11.5[a]	2.06
± SE	13,157	6	60	2.2	1.4	0.01
% change from C	↑ 29	↑ 41	↓ 11	↓ 7	↑ 58	↑ 3
C (n = 5)						
Mean	41,387	138	300	19.3	7.3	2.00
± SE	6,281	5	43	1.4	0.5	0.02

[a]Indicates $p < 0.01$ vs. C.
L/W, length/width. C, unsuitable donors with patent coronary arteries and non-failing, non-dilated ventricles;

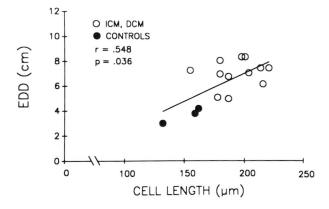

FIG. 1. Left ventricular end-diastolic diameter (EDD) versus cell length.

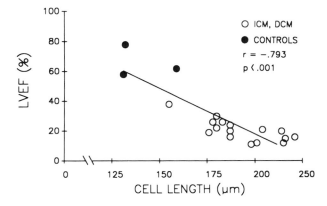

FIG. 2. Left ventricular ejection fraction (LVEF) versus cell length.

diastolic diameter measurements (Fig. 1) from previous and current patients are reported for the first time.

DISCUSSION

In the process of ventricular dilatation leading to heart failure, a concept has emerged that progressive dilatation is associated with a decline in ventricular systolic performance. This association has been described in humans for left ventricular ejection fraction (10) and for mechanical variables such as wall stress (11,12). Similar observations have been made in a canine model of progressive ventricular dilatation leading to heart failure (13). The findings in this chapter are the first to relate cellular size and shape changes to functional and anatomical alterations occurring at the ventricular level in humans. To summarize, longer myocytes are associated with increased left ventricular chamber diameters and left ventricular systolic dysfunction in congestive heart failure.

Cellular changes suggest that lengthening of myocytes can account for the chamber dilatation. Under this concept, cell slippage need not play a major role in the dilation process. The apparent complex linkage of individual cardiac myocytes to their adjacent neighboring myocytes (14) lends further support that a lengthening process rather than slippage may be the primary event leading to ventricular dilatation. It should be stressed, however, that potential contributions of myocyte slippage to chamber dilation were not examined here and cannot be assessed with the techniques employed in this study.

Subjects with congestive failure were divided into two groups in this study: DCM (idiopathic) and ICM. Data were also collected from hearts obtained from five unsuitable donors (controls).

Compared to data from nonfailing "controls," dimensions of cardiac myocytes from subjects with DCM and ICM were altered in a similar manner. Myocyte length and myocyte length:width ratios were significantly greater in subjects with DCM and ICM. Cell lengthening was likely due to addition of new sarcomeres in series, because sarcomere length was not changed in isolated myocytes from subjects with either disease. Sarcomere registration also appeared normal in isolated myocytes from several failing hearts examined using rhodamine–phalloidin labeling of actin or polarizing light. The changes in myocyte dimensions noted in subjects with ICM in this study are virtually identical to similar data from six other subjects with ICM reported in 1992 (6).

The relative change in myocyte length in subjects with DCM and ICM corresponds closely to the increase in chamber diameter typically reported for subjects with these diseases (e.g., an increase from 5 to 7 cm) (2,3). Although clinical data are limited at this time, a significant correlation was noted between end-diastolic diameter and cell length. Increased cell length was also associated with a decline in systolic ventricular function (e.g., ejection fraction). The increase in myocyte length:width ratio also reflects the characteristic alteration in chamber radius:wall thickness ratio observed in subjects with ICM and DCM. Thus, adverse changes in wall stress during ventricular dilation due to heart failure, as calculated by the LaPlace equation, may be due primarily to the observed change in cardiac myocyte shape.

The precise mechanism by which alterations in mechanical stress result in either series or parallel addition of new contractile units is unknown. Grossman et al. (15) and others (16,17) have proposed that myocytes remodel in a manner that reflects gross changes in ventricular anatomy associated with specific alterations in wall stress. Consequently, it is believed that concentric hypertrophy (e.g., due to hypertension) is due solely to an increase in myocyte cross-sectional area, while eccentric hypertrophy (e.g., due to volume overloading) is characterized by a proportional increase in cell length and diameter. Although it is difficult to reach such a conclusion based on data published prior to 1985 (mostly morphometric data collected from whole-tissue sections), results from experimental animal studies using isolated myocytes strongly agree with this theory (18–22).

The absence of a compensatory increase in myocyte diameter is noteworthy because such a response would help restore ventricular function and reduce wall stress. Systolic wall stress, believed to be the signal for increased transverse growth of the myocyte, is typically increased in subjects with ICM and DCM. Thus, it appears that myocytes are not responding appropriately to the signal for adaptive growth in congestive failure. In contrast to the situation with myocyte width in congestive failure, a substantial increase in myocyte length occurred presumably as a result of new sarcomere formation. The most likely stimulus for new sarcomere formation is increased end-diastolic wall stress, which is dramatically elevated in congestive heart failure (15). An increase in myocyte length and length:width ratio was also observed in surviving left ventricular myocytes 1 month after a transmural infarction in rats (23).

It is possible that the signal for increased myocyte diameter is mediated by mechanical structures alone. Within cardiac myocytes, cytoskeletal proteins such as talin, vinculin, and desmin connect the sarcolemma to the nucleus via other proteins associated with the Z lines (e.g., α-actinin) (24). Thus, a mechanism exists for radial transmission of mechanical stress from the sarcolemma to the nucleus. Because mechanical stress is transmitted between myocytes by extracellular collagen struts (25), which insert into the sarcolemma at the level of the Z line, it is likely that physical stresses within the myocardium can directly affect the myocyte nucleus. This process could also lead to up-regulation of specific genes, because it has been demonstrated that increased messenger RNA synthesis occurs in isolated cardiac myocyte nuclei subjected to increased hydrostatic pressure (26). Alterations in cytoskeletal proteins within myocytes, in collagen struts between myocytes, or in collagen-binding integrins (27) could potentially disrupt the mechanical signal for transverse myocyte growth in subjects with ICM and DCM. A few years ago, changes in the amount and distribution of desmin and vinculin were reported in cardiac myocytes from subjects with dilated cardiomyopathy (28). Dilated cardiomyopathy and other pathological conditions, such as tachycardia and myocardial infarction, may also lead to disruption of intermyocyte collagen struts (29–31).

Acquisition of fresh myocardium from subjects with no sign of cardiovascular disease (e.g., controls) is a recognized problem in studies of this type. Fortunately, data from five suitable controls (e.g., nondilated, nonfailing ventricles with normal ejection fraction and widely patent coronary arteries) were obtained. Two of these hearts were excellent controls because the individuals (one male, one female) had no history of hypertension or other diseases before death. It should be noted that cell size data from these subjects are indistinguishable from comparable data collected from rats with the same method (32). The other three control hearts were not dilated but had a moderate increase in wall thickness due to hypertension.

Myocyte length:width ratio is an internal parameter that is affected minimally, if at all, by genetic variability in myocyte size, physiological growth, or compensated hypertrophy (18–21). This parameter is very similar in all adult mammals, male or female, examined with these methods to this point (7,32–34). Unlike myocyte slippage, myocyte length:width ratio is easy to quantify. Finally, increased myocyte length:width ratio appears to be specific for heart failure because no overlapping data were observed in isolated myocyte preparations from nonfailing ventricles.

We have observed previously that myocyte length:width ratio is unusually high in hearts from neonatal rats undergoing nuclear and cellular division (35). Thus, dilation in congestive heart failure may result from reexpression of specific genes affecting cardiac myocyte shape that are normally expressed in fetal and early postnatal growth. It is critical that the underlying mechanism of this cellular change be defined and targeted for potential new interventions. Recent evidence suggesting that angiotensin-converting enzyme inhibitors produce beneficial ventricular remodeling in patients with heart failure underscores the importance of additional work in this area (36,37).

SUMMARY

Myocyte shape was examined in isolated myocytes from explanted hearts from patients with DCM and ICM. Myocytes from nonfailing, unsuitable donors (C) were also examined. Cell volume was $41,387 \pm 6,281$ μm^3; cell length was 138 ± 5 μm; cell width was 19.3 ± 1.4 μm; cell length:width ratio was 7.3 ± 0.5; and sarcomere length was 2.00 ± 0.02 μm in C. Compared with C, cell length was 41% longer ($p < 0.01$) and cell length:width ratio was 49% greater ($p < 0.01$) in DCM. Cell length was 41% longer ($p < 0.01$) and cell length:width ratio was 58% greater ($p < 0.01$) in ICM. Thus, myocyte length and myocyte length:width ratio were increased to a similar extent in DCM and ICM when compared with values from C. These changes mirror alterations in chamber radius and chamber radius/wall thickness typical of these diseases. Results suggest that chamber dilation due to ICM and

DCM may involve a final common pathway characterized by a specific change in myocyte shape that appears to be maladaptive.

ACKNOWLEDGMENTS

The authors are grateful to Lawrence Miller, Lee Langley, Trish Carroll, and Tom Nolte from Lifelink of Florida (Tampa) for their valuable assistance in obtaining cardiac tissue, and to Krystyna Malec, Linda Clark, and Roney Francois for their technical assistance. This protocol was approved by the University of South Florida Health Sciences Center Institutional Review Board and the Institutional Review Board of Tampa General Hospital. Informed consent was obtained from individuals prior to transplantation or from next of kin (unsuitable donor hearts). Scott E. Kellerman was supported by a Medical Student Research Fellowship from the American Heart Association.

REFERENCES

1. Roberts WC, Ferrans VJ. Pathologic anatomy of the cardiomyopathies. *Hum Pathol* 1975;6:287–342.
2. Hayakawa M, Inoh T, Fukuzaki H. Dilated cardiomyopathy: an echocardiographic follow-up of 50 patients. *Jpn Heart J* 1984;25:955–968.
3. Corya BC, Feigenbaum H, Rasmussen S, Black MJ. Echocardiographic features of congestive cardiomyopathy compared with normal subjects and patients with coronary artery disease. *Circulation* 1974;49:1153–1159.
4. Linzbach AJ. Heart failure from the point of view of quantitative anatomy. *Am J Cardiol* 1960;5:370–382.
5. Rousseau MF, Pouleur H. Remodeling in chronic ischemic heart disease: acute and long-term intervention. *J Mol Cell Cardiol* 1991;23[Suppl 5]:S45(abst).
6. Gerdes AM, Kellerman SE, Moore JA, et al. Structural remodeling of cardiac myocytes in patients with ischemic cardiomyopathy. *Circulation* 1992;86:426–430.
7. Gerdes AM, Moore JA, Hines JM, Kirkland PA, Bishop SP. Regional differences in myocyte size in normal rat heart. *Anat Rec* 1986;215:420–426.
8. Gerdes AM, Kriseman J, Bishop SP. Morphometric study of cardiac muscle: the problem of tissue shrinkage. *Lab Invest* 1982;46:271–274.
9. Wallenstein S, Zucker CL, Fleiss JL. Some statistical methods useful in circulation research. *Circ Res* 1980;47:1–9.
10. Field BJ, Baxley WA, Russell RO Jr, et al. Left ventricular function and hypertrophy in cardiomyopathy with depressed ejection fraction. *Circulation* 1973;47:1022–1031.
11. Dodge HT, Stewart DK, Frimer M. Implications of shape, stress and wall dynamics in clinical heart disease. In: Fishman AP, ed. *Heart failure*. Washington, DC: Hemisphere; 1978:43–54.
12. Lasey WK, Sutton MSJ, Zeevi G, Hirshfield JW, Reicheck N. Left ventricular mechanics in dilated cardiomyopathy. *Am J Cardiol* 1984;54:620–625.
13. Sabbah HN, Kono T, Stein PD, Mancini GBJ, Goldstein S. Left ventricular shape changes during the course of evolving heart failure. *Am J Physiol* 1992;263:H266–H270.
14. Hoyt RH, Cohen ML, Saffitz JE. Distribution and three-dimensional structure of intercellular junctions in canine myocardium. *Circ Res* 1989;64:563–574.
15. Grossman W, Jones D, McLaurin LP. Wall stress and patterns of hypertrophy in the human left ventricle. *J Clin Invest* 1975;56:56–64.
16. Ford LE. Heart size. *Circ Res* 1976;39:297–303.
17. Grant C, Green DG, Bunnell IL. Left ventricular enlargement and hypertrophy: a clinical and angiocardiographic study. *Am J Med* 1965;39:895–904.

18. Smith SH, Bishop SP. Regional changes in compensated right ventricular hypertrophy in the ferret. *J Mol Cell Cardiol* 1985;17:1005–1011.
19. Liu Z, Hilbelink DR, Crockett WB, Gerdes AM. Regional changes in hemodynamics and cardiac myocyte size in rats with aortocaval fistulas. I. Developing and established hypertrophy. *Circ Res* 1991;69:52–58.
20. Liu Z, Hilbelink DR, Gerdes AM. Regional changes in hemodynamics and cardiac myocyte size in rats with aortocaval fistulas. II. Long-term effects. *Circ Res* 1991;69:59–65.
21. Gerdes AM, Moore JA, Hines JM. Regional changes in myocyte size and number in propranolol-treated hyperthyroid rats. *Lab Invest* 1987;57:708–713.
22. Gerdes AM. The use of isolated myocytes to evaluate myocardial remodeling. *Trends Cardiovasc Med* 1992;2:152–155.
23. Zimmer HG, Gerdes AM, Lortet S, Mall G. Changes in heart function and cardiac cell shape in rats with chronic myocardial infarction. *J Mol Cell Cardiol* 1990;22:1231–1243.
24. Terracio L, Borg TK. Factors affecting cardiac cell shape. *Heart Failure* 1988;4:114–124.
25. Robinson TF, Cohen-Gould L, Factor SM. Skeletal framework of mammalian heart muscle. Arrangement of inter- and pericellular connective tissue structures. *Lab Invest* 1983;49:482–498.
26. Schreiber SS, Oratz M, Rothschild MA, Reff R. Effect of hydrostatic pressure on isolated cardiac nuclei: stimulation of RNA polymerase II activity. *Cardiovasc Res* 1978;12:265–268.
27. Terracio L, Rubin K, Gullberg D, et al. Expression of collagen binding integrins during cardiac development and hypertrophy. *Circ Res* 1991;68:734–744.
28. Schaper J, Froede R, Hein S, et al. Impairment of myocardial ultrastructure and changes of the cytoskeleton in dilated cardiomyopathy. *Circulation* 1991;83:504–514.
29. Weber KT, Pick R, Janicki JS, Gadodia G, Lakier LB. Inadequate collagen tethers in dilated cardiomyopathy. *Am Heart J* 1988;116:1641–1646.
30. Zellner JL, Spinale FG, Eble DM, Hewett KW, Crawford FA Jr. Alterations in myocyte shape and basement membrane attachment with tachycardia-induced heart failure. *Circ Res* 1991;69:590–600.
31. Whittaker P, Boughner DR, Kloner RA. Role of collagen in acute myocardial infarct expansion. *Circulation* 1991;84:2123–2134.
32. Bai S, Campbell SE, Moore JA, Morales MC, Gerdes AM. Influence of aging, growth, and sex on cardiac myocyte size and number. *Anat Rec* 1990;226:207–212.
33. Campbell SE, Gerdes AM, Smith TD. Comparison of regional differences in cardiac myocyte dimensions in rats, hamsters, and guinea pigs. *Anat Rec* 1987;219:53–59.
34. Kozlovskis PL, Gerdes AM, Smets M, et al. Regional increase in myocyte volume after healing of myocardial infarction in cats. *J Mol Cell Cardiol* 1991;23:1459–1466.
35. Alvarez MA, Clark LC, Moore JA, Morales MC, Gerdes AM. Results of prenatal alcohol exposure on the dimensions and binucleation of cardiac myocytes in neonatal and weanling rats. *Teratology* 1991;44:395–404.
36. SOLVD Trial Study Group. Effects of the angiotensin converting enzyme inhibitor enalapril on the long-term progression of left ventricular dysfunction in patients with heart failure. *Circulation* 1992;86:431–438.
37. CONSENSUS Trial Study Group. Effects of enalapril on mortality in severe congestive heart failure: results of the Cooperative North Scandinavian Enalapril Survival Study. *N Engl J Med* 1987;316:1429–1435.

The Failing Heart, edited by N. S. Dhalla,
R. E. Beamish, N. Takeda, and M. Nagano.
Lippincott-Raven Publishers, Philadelphia © 1995.

17

Structural and Functional Consequences of Angiotensin-Converting Enzyme Inhibition and Angiotensin Type 1 Receptor Inhibition following Myocardial Infarction in Rats

Robert C.J.J. Passier, *Mat J.A.P. Daemen, and Jos F.M. Smits

*Departments of Pharmacology and *Pathology, Cardiovascular Research Institute Maastricht, University of Limburg, 6200 MD Maastricht, The Netherlands*

MYOCARDIAL INFARCTION: HEMODYNAMIC, NEUROHUMORAL, AND STRUCTURAL CHANGES

The primary loss of viable myocardium in myocardial infarction triggers a large number of hemodynamic, neural, and hormonal events (1). The decrease in cardiac mass decreases stroke volume and cardiac output, resulting in a decrease of blood pressure. Reductions in cardiac output and blood pressure trigger sympathetic activity through the sinoaortic baroreceptors. Furthermore, both this increase in sympathetic activity and the decrease in blood pressure and cardiac output per se increase the activity of the renin-angiotensin-aldosterone system. Although virtually all systems that are involved in cardiovascular homeostasis are activated in the process of maintaining an adequate circulation following myocardial infarction, they will not be discussed in the context of this chapter.

In addition to these hemodynamic and neurohumoral processes, myocardial infarction also triggers a number of structural changes in the heart that are generally referred to as *remodeling*. Several aspects may be distinguished in the remodeling response, that is, remodeling of infarcted versus viable myocardium, and the cell types involved.

In the infarct area, cardiomyocyte edema and necrosis are observed. Following myocyte necrosis, a wound healing response occurs, which involves a local inflammatory reaction, excessive extracellular matrix deposition, angiogenesis, and the appearance of myofibroblasts to increase the tensile strength of the infarct (2,3).

Dilatation and thinning, also called *infarct expansion* (4), are the most important architectural changes of the infarcted tissue; this is caused not only by myocyte necrosis but also by myocyte slippage (5). Infarct expansion, which can lead ultimately to a ventricular aneurysm, is limited to the first weeks after myocardial infarction.

The most prominent changes in the noninfarcted myocardium are dilatation and hypertrophy (2). Ventricular dilatation, which is initially beneficial to maintain stroke volume, however, also increases ventricular wall stress, which stimulates further ventricular enlargement, resulting in a vicious circle (2). The changes in myocyte mass do not compensate fully for the loss of viable tissue and for the loss of function. A possible explanation for this apparent paradox (i.e., more cardiac mass without an increased cardiac function) is that cardiac hypertrophy is associated with alterations in the quantity and quality of the expression of contractile, cytoskeletal, and neurohormonal genes. For instance, the expression of the gene of the heavy chain of the contractile protein myosin changes from the α to the β chain, which contracts more slowly, but is less energy consuming (6).

Although the bulk of the mass of the heart is comprised of cardiomyocytes, the majority of the cells are found in the interstitium (7). In an animal model for myocardial infarction, the rat following ligation of the left coronary artery, we have documented extensively the response of the interstitium to this insult (8). Using incorporation of 5-bromo-2′-deoxyuridine (BrdU) as a marker for DNA synthesis, we observed an increase of DNA synthesis in both ventricles, which peaked between the first and second week after infarction and was back at control levels at 5 weeks after infarction (8) (Fig. 1). In contrast to cardiomyocytes, which were only sporadically found to be positive for DNA synthesis, both endothelial cells and fibroblasts were found to exhibit increased DNA synthesis, with endothelium comprising approximately 25% of BrdU-positive cells (9).

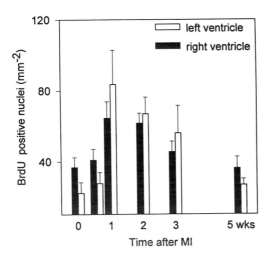

FIG. 1. Numbers of BrdU-positive nuclei per mm² in left and right (uninfarcted) ventricles as a function of time following myocardial infarction (MI). Altered from Van Krimpen et al. (8).

The increased DNA synthesis in cardiac fibroblasts was associated with increased deposition of collagen, as evidenced by increased concentrations in both ventricles (Fig. 2), as well as increased levels of mRNA for both collagen I and III (10). In rat hearts, the increase in collagen volume fraction is maintained over a prolonged period of time (Fig. 2). Similarly, we have observed increased collagen deposition in postmortem samples from human hearts with old infarcts (11). The fibrillar collagens, type I and type III, are the major components of the cardiac extracellular matrix. The amount and distribution of these fibrillar collagens in the myocardium are important denominators of cardiac function, and changes in the amount and/or distribution of collagen can affect the function of the heart. For instance, an increased collagen fraction increases the stiffness of the heart, leading to a decreased compliance and diminished diastolic filling. Increased intercellular and pericellular collagen fibers may limit myocyte motion and decrease the compliance of the ventricle.

The amount of fibronectin, which provides the scaffold for the deposition of

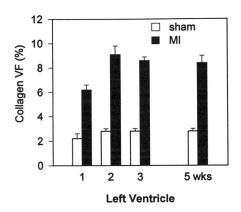

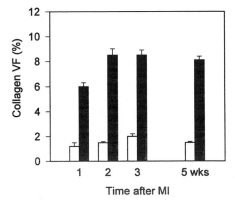

FIG. 2. Collagen volume fraction (CVF) in sham-operated and infarcted rats, measured in right (*top*) and left (*bottom*) uninfarcted ventricle as a function of time after myocardial infarction (MI). Altered from Van Krimpen et al. (8).

collagen, also increases shortly after the induction of cardiac hypertrophy by myocardial infarction (12) or pressure overload (13).

The aforementioned increase in endothelial cell DNA synthesis is indicative of
vascular outgrowth. Although there is a substantial growth in the number and length
of capillaries in the noninfarcted myocardium, this increase is insufficient to meet
the increase in cardiomyocyte hypertrophy and capillary to cardiomyocyte fiber
ratio decreases during ventricular remodeling after myocardial infarction (14). The
increase in distance between capillaries and the decrease in density of capillary
profiles during ventricular remodeling leads to a relative energy starvation (15). The
expression of less-energy-consuming phenotypes (see previous discussion) may be
seen as an adaptation to the energy starvation of the hypertrophied cardiomyocyte,
but is detrimental for contractility (15).

THE ROLE FOR THE RENIN–ANGIOTENSIN SYSTEM IN THE STRUCTURAL RESPONSES TO MYOCARDIAL INFARCTION

The mechanisms that govern the previously described remodeling response of the
heart following myocardial infarction are still largely obscure. Obviously, one important factor may be the mechanical stress imposed on the remnant ventricle. The
observation that the response is not limited to the left ventricle, however, suggests
that other factors may be involved. In this respect, the renin-angiotensin-aldosterone system has received ample attention.

There is now good evidence that several tissues, including the heart, express all
components that comprise local renin–angiotensin systems (for a review, see Lee
and Lindpaintner [16]). Expression of angiotensinogen, renin, and angiotensin-I
converting enzyme (ACE) has been demonstrated at the mRNA as well as the protein level in cardiac myocytes as well as cardiac fibroblasts. Of special interest are
the observations that expression of angiotensinogen mRNA (17) and ACE mRNA
(18) are increased in the remnant myocardium following myocardial infarction in
rats. Similarly, increased ACE mRNA expression was observed in failing human
hearts (19). In rats, the increased wall stress in this situation correlated with angiotensinogen expression (17), and similarly ACE expression correlated with the
extent of myocardial infarction (18), suggesting local regulation of the activity of
the cardiac renin–angiotensin system. In a recent study, we noted the highest degree of
ACE mRNA expression and protein concentrations in the border zone of the myocardial infarct in rats; the fact that expression occurred mainly in endothelial cells implies
that it may be associated with formation of blood vessels in this area (20).

In a relatively recent paper, the possible functional role of tissue renin–angiotensin systems was reviewed (21). Angiotensin II not only may influence cardiac inotropy and chronotropy, but also may contribute to the cellular responses described
earlier. The functional and structural effects could be indirect (i.e., through pre-
synaptic activation of the sympathetic nervous system). With respect to the cellular
responses, α-adrenoceptor stimulation has been shown to stimulate hypertrophy in

neonatal rat cardiac myocytes (22). Alternatively, angiotensin II could have direct effects on cardiac cells. Angiotensin II has been shown to have blood pressure–independent trophic effects on cardiac myocytes, including the trophic response to stretch (23). The trophic effect in vivo is mediated entirely through AT$_1$-angiotensin receptors (24). The fact that losartan completely blocked the hypertrophic response following myocardial infarction in our rat model suggests a role for these receptors in myocyte growth in this circumstance as well (25,26).

In contrast to cardiomyocytes, endothelial cells and fibroblasts are capable of replicating. Cardiac fibroblasts exhibit a mitogenic response to angiotensin II in cell culture (27). Again, this response was mediated by AT$_1$-receptors.

In vivo, following myocardial infarction in rats, we noted that captopril completely abolished the structural response of the interstitium: DNA synthesis as well as collagen deposition were normalized when captopril was administered in the first 2 weeks after infarction, i.e., the period in which these processes were activated (Fig. 3) (8). In accordance with the aforementioned role for AT$_1$-receptors in the

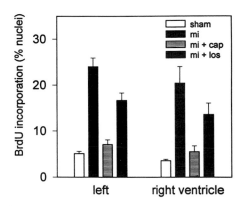

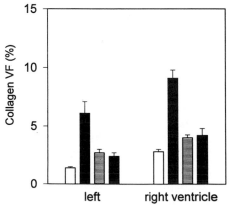

FIG. 3. Effects of myocardial infarction (MI; 14 days post-MI) and early (0–14 days) treatments with captopril (cap; 12 mg/kg/d) and losartan (los; 15 mg/kg/d) on BrdU incorporation (*top*) and collagen volume fraction (VF) in left and right ventricle. Altered from data in Van Krimpen et al. (8) and Smits et al. (26).

effect of angiotensin II on cardiac fibroblast growth, we found that losartan was equally well capable of reducing collagen deposition following infarction as was captopril (Fig. 3) (26). Losartan only partly reduced DNA synthesis following infarction (Fig. 3), however, suggesting a dissociation of these two phenomena.

We propose that the endothelial response may be spared by losartan, and, thus, be mediated by another pathway. Interestingly, in a model for vascular neogenesis, the chick chorioallantoic membrane, angiotensin II induces a potent neovascularization response that is resistant to losartan and the nonpeptidic AT_2-antagonist PD 123319, but may be completely inhibited by the peptidic AT_2-antagonist CGP42112A (28). This also suggests involvement of a non–AT_1-receptor in the neovascularization response.

HEMODYNAMIC EFFECTS OF ANGIOTENSIN-CONVERTING ENZYME INHIBITION AND AT₁-RECEPTOR INHIBITION FOLLOWING MYOCARDIAL INFARCTION

In 1985, Pfeffer and co-workers were the first to demonstrate the effect of long-term captopril treatment in rats following myocardial infarction, not only on cardiac function (29), but also on survival (30). Because enalapril similarly improves survival, this suggests a class effect for ACE inhibitors (31). The functional improvement was not the result of decreased afterload because it cannot be mimicked by hydralazine in the same animal model at a dose that reduced blood pressure to a similar extent (32). The authors of the latter study suggested that the difference in response depends on differential effects on preload, based on measurements of venous capacitance. This concept has been corroborated in studies comparing the effects of enalapril and combined hydralazine/nitrate treatment in humans with heart failure (33); both treatments improved survival, although enalapril was more effective than the combined vasodilator treatment.

For captopril, the functional improvement was associated with inhibition of cardiac hypertrophy and dilatation, whereas cardiac stiffness did not increase (29). The latter would be in keeping with a reduction of collagen as discussed earlier. Because both captopril and losartan had similar effects on collagen deposition, it became of interest to compare both substances with respect to their functional effects. In these studies, we made a distinction between treatments during the period of structural adaptations (0–3 weeks; see Figs. 1 and 2) and after completion of this healing phase. In accordance with the observations by Pfeffer et al. (29), captopril was found to improve cardiac function following myocardial infarction if treatment was started after the healing phase (34) (Fig. 4). In contrast, losartan, given during the same period and in a dose that inhibited the renin–angiotensin system to a similar degree, did not affect cardiac function (26) (Fig. 4). This indicates that AT_1-receptors are not involved in the improvement of cardiac function by captopril.

It is not clear whether an effect on collagen deposition is involved in the late beneficial effect of captopril, because collagen levels in rats treated from 3 to 5

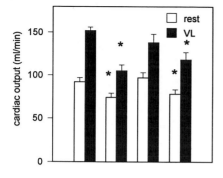

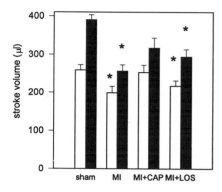

FIG. 4. Effects of myocardial infarction (MI) and late (21–35 days post-MI) treatments with captopril (cap; 12 mg/kg/d) and losartan (los; 15 mg/kg/d) on cardiac output (*top*) and stroke volume (*bottom*) at rest and during rapid volume loading (VL). *$p < 0.05$ as compared to sham-operated animals. Altered from Schoemaker et al. (34) and Smits et al. (26).

weeks after infarction were not affected by captopril (8). This period may have been too brief for a clear regression of structural changes other than hypertrophy. Litwin et al. (35) treated rats with captopril from 3 to 6 weeks after infarction and also did not note an effect on collagen deposition or cardiac stiffness. In contrast, Michel et al. (36) found that 2 months of perindopril treatment was associated with diminution of collagen deposition and cardiac stiffening. This discrepancy may be related to the long half-life of cross-linked collagens. We have not yet studied the effect of losartan on late collagen deposition. Thus, a contribution of collagen reduction and a possible later effect of losartan on cardiac function that could be attributed to such an effect cannot be eliminated.

Captopril treatment during the healing phase resulted in a completely different effect on hemodynamics. In this situation, cardiac function decreased rather than increased (34) (Fig. 5). This was especially clear from a reduction of resting stroke volume and stroke volume on maximal volume loading (34). Increased heart rate maintained cardiac output. Again, losartan did not mimic this effect (26) (Fig. 5). This indicates that the reduction of collagen, which occurred to a similar extent with both substances, is not crucial for the reduction in function. Rather, the inhibition of endothelial cell proliferation, that we suggested earlier to be specific for captopril

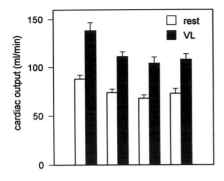

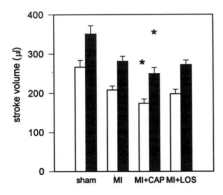

FIG. 5. Effects of myocardial infarction (MI) and early (0–21 days post-MI) treatments with captopril (cap; 12 mg/kg/d) and losartan (los; 15 mg/kg/d) on cardiac output (*top*) and stroke volume (*bottom*) at rest and during rapid volume loading (VL). *$p<0.05$ as compared to sham-operated animals. Altered from Schoemaker et al. (34) and Smits et al. (26).

over losartan, might explain the reduction of function as well as the divergence of the effects of losartan and captopril during early treatment.

The effects of captopril could also be due to the increased bradykinin levels rather than decreased angiotensin II levels, because ACE inhibitors also prevent the degradation of this peptide (37). This possibility is supported by observations in the dog, where the bradykinin antagonist HOE 140 blocked the effects of the ACE inhibitor ramiprilat on infarct size (38). Further studies on the effects of bradykinin on cardiac remodeling following myocardial infarction are, however, not available.

Alternatively, the effects of captopril could be mediated through inhibition of stimulation of AT_2-receptors. Certainly, evidence from studies on neovascularization as cited previously (28) corroborates this hypothesis. At present, involvement of AT_2-receptors in the late response also cannot be discounted. Studies to test this hypothesis are ongoing.

SUMMARY

Myocardial infarction triggers a number of structural and hemodynamic events in the rat. The early structural events, which can be inhibited completely by captopril, seem to be physiological rather than pathological, because their inhibition is associated with a reduction of cardiac function. Our animal experimental data indicating a discrepancy between the hemodynamic effects of early and delayed treatment with ACE inhibitors have been confirmed in trials in patients (39).

Losartan did not exhibit an early detrimental effect. The observation that losartan does not reduce total labeling, but does reduce collagen content following myocardial infarction, indicates that the endothelial response may be be resistant to AT_1-receptor blockade. Combination of structural and functional observations suggests that inhibition of proliferation of endothelial cells, rather than fibroblasts, may be detrimental. Thus, the early effects of captopril and losartan differ. Also, the late functional effects of captopril, which were beneficial, were not mimicked by losartan. This suggests that mechanisms other than AT_1-receptor inhibition mediate the effects of captopril following myocardial infarction.

REFERENCES

1. Remme WJ. Congestive heart failure. Pathophysiology and medical treatment. *J Cardiovasc Pharmacol* 1986;8[Suppl 1]:36–52.
2. Vracko R, Thorning D. Contractile cells in rat myocardial scar tissue. *Lab Invest* 1991;65:221–227.
3. Willems IEMG, Havenith MG, DeMey JGR, Daeman MJAP. The alpha-smooth muscle actin-positive cells in healing human myocardial scars. *Am J Pathol* 1994;145:868–875.
4. Pfeffer MA, Braunwald E. Ventricular remodeling after myocardial infarction. Experimental observations and clinical implications. *Circulation* 1990;81:1161–1172.
5. Tsutsui H, Ishihara K, Cooper G 4th. Cytoskeletal role in the contractile dysfunction of hypertrophied myocardium. *Science* 1993;260:682–687.
6. Schwartz K, Boheler KR, De La Bastie D, Lompre AM, Mercadier JJ. Switches in cadiac muscle gene expression as a result of pressure and volume overload. *Am J Physiol* 1992;262:R364–R369.
7. Weber KT, Brilla CG. Pathological hypertrophy and cardiac interstitium. *Circulation* 1991;83: 1849–1865.
8. Van Krimpen C, Smits JFM, Cleutjens JPM, et al. DNA synthesis in the non-infarcted cardiac interstitium is increased after left coronary artery ligation in the rat: effects of captopril. *J Mol Cell Cardiol* 1991;23:1245–1253.
9. Kuizinga MC, Cleutjens JPM, Smits JFM, Daemen MJAP. Griffonia simplicifolia I (GSI): a suitable rat cardiac microvascular marker on paraffin embedded tissue. *J Mol Cell Cardiol* 1992;24 [Suppl V]:S57.
10. Cleutjens JPM, Smits JFM, Daemen MJAP. Type I and III collagen mRNA and protein increase in the infarcted and non-infarcted rat heart after myocardial infarction. *J Mol Cell Cardiol* 1992;24 [Suppl V]:S50.
11. Volders PGA, Willems IEMG, Cleutjens JPM, Arends JW, Havenith MG, Daemen MJAP. Interstitial collagen is increased in the non-infarcted myocardium after myocardial infarction. *J Mol Cell Cardiol* 1993;25:317–323.
12. Shekhonin BV, Guriev SB, Irgashev SB, Koteliansky VE. Immunofluorescence identification of fibronectin and fibrinogen/fibrin in experimental myocardial infarction. *J Mol Cell Cardiol* 1990;22: 533–541.
13. Samuel JL, Barrieux A, Dufour S, et al. Accumulation of fetal fibronectin mRNAs during the development of rat cardiac hypertrophy induced by pressure overload. *J Clin Invest* 1991;88:1737–1746.
14. Olivetti G, Anversa P. Long term pressure induced cardiac hypertrophy: capillary and mast cell production. *Am J Physiol* 1989;257:H1766–H1772.
15. Katz A. Cardiomyopathy of overload. *N Engl J Med* 1990;322:100–110.
16. Lee YA, Lindpaintner K. The cardiac renin angiotensin system; from basic research to clinical relevance. *Drug Res* 1993;43:201–206.
17. Lindpaintner K, Lu W, Neidermajer N, et al. Selective activation of cardiac angiotensinogen gene

expression in post-infarction ventricular remodeling in the rat. *J Mol Cell Cardiol* 1993;25:133–143.

18. Hirsch AT, Talsness CE, Schunkert H, Paul M, Dzau VJ. Tissue-specific activation of cardiac angiotensin converting enzyme in experimental heart failure. *Circ Res* 1991;69:475–482.

19. Studer R, Reinecke H, Müller B, Holtz J, Just H, Drexler H. Increased angiotensin I converting enzyme gene expression in the failing human heart. *J Clin Invest* 1994;94:301–310.

20. Passier RCJJ, Smits JFM, Daemen MJAP. Localization of angiotensin converting enzyme in the rat heart after myocardial infarction. *Can J Physiol Pharmacol* 1994;72[Suppl 1]:173.

21. Dzau VJ. Tissue renin-angiotensin system in myocardial hypertrophy and failure. *Arch Intern Med* 1993;153:937–942.

22. Simpson P. Stimulation of hypertrophy of cultured neonatal rat heart cells through an alpha 1-adrenergic receptor and induction of beating through an alpha 1- and beta 1-adrenergic receptor interaction. Evidence for independent regulation of growth and beating. *Circ Res* 1985;56:884–894.

23. Sadoshima J, Xu J, Slayter HS, Izumo S. Autocrine release of angiotensin II mediates stretch induced hypertrophy of cardiac myocytes in vitro. *Cell* 1993;75;977–984.

24. Dostal DE, Baker KM. Angiotensin II stimulation of left ventricular hypertrophy in adult rat heart. Mediation by the AT1 receptor. *Am J Hypertens* 1992;5:276–280.

25. Schieffer B, Wirger A, Meybrunn M, et al. Comparative effects of chronic angiotensin-converting enzyme inhibition and angiotensin II type 1 receptor blockade on cardiac remodeling after myocardial infarction in the rat. *Circulation* 1994;89:2273–2282.

26. Smits JF, van Krimpen C, Schoemaker RG, Cleutjens JP, Daemen MJ. Angiotensin II receptor blockade after myocardial infarction in rats: effects on hemodynamics, myocardial DNA synthesis, and interstitial collagen content. *J Cardiovasc Pharmacol* 1992;20:772–778.

27. Schorb W, Booz GW, Dostal DE, Conrad KM, Chang KC, Baker KM. Angiotensin II is mitogenic in neonatal rat cardiac fibroblasts. *Circ Res* 1993;72:1245–1254.

28. Le Noble FA, Schreurs NH, van Straaten HW, et al. Evidence for a novel angiotensin II receptor involved in angiogenesis in chick embryo chorioallantoic membrane. *Am J Physiol* 1993;264:R460–R465.

29. Pfeffer JM, Pfeffer MA, Braunwald E. Influence of chronic captopril therapy on the infarcted left ventricle of the rat. *Circ Res* 1985a;57:84–95.

30. Pfeffer MA, Pfeffer JM, Steinberg C, Finn P. Survival after an experimental myocardial infarction: beneficial effects of long-term therapy with captopril. *Circulation* 1985b;72:406–412.

31. Sweet CS, Emmert SE, Stabilito II, Ribeiro LG. Increased survival in rats with congestive heart failure treated with enalapril. *J Cardiovasc Pharmacol* 1987;10:636–642.

32. Raya T, Gay R, Aguirre M, Goldman S. Importance of venodilatation in prevention of left ventricular dilatation after chronic large myocardial infarction in rats; a comparison of captopril and hydralazine. *Circ Res* 1989;64:330–337.

33. Cohn JN, Archibald DG, Ziesche S, et al. Effect of vasodilator therapy on mortality in chronic congestive heart failure. Results of a Veterans Administration cooperative study. *N Engl J Med* 1986;314:1547–1552.

34. Schoemaker RG, Debets JJM, Struyker-Boudier HAJ, Smits JFM. Delayed but not immediate captopril therapy improves cardiac function in conscious rats, following myocardial infarction. *J Mol Cell Cardiol* 1991;23:187–197.

35. Litwin SE, Litwin CM, Raya TE, Warner AL, Goldman S. Contractility and stiffness of noninfarcted myocardium after coronary ligation in rats. Effects of chronic angiotensin converting enzyme inhibition. *Circulation* 1991;83:1028–1037.

36. Michel J, Lattion A, Salzmann J, et al. Hormonal and cardiac effects of converting enzyme inhibition in rat myocardial infarction. *Circ Res* 1988;62:641–650.

37. Martorana PA, Scholkens BA. Does bradykinin play a role in the cardiac antiischemic effect of the ACE-inhibitors? *Basic Res Cardiol* 1991;86:293–296.

38. Martorana P, Kettenbach B, Breipohl G, Linz W, Scholkens B. Reduction of infarct size by local angiotensin converting enzyme inhibition is abolished by a bradykinin antagonist. *Eur J Pharmacol* 1990;182:395–396.

39. Swedberg K, Held P, Kjekdhus J, et al. Effects of the early administration of enalapril on mortalility in patients with acute myocardial infarction—results of the cooperative New Scandinavian Enalapril Survival study (CONSENSUS II). *N Engl J Med* 1992;327:678–684.

The Failing Heart, edited by N. S. Dhalla,
R. E. Beamish, N. Takeda, and M. Nagano.
Lippincott-Raven Publishers, Philadelphia © 1995.

18

Remodeling of Cardiac Membranes During the Development of Congestive Heart Failure Due to Myocardial Infarction

Ian M.C. Dixon, *Nasir Afzal, †Nobuakira Takeda,
‡Makoto Nagano, and §Naranjan S. Dhalla

*Departments of Physiology and §Cardiovascular Sciences, Faculty of Medicine,
University of Manitoba, St. Boniface General Hospital Research Centre, Winnipeg,
Manitoba R2H 2A6 Canada; *Department of Pathology, University of Manitoba, Health
Sciences Centre, Winnipeg, Manitoba R2N 3JI Canada; †Department of Internal Medicine,
Aoto Hospital, Jikei University, School of Medicine, Tokyo 125 Japan; and
‡Jikei University, School of Medicine, Tokyo 150 Japan*

By virtue of their properties that raise and lower the concentration of intracellular Ca^{2+} on a beat-to-beat basis, the cardiac sarcolemma (SL) and sarcoplasmic reticulum (SR) are involved in the regulation of heart function and metabolism (1–3). Recent work in the field of cardiac excitation–contraction coupling has lead to the general belief that depolarization of the cardiac cell activates L-type Ca^{2+} channels in the SL membrane to permit the entry of a relatively small amount of Ca^{2+} into the cell. Other work has suggested that some Ca^{2+} may also enter the cytoplasm via the SL Na^+-Ca^{2+} exchange mechanism upon cellular depolarization. The initial Ca^{2+} entry from extracellular sources is not sufficient to cause contraction but results in the secondary release of an additional relatively large quantity of Ca^{2+} from the intracellular SR compartment via the recently identified Ca^{2+}-release channel. The increased level of cytoplasmic free Ca^{2+} promotes the binding of Ca^{2+} with troponin, relieves the inhibitory effect of the troponin–tropomyosin complex on actin and myosin, and results in the sliding of thin and thick filaments for the generation of contractile force. The Ca^{2+} pump present in the SR as well as the SL Ca^{2+} pump and SL Na^+-Ca^{2+} exchange system lower the cytoplasmic level of free Ca^{2+} and allow the troponin–tropomyosin complex to exert an inhibitory effect on actin and myosin, yielding net relaxation of the myofibrils. Sarcolemmal Na^+-K^+ ATPase maintains the intracellular concentration of Na^+ at a relatively low level, but whenever the activity of this enzyme is depressed, the intracellular concentration of Na^+ will rise, and this would favor the increased entry or retention of Ca^{2+} through the Na^+-Ca^{2+} exchange system. Although mitochondria may also accumulate Ca^{2+}, the low rate of mitochondrial Ca^{2+} flux limits their contribution to regulation of intracellular Ca^{2+} levels in physiologic conditions. Thus, it is evident that the functional integrity of SL and SR is crucial for maintenance of proper function of the heart, and any change in the behavior of these organelles can be seen to be associated with the development of heart dysfunction under pathologic conditions. Although other subcellular mechanisms, such as changes in myofibrillar activity, are believed to be important for the development of heart failure, we will focus on organelles involved in transport of cations in the infarcted hearts. Thus, it is not our intention to rule out other subcellular abnormalities that may occur in pathogenesis of congestive heart failure. We will review the existing information on the development of congestive heart failure in the rat myocardial infarction model.

PATHOPHYSIOLOGY OF HEART DYSFUNCTION IN THE RAT MODEL OF CHRONIC INFARCTION

A wide variety of alterations in subcellular organelles have been reported in various types of heart disease, including in the experimental model of hypertrophy and congestive heart failure after myocardial infarction in rats (4). This model was pioneered by Johns and Olson (5) who used a surgical method for producing reproducible myocardial infarct size. It should be noted that the rat heart lacks collateral arterioles and is therefore dissimilar from the human heart; this feature of myocardial architecture is deemed useful by virtue of reproducibility of infarct size. Although measurement of scar size is a valuable relative indicator of the extent of myocardial damage, the first study to assess left ventricular function in rats with large myocardial infarction appeared in 1979, wherein baseline and volume-loaded hemodynamic parameters were assessed in rats 21 days after infarction (6). These authors discovered that animals with large infarcts (>45% of the left ventricle inferred by planometric measurement of transmural scar size) had overt heart failure characterized by elevated filling pressures, reduced cardiac output, and little ability to respond to pre- and afterload stress. Indeed, graded left ventricular dysfunction has been shown to be closely related to the extent of the healed myocardial infarction (7,8). The most common cause of right-sided cardiac failure and pulmonary hypertension is left-sided cardiac failure (9,10). Likewise, right ventricular hypertrophy was consistently present in experimental rats showing elevated left ventricular filling pressures (6–8). It thus appears that left ventricular dysfunction may eventually cause severe right ventricular overload and dysfunction such that the right ventricle becomes a limiting factor in heart failure in rats with infarction.

Relatively little is known of biochemical parameters such as myofibrillar ATPase activity, myosin isozyme composition, myocardial high-energy phosphate content, as well as SR and SL membrane functions in the viable myocardium of rat heart with myocardial infarction. Significant reduction of myofibrillar ATPase activity was found in hearts of infarcted animals (11) and was associated with a V_1 to V_3 shift in myosin heavy-chain isozyme content (12). Two days following infarction, the adenosine triphosphate (ATP)-content of viable myocardium was found to be significantly lower than control values; however, ATP levels in these hearts were not different from control at 4 days after occlusion of the left coronary artery (13). Although other investigators confirmed that ATP and total adenine nucleotide contents were normal in viable tissue of hearts at 1 or 3 weeks after the induction of myocardial infarction, they observed that the tissue concentrations of creatine phosphate and free creatine were decreased (14). Very few studies to assess SR and SL functions directly or indirectly have been attempted in this model. We have hypothesized that the occurrence of intracellular Ca^{2+} deficiency may be crucial in the development of progressive contractile failure following myocardial infarction. This hypothesis was substantiated by the finding that the sensitivity of the surviving myocardium to verapamil was increased when compared to control (14), and that hearts were less sensitive to extracellular Ca^{2+} 1 to 3 weeks after myocardial infarction. Furthermore, these authors suggested that inward Ca^{2+} channel activity may be depressed in the infarcted hearts. It is pointed out, however, that the SL membrane is only one organelle that may contribute to a loss of intracellular Ca^{2+} homeostasis in heart failure; the SR has long been the focus of studies to elucidate mechanisms for heart failure (15). These efforts have revealed that Ca^{2+} transients of muscles from failing hearts are markedly prolonged and show a diminished capacity to restore low resting Ca^{2+} levels during diastole, which is consistent with a reduced rate of sequestration of Ca^{2+} in these hearts (16,17). It has been suggested that impaired rate of uptake of Ca^{2+} by SR results in a rise in resting tension, leading to diastolic cardiac dysfunction (17). Although all of these studies suggest impaired function of SL and SR, the sequence of changes in these subcellular organelles during the development of congestive heart failure due to myocardial infarction has not been clearly established. Because it appears that the development of heart failure in this model is time-dependent (18), it was considered of interest to examine the time course of alterations in SL and SR membranes to gain information regarding the cause–effect relationship with the degree of congestive heart failure.

SARCOLEMMAL AND SARCOPLASMIC RETICULAR CHANGES DURING THE DEVELOPMENT OF CONGESTIVE HEART FAILURE

To investigate the status of SL and SR membranes during the development of congestive heart failure, we surgically ligated the left coronary artery in male Sprague-Dawley rats (200–250 g), which yielded large (transmural scar ≥35% of the total left ventricular circumference) reproducible infarcts in experimental animals. Examination of general characteristics and hemodynamic parameters in experimental animals with large myocardial infarction revealed that experimental animals exhibited signs of graded cardiac dysfunction with time (18–21). From the results shown in Fig. 1, it can be seen that accumulation of fluid (ascites) in the abdominal cavity was evident at 4, 8, and 16 weeks, whereas lung congestion, as noted from the wet to dry lung weight ratio, became apparent in the 8-week and 16-week experimental groups. Control and experimental animals were anesthetized (50 mg/kg pentobarbitol sodium; i.p.) and studied for hemodynamic characteristics by

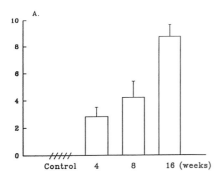

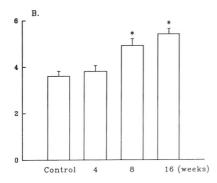

FIG. 1. (A) Incidence of ascites and (B) lung wet/dry weight ratio in control and experimental animals at 4, 8, and 16 weeks after infarction. Data are expressed as mean ± SE of eight experiments. *$p < 0.05$.

catheterization of the left ventricle by a microtip pressure transducer (model SPR-249, Millar Instruments, Houston, TX), which was introduced via the right carotid artery. Readings were taken from a Dynograph recorder (model R511A, Beckman, Fullerton, CA). The data in Fig. 2 revealed that a significant decrease in left ventricular systolic pressure (LVSP) was significantly decreased only in the 16-week experimental group, whereas left ventricular end-diastolic pressure (LVEDP) was markedly increased 4 weeks after induction of myocardial infarction and remained elevated in 8-week and 16-week experimental groups. The results shown in Fig. 3 indicate that rate of contraction ($+ dP/dt$) and rate of relaxation ($- dP/dt$) of experimental hearts were both significantly depressed in 4-, 8-, and 16-week groups. Although scar weights in the 4-, 8-, and 16-week experimental groups were not different from each other (Fig. 4), a significant increase in the viable (noninfarcted) left ventricular tissue was evident in the 16-week experimental animals when compared with the respective sham control rats (data not shown). A progressive increase in the muscle mass (normalized hypertrophy) of the viable left ventricle was seen in experimental animals. These observations regarding changes in general characteristics and hemodynamic parameters are similar to those described earlier from our laboratory using the same experimental model (18–22). It should also be indicated that an increase in right ventricular muscle mass after 4, 8, and 16 weeks has been reported previously (18–20,22). On the basis of these find-

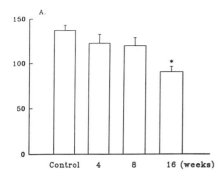

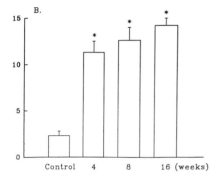

FIG. 2. Hemodynamic characteristics of control and experimental animals at 4, 8, and 16 weeks after infarction. (**A**) Left ventricular systolic pressure (LVSP). (**B**) Left ventricular end-diastolic pressure (LVEDP). All measurements were made on a Beckman dynograph using a Millar microcatheter; the catheter was inserted in the left ventricle via cannulation of the right carotid artery. Data are expressed as mean ± SE of eight experiments. *$p < 0.05$.

ings, the rats with chronic myocardial infarction were considered to be in prefailure, moderate failure, and severe congestive heart failure at 4, 8, and 16 weeks respectively. It is understood that this classification and division of experimental animals into these stages is arbitrary and intended for comparison of hemodynamic and clinical changes with biochemical parameters. Because we and others have demonstrated that the induction of relatively large myocardial infarction is critical for development of heart failure, we monitored scar size in the experimental animals and used only those animals with large (>35% of left ventricular circumference) myocardial infarction for the current study.

For the isolation of different subcellular organelles, the viable left ventricle from three to five experimental animals in each group were pooled; control (sham-operated) animals of the same age group were used for comparison. Because the data from the sham control preparations at 4, 8, and 16 weeks of operation were not different ($p > 0.05$) from one group to another, the results were pooled together and represented in all figures as "control." Purified SR and SL fractions were isolated in each batch according to methods described elsewhere (23,24). The SR ATP-dependent Ca^{2+}- uptake and Ca^{2+}-stimulated ATPase activities were determined according to the methods of Alto and Dhalla (25). All techniques for measuring SL Mg^{2+} ATPase, Na^{+}-Ca^{2+} ATPase, and Na^{+}-dependent Ca^{2+} uptake, dihydropyridine binding, and ATP-dependent Ca^{2+} uptake were the same as those described earlier

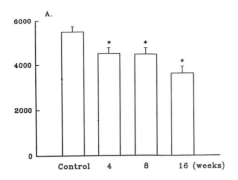

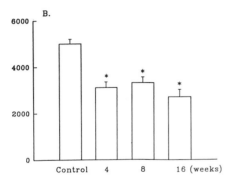

FIG. 3. Rates of (**A**) cardiac contraction (+dP/dt) and (**B**) cardiac relaxation (−dP/dt) in control and experimental hearts at 4, 8, and 16 weeks after infarction. Data are expressed as mean ± SE of eight experiments. *$p<0.05$.

(18–20). The results were analyzed using Student's t test (one-tailed) and presented as mean ± SE, and the difference between control and experimental preparations was considered significant when $p \leq 0.05$.

The ATP-dependent Ca^{2+} uptake in the SR vesicles was determined in the presence of a permeant anion, oxalate, and the results are shown in Fig. 5. These data revealed that a significant reduction in SR Ca^{2+} uptake occurred in experimental hearts at 4, 8, and 16 weeks after induction of myocardial infarction when compared with control values. Likewise, SR Ca^{2+}-stimulated ATPase activity was significantly depressed at all stages of failure. These results suggest that the cardiac SR membrane is altered early in the development of congestive heart failure after myocardial infarction, and remains depressed throughout the course of the progression of heart failure in experimental animals. Thus, it appears that reduced sequestration of Ca^{2+} from the cytosol to the lumen of the SR may be a primary defect leading to incomplete removal of Ca^{2+} from the cytosol during diastole, which may explain impaired relaxation in these hearts. On the other hand, because the degree of Ca^{2+} loading of the SR has a direct bearing on the amount of Ca^{2+} available for subsequent cardiac contraction, it can be seen that reduced SR Ca^{2+} pump activity may eventually lead to reduced availability of Ca^{2+} for beat-to-beat contraction, and therefore to reduced force of contraction. This may explain the significant reduction in the rate of cardiac contraction that was seen in experimental hearts.

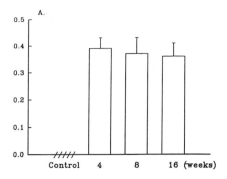

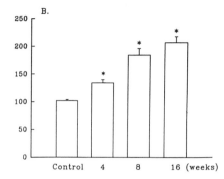

FIG. 4. (**A**) Scar weight and (**B**) percent increase in myocardial mass (normalized hypertrophy) in control and experimental animals at 4, 8, and 16 weeks after infarction. For the determination of degree of hypertrophy, the percentage of the infarcted left ventricle was estimated 3 weeks after coronary artery ligation by planimetric techniques; this percentage was extrapolated to the respective experimental groups. Data are expressed as mean ± SE of eight experiments. *$p < 0.05$.

The data in Fig. 6 show SL Na^+-K^+ ATPase activities in experimental hearts at different stages of congestive heart failure. Although SL Na^+-K^+ ATPase was depressed only in moderate and severe stages, sarcolemmal Mg^{2+} ATPase activity was significantly depressed at all stages of heart failure (control 4 weeks; 86.6 ± 3.2 vs. 4-week experimental; $71.5 \pm 3.21^*$: control 8 weeks; 81.3 ± 4.2 vs. 8-week experimental; $58.3 \pm 3.0^*$: control 16 weeks; 80.5 ± 2.9 vs. 16-week experimental; $55.6 \pm 3.3^*$). All activities were expressed as μmol Pi/mg protein/h). Because the SL Na^+-K^+ ATPase activity in 4-week experimental preparations was not altered, it appears that the observed depression of enzyme activity at moderate and severe stages of heart failure is a consequence of events occurring during the development of congestive heart failure. The possibility must be considered that the alterations observed in the Na^+-K^+ ATPase activity were not specific for the development of congestive heart failure, but were related to hypertrophy of the myocardium in experimental animals. It should be noted, however, that no alteration of Na^+-K^+ ATPase activities was found in SL preparations from hypertrophied rabbit hearts due to pressure overload (26). Furthermore, about 35% hypertrophy of the left ventricle in 4-week experimental animals was not associated with any change in SL Na^+-K^+ ATPase activity in the current study. Thus myocardial hypertrophy of the left ventricle cannot explain the observed alteration of Na^+-K^+ ATPase activity in congestive heart failure.

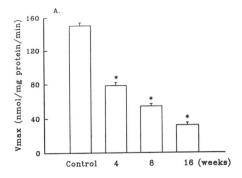

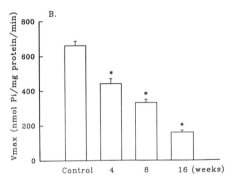

FIG. 5. (A) ATP-dependent sarcoplasmic reticular Ca^{2+} uptake and **(B)** sarcoplasmic reticular Ca^{2+}-stimulated ATPase activity in the viable left ventricle at 4, 8, and 16 weeks after infarction. Data are expressed as mean ± SE of eight experiments. *$p < 0.05$.

Because the cardiac Na^+-K^+ ATPase is an essential part of the Na^+ pump, which is suggested to participate in the maintenance of cellular resting potential (27), a decline of Na^+-K^+ ATPase activity can cause disturbance in the electrical behavior of the failing myocardium. Thus, it is conceivable that depressed SL Na^+-K^+ pump activity could lead to decreased maximum diastolic potential across the SL membrane in surviving myocardium of animals with moderate and severe congestive heart failure. Subsequent partial inactivation of fast Na^+ channels in these hearts may occur and could reduce the magnitude of Na^+ current to the myocardium, known to be involved in release of intracellular Ca^{2+} from SR stores (28). Such a change in SL Na^+-K^+ ATPase in failing heart was not seen in the early stages of congestive heart failure and thus cannot be considered to be the cause of contractile failure in this experimental model. On the other hand, inhibition of SL Na^+-K^+ ATPase in failing heart can be considered to augment contractile force development in a manner similar to that proposed for cardiac glycosides (29,30). Such an augmentation of contractile force would tend to maintain the ability of cardiac muscle to pump blood in moderate congestive heart failure stage, and in this context the observed depression in Na^+-K^+ ATPase may be adaptive in nature.

The results shown in Fig. 7 indicate a significant depression in the V_{max} values for the SL Na^+-Ca^{2+} exchange activities in preparations from experimental hearts at all stages of congestive heart failure. Because SL Na^+-Ca^{2+} exchange has been

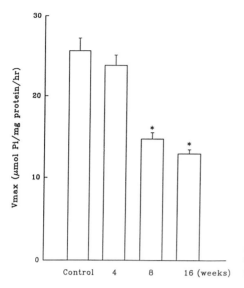

FIG. 6. Sarcolemmal Na^+-K^+ ATPase activity in the viable left ventricle at 4, 8, and 16 weeks after infarction. Data are expressed as mean $\pm$ SE of eight experiments. $^*p<0.05$.

suggested to participate in the efflux of Ca^{2+} from the cytosolic space and thus contribute to the maintenance of low diastolic cytosolic Ca^{2+} concentration, depressed relaxation of the myocardium in early, moderate, and severe failure may be partly explained. On the other hand, some work has shown that depolarization of membranes elicited release of Ca^{2+} from stores in the SR that was dependent on extracellular Ca^{2+} concentration (28), even when Ca^{2+} entry through voltage-dependent

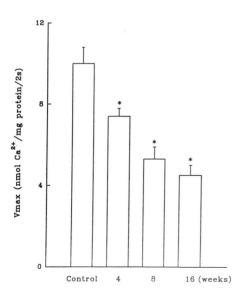

FIG. 7. Sarcolemmal Na^+-Ca^{2+} exchange activity (Na^+-dependent Ca^{2+} uptake) in the viable left ventricle at 4, 8, and 16 weeks after infarction. Data are expressed as mean $\pm$ SE of eight experiments. $^*p<0.05$.

Ca^{2+} channels was blocked. It was suggested by these authors that the Na^+-Ca^{2+} exchange mechanism may contribute to Ca^{2+} entry to the myocardium, which serves to trigger release of relatively greater quantities of so-called activator Ca^{2+} from the SR. Therefore, a reduction of SL Ca^{2+} influx by depressed Na^+-Ca^{2+} exchange activity could lead to decreased contractility in the myocardium. The possibility must be considered that the alterations observed in Na^+-dependent Ca^{2+} uptake were not specific for events occurring during the development of congestive heart failure, but were directly related to hypertrophy of the experimental hearts. Because reports from our group and others have noted that other experimental models of cardiac hypertrophy and failure were associated with no change or an increase in Na^+-dependent Ca^{2+} uptake (26,31), it seems unlikely that the mechanism for depression of Na^+-Ca^{2+} exchange activity in congestive heart failure can be explained by myocardial hypertrophy.

To gain information on other SL mechanisms for Ca^{2+} entry and efflux in the failing myocardium, we sought to determine the status of SL Ca^{2+} channels and SL Ca^{2+} pump activity. Using $[^3H]$-nitrendipine to assay the density of SL voltage-sensitive Ca^{2+} channels in the surviving left ventricular myocardium of experimental animals, it was revealed that the density (B_{max}) of these channels was significantly reduced in moderate and severe congestive heart failure stages, but not in prefailure stage when compared with control values (Fig. 8). The dissociation

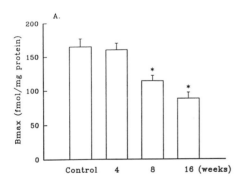

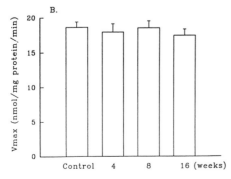

FIG. 8. (A) Binding density of ^{3}H-nitrendipine and (B) sarcolemmal ATP-dependent Ca^{2+} uptake in SL preparations from the viable left ventricle at 4, 8, and 16 weeks after infarction. Data are expressed as mean ± SE of eight experiments. *$p < 0.05$.

constant (Kd) for binding of ^{3}H-nitrendipine was unchanged at any stage of failure when compared with control preparations (data not shown). The SL Ca^{2+} channels are considered to play a critical role in the movement of relatively small quantities of Ca^{2+} into the myocardium at the plateau of the cardiac action potential. As the movement of so-called trigger Ca^{2+} is believed to play a crucial role for Ca^{2+}-induced Ca^{2+} release in the myocardium from SR stores, reduced density of SL Ca^{2+} channels could be seen to contribute to a decrease in the availability of Ca^{2+} in the myocardium. Because these channels were altered only in the latter stages of congestive heart failure, it is apparent that the observed changes were similar to those with Na^+-K^+ ATPase activity insofar as they are likely a consequence of events occurring during the progression of disease. To examine the possibility of altered SL Ca^{2+} pump activity, ATP-dependent Ca^{2+} accumulation was assayed in control and experimental preparations (Fig. 8). Sarcolemmal vesicles prepared from experimental (4, 8, and 16 weeks after myocardial infarction) hearts showed no changes in ATP-dependent Ca^{2+} accumulation when compared with control preparations. It should be noted that ATP-dependent uptake was not augmented in the presence of 2 mM of oxalate, which is known to increase the ATP-dependent Ca^{2+} accumulation in the SR, and therefore our SL preparation was free of contamination by this subcellular organelle. As the SL Ca^{2+} pump is known to bind Ca^{2+} with high affinity and transport Ca^{2+} from the cytosolic space with a relatively slow turnover rate, it has been suggested that the sarcolemmal Ca^{2+} pump is important for maintaining diastolic cytosolic Ca^{2+} concentration below 10^{-6} M. Normal SL Ca^{2+} pump activities indicate that removal of cytoplasmic Ca^{2+} from cardiac myocytes was intact by this mechanism, and in light of depressed mechanisms for Ca^{2+} influx, this system may contribute toward decreasing the availability of Ca^{2+} for contraction in the failing myocardium.

From the foregoing discussion of the results in the rat model of congestive heart failure after large myocardial infarction, the sequence of membrane alterations in the failing myocardium seems clear. The prefailure stage in this experimental model was associated with depressed activities of cardiac SR Ca^{2+} pump and SL Na^+-Ca^{2+} exchange; these may be primary defects causing the reduction of availability of Ca^{2+} for contraction (Ca^{2+} deficiency). Although both of these mechanisms are believed to play a role in the removal of Ca^{2+} from the cytosolic space following myocardial contraction, and thereby may contribute to impaired myocardial relaxation, it needs to be pointed out that (a) a steady-state reduction in Ca^{2+} loading of the SR by impaired Ca^{2+} sequestration is a likely consequence of depressed SR pump function and (b) reduced sarcolemmal Ca^{2+}-influx trigger Ca^{2+} is possible by depressed SL Na^+-Ca^{2+} exchange activity. Thus, a depression in these activities may explain reductions in rate of contraction and relaxation in prefailure-stage hearts. The moderate and severe stages of congestive heart failure were associated with decreased SL Na^+-K^+ ATPase activity and SL Ca^{2+} channel density in addition to depressed SR Ca^{2+} pump function and SL Na^+-Ca^{2+} exchange activity. Although reduced density of SL Ca^{2+} channels can be seen to contribute to cytosolic Ca^{2+} deficiency in experimental hearts at moderate and severe stages of congestive heart failure, depressed SL Na^+-K^+ ATPase activity was considered to serve as an adaptive mechanism because it can be seen to increase the entry of Ca^{2+}, thereby reducing the extent of intracellular Ca^{2+} deficiency in the cardiac myocytes of the experimental animals. As sarcolemmal Ca^{2+} pump function was normal at all stages of failure, removal of Ca^{2+} from the cytoplasm by this mechanism may assist in reducing the availability of Ca^{2+} for the contractile apparatus during the development of congestive heart failure. Thus, it appears that a remodeling of cardiac SL and SR occurs, and alterations in the function of these membranes may lead to the development of congestive heart failure in rats after large myocardial infarction.

SUMMARY

Depressed cardiac pump function is the hallmark of congestive heart failure, and it is suggested that abnormal Ca^{2+} handling by the cardiac myocyte is responsible for depressed contractility. As SL Ca^{2+} channels, Na^+-K^+ ATPase, Na^+-Ca^{2+} exchange, and Ca^{2+} pump, as well as SR Ca^{2+} pump, are known to be involved in transsarcolemmal Ca^{2+} movements, these mechanisms were examined to identify Ca^{2+} handling defects in failing myocardium by using the rat model of congestive heart failure at 4, 8, and 16 weeks after myocardial infarction. Hemodynamic assessment with respect to the left ventricular pressures, as well as rates of contraction and relaxation, and clinical signs such as abdominal ascites and lung congestion revealed that experimental animals at 4, 8, and 16 weeks were at early, moderate, and severe stages of congestive heart failure. The SR ATP-dependent Ca^{2+} uptake and Ca^{2+}-stimulated ATPase activities were significantly depressed in the viable left ventricles of all experimental groups when compared with control values. On the other hand, SL Na^+-K^+ ATPase activity was found to be depressed in moderate and severe stages of congestive heart failure, but was unchanged in the prefailure stage when compared with control values. Sarcolemmal Na^+-Ca^{2+} exchange activity (Na^+-dependent Ca^{2+} uptake) was depressed in 4-, 8-, and 16-week experimental animals. [³H]-nitrendipine binding assay revealed that the density of SL Ca^{2+} channels was decreased in the viable failing left ventricle at 8 and 16 weeks, whereas SL ATP-dependent Ca^{2+} uptake was unchanged in experimental hearts at any stage of failure when compared with control. These results suggest that cardiac membranes are remodeled with respect to Ca^{2+} handling, and these changes may cause an overall reduction in the availability of Ca^{2+} for the contractile apparatus; this may play a crucial role for depressed contractility in this model of congestive heart failure.

ACKNOWLEDGMENT

The research reported in this chapter was supported by a grant from the Medical Research Council of Canada under the MRC Group in Experimental Cardiology.

REFERENCES

1. Dhalla NS, Das PK, Sharma GP. Subcellular basis of cardiac contractile failure. *J Mol Cell Cardiol* 1978;10:363–385.
2. Dhalla NS, Pierce GN, Panagia V, Singal PK, Beamish RE. Calcium movements in relation to heart failure. *Basic Res Cardiol* 1982;77:117–139.
3. Dhalla NS, Dixon IMC, Beamish RE. Biochemical basis of heart function and contractile failure. *J Appl Cardiol* 1991;6:7–30.
4. Pfeffer JM, Pfeffer MA, Fletcher PH, Braunwald E. Ventricular performance in rats with myocardial infarction and failure. *Am J Med* 1984;76:99–103.
5. Johns TNP, Olson BJ. Experimental myocardial infarction. I. A method of coronary occlusion in small animals. *Ann Surg* 1984;140:675–682.
6. Pfeffer MA, Pfeffer JM, Fishbein MC, et al. Myocardial infarct size and ventricular function in rats. *Circ Res* 1979;44:503–512.
7. Fletcher PJ, Pfeffer JM, Pfeffer MA, Braunwald E. Left ventricular diastolic pressure-volume relations in rats with healed myocardial infarction: effects on systolic function. *Circ Res* 1981;49:618–626.
8. Fletcher PJ, Pfeffer JM, Pfeffer MA, Braunwald E. Effects of hypertension on cardiac performance in rats with myocardial infarction. *Am J Cardiol* 1982;50:488–496.
9. Bloomfield RA, Lauson HD, Cournand A, Brecel ES, Richards DW Jr. Recording of right heart pressures in normal subjects and in patients with chronic pulmonary disease and various types of cardio-circulatory disease. *J Clin Invest* 1946;25:639–664.
10. Parmley WW. Pathophysiology of congestive heart failure. *Am J Cardiol* 1985;55(2):9A-14A.
11. Geenen DL, White TP, Lampman RM. Papillary mechanics and cardiac morphology of infarcted rat hearts after training. *J Appl Physiol* 1987;63:92–96.
12. Mercadier JJ, Lompre AM, Wisnewsky C, et al. Myosin isoenzymic changes of several models of rat cardiac hypertrophy. *Circ Res* 1981;49:525–532.
13. Zimmer H-G, Mortias PA, Morschner G. Myocardial infarction in rats: effects of metabolic and pharmacologic interventions. *Basic Res Cardiol* 1989;84:332–343.
14. Fellenius E, Hansen CA, Mjos O, Neely JR. Chronic infarction decreases maximum cardiac work and sensitivity of the heart to extracellular calcium. *Am J Physiol* 1985;249:H80–H87.
15. Grossman W. Diastolic dysfunction and congestive heart failure. *Circulation* 1990;81[Suppl III]:1–7.
16. Gwathmey JK, Morgan JP. Altered calcium handling in experimental pressure-overload hypertrophy in the ferret. *Circ Res* 1985;57:836–843.
17. Morgan JP, Emy R, Allen PD, Grossman W, Gwathmey JK. Abnormal intracellular Ca^{2+} handling, a major cause of systolic and diastolic dysfunction in ventricular myocardium from patients with heart failure. *Circulation* 1990;81[Suppl III]:21–32.
18. Dixon IMC, Lee SL, Dhalla NS. Nitrendipine binding in congestive heart failure due to myocardial infarction. *Circ Res* 1990;66:782–788.
19. Dixon IMC, Hata T, Dhalla NS. Sarcolemmal ATPase activity in congestive heart failure due to myocardial infarction. *Am J Physiol* 1992;262:C664–C671.
20. Dixon IMC, Hata T, Dhalla NS. Sarcolemmal Ca^{2+}-transport in congestive heart failure due to myocardial infarction in rats. *Am J Physiol* 1992;262:H1387–H1394.
21. Dhalla NS, Dixon IMC, Rupp H, Barwinsky J. Experimental congestive heart failure due to myocardial infarction: sarcolemmal receptors and cation transporters. In: Gulch RW, Kissling G, eds. *Current topics in heart failure*. Darmstadt: Steinkopff Verlag; 1991:13–23.
22. Afzal N, Dhalla NS. Differential changes in left and right ventricular SR calcium transport in congestive heart failure. *Am J Physiol* 1992;262:H864–H874.
23. Harigaya S, Schwartz A. Rate of calcium binding and uptake in normal animals and failing human cardiac muscle membrane vesicles (relaxing system) and mitochondria. *Circ Res* 1969;25: 781–794.
24. Pitts BJR. Stoichiometry of sodium-calcium exchange in cardiac sarcolemmal vesicles. *J Biol Chem* 1979;254:6232–6235.
25. Alto LE, Dhalla NS. Role of change in microsomal calcium uptake in the effects of reperfusion of Ca^{2+}-deprived rat hearts. *Circ Res* 1981;48:17–24.
26. Heyliger CE, Takeo S, Dhalla NS. Alterations in sarcolemmal Na^{+}-Ca^{2+} exchange and ATP-dependent Ca^{2+} binding in hypertrophied heart. *Can J Cardiol* 1985;1:328–339.

27. Glitsch HG. Characteristics of active Na support in intact cardiac cells. *Am J Physiol* 1979;236: H189–H199.
28. LeBlanc N, Hume JR. Sodium current-induced release of calcium from cardiac sarcoplasmic reticulum. *Science* 1990;248:372–376.
29. Schuurmans-Stekhoven F, Bonting SL. Transport adenosine triphosphatases: properties and functions. *Physiol Rev* 1981;61:2–76.
30. Schwartz A, Lindenmayer GE, Allan JC. The sodium-potassium adenosine triphosphatase: pharmacological, physiological and biochemical aspects. *Pharmacol Rev* 1975;27:3–134.
31. Nakanishi H, Makino N, Hata T, Matsui H, Yano K, Yanaga T. Sarcolemmal Ca^{2+} transport activities in cardiac hypertrophy caused by pressure overload. *Am J Physiol* 1989;245:C241–C247.

The Failing Heart, edited by N. S. Dhalla,
R. E. Beamish, N. Takeda, and M. Nagano.
Lippincott-Raven Publishers, Philadelphia © 1995.

19

Modification of Left Ventricular Remodeling After Myocardial Infarction

Bodh I. Jugdutt

*Department of Medicine, University of Alberta Hospitals,
Edmonton, Alberta, T6G 2R7 Canada*

Left ventricular remodeling after myocardial infarction has sinister implications, especially in patients with large anterior transmural infarction (1,2). It is now recognized as a major mechanism for disability and death postinfarction. It occupies a central position in the cascade to ventricular dilation, congestive heart failure, more ventricular dysfunction, and end-stage heart disease (Table 1). There is increasing evidence that left ventricular remodeling is progressive in survivors (3–7) and that the vicious cycle can be interrupted or even prevented (8–24). Because myocardial infarction and congestive heart failure are major causes of suffering and death, a major health care research initiative has been the development (27–33) and testing (34–40) of therapeutic strategies to minimize harmful aspects of remodeling (Tables 2 and 3). The focus of this chapter is the pharmacologic modification of left ventricular remodeling after infarction.

QUANTITATION

In broad terms, ventricular remodeling refers to the structural and shape changes associated with myocardial damage. The definitions of remodeling in *The Oxford English Dictionary* and *Webster's English Dictionary* emphasize structure, shape, and three-dimensional (3D) reconstruction (Table 4). Acute infarction results in a cycle of dysfunction, shape distortion, and more dysfunction. Repair that follows myocardial infarction attempts to restore shape and function (Table 5) and involves considerable remodeling over weeks and months (2). To understand how to modify remodeling and preserve shape and function, it is necessary to quantify structure, shape, and function repeatedly during life. Two-dimensional echocardiography (2D-Echo) is a widely available diagnostic tool that can be applied for serial interrogations of the remodeling process in vivo (5,6,12,24–26). It allows quantitation of at least three sets of parameters: (a) regional dilation, extent of asynergy, elonga-

TABLE 1. *Results of left ventricular remodeling after myocardial infarction*

Ventricular remodeling
Infarct expansion and thinning
Aneurysm formation
Progressive ventricular dilation
Ventricular rupture: free wall, septum
Progressive ventricular dysfunction
Congestive heart failure
Volume overload
Hypertrophy
Arrhythmias
Increased morbidity
Increased mortality

Modified from Jugdutt (2).

TABLE 2. *Thirteen randomized trials pertinent to remodeling after myocardial infarction*

Ref./year	No. of patients	Onset of therapy	Duration of therapy	Outcome
Flaherty et al. (27)/1985	10 placebo 10 NTG + IABP	<12 h	4–5 d	Less LV dilation Function: no change
Gottlieb et al. (28)/1988	68 placebo 64 nifedipine	<12 h	6 wk	Less expansion Function: no change
Jugdutt and Warnica (12)/1988	156 placebo 154 NTG	<12 h	48 h	Less LV remodeling Improved function Fewer deaths
Tymchak et al. (29)/1988	16 placebo 16 NTG 18 NTG + RP	<6 h	48 h	Less expansion Function improved early
Sharpe et al. (30)/1988	20 placebo 20 furosemide 20 captopril	1 wk	12 mo	Less LV dilation Improved function
Pfeffer et al. (13)/1988	29 placebo 30 captopril	11–31 d	12 mo	Less dilation
Touchstone et al. (31)/1989	No controls Streptokinase	<4 h	acute	Less expansion
Michorowski et al. (21)/1990	25 placebo 25 buccal NTG	48 h + NTG <12 h	6 wk	Less LV remodeling Improved function
Jugdutt et al. (22)/1990	20 placebo 20 captopril 20 NTG 20 captopril + NTG	48 h + NTG <12 h	6 wk	Less LV remodeling Improved function
Nabel et al. (32)/1991	18 placebo + rtPA 20 captopril + rtPA	>3 h	3 mo	Less LV dilation Function: no change
Oldroyd et al. (15)/1991	50 placebo 49 captopril	<24 h	2 mo	Less expansion Volume: no change
St. John Sutton et al. (24)/1994	259 placebo 253 captopril	3–16 d	12 mo	Fewer events Less LV dilation
Foy et al. (33)/1994	75 placebo 75 captopril 75 enalapril	<24 h	3 mo	Less LV dilation

Modified from Jugdutt (2).

IABP, intraaortic balloon pumping; LV, left ventricular; NTG, nitroglycerin; RP, reperfusion (streptokinase ± angioplasty); rtPA, recombinant tissue plasminogen activator.

TABLE 3. *Six large clinical trials of ACE inhibitors after myocardial infarction*

Trial	Full name (ref.)	Onset of therapy	Duration of therapy
SOLVD	Studies of Left Ventricular Dysfunction		
	Treatment (34)	>1 mo	41 mo
	Prevention (35)	>1 mo	37 mo
SAVE	Survival and Left Ventricular Enlargement (36)	3–16 d	42 mo
CONSENSUS II	Cooperative New Scandinavian Enalapril Survival Study II (37)	≤24 h	6 mo
AIRE	Acute Infarction Ramipril Efficacy (38)	3–10 d	15 mo
GISSI-3	Gruppo Italiano per lo Studio della Sopravvivenza nell' Infarcto Miocardico (39)	≤24 h	6 wk
ISIS-4	Fourth International Study of Infarct Survival (40)	≤24 h	30 d

tion and thinning of infarct segments in short axis, (b) bulging in antero-apical or infero-basal regions on the long axis, and (c) the endocardial surface area of regional asynergy, volumes, and ejection fraction from 3D reconstruction algorithms (Fig. 1). A host of useful regional and global shape indexes (6,25,41–44) and a sphericity index (45) can be measured.

PATHOPHYSIOLOGIC CONSIDERATIONS

Therapy should be aimed at the major determinants of remodeling, namely infarction, healing, mechanical deformation forces, the supporting matrix, and progressive dilation (Table 6). It is now clear from studies using serial quantitative 2D-Echo in patients that remodeling begins very early during infarction, with infarct expansion, or a stretching, thinning, and bulging of the infarct area (6,12,46). Similar studies performed during healing over 6 weeks after infarction in the canine model (47) indicate that further remodeling occurs during healing, with late infarct thinning after the infarct collagen plateau is reached at about 2 weeks (48). In fact, the major proportion of remodeling appears to occur during infarction and healing. Therefore, early and prolonged therapy spanning the infarction and healing phases

TABLE 4. *Definition: remodel*

Webster's Dictionary: to alter the structure of; remake
The Oxford Dictionary: to model again or differently; to reconstruct or reorganize (model n: representation in 3 dimensions of proposed structure; vb: fashion, shape)

TABLE 5. *Definition: repair*

Webster's Dictionary: vb: to restore, fix, renew, make good, mend, remedy; n: replacement of destroyed cells or tissues by new formations

The Oxford Dictionary: vb: to restore to good condition after damage or wear, to set right, to fix, renovate, refix

---

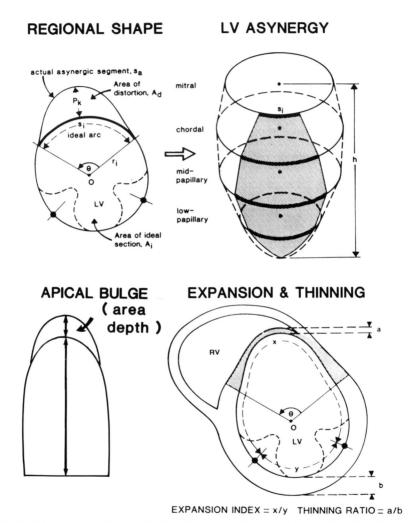

EXPANSION INDEX = x/y   THINNING RATIO = a/b

FIG. 1. Echocardiographic quantitation of left ventricular remodeling and function after myocardial infarction. **Upper left:** Measurement of regional bulging on end-diastolic outlines in short-axis 2D Echos. P_k, peak distortion equals depth of bulge; θ, angular extent of asynergy. **Upper right:** 3D reconstruction algorithm for endocardial shell and surface area of left ventricular asynergy and volumes. h, height derived from average long-axis length of the apical four- and two-chamber views. **Lower left:** Measurement of regional bulging in the apical four-chamber view. **Lower right:** Measurement of elongation and thinning of the infarct segment. Modified from Jugdutt (6) and Jugdutt et al. (41).

TABLE 6. *Major targets for limiting left ventricular remodeling and preserving function in myocardial infarction*

Infarction process
Healing process
Deformation process
Disruption of the supporting matrix
Progressive dilation

Modified from Jugdutt (2).

sounds logical, but questions regarding how soon and for how long remain unanswered.

The temporal pathophysiologic staging of the remodeling process provides some guidance on timing and duration of therapy (2) (Table 7). Very early therapy seems justified in view of the fact that very early remodeling involving infarct expansion (5,6,46), early regional diastolic bulging (6,42), myocyte slippage (49), collagen matrix disruption, and increased regional distensibility (50,51), occurs in the first few hours after infarction. Although healing after infarction generally takes 6 weeks in dogs (48), autopsy studies have shown that healing might take up to 6 months with large human infarcts (52), during which time significant remodeling can be expected. In addition, clinicopathologic studies suggest that the rate of healing can be modified by concomitant therapy. Thus, healing is delayed by corticosteroids (53). Delayed healing has been confirmed experimentally with steroidal (54) and nonsteroidal (55–57) antiinflammatory agents. In contrast, reperfusion, by opening the culprit coronary lesion, not only interrupts the march to necrosis, decreases infarct size (58), and reduces expansion and thinning (19), but also is associated with disruption of the extracellular collagen matrix (59) and more rapid healing (60). Late reperfusion, however, results in delayed recovery of function, so that the algorithm "decrease in infarct size→limitation of remodeling→improvement of function" might not hold true when thrombolytic agents are used. In fact, Gaudron et al. (7) recently documented that progressive global left ventricular dilation occurs up to 3 years after infarction in some patients from the thrombolytic era.

Clinical evidence suggests that early regional dilation is a precursor to late dila-

TABLE 7. *Temporal staging of postinfarction ventricular remodeling as a guide for timing of therapy*

Timing	Pathophysiologic process
Very early: first 24 h	Acute evolution and completion of myocardial infarction
Early: Day 2 to 2 wk	Healing before infarct collagen plateau
Late: 3 to 6 wk (up to 6 mo)	Healing after infarct collagen plateau
Very late: after 1.5 mo (up to 12 mo)	Late postinfarct healing

Modified from Jugdutt (2).

TABLE 8. *Therapeutic principles for modifying ventricular remodeling in acute myocardial infarction*

Prevent infarction of ischemic myocardium
Limit infarction size by early reperfusion
Reduce infarct transmurality
Limit early infarct expansion and bulging
Prevent or limit reperfusion injury
Ensure judicious LV unloading during infarction
Avoid hypotension and the paradoxical J-curve effect
Prevent or limit early infarct thinning

Modified from Jugdutt (2).
LV, left ventricular.

tion (5,6,61), and a gradient in regional wall stress caused by the early bulge is the driving force for global dilation and the more globular shape (62). Experimental evidence suggests that progressive chamber dilation may partly involve collagenase activation (63), in addition to matrix disruption and side-to-side slippage in noninfarct zones (59,64), and matrix disruption due to ischemia or necrosis (65,66). Because marked early bulging on 2D-Echo identifies patients with Q-wave infarction who are prone to marked infarct expansion and global dilation (6) or ventricular septal rupture (67), early therapy appears to be a potentially powerful strategy for prevention (Table 8). Furthermore, the connection between early infarct expansion and subsequent chamber dilation supports the idea of therapy spanning the infarction and healing phases and extending beyond (Tables 9 through 11).

INFARCT COLLAGEN PLATEAU

Another consideration is that ventricular remodeling is associated with profound changes at cellular, biochemical, molecular, and genetic levels in the heart, and adaptive changes are triggered in the heart and neurohumoral milieu. Some of these changes impact negatively on left ventricular function.

TABLE 9. *Therapeutic principles for ventricular remodeling during healing after acute myocardial infarction*

Promote normal infarct healing
Ensure LV unloading during healing
Maintain infarct-related artery patency
Increase nutrient collateral flow to infarct zone
Maintain noninfarct-related artery patency
Preserve collagen matrix in noninfarct tissue
Preserve architectural framework
Prevent or limit scar thinning

Modified from Jugdutt (2).
LV, left ventricular.

TABLE 10. *Therapeutic targets during ventricular remodeling and repair after myocardial infarction*

Decrease mechanical deformation forces
    Ensure LV unloading during infarction, healing, and beyond
    Decrease chamber size, diastolic wall stress
    Decrease systolic wall stress
    Preserve shape, prevent bulging, limit sphericity
    Decrease thinning
Protect the supporting matrix
    Collagen and other matrix proteins in infarct, border, and noninfarct tissue
    Collagen promoters vs. disrupters
Prevent matrix disruption
    Mechanical
    Metabolic
    Pharmacologic

Modified from Jugdutt (2).
LV, left ventricular.

Because remodeling and healing after infarction are two dynamic processes that progress in parallel, therapeutic agents may differ in their effects on the rate of progression or different components of the substrate and produce different interactions depending on timing. They may differ in their effects on acute and chronic inflammation that occur in the first 2 weeks or the connective tissue proliferation and infarct collagen deposition that occur in the third week onward (48,52,68). As discussed earlier, they may influence the rate of healing, which differs among species, being slower in humans (3 to 6 months) than dogs (6 weeks), rabbits (4 weeks), or rats (3 weeks) (48). They may differ in effects on the early remodeling that occurs after infarction and before the collagen plateau occurs (in the first 2 weeks in dogs), with further expansion of the infarct segment and disruption of the matrix in the noninfarct segment (2). They may also differ in effects on the late remodeling that occurs after the infarct collagen plateau (up to 6 weeks in dogs). This late remodeling involves compaction of infarct collagen, late thinning, hypertrophy of the noninfarct segment, and left ventricular dilation due to the distension of both infarct and noninfarct segments, further increase in diastolic wall stress and left ventricular hypertrophy, formation of connections between collagen fibrils in

TABLE 11. *Therapeutic principles for ventricular remodeling to limit progressive dilation after infarction and healing*

Limit progressive chamber dilation
Prolong LV unloading
Prevent inappropriate hypertrophy
Protect architectural framework and matrix
Preserve shape and prevent sphericity
Preserve perfusion to noninfarct zones

Modified from Jugdutt (2).
LV, left ventricular.

the infarct zone and adjacent live myocytes, and disruption of the matrix in the noninfarct segment (48,50).

Experimental studies in the dog (48) indicate that deposition of collagen in an already expanded infarct segment seems to make the regional shape distortion permanent with aneurysm formation, so that remodeling before and after infarct collagen plateaus might have a bearing on the timing and duration of therapy (2, 47,48). More importantly, it appears that the potential for preventing remodeling is greater with therapy before the infarct collagen plateau (26,47).

CELLULAR AND METABOLIC EVENTS

Pharmacologic modification of cellular and metabolic events during early infarction can be expected to influence subsequent healing. Even short-term early therapy might have marked delayed effects on remodeling via different mechanisms (10,12,42). The nonsteroidal antiinflammatory agents ibuprofen and indomethacin both impair healing and cause scar thinning (55,56) despite divergent effects on infarct size (69,70). In contrast, nitroglycerin increases infarct collagen and preserves scar thickness (10). Clinically, indomethacin and ibuprofen, given for postinfarction pericarditis, were associated with a higher frequency of infarct expansion and deaths (42), while nitroglycerin postinfarction prevented infarct expansion and improved survival (12). Although the angiotensin-converting enzyme (ACE) inhibitor captopril has antiinflammatory properties, it was found to attenuate left ventricular dilation and functional deterioration over the first 3 months after infarction in rats (8) and improve survival (9). Clinically, ACE inhibitors have been found to reduce ventricular dilation (13–15,24,30,32,45) and improve survival in selected patients (36,38–40). The effect of ACE inhibitors on infarct collagen and the extracellular collagen matrix, however, has not received much attention.

COLLAGEN MATRIX AND INFARCT COLLAGEN

The importance of the extracellular collagen matrix in the supporting myocardial framework has been emphasized by Caulfield and Borg (71). The role of infarct collagen in infarct stiffness and resistance to rupture has been documented in rabbit (72) and dog (47) hearts. Increase in collagen concentration and collagen cross-linking has been documented in both pressure and volume-overload hypertrophy, and damage to the collagen weave has been correlated with aneurysm development (73). Because tissue ACE promotes fibroblast activity and collagen deposition, ACE inhibition has the potential for inhibiting fibroblast activity and collagen deposition after infarction, causing harm. In large rat infarctions, late captopril given between 3 and 6 weeks (i.e., after healing is completed) decreases left ventricular hypertrophy but does not influence noninfarct collagen (74). Early captopril, however, within 3 weeks of infarction inhibited noninfarct collagen deposition and DNA synthesis in the rats (74,75) and caused hemodynamic deterioration (76).

Another ACE inhibitor, perindopril, given 1 week after infarction also decreased noninfarct collagen in the rat (77). Interestingly, complete inhibition of noninfarct collagen was observed in the rat with the angiotensin II antagonist losartan (78). In rats with genetic hypertension but no infarction, the ACE inhibitor lisinopril caused regression of left ventricular hypertrophy, decrease in interstitial fibrosis, medial thickening of coronary arteries, and myocardial collagen (79). In the canine model of small myocardial infarctions, enalapril was found recently to decrease collagen deposition in the infarct scar, but no significant adverse effects on ventricular dilation or function were detected (80). Although the effect of enalapril in large infarctions was not studied, the possibility that ACE inhibition in that setting might decrease infarct collagen and promote dilation and dysfunction should be considered.

REPERFUSION AND REPERFUSION INJURY

In subendocardial infarcts, as commonly seen after early reperfusion, the epicardial rim of normal myocardium and collagen matrix (66) acts as a scaffold that resists bulging (2). As the epicardial rim later undergoes hypertrophy, it not only preserves regional wall thickness (81), but also might restrain bulging even more (2). The development of connections between collagen fibrils and live myocytes, and phenotypic conversion of fibroblasts to myofibroblasts containing actin and capable of contraction (50), might also play a role in resisting regional distension.

Although late reperfusion preserves infarct wall thickness (19,81), it might cause structural disruption of the extracellular collagen matrix, disrupt mechanical coupling, and contribute to mechanical dysfunction (82,83). Oxygen free-radical accumulation (82–84) or other biochemical abnormalities, such as calcium overload (85), likely mediate these effects so that free-radical scavengers (82,84) and calcium channel blockers (85) might be beneficial.

THERAPEUTIC STRATEGIES

In general, ideal therapy to limit remodeling should consider the infarct and noninfarct zones as well as the entire ventricle (Fig. 2). There should be at least five goals: First, to decrease infarct size and transmurality; second, to promote healing and preserve nutrient flow; third, to protect the collagen matrix, avoid decreasing infarct collagen, and avoid infarct thinning; fourth, to decrease deformation forces (such as high afterload and preload, large ventricular size, high heart rate, increased contractility, and increased wall stress); and fifth, to prevent continuing ventricular dilation, excessive hypertrophy, and further necrosis. With late reperfusion, left ventricular dysfunction due to myocardial stunning, hibernation, and reperfusion injury should be prevented (86). Some specific major therapeutic approaches are depicted in Table 12.

Because vasodilator therapy (e.g., nitrate) and ACE-inhibitor therapy (e.g., cap-

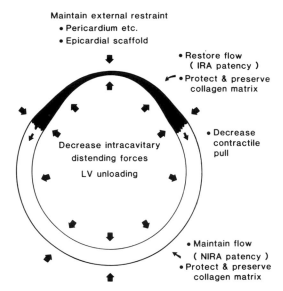

Maintain external restraint
- Pericardium etc.
- Epicardial scaffold

- Restore flow
  (IRA patency)
- Protect & preserve
  collagen matrix

Decrease intracavitary
distending forces

LV unloading

- Decrease
  contractile
  pull

- Maintain flow
  (NIRA patency)
- Protect & preserve
  collagen matrix

FIG. 2. Major therapeutic approaches for modification of left ventricular remodeling after myocardial infarction. Short-axis section of the left ventricle showing the diastolic bulge in the infarct segment (*darkened*). IRA, infarct-related artery; LV, left ventricle; NIRA, noninfarct-related artery.

topril) postinfarction can potentially (a) decrease left ventricular load, wall stress, chamber size, and expansion; (b) limit left ventricular hypertrophy; and (c) improve myocyte energetics, metabolism, and coronary artery reactivity, these agents were proposed and tested for prevention in selected patients with suspected infarction (39,40). Although prolonged left ventricular unloading to decrease wall stress with nitrates and ACE inhibitors (2,18) might be very effective in preventing ventricular dilation, thereby preserving the matrix, very early ACE inhibition can decrease infarct and noninfarct collagen, promote infarct thinning and bulging, and disrupt the matrix. Both nitrates and ACE inhibitors can potentially also cause excessive hypotension and extension of necrosis during acute infarction, so they should be used judiciously in early infarction (12,18). Because prolonged nitrate use is associated with development of tolerance (18), strategies to minimize tolerance should be

TABLE 12. *Some potential pharmacologic therapies for limiting remodeling after acute myocardial infarction*

Mechanism	Potential therapy
Decrease infarct size	Reperfusion; nitrate
Decrease preload	Nitrate; ACE inhibitor
Decrease afterload	Nitrate; nifedipine; ACE inhibitor
Decrease chamber size	Nitrate; ACE inhibitor
Decrease heart rate	Beta blocker; calcium blocker
Decrease contractility	Beta blocker; calcium blocker
Increase collateral flow	Nitrate
Decrease reperfusion injury	Calcium blocker; SOD; ACE inhibitor (?); nitrate (?)

Modified from Jugdutt (2).
SOD, superoxide dismutase.

used (26). Thus, the final outcome of anti-remodeling therapy represents a balance of effects. In general, remodeling studies show good correlation between limitation of remodeling parameters and improved prognosis (12,44). Because large anterior transmural infarctions are especially prone to severe remodeling and poor outcome, this high-risk group should be considered for aggressive anti-remodeling therapy.

SUMMARY

In conclusion, myocardial infarction is associated with remodeling of both in-farcted and noninfarcted myocardium over weeks to months, resulting in progressive ventricular dilatation, hypertrophy, and dysfunction. Major determinants of in-farct remodeling are infarct size and transmurality, the efficacy of infarct healing, and the magnitude of mechanical deformation forces, such as the degree of ventricular loading and magnitude of ventricular wall stress. These factors also influence remodeling of noninfarcted myocardium. In addition, two other factors that play major roles in remodeling of noninfarcted myocardium are the patency of the noninfarct-related coronary artery and the integrity of the collagen matrix. Limitation of remodeling involves efforts to decrease infarct size and transmurality, reduce ventricular loading and wall stress, promote healing, preserve the supporting collagen matrix, and restore patency of the infarct- and noninfarct-related arteries. Outcome depends critically on timing and duration of therapy with attention to the pathophysiologic stage of the remodeling process. Maximum benefit from unloading therapy is achieved when it is begun very early, spans the healing process and extends beyond, and avoids the paradoxical J-curve effect. Strategies targeted at restoring ventricular function in viable but stunned or hibernating myocardium and preserving the collagen matrix need to be developed.

ACKNOWLEDGMENTS

This work was supported in part by grants from the Medical Research Council and the Heart and Stroke Foundation of Canada, Ottawa, Ontario. The work was done during the tenure of Dr. Jugdutt as a Scientist of the Alberta Heritage Foundation for Medical Research. The author is grateful to Catherine Jugdutt for typing the manuscript.

REFERENCES

1. Pfeffer MA, Braunwald E. Ventricular remodeling after myocardial infarction. Experimental observations and clinical implications. *Circulation* 1990;81:1161–1172.
2. Jugdutt BI. Prevention of ventricular remodelling post myocardial infarction: timing and duration of therapy. *Can J Cardiol* 1993;9:103–114.
3. Hutchins GM, Bulkley BH. Infarct expansion versus extension: two different complications of acute myocardial infarction. *Am J Cardiol* 1978;41:1127–1132.
4. Roberts CS, Maclean D, Maroko P, Kloner RA. Early and late remodeling of the left ventricle after acute myocardial infarction. *Am J Cardiol* 1984;54:407–410.

5. Erlebacher JA, Weiss JL, Eaton LW, Kallman C, Weisfeldt ML, Bulkley BH. Late effects of acute infarct dilation on heart size: a two-dimensional echocardiographic study. *Am J Cardiol* 1982;49: 1120–1126.
6. Jugdutt BI. Identification of patients prone to infarct expansion by the degree of regional shape distortion on an early two-dimensional echocardiogram after myocardial infarction. *Clin Cardiol* 1990; 13:28–40.
7. Gaudron P, Eilles C, Kugler I, Ertl G. Progressive left ventricular dysfunction and remodeling after myocardial infarction. Potential mechanisms and early predictors. *Circulation* 1993;87:755–763.
8. Pfeffer JM, Pfeffer MA, Braunwald E. Influence of chronic captopril therapy on the infarcted left ventricle of the rat. *Circ Res* 1985;57:84–95.
9. Pfeffer MA, Pfeffer JM, Steinberg C, Finn P. Survival after an experimental myocardial infarction: beneficial effects of long-term therapy with captopril. *Circulation* 1985;72:406–412.
10. Jugdutt BI. Delayed effects of early infarct-limiting therapies on healing after myocardial infarction. *Circulation* 1985;72:907–914.
11. Jugdutt BI. Effect of nitroglycerin and ibuprofen on left ventricular topography and rupture threshold during healing after myocardial infarction in the dog. *Can J Physiol Pharmacol* 1988;66:385–395.
12. Jugdutt BI, Warnica JW. Intravenous nitroglycerin therapy to limit myocardial infarct size, expansion, and complications. Effect of timing, dosage, and infarct location. *Circulation* 1988;78:906–916.
13. Pfeffer MA, Lamas GA, Vaughan DE, Parisi AF, Braunwald E. Effect of captopril on progressive ventricular dilatation after anterior myocardial infarction. *N Engl J Med* 1988;319:80–86.
14. Sharpe N, Smith H, Murphy J, et al. Early prevention of left ventricular dysfunction after myocardial infarction with angiotensin-converting-enzyme inhibition. *Lancet* 1991;337:872–876.
15. Oldroyd KG, Pye MP, Ray SG, et al. Effects of early captopril administration on infarct expansion, left ventricular remodelling and exercise capacity after acute myocardial infarction. *Am J Cardiol* 1991;68:713–718.
16. Jugdutt BI, Schwarz-Michorowski BL, Khan MI. Effect of long-term captopril therapy on left ventricular remodeling and function during healing and canine myocardial infarction. *J Am Coll Cardiol* 1992;19:713–721.
17. Jugdutt BI, Humen DP, Khan MI, Schwarz-Michorowski BL. Effect of left ventricular unloading with captopril on remodelling and function during healing of anterior transmural myocardial infarction in the dog. *Can J Cardiol* 1992;8:151–163.
18. Jugdutt BI. Intravenous nitroglycerin unloading in acute myocardial infarction. *Am J Cardiol* 1991; 68:52D–63D.
19. Hochman JS, Choo H. Limitation of myocardial expansion by reperfusion independent of myocardial salvage. *Circulation* 1987;75:299–306.
20. Flaherty JT, Becker LC, Bulkley BH, et al. A randomized prospective trial of intravenous nitroglycerin in patients with acute myocardial infarction. *Circulation* 1983;68:576–588.
21. Michorowski BL, Tymchak WJ, Jugdutt BI. Improved left ventricular function and topography by prolonged nitroglycerin therapy after acute myocardial infarction. *Circulation* 1987;76[Suppl IV]: IV-128(abst).
22. Jugdutt BI, Tymchak WJ, Humen DP, Gulamhusein S, Tang SB. Effect of thrombolysis and prolonged captopril and nitroglycerin on infarct size and remodeling in transmural myocardial infarction. *J Am Coll Cardiol* 1992;19:205A(abst).
23. McDonald KM, Francis GS, Matthews J, Hunter D, Cohn JN. Long-term oral nitrate therapy prevents chronic ventricular remodeling in the dog. *J Am Coll Cardiol* 1993;21:514–522.
24. St. John Sutton M, Pfeffer MA, Plappert T, et al. Quantitative two-dimensional echocardiographic measurements are major predictors of adverse cardiovascular events after acute myocardial infarction. The protective effects of captopril. *Circulation* 1994;89:68–75.
25. Johnston BJ, Blinston GE, Jugdutt BI. Overestimation of myocardial infarct size on two-dimensional echocardiograms due to remodelling of the infarct zone. *Can J Cardiol* 1994;10:77–86.
26. Jugdutt BI, Khan MI. Effect of prolonged nitrate therapy on left ventricular remodeling after canine acute myocardial infarction. *Circulation* 1994;89:2297–2307.
27. Flaherty JT, Becker LC, Weiss JL, et al. Results of a randomized prospective trial of intraaortic balloon counterpulsation and intravenous nitroglycerin in patients with acute myocardial infarction. *J Am Coll Cardiol* 1985;6:434–446.
28. Gottlieb SO, Becker LC, Weiss JL, et al. Nifedipine in acute myocardial infarction: an assessment

of left ventricular function, infarct size, and infarct expansion. A double blind, randomised, placebo controlled trial. *Br Heart J* 1988;59:411–418.

29. Tymchak WJ, Michorowski BL, Burton JR, Jugdutt BI. Preservation of left ventricular function and topography with combined reperfusion and intravenous nitroglycerin in acute myocardial infarction. *J Am Coll Cardiol* 1988;11:90A(abst).

30. Sharpe N, Murphy J, Smith H, Hannon S. Treatment of patients with symptomless left ventricular dysfunction after myocardial infarction. *Lancet* 1988;i:255–259.

31. Touchstone DA, Beller GA, Nygaard TW, Tedesco C, Kaul S. Effects of successful intravenous reperfusion therapy on regional myocardial function and geometry in humans: a tomographic assessment using two-dimensional echocardiography. *J Am Coll Cardiol* 1989;13:1506–1513.

32. Nabel EG, Topol EJ, Galaena A, et al. A placebo-controlled trial of combined early intravenous captopril and recombinant tissue-type plasminogen activator in acute myocardial infarction. *J Am Coll Cardiol* 1991;17:467–473.

33. Foy SG, Crozier IG, Turner JG, et al. Comparison of enalapril versus captopril on left ventricular function and survival three months after acute myocardial infarction (the "Practical" Study). *Am J Cardiol* 1994;73:1180–1186.

34. Yusuf S, the SOLVD Investigators. Effect of enalapril on survival in patients with reduced left ventricular ejection fractions and congestive heart failure. *N Engl J Med* 1991;325:293–302.

35. Yusuf S, the SOLVD Investigators. Effect of enalapril on mortality and the development of heart failure in asymptomatic patients with reduced left ventricular ejection fractions. *N Engl J Med* 1992; 327:685–691.

36. Pfeffer MA, Braunwald E, Moyé LA, et al., on behalf of the SAVE Investigators. Effect of captopril on mortality and morbidity in patients with left ventricular dysfunction after myocardial infarction. *N Engl J Med* 1992;327:669–677.

37. Swedberg K, Held P, Kjekshus J, Rasmussen K, Ryden L, Wedel H, for the CONSENSUS II Study Group. Effects of early administration of enalapril on mortality in patients with acute myocardial infarction. Results of the co-operative New Scandinavian Enalapril Survival Study II (CONSENSUS II). *N Engl J Med* 1992;327:678–684.

38. Ball SG, The Acute Infarction Ramipril Efficacy (AIRE) Study Investigators. Effect of ramipril on mortality and morbidity of acute myocardial infarction with clinical evidence of heart failure. *Lancet* 1993;342:821–828.

39. Gruppo Italiano per lo Studio della Sopravvivenza nell' Infarto Miocardico. GISSI-3: effects of lisinopril and transdermal glyceryl trinitrate singly and together on 6-week mortality and ventricular function after acute myocardial infarction. *Lancet* 1994;343:1115–1122.

40. ISIS-4 Collaborative Group. Fourth International Study of Infarct Survival: protocol for a large simple study of the effects of oral mononitrate, of oral captopril, and of intravenous magnesium. *Am J Cardiol* 1991;68:87D–100D.

41. Jugdutt BI, Michorowski BL, Kappagoda TC. Exercise training after Q-wave myocardial infarction: importance of regional left ventricular function and topography. *J Am Coll Cardiol* 1988;12:363–372.

42. Jugdutt BI, Basualdo CA. Myocardial infarct expansion during indomethacin or ibuprofen therapy for symptomatic post-infarction pericarditis. Influence of other pharmacologic agents during early remodeling. *Can J Cardiol* 1989;5:211–221.

43. Douglas PS, Morrow R, Ioli A, Reichek N. Left ventricular shape, afterload and survival in idiopathic dilated cardiomyopathy. *J Am Coll Cardiol* 1989;13:311–315.

44. Picard MH, Wilkins GT, Ray PA, Weyman AE. Progressive changes in ventricular structure and function during the year after acute myocardial infarction. *Am Heart J* 1992;124:24–31.

45. Lamas GA, Vaughan DE, Parisi AF, Pfeffer MA. Effects of left ventricular shape and captopril therapy on exercise capacity after anterior wall acute myocardial infarction. *Am J Cardiol* 1989;63:1167–1173.

46. Eaton LW, Weiss JL, Bulkley BH, Garrison JB, Weisfeldt ML. Regional cardiac dilatation after acute myocardial infarction. *N Engl J Med* 1979;300:57–62.

47. Jugdutt BI. Left ventricular rupture threshold during the healing phase after myocardial infarction in the dog. *Can J Physiol Pharmacol* 1987;65:307–316.

48. Jugdutt BI, Amy RWM. Healing after myocardial infarction in the dog: changes in infarct hydroxyproline and topography. *J Am Coll Cardiol* 1986;7:91–102.

49. Weisman HF, Bush DE, Mannisi JA, Weisfeldt ML, Healy B. Cellular mechanisms of myocardial infarct expansion. *Circulation* 1988;78:186–201.

50. Whittaker P, Boughner DR, Kloner RA. Analysis of healing after myocardial infarction using polarized light microscopy. *Am J Pathol* 1989;34:879–893.
51. Whittaker P, Boughner DR, Kloner RA. Role of collagen in acute infarct expansion. *Circulation* 1991;84:2123–2124.
52. Mallory GK, White PD, Salcedo-Salgar J. The speed of healing of myocardial infarction: a study of the pathological anatomy in 72 cases. *Am Heart J* 1939;18:647–671.
53. Bulkley BH, Roberts WC. Steroid therapy during acute myocardial infarction: a cause of delayed healing and of ventricular aneurysm. *Am J Med* 1974;56:244–250.
54. Hammerman H, Kloner RA, Hale S, Schoen FJ, Braunwald E. Dose-dependent effects of short-term methylprednisolone on myocardial infarct extent, scar formation, and ventricular function. *Circulation* 1983;68:446–452.
55. Brown EJ, Kloner RA, Schoen FJ, Hammerman H, Hale S, Braunwald E. Scar thinning due to ibuprofen administration following experimental myocardial infarction. *Am J Cardiol* 1983;51:877–883.
56. Hammerman H, Kloner RA, Schoen FJ, Brown EJ, Hale S, Braunwald E. Indomethacin-induced scar thinning following experimental infarction. *Circulation* 1983;67:1290–1295.
57. Hammerman H, Schoen FJ, Braunwald E, Kloner RA. Drug-induced expansion of infarct: morphologic and functional correlations. *Circulation* 1984;69:611–617.
58. Reimer KA, Jennings RB. The "wavefront phenomenon" of myocardial ischemic cell death. II. Transmural progression of necrosis within the framework of ischemic bed size (myocardium at risk) and collateral flow. *Lab Invest* 1979;40:633–644.
59. Zhao M, Zhang H, Robinson TF, et al. Profound structural alterations of the extracellular collagen matrix in postischemic dysfunctional ("stunned") but viable myocardium. *J Am Coll Cardiol* 1987; 10:1322–1334.
60. Boyle MP, Weisman HF. Limitation of infarct expansion and ventricular remodeling by late reperfusion. Study of time course and mechanism in a rat model. *Circulation* 1993;88:2872–2883.
61. Erlebacher JA, Weiss JL, Weisfeldt ML, Bulkley BH. Early dilation of the infarcted segment in acute transmural myocardial infarction: role of infarct expansion in acute left ventricular enlargement. *J Am Coll Cardiol* 1984;4:201–208.
62. Jugdutt SJ, Khan MI, Blinston GE, Jugdutt BI. Progressive changes in regional and global left ventricular dilation during remodeling post-myocardial infarction. *Clin Res* 1994;42:194A(abst).
63. Armstrong PA, Moe GW, Howard RJ, Grima EA, Cruz TF. Structural remodelling in heart failure: gelatinase induction. *Can J Cardiol* 1994;10:214–220.
64. Olivetti G, Capasso JM, Sonnenblik EH, Anversa P. Side-to-side slippage of myocytes participates in ventricular remodeling acutely after myocardial infarction in rats. *Circ Res* 1990;67:23–34.
65. Fujiwara H, Ashraf M, Sato S, Millard R. Transmural cellular damage and blood flow distribution in early ischemia in pig heart. *Circ Res* 1982;51:683–693.
66. Jugdutt BI, Tang S-B, Khan MI, Basualdo CA. Functional impact of remodeling during healing after non–Q wave versus Q wave anterior myocardial infarction in the dog. *J Am Coll Cardiol* 1992; 20:722–731.
67. Jugdutt BI, Michorowski BL. Role of infarct expansion in rupture of the ventricular septum after acute myocardial infarction: a two-dimensional echocardiographic study. *Clin Cardiol* 1987;10: 641–652.
68. Fishbein MC, Maclean D, Maroko PR. The histopathologic evolution of myocardial infarction. *Chest* 1978;73:843–849.
69. Jugdutt BI, Hutchins GM, Bulkley BH, Pitt B, Becker LC. Effect of indomethacin on collateral blood flow and infarct size in the conscious dog. *Circulation* 1979;59:734–743.
70. Jugdutt BI, Hutchins GM, Bulkley BH, Becker LC. Salvage of ischemic myocardium by ibuprofen during infarction in the conscious dog. *Am J Cardiol* 1980;46:74–82.
71. Caulfield JB, Borg TK. The collagen network of the heart. *Lab Invest* 1979;40:364–372.
72. Lerman RH, Apstein CS, Kagan MH, et al. Myocardial healing and repair after experimental infarction in the rabbit. *Circ Res* 1983;53:378–388.
73. Covell JW. Factors influencing diastolic function. Possible role of the extracellular matrix. *Circulation* 1990;81[Suppl III]:III-115–III-158.
74. Litwin SE, Litwin CM, Raya TE, Warner AL, Goldman S. Contractility and stiffness of noninfarcted myocardium after coronary ligation in rats. Effects of chronic angiotensin converting enzyme inhibition. *Circulation* 1991;83:1028–1037.
75. van Krimpen C, Schoemaker RG, Cleutjens JPM, et al. Angiotensin I converting enzyme inhibitors and cardiac remodeling. *Basic Res Cardiol* 1991;86:149–155.

76. Schoemaker RG, Debets JJM, Struyker-Boudier HAJ, Smits JFM. Delayed but not immediate captopril therapy improves cardiac function in conscious rats, following myocardial infarction. *J Mol Cell Cardiol* 1991;23:187–197.

77. Michel JB, Lattion AL, Salzmann JL, et al. Hormonal and cardiac effects of converting enzyme inhibition in rat myocardial infarction. *Circ Res* 1988;62:641–650.

78. Smits JFM, van Krimpen C, Schoemaker RG, Cleutjens JPM, Daemen MJAP. Angiotensin II receptor blockade after myocardial infarction in rats: effects on hemodynamics, myocardial DNA synthesis, and interstitial collagen content. *J Cardiovasc Pharmacol* 1992;20:772–778.

79. Brilla CG, Janicki JS, Weber KT. Cardioreparative effects of lisinopril in rats with genetic hypertension and left ventricular hypertrophy. *Circulation* 1991;83:1771–1779.

80. Jugdutt BI, Khan MI, Jugdutt SJ, Blinston GE. Effect of enalapril on ventricular remodeling and function during healing after anterior myocardial infarction in the dog. *Circulation* 1995;91:802–812.

81. Kambayashi M, Miura T, Oh B-H, et al. Myocardial cell hypertrophy after myocardial infarction with reperfusion in dogs. *Circulation* 1992;86:1935–1944.

82. Przyklenk K, Kloner RA. Superoxide dismutase plus catalase improve contractile function in the canine model of the stunned myocardium. *Circ Res* 1986;58:148–156.

83. Kloner RA, Przyklenk K, Whittaker P. Deleterious effects of oxygen radicals in ischemia/reperfusion: resolved and unresolved issues. *Circulation* 1989;80:1115–1127.

84. Ambrosio G, Becker LC, Hutchins GM, Weisman HF, Weisfeldt ML. Reduction in experimental infarct size by recombinant human superoxide dismutase: insights into pathophysiology of reperfusion injury. *Circulation* 1986;74:1424–1433.

85. Przyklenk K, Kloner RA. Effect of verapamil on postischemic "stunned" myocardium: importance of timing of treatment. *J Am Coll Cardiol* 1988;11:614–623.

86. Braunwald E. Myocardial reperfusion, limitation of infarct size, reduction of left ventricular dysfunction, and improved survival: should the paradigm be expanded? *Circulation* 1989;79:441–442.

The Failing Heart, edited by N. S. Dhalla,
R. E. Beamish, N. Takeda, and M. Nagano.
Lippincott-Raven Publishers, Philadelphia © 1995.

20

Pharmacologic Interventions in Experimental Remodeling: Angiotensin-Converting Enzyme Inhibitors and Angiotensin II Subtype I Receptor Blockers

Gary S. Francis, Kenneth McDonald, and *Jay N. Cohn

*Department of Medicine, *Cardiovascular Division, University of Minnesota Medical School, Minneapolis, Minnesota 55455 United States*

Heart failure clearly has emerged as a recognized public health problem in the Western world. The magnitude of the problem is growing, even if one adjusts for the aging population (1,2). In the United States, the most common cause of congestive heart failure is coronary artery disease (3), although a substantial proportion of cases are due to dilated cardiomyopathy.

An understanding of the pathophysiology is traced back to seminal studies by Frank and Starling performed at the turn of the twentieth century, but the fundamental underpinnings of precisely how the heart enlarges progressively has escaped our full understanding. There remains considerable uncertainty regarding the pathophysiologic cellular mechanisms operative in the failing heart (4). Despite these uncertainties, several important observations have helped to clarify the natural history of heart failure. The end-diastolic, particularly the end-systolic volume (i.e., the size of the heart), remains one of the most important prognostic features associated with survival (5). Once the heart has substantially enlarged, the influence of pharmacologic therapy remains somewhat limited, although recent advances have been made in large clinical trials. Therefore, an understanding of how the heart enlarges progressively has been a focus of intense interest in many research laboratories.

Our laboratory has been working from the premise that heart failure is characterized by a response to an index injury event. Such injury often takes the form of acute myocardial necrosis or possibly a less defined insult, either one leading to a dilated cardiomyopathic state (6,7). The response to injury, which is characterized in part by an increase in myocardial cell size (8,9), is presumably adaptive in a teleologic sense, as it serves to maintain myocardial performance in remaining viable cells so that the organ functions sufficiently to maintain perfusion to vital organs. Loss of myocardial mass or contractile tissue is offset by a process of hypertrophy and dilatation, often referred to in a generic sense as left ventricular *remodeling* (10). Although the remodeling process may contribute early on to maintenance of stroke volume and myocardial performance, the long-term consequences of cardiomegaly are highly detrimental (11,12). We now know that patients with left ventricular hypertrophy from any cause are at considerable risk for cardiac arrhythmias, sudden death, and a foreshortened survival (13). When hypertrophy and dilatation coexist, the prognosis is seemingly even worse, as depicted by the foreshortened survival of patients with end-stage heart failure (14).

Ventricular remodeling after myocardial infarction is characterized by both an increase in mass and left ventricular dilation (15–18). These structural changes, although not completely understood, probably result from a combination of factors, including myocyte hypertrophy (4), cell dropout (17,19), slippage of muscle bundles (20), and alterations in the cardiac interstitium (21–23). The long-term effects of remodeling on prognosis are clearly detrimental (5). Within the past 10 years there have been a number of experimental (24–27) and clinical (28–35) studies designed to examine the influence of pharmacologic therapy on left ventricular remodeling changes. Among the pharmacologic agents that attenuate left ventricular remodeling, the angiotensin-converting enzyme (ACE) inhibitors have consistently demonstrated a favorable effect (28–35). The mechanism whereby ACE inhibitors prevent left ventricular remodeling following acute myocardial damage, however, remains incompletely understood.

METHODS

Our group has developed a model of discrete myocardial damage that has been very useful in characterizing the initial increase in mass and subsequent left ventricular dilation that occurs in response to injury (36). With this technique, which was first developed by Jay Cohn and subsequently refined by Kenneth McDonald, anesthetized dogs are placed in the right lateral position and a pigtail catheter is advanced across the aortic valve. A premeasured soft metalic guidewire is then passed through the catheter and approximately 5 mm of wire is extended beyond the catheter tip into the left ventricular cavity. One electrode paddle is then placed over the shaved area on the left chest and the second electrode is connected to the proximal end of the guidewire that has been placed in the left ventricle. Shocks of 80 J are delivered at 25- to 60-second intervals for a total of one shock per kilogram of body weight. The mortality is now less than 5%. Our experience with this protocol has indicated that a moderate-sized area of myocardial damage involving on average $17\% \pm 6\%$ of the left ventricle is produced. Using magnetic resonance imaging (MRI), McDonald and colleagues from our group have demonstrated that surviving dogs demonstrate an early increase in left ventricular mass followed by a subsequent increase in left ventricular volume (37). We have used this model extensively to examine the role of the renin–angiotensin system in the role of left ventricular remodeling.

RESULTS

Because the renin–angiotensin system is believed to importantly participate in the left ventricular postmyocardial damage-remodeling process (38), we and many others have reasoned that the use of ACE inhibitors would attenuate subsequent remodeling in response to discrete myocardial injury. McDonald and colleagues have demonstrated that introduction of ACE inhibitors within 24 hours after onset of acute myocardial damage attenuates the expected increase in ventricular mass and volume (39). This has been demonstrated with both the sulfhydryl-containing ACE inhibitor zofenopril and the nonsulfhydryl ACE inhibitor ramipril. Contrary to findings with the rat-coarctation model (40), however, we have been unable to demonstrate inhibition of ventricular remodeling with low-dose (non–blood pressure altering dose) ramipril (39).

McDonald and colleagues have also demonstrated that the alpha-adrenergic blocking agent terazosin tends to block the early increase in myocardial mass in response to acute injury (39), but that remodeling subsequently ensues. However, 5-mononitrate therapy appears to be as effective as ACE inhibitor in the prevention of remodeling in this canine paradigm (41).

The angiotensin II receptor blocker DUP 753 has previously been shown in the rat myocardial infarction model to attenuate left ventricular remodeling (42). This particular experimental myocardial infarction model, however, causes large infarction and is associated with an activated systemic renin–angiotensin system. It is, therefore, not unexpected that blocking the angiotensin II receptor might abrogate the remodeling process in the rat with myocardial infartion. Using the canine paradigm of acute myocardial damage and left ventricular remodeling, McDonald and colleagues have demonstrated that the angiotensin II receptor DUP 532 fails to block left ventricular remodeling (39). DUP 532 is a noncompetitive receptor blocker that is an analog of the DUP 753, a more commonly used angiotensin II receptor competitive antagonist. DUP 532, however, lacks carboxyl group at the 5′ position of the imidazole ring. Failure of the specific angiotensin II receptor blocker DUP 532 to attenuate left ventricular remodeling would suggest that alternative pharmacologic mechanisms of ACE inhibitor therapy may be operative in the attenuation of left ventricular remodeling. For example, it is possible that the local increment in bradykinin produced by the use of ACE inhibitor (due to the inhibition of kininase II or converting enzyme) may have an antigrowth or antihypertrophy influence. The local increment in bradykinin may stimulate intracellular nitric oxide (NO) to produce cyclic GMP, a known inhibitor of cellular growth (43). Although purely speculative, it is certainly possible that ACE inhibitors benefit left ventricular remodeling through mechanisms unrelated to angiotensin II or the angiotensin II

(AT$_1$) receptor. This concept is currently being explored in our model with the use of a bradykinin-2 receptor blocker HOE 140 (44).

SUMMARY

Left ventricular remodeling following myocardial injury has emerged as an area of intense interest in both basic science and clinical research arenas. Both scientists and clinicians have produced ample evidence that angiotensin-converting enzyme inhibitors have the clear potential to block left ventricular remodeling following myocardial injury (24–35). In principle, such therapy may forestall the onset of heart failure and dramatically reduce the mortality and morbidity of patients destined to develop heart failure as a consequence of acute myocardial injury. Although the use of animal models will never replace clinical investigation in patients, such models do afford investigators the opportunity to understand mechanisms and to develop new concepts regarding fundamental biologic processes and pharmacologic interventions. The canine model of discrete myocardial injury, which is characterized by early and progressive left ventricular remodeling, has been particularly rewarding in this regard. The use of this model has allowed the exploration of numerous therapeutic strategies designed to block left ventricular remodeling, some of which have been brought to the clinical forefront. More importantly, the use of this model has underscored the complexities of left ventricular remodeling and has allowed for the emergence of new concepts that may lead to exciting and improved treatment strategies.

REFERENCES

1. Ghali JK, Cooper R, Ford E. Trends in hospitalization rates for heart failure in the United States, 1973–1986. Evidence for increasing population prevalence. *Arch Intern Med* 1990;150:769–773.
2. Ho KKL, Pinskey JL, Kannel WB, Levy D. The epidemiology of heart failure: The Framingham Study. *J Am Coll Cardiol* 1993;22[Suppl A]:6A–13A.
3. Bourassa MG, Gurne O, Bangdiwalla SI, et al. Natural history and patterns of current practice in heart failure. *J Am Coll Cardiol* 1993;22[Suppl A]: 14A–19A.
4. Katz, AM. Cardiomyopathy of overload. A major determinant of prognosis in congestive heart failure. *N Engl J Med* 1990;322:100–110.
5. White HD, Norris RM, Brown MA, Brandt PWT, Whitlock RML, Wild CJ. Left ventricular end-systolic volume as the major determinant of survival after recovery from myocardial infarction. *Circulation* 1987;76:44–51.
6. Francis GS, McDonald KM. Left ventricular hypertrophy: an initial response to myocardial injury. *Am J Cardiol* 1992;69:3G–9G.
7. Francis GS, McDonald KM, Cohn JN. Neurohumoral activation in preclinical heart failure. *Circulation* 1993;87[Suppl IV]:IV-90–IV-96.
8. Gerdes AM, Kellerman SE, Moore JA, et al. Structural remodeling of cardiac myocytes in patients with ischemic cardiomyopathy. *Circulation* 1992;86:426–430.
9. Gerdes AM. The use of isolated myocytes to evaluate myocardial remodeling. *Trends Cardiovasc Med* 1992;2:152–155.
10. Pfeffer MA, Braunwald E. Ventricular remodeling after myocardial infarction. Experimental observations and clinical implications. *Circulation* 1990;81:1161–1172.

11. Pfeffer MA, Braunwald, E. Ventricular enlargement following infarction is a modifiable process. *Am J Cardiol* 1991;68:127D–131D.

12. Lee TH, Hamilton MA, Stevenson LW, et al. Impact of left ventricular cavity size on survival in advanced heart failure. *Am J Cardiol* 1993;72:672–676.

13. Levy D, Garrison RJ, Savage DD, Kannel WB, Castelli WP. Prognostic implications of echocardiographically determined left ventricular mass in the Framingham heart study. *N Engl J Med* 1990; 322:1561–1566.

14. Francis GS, Kubo SH. Prognostic factors affecting diagnosis and treatment of congestive heart failure. *Curr Probl Cardiol* 1989;11:629–671.

15. Gold KL, Lipscomb K, Hamilton GW, Kennedy JW. Left ventricular hypertrophy in coronary artery disease. *Am J Med* 1973;55:595–601.

16. Benjamin IJ, Schuster EH, Bulkley BH. Cardiac hypertrophy in idiopathic dilated congestive cardiomyopathy: a clinicopathologic study. *Circulation* 1981;64:442–447.

17. Anversa P, Sonnenblick EH. Ischemic cardiomyopathy: pathophysiologic mechanisms. *Prog Cardiovasc Dis* 1990;33:49–70.

18. Anversa P, Capasso JM. Cardiac hypertrophy and venrtricular remodeling. *Lab Invest* 1991;64:441–445.

19. Anversa P, Li P, Zhang X, Olivetti G, Capasso JM. Ischemic myocardial injury and ventricular remodeling. *Cardiovasc Res* 1993;27:145–157.

20. Olivetti G. Capasso JM, Sonnenblick EH, Anversa P. Side-to-side slippage of myocytes participates in ventricular wall remodeling acutely after myocardial infarction in rats. *Circ Res* 1990;67:23–34.

21. Weber KT, Janicki JS. Angiotensin and the remodeling of the myocardium. *Br J Clin Pharm* 1989; 28:141S–150S.

22. Weber KT. Cardiac interstitium in health and disease: the fibrillar collagen network. *J Am Coll Cardiol* 1989;13:1637–1652.

23. Weber KT, Brilla CG. Pathological hypertrophy and cardiac interstitium. Fibrosis and renin-angiotensin-aldosterone system. *Circulation* 1991;83:1849–1865.

24. Pfeffer JM, Pfeffer MA, Braunwald E. Influence of chronic captopril therapy on the infarcted left ventricle of the rat. *Circ Res* 1985;57:84–95.

25. Pfeffer MA, Pfeffer JM, Steinberg C, Finn P. Survival after an experimental myocardial infarction: beneficial effects of long-term therapy with captopril. *Circulation* 1985;406–412.

26. Raya TE, Gay RG, Aguirre M, Goldman S. Importance of venodilation in prevention of left ventricular dilation after chronic large myocardial infarction in rats. A comparison of captopril and hydralazine. *Circ Res* 1989;64:330–337.

27. Litwin SE, Raya TE, Anderson PG, Litwin CM, Bressler R, Goldman S. Induction of myocardial hypertrophy after coronary ligation in rats decreases ventricular dilatation and improves systolic function. *Circulation* 1991;84:1819–1827.

28. Pfeffer MA, Lamas GA, Vaughan DE, Parisi AF, Braunwald E. Effect of captopril on progressive ventricular dilatation after anterior myocardial infarction. *N Engl J Med* 1988;319:80–86.

29. Pfeffer MA, Pfeffer JM. Ventricular enlargement and reduced survival after myocardial infarction. *Circulation* 1987;75[Suppl IV]:IV93–IV97.

30. Pfeffer MA, Braunwald E. Ventricular enlargement following infarction is a modifiable process. *Am J Cardiol* 1991;68:127D–131D.

31. Konstam MA, Kronenberg MW, Rousseau MF, et al., for the SOLVD Investigators. Effects of the angiotensin converting enzyme inhibitor enalapril on the long-term progression of left ventricular dilatation in patients with asymptomatic systolic dysfunction. *Circulation* 1993;88:2277–2283.

32. Sutton JSJ, Pfeffer MA, Plappert T, et al., for the SAVE Investigators. Quantitative two-dimensional echocardiographic measurements are major predictors of adverse cardiovascular events after acute myocardial infarction. The protective effects of captopril. *Circulation* 1994;89:68–75.

33. Oldroyd KG, Pye MP, Ray SG, et al. Effects of early captopril administration on infarct expansion, left ventricular remodeling and exercise capacity after acute myocardial infarction. *Am J Cardiol* 1991;68:713–718.

34. Bonarjee VVS, Carstensen S, Caidahl K, Nilsen DWT, Edner M, Berning J. Attenuation of left ventricular dilatation after acute myocardial infarction by early initiation of enalapril therapy. *Am J Cardiol* 1993;72:1004–1009.

35. Foy SG, Crozier IG, Turner JG, et al. Comparison of enalapril versus captopril on left ventricular function and survival three months after acute myocardial infarction (the "PRACTICAL" study). *Am J Cardiol* 1994;73:1180–1186.

36. Mehta J, Runge W, Cohn JN, Carlyle P. Myocardial damage after repetitive direct current shock in the dog: correlation between left ventricular end-diastolic pressure and extent of myocardial necrosis. *J Lab Clin Med* 1978;91:272–279.
37. McDonald KM, Francis GS, Carlyle PF, Matthews J, Hunter DW, Cohn JN. Hemodynamic, left venrtricular structural and hormonal changes after discrete myocardial damage in the dog. *J Am Coll Cardiol* 1992;19:460–467.
38. Lindpaintner K, Lu W, Niedermajer N, et al. Selective activation of cardiac angiotensinogen gene expression in post-infarction ventricular remodeling in the rat. *J Mol Cell Cardiol* 1993;25:133–143.
39. McDonald KM, Garr M, Carlyle PF, et al. The relative effects of alpha-1 adrenoceptor blockade, converting enzyme inhibitor therapy and angiotensin II sub-type 1 receptor blockade on ventricular remodeling in the dog. *Circulation* 1994;90:3034–3046.
40. Linz W, Scholkens BA, Ganten D. Converting enzyme inhibition specifically prevents the development and induces regression of cardiac hypertrophy in rats. *Clin Exp Hypertens* 1989;A11(7):1325–1350.
41. McDonald KM, Francis GS, Mathews J, Hunter D, Cohn JN. Long-term oral nitrate therapy prevents chronic ventricular remodeling in the dog. *J Am Coll Cardiol* 1993;21:514–522.
42. Raya TE, Fonken SJ, Lee RW, et al. Hemodynamic effects of direct angiotensin II blockade compared to converting enzyme inhibition in a rat model of heart failure. *Am J Hypertens* 1991;4:334S–340S.
43. Garg UC, Hassis A. Nitric oxide-generating vasodilators and 8-bromo-cyclic guanosine monophosphate inhibit mitogenesis and proliferation of cultured rat vascular smooth muscle cells. *J Clin Invest* 1989;83:1774–1777.
44. McDonald KM, Mock J, D'Aloia A, Parrish T, Hauer K, Francis GS, Stillman A, Cohn JN. Bradykinin antagonism inhibits the antigrowth effect of converting enzyme inhibition in the dog myocardium after discrete transmural myocardial necrosis. *Circulation* 1995;91:2043–2048.

The Failing Heart, edited by N. S. Dhalla,
R. E. Beamish, N. Takeda, and M. Nagano.
Lippincott-Raven Publishers, Philadelphia © 1995.

21

Angiotensin II Receptor Blockade E-4177 Induces Regression of Pressure-Overload Left Ventricular Hypertrophy

Naoki Makino, Tomoji Hata, Masahiro Sugano, Hirosuke Matsui, Sachiyo Taguchi, and Takashi Yanaga

Department of Bioclimatology and Medicine, Medical Institute of Bioregulation, Kyushu University, Beppu, Oita 874 Japan

There is increasing evidence that, in response to pressure overload, the renin–angiotensin system may play an important role in modulating the adaptive growth pattern in cardiac hypertrophy (1). Evidence supporting the presence of this system in cardiac tissue includes the demonstrating of angiotensinogen and renin mRNA (2,3) and the biochemical identification of renin–angiotensin-converting enzyme (ACE) (4) and angiotensin (Ang) II (5) as well as its receptor (6) in the heart. Studies in the early 1990s demonstrated ACE inhibitor–induced regression of left ventricular (LV) hypertrophy, both in experimental animal models (7,8) and in hypertensive patients (9). Ang II-receptor antagonist TCV-116 also induced regression of cardiac hypertrophy and had cardioprotective effects on hypertrophied myocardium in vitro and in vivo (10).

Two distinct subtypes of Ang II receptors have been identified (11). A standard nomenclature for Ang II-receptor subtypes has been proposed in which the Ang II receptors inhibited by losartan, a prototypic AT_1-receptor antagonist, are designated AT_1 receptors; those inhibited by PD123177, PD123319, or CGP42112A are designated as AT_2 receptors (12). AT_1 receptors are believed to be responsible for known biological actions of Ang II, but the function of AT_2 receptors is not clear at present (13). A competitive-type AT_1 antagonist, E14177, was recently developed. Its pharmacological properties (14) have an affinity twice as potent as losartan in human arteries.

In the present study, we compared ACE blockade using enalapril with AT_1-receptor antagonist E-4177 for cardiac regression from hypertrophy of rats in order to test effects of specific intervention at ACE and Ang II–receptor levels in the renin–angiotensin cascade. The regression of cardiac hypertrophy was examined in rats subjected to aortic banding.

METHODS

Animal Model

Adult male Wistar rats (150–180 g) were fasted for 12 hours before the experiments. Left ventricular hypertrophy was produced by banding the abdominal aorta in rats anesthetized with sodium pentobarbital (40 mg/kg of body weight; i.p.). The abdominal aorta was surgically isolated above the renal arteries and was constricted with a blunt 21-gauge needle (0.8 mm in outer diameter) as a guide (15).

Experimental Protocol

Cardiac hypertrophy was induced 6 weeks after aortic banding. At this time, the ACE inhibitor enalapril or AT_1-receptor antagonist E-4177 was added to drinking water, and the solution was given ad libitum for an additional 6 weeks. Tap water was given to the sham-operated control rats. It was estimated that each treated rat received about 10 mg/kg of enalapril or 7.5 mg/kg of E-4177 daily by oral intake. The number of rats used for the study was eight to ten in each group. All animals were kept under similar conditions and fed rat chow. At the end of 6-week treatment with enalapril or E-4177, the blood pressure was measured through the carotid artery by introducing a transducer-tipped no. 2 catheter (Millar, Houston, TX). After the blood pressure measurement, the rats were killed by decapitation, and the LV was immediately removed, cleaned, weighed, and prepared for the determination of ACE activity, collagen concentrations, and the RNA isolation.

Measurement of Angiotensin-Converting Enzyme Activity

Myocardial ACE activity was measured as the rate of generation of His-Leu from a Hip-His-Leu substrate by using the fluorometric assay described by Cushman and Cheung (16). Tissue was homogenated in ice-cold 50-mM potassium phosphate buffer, pH 7.5. An aliquot of the homogenized sample was then incubated with 12.5-mM Hip-His-Leu for 10 min at 37° C in a shaking water bath. The reaction was stopped by adding 280 mM of NaOH, pH 8.5. The His-Leu product was then tagged with 0.1% phthaldialdehyde and quantified fluorometrically at an excitation wavelength of 386 nm and an emission wavelength of 436 nm. This assay was linear between 0.02 and 15 mM of His-Leu product.

Measurement of Collagen Concentration

The myocardial collagen concentration was measured by determining the hydroxyproline concentration of the LV (100–150 mg) (17). After drying the heart for 24 hours, the specimens were hydrolyzed in 6 N hydrogen chloride solution at 100°C.

After resolution in buffer at pH 7.0, p-dimethylaminobenzaldehyde was added to form a complex with hydroxyproline. The collagen concentration was measured by a spectrophotometric analysis at a wavelength of 558 nm and estimated by multiplying the hydroxyproline content by a factor of 8.2. This was expressed as milligram of collagen per gram dry weight.

Angiotensin II–Binding Assay

Ventricular membranes from rats were prepared using a slight modification of the method by Baker et al. (11). A tissue homogenate was prepared with 0.25 M sucrose and 25 mM Tris, pH 7.5, containing 0.5 mmol EDTA, 0.5 mmol phenylmethylsulfonyl fluoride (PMSF), 10 mg/l bacitracin, 4 μg/ml leupeptin, 4 μg/ml pepstatin, and 40 U/ml trasylol with a Polytron (twice for 30 second each) at half-maximal speed. The homogenate was sedimented at 10,000 g for 20 min (twice), and supernatant was centrifuged at 45,000 g for 30 min. The pellet was resuspended in 0.6 M KCl and 30 mmol histidine at pH 7.0, containing 0.5 mmol EDTA, 0.5 mmol PMSF, 10 mg/l bacitracin, 4 μg/ml leupeptin, 4 μg/ml pepstatin, and 40 U/ml trasylol, and resedimented at 45,000 g for 30 min. The pellets obtained from the final centrifugation were washed three times and resuspended in 25 nnol/l Tris, pH 7.5, containing 10 mmol/l $MaCl_2$, 0.5 mmol PMSF, 10 mg/l bacitracin, 4 μg/ml leupeptin, 4 μg/ml pepstatin, and 40 U/ml trasylol using a hand-driven glass/glass homogenizer. All centrifugations were performed at 4°C. The membrane preparations were frozen immediately in liquid nitrogen and held in aliquots at $-80°C$ until used. The yield was approximately 1 mg protein per gram of heart. The assay buffer was 25 mmol/l Tris, pH 7.5, containing 10 mmol/l $MaCl_2$, 2 g/l bovine serum albumin (BSA), 10 mg/l bacitracin, and peptidase inhibitors antipan, phosphoramidon, leupeptin, pepstatin, and amastatin, each at 1 μg/ml, and 0.5 mmol/l PMSF (18). Membrane protein (120–140 μg) were incubated with increasing concentrations of the radiolabeled Ang II antagonist ^{125}I-[Sar^1,Ile^8]Ang II (sp. act., 2,200 Ci/mmol; New England Nuclear, Mississauga, Ontario). The incubation mixture was composed of the assay buffer ^{125}I-[Sar^1,Ile^8]Ang II and a competing unlabeled Ang II antagonist. The reaction was initiated by the addition of membrane protein and continued for 60 min at 37°C. Saturation isotherms with increasing concentrations of ^{125}I-[Sar^1,Ile^8]Ang II between 0.1 and 2 nM were obtained. Binding assays were done in duplicate or triplicate. Specific binding was defined as the portion of total counts displayed by 1 μmol [Sar^1,Ile^8]Ang II. At ligand concentrations equivalent to the affinity of the receptor for the radioligand (Kd), specific binding averaged 85%.

Quantitative Reverse Transcriptase Polymerase Chain Reaction

This methodology was used to detect ACE and Ang II–receptor mRNA in ventricular tissue of experimental rats. Total RNA was isolated by a modification of the acid guanidine thiocyanate technique (RNAzol, Cinna/Biotecx, Houston, TX). Detail of reactions used are given by others (19). First-strand cDNA was synthesized from total RNA, as reported for AT_1-receptor mRNA in rat ventricle (20). Two oligonucleotides (5'-GATTTCGAATAGTGTCTGAGACC-3 and 5'-TTGAACC-TGTCACTCCACCTCAA-3') were synthesized on a synthesizer (Model 352 and 394 DNA/RNA Synthesizers, Applied Biosystems, Mississauga, Ontario) and purified by high-performance liquid chromatography. These oligonucleotides were used to amplify, by the polymerase chain reaction (PCR), an 1131-bp fragment (nucleotides 44-1089) of cDNA encoding rat AT_1 receptor. The conditions for the PCR were 94°C for 1 min, 55°C for 2 min, and 72°C for 3 min, repeated for 25 cycles. Specificity of gene amplification was continued by correspondence of the size of PCR products that were predicted from the cDNA sequence and by the restriction digestion pattern. Oligonucleotide sequences used to prime the PCR and the probe for rat ACE are as follows: 5'-CGCAGACCTGGTCCAACATC-3' and 5'-AACT-GGATGATGAAGCTGAC-3'. The oligonucleotides were used to amplify by PCR a 755-bp fragment of cDNA encoding rat ACE. The conditions for PCR were 94°C for 1 min, 55°C for 2 min, and 72°C for 3 min, repeated for 25 cycles. As an internal control for input RNA, PCR oligonucleotide primers (two oligonucleotides: 5'-CATGGTCTACATGTTCCAGT-3' and 5'-GGCTAAGCAGTTGGTGGTGC-3') for glyceraldehyde-3-phosphate-dehydrogenase (GAPDH) chosen were 343 bp in length from rat DNA sequence between positions -495 and -151 (19).

Statistical Analysis

Student's t test was employed to determine the statistically significant difference between the two groups. For more than two groups, a multiple analysis of variance was performed, and Duncan's new multiple range test was used to determine the significance. All values were expressed as the means $\pm$ SEM, and $p < 0.05$ was considered a significant difference.

RESULTS

Each of the eight animals subjected to aortic banding exhibited cardiac hypertrophy on examination after 12 weeks postsurgery in comparison with sham-operated rats (Table 1). The LV weight in banded rats increased significantly from the first week after surgery ($p < 0.05$) (15). The data in Table 1 indicate that the administration of enalapril or E-4177 significantly reduced the LV weight, the LV to body weight ratio, and the systolic blood pressure in aortic-banding rats compared with untreated aortic-banding rats. Thus, it was observed that antihypertensive treatment for 6 weeks reversed cardiac hypertrophy with significant reduction in blood pressure.

The LV collagen concentration and ACE activity are shown in Table 2. Both were significantly increased in 6-week aortic-banding rats compared with sham-operated

TABLE 1. *General characteristics in experimental groups*

	LV weight (g)	LV/body weight (10^{-3})	Systolic blood pressure (mm Hg)
Sham	0.73 ± 0.02	1.8 ± 0.2	130 ± 7
AB (untreated)	1.16 ± 0.05^a	2.6 ± 0.3^a	182 ± 8^a
AB + enalapril	$0.96 \pm 0.03^{a,b}$	$2.0 \pm 0.2^{a,b}$	144 ± 6^b
AB + E-4177	$0.92 \pm 0.07^{a,b}$	$2.1 \pm 0.2^{a,b}$	138 ± 8^b
AB ± PD123319	1.12 ± 0.06^a	2.5 ± 0.3^a	160 ± 12^a

Values are mean ± SE of six experiments. Enalapril (10 mg/kg/d) or E-4177 (7.5 mg/kg/d) was administered to aortic-banding rats for 6 weeks starting 6 weeks after the operation. Data of untreated AB rats were obtained at 12 weeks after the operation.
$^a p < 0.05$, compared with sham-operated rats.
$^b p < 0.05$, compared with untreated AB rats.
LV, left ventricle; AB, aortic banding.

rats. When enalapril at 10 mg/kg was administered to aortic-banding rats for 6 weeks, the LV collagen concentration decreased significantly by 25%, compared with untreated aortic-banding rats. In addition, the administration of E-4177 at 7.5 mg/kg also significantly decreased LV collagen concentration. In myocardial ACE activity, enalapril showed a significant reduction in aortic-banding rats, but not in banding rats administered with E-4177.

The data in binding of [^{125}I]Ang II to the ventricular membranes demonstrated the presence of specific sites with high affinity but limited density for Ang II in the presence of protease inhibitors. Analysis of the Scatchard plot suggests the single class of receptors with Kd of 0.9 ± 0.2 nmol/l and B_{max} of 16 ± 0.7 fmol/mg protein (n = 4).

As shown in Fig. 1, Ang II–receptor densities estimated by B_{max} (fmol/mg protein) were higher (more than 40%; $p < 0.05$) in heart membranes from aortic-banding rats as compared with sham-operated rats, whereas Kd values did not change significantly between these two samples (0.9 ± 0.16 nm/l vs. 1.0 ± 0.14 nmol/l, respectively; $p > 0.05$). Treatment with E-4177 (7.5 mg/kg) for 6 weeks signifi-

TABLE 2. *Left ventricular collagen contents and angiotensin-converting enzyme activites after treatment with enalapril or E-4177*

	LV collagen content (mg/g)	ACE activity (nmol/min/g)
Sham	1.32 ± 0.06	24.0 ± 0.8
AB (untreated)	1.74 ± 0.10^a	36.6 ± 1.3^a
AB + enalapril × 3.0 mg/kg/d	1.48 ± 0.10^b	33.6 ± 1.1^a
10.0 mg/kg/d	1.30 ± 0.11^b	$19.4 \pm 1.2^{a,b}$
AB + E-4177 × 2.5 mg/kg/d	1.75 ± 0.12^a	36.4 ± 1.4^a
10.0 mg/kg/d	$1.51 \pm 0.11^{a,b}$	38.8 ± 1.6^a

Values are mean ± SE of six experiments. Experimental conditions are the same as in Table 1.
$^a p < 0.05$, compared with the sham-operated rats.
$^b p < 0.05$, compared with untreated AB rats.
LV, left ventricle; AB, aortic banding.

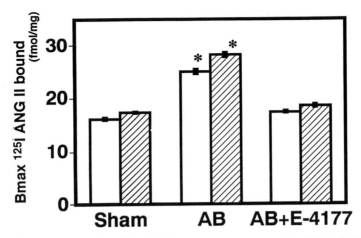

FIG. 1. Ang II–receptor densities (B_{max}) in the heart membranes isolated from sham-operated (*sham*), aortic-banding (*AB*), and E-4177 treated rats. The data of three groups were obtained at 4 and 6 weeks after the administration of E-4177 (7.5 mg/kg; p.o.). Each bar represents mean ± SEM of five experiments. *$p < 0.05$, compared with B_{max} in sham-operated rats.

cantly decreased Ang II–receptor densities to the level of those in sham-operated rats.

Angiotensin-converting enzyme mRNA and AT_1 mRNA were detected in LV myocardium of aortic-banding rats and sham-operated rats by reverse transcriptase PCR (RTPCR). Similar analyses were performed in preparations from ventricular tissue with enalapril or E-4177 treatment. These results are illustrated in Fig. 2. These approaches were used to establish the validity of the quantitative aspect of RTPCR. Increasing amounts of RNA, ranging from 0.2 to 2.0 μg, were amplified by RTPCR (20 and 28 cycles) and subsequently hybridized with the ACE or AT_1 probe. By this approach, it was possible to document the difference in the expression of ACE mRNA and AT_1 mRNA in LV tissue. An apparent increase in ACE mRNA and AT_1 mRNA levels was seen in aortic-banding rat heart (middle lane), whereas the GAPDH signals used as internal controls appeared to be unchanged in these experimental rats. Fig. 2 also illustrates that expressions in both ACE mRNA and AT_1 mRNA were reduced in banding rat heart by enalapril. The hybridization signals in both ACE and AT_1 mRNA, however, were decreased markedly in myocardium treated with enalapril in comparison with untreated banding rats.

DISCUSSION

This study has two major findings: (a) In pressure-overload–induced cardiac hypertrophy, the AT_1 antagonist E-4177 and the ACE inhibitor enalapril reduced LV weight similarly and in parallel to systolic pressure reduction. (b) In the molecular

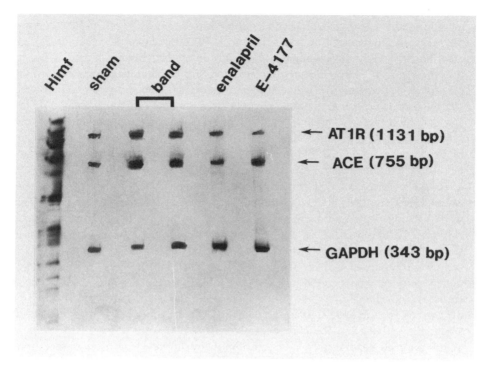

FIG. 2. Results of mRNA expression of ACE and Ang II receptor by reverse transcriptase polymerase chain reaction. **Left lane:** Sham-operated rat; **middle lanes:** untreated aortic-banding rat; **right lanes:** enalapril- and E-4177–treated rats. Himf, RNA marker.

and biochemical analysis, those antihypertensive drugs reduced Ang II–receptor densities and AT_1–receptor mRNA expression.

Regression of cardiac hypertrophy might be due to the reduction in cardiac load by antihypertensive drugs, but the sympathetic nervous system or the renin–angiotensin system may also contribute to regression (21). Angiotensin-converting enzyme inhibition can cause regression of vascular and cardiac hypertrophy and an increase in vascular flow reserve (22), perhaps by increasing the local concentration of peptides such as the vasodilative kinins, especially bradykinin (23). In this study, chronic treatment with enalapril or E-4177 caused regression of cardiac hypertrophy and a reduction in blood pressure. It is therefore assumed that the effect of these drugs on regression might be attributed not only to afterload reduction, but also to nonhemodynamic effects.

The involvement of the renin–angiotensin system in remodeling of the heart differs between different models of pressure-overload–induced cardiac hypertrophy and may even differ within the same model for development versus maintenance of cardiac hypertrophy. The ACE inhibitor quinapril did not prevent development of cardiac hypertrophy after ascending aorta banding (22). In addition, quinapril administered for 6 weeks after aortic banding caused regression of cardiac hypertrophy (22). In rats induced by abdominal aorta banding above the renal artery, enalapril prevented the development and caused complete regression of cardiac hypertrophy (24). In this present study, constriction of the abdominal aorta between the origins of the renal arteries induced hypertension and cardiac hypertrophy associated with increases in plasma Ang II concentrations (24). This is explained by the low perfusion pressure in the left kidney, which stimulates renin release and consequently Ang II production. In the view of cardiac regression, Ang II–receptor blockades losartan and TCV-116 also have been reported to induce regression of cardiac hypertrophy (10,25,26).

To elucidate the molecular mechanisms by which ACE or AT_1-receptor gene expression is regulated at the transcriptional level, we have demonstrated that those mRNA expressions were increased in the hearts of the pressure-overload–induced cardiac hypertrophy. These results are consistent with the previous observation in spontaneously hypertensive rats (26). In Ang II–receptor binding analysis, E-4177 significantly reduced the Ang II–receptor numbers to the control levels and completely reversed the increased levels of AT_1 mRNA levels. Enalapril also produced the same observation in both the AT_1-receptor numbers and Ang II–receptor mRNA, as seen in E-4177 (data not shown). On the other hand, in the enalapril study, the activity and the gene expression for ACE were observed to decrease significantly in banding rats. These results were supported by other observations (24). Both blockers decreased LV mass in parallel with their effect on afterload. Thus, it is suggested that in the heart, Ang II action that is mediated through the AT_1 receptor may be more important in cardiac growth and the development of pressure-overload hypertrophy. Further investigation, however, is necessary to clarify the precise molecular mechanisms by which the AT_1-receptor antagonist prevents and reduces cardiac hypertrophy–produced pressure overload.

SUMMARY

Numerous studies suggest that the renin–angiotensin system is involved in the development of cardiac hypertrophy. In this chapter, we produced cardiac hypertrophy in rats subjected to abdominal aortic banding and induced cardiac regression by an ACE inhibitor, enalapril (10 mg/kg/d), or an Ang II–receptor antagonist, E-4177 (7.5 mg/kg/d). Each drug was administered into rats for 4 or 6 weeks, starting 6 weeks after aortic banding. The systolic blood pressure was significantly decreased after each treatment. Compared with untreated aortic-banding rats, the LV collagen concentration in treated rats was significantly decreased by enalapril or E-4177, and the ACE activity in those rats was decreased significantly only by enalapril administration. The Scatchard analysis for [^{125}I]Ang II–receptor binding showed that the densities were increased significantly in heart membranes of aortic-banding rats and were significantly decreased in heart membranes treated with E-4177. Using RTPCR, we examined mRNA expression for the ACE and type-1 Ang II receptor

(AT_1) in rat hearts. In the LV of aortic-banding rats, enhanced mRNA expressions for ACE and AT_1 were found. These observations were inhibited by E-4177, but only ACE mRNA was reduced by enalapril. These results indicate that the Ang II antagonist E-4177, as well as the ACE inhibitor enalapril, had produced regression in pressure-overload cardiac hypertrophy of rats through the inhibition of the renin–angiotensin system, which we suggest plays a crucial role in the regression of pressure-overload hypertrophy.

REFERENCES

1. Baker KM, Booz GW, Dostal DE. Cardiac actions of angiotensin II: role of an intracardiac renin-angiotensin system. *Annu Rev Physiol* 1992;54:227–241.
2. Jin M, Markus JW, Lang RE, Unger T, Lindpaintner K, Ganten D. Endogeneous tissue renin-angiotensin system. *Am J Med* 1988;84:28–36.
3. Kanapuli SP, Kumar A. Molecular cloning of human angiotensinogen cDNA and evidence for the presence of its mRNA in rat heart. *Circ Res* 1987;60:786–790.
4. Chunkert H, Dzau VJ, Tang SS, Hirsch AT, Apstein CS, Lorell BH. Increased rat cardiac angiotensin converting enzyme activity and mRNA expression in pressure overload left ventricular hypertrophy. *J Clin Invest* 1990;36:1913–1920.
5. Baker KM, Aceto JF. Angiotensin II stimulation of protein synthesis and cell growth in chick heart cell. *Am J Physiol* 1990;259:H610–H618.
6. Suzuki J, Matsubara H, Urakami M, Inada M. Rat angiotensin II (type 1A) receptor mRNA regulation and subtype expression in myocardial growth and hypertrophy. *Circ Res* 1993;73:439–447.
7. Makino N, Matsui H, Masutomo K, Hata T, Yanaga T. Effect of angiotensin converting enzyme inhibitor on regression in cardiac hypertrophy. *Mol Cell Biochem* 1993;119:23–28.
8. Zierhut WH, Zimmer HG, Gerdes AM. Effects of angiotensin converting enzyme inhibition on pressure-induced left ventricular hypertrophy in rats. *Circ Res* 1991;69:609–617.
9. Dunn FG, Oigman W, Ventura HO, Messeri FH, Kobrin I, Frohlich ED. Enalapril improves systemic and renal hemodynamics and allows regression of left ventricular mass in essential hypertension. *Am J Cardiol* 1984;53:1044–1049.
10. Kojima M, Shiojima I, Yamazaki T, et al. Angiotensin II receptor antagonist TCV-116 induces regression of hypertensive left ventricular hypertrophy in vivo and inhibits the intracellular signaling pathway of stretch-mediated cardiomyocytes hypertrophy in vitro. *Circulation* 1994;89:2204–2211.
11. Baker KM, Campanile CP, Trachte GJ, Peach MJ. Identification and characterization of rabbit angiotensin II myocardial receptor. *Circ Res* 1984;54:286–293.
12. Bumps FM, Catt KJ, Chiu AT, et al. Nomenclature for angiotensin receptors: a report of the nomenclature committee of the council for high blood pressure research. *Hypertension* 1991;17:720–721.
13. Wong PC, Hart SD, Zaspel AM, et al. Functional studies of nonpeptide angiotensin II receptor subtype-specific ligands: Dup753(AII-1) and PDi23177 (AII-2). *J Pharmacol Exp Ther* 1990;255:584–592.
14. Okunishi H, Song K, Oka Y, et al. In vitro pharmacology of a novel non-peptide angiotensin II-receptor antagonist, E-4177. *Jpn J Pharmacol* 1993;62:239–244.
15. Nakanishi H, Makino N, Hata T, Matsui H, Yano K, Yanaga T. Sarcolemnal Ca^{2+} transport activities in cardiac hypertrophy caused by pressure overload. *Am J Physiol* 1989;257(*Heart Circ Physiol* 26):H349–H356.
16. Cushman DW, Cheung HS. Concentrations of angiotensin-converting enzyme in tissues of the rat. *Biochim Biophys Acta* 1971;250:261–265.
17. Bergman J, Loxley R. Two improved and simplified methods for the spectrophotometric determination of hydroxyproline. *Anal Chem* 1963;36;1961–1965.
18. Rogg H, Schmid A, de Gaspano M. Identification and characterization of angiotensin II receptor subtypes in rabbit ventricular myocardium. *Biochem Biophys Res Commun* 1990;173:416–422.
19. Reiss K, Capasso JM, Huang HE, Meggs LG, Li P, Anversa P. ANG II receptors, c-mic, and c-jun in myocytes after myocardial infarction and ventricular failure. *Am J Physiol* 1993;264:H760–H769.

20. Murphy TJ, Alexander RW, Griendling KK, Runge MS, Bernstein KE. Isolation of a cDNA encoding the vascular type-1 angiotensin II receptor. *Nature* 1991;351:233–236.
21. Frohlich ED, Tarazi RC. Is arterial pressure the sole factor responsible for hypertensive cardiac regression? *Am J Cardiol* 1979;44:959–963.
22. Kromer EP, Rigger GAJ. Effects of long-term angiotensin converting enzyme inhibition on myocardial hypertrophy in experimental aortic stenosis in the rat. *Am J Cardiol* 1988;62:161–163.
23. Wiemer G, Scholkens BA, Beker RHA, Busse R. Ramiprilat enhances endothelial autacoid formation by inhibiting breakdown of endothelium-derived bradykinin. *Hypertension* 1991;18:558–563.
24. Linz W, Scholkens BA, Ganten D. Converting enzyme inhibition specifically prevents the development and induces regression of cardiac hypertrophy in rats. *Clin Exp Hypertens* 1989;A11:1325–1350.
25. Ruzicka M, Yuan B, Leenen FHH. Effects of enalapril versus losartan on regression of volume overload-induced cardiac hypertrophy in rats. *Circulation* 1994;90:484–491.
26. Suzuki J, Matsubara H, Urakami M, Inada M. Rat angiotensin II (type 1A) receptor mRNA regulation and subtype expression in myocardial growth and hypertrophy. *Circ Res* 1993;73:439–447.

The Failing Heart, edited by N. S. Dhalla,
R. E. Beamish, N. Takeda, and M. Nagano.
Lippincott-Raven Publishers, Philadelphia © 1995.

22

The Renin–Angiotensin System and Angiotensin-Converting Enzyme Inhibitors in Heart Failure

Robert S. McKelvie and Salim Yusuf

Department of Medicine, Division of Cardiology, McMaster University, Hamilton General Hospital, Hamilton, Ontario, L8L 2X2 Canada

Congestive heart failure (CHF) is a major and growing public health problem. More than two million individuals in the United States suffer from CHF, and the proportion may be 10 to 15 times this number worldwide (1). The number of patients with CHF is expected to increase over the next few decades, partly due to the survival of high-risk patients following myocardial infarction (MI) and hypertension, to the extension in survival of individuals with CHF, and to the aging population.

Based on the Framingham Heart Study results published some 20 years ago, the 1-year mortality in patients with CHF was reported to be approximately 15% to 20% (2). More recent data from the Framingham study, however, indicate that as the population has aged, mortality in patients with heart failure in the community at 1 year is approximately twice what was originally estimated (3). In the United States and Canada, CHF is the most common cause of hospitalization in individuals over the age of 65 years (1). Based on the Studies of Left Ventricular Dysfunction (SOLVD) registry, it appears that approximately 30% of patients are admitted to a hospital each year, and of these, approximately one-third are rehospitalized more than once during the year (4). The most common cause of death or hospitalization in these patients is worsening heart failure, which accounts for 40% to 50% of all deaths (5). A further significant proportion of mortality/morbidity is due to arrhythmic or ischemic events (5–7). In addition, patients with CHF are at higher risk of developing stroke or suffering major thromboembolic events, such as pulmonary embolism or peripheral embolic events. A higher incidence of developing lung infections, such as pneumonia and bronchitis, has also been found in patients with CHF, who have not only high annual mortality and hospitalization rates, but also significant impairments of quality of life, functional capacity, activities of daily living, and more often manifest depression, anxiety, and reduced life expectations.

These varied clinical complications and psychological states result in numerous reasons for hospitalization and death and, therefore, indicate that a multifactorial approach is needed to treat patients with heart failure. A comprehensive discussion of CHF treatment is beyond the scope of this chapter. We will, however, briefly review the pathophysiologic changes in the renin–angiotensin system in patients with left ventricular (LV) dysfunction and the way its response is altered during the development of CHF. Against this background, the major clinical trials that have examined the effects of angiotensin-converting enzyme (ACE) inhibitors in patients with different severities of LV dysfunction will also be reviewed.

RENIN–ANGIOTENSIN SYSTEM

Activation of the renin–angiotensin system results in the production of angiotensin II (8). Angiotensinogen is synthesized by the liver and is the precursor to angiotensin II. Renin, which is produced mainly by the kidney and released into the blood, is an enzyme that catalyzes the conversion of angiotensinogen to angiotensin I. Angiotensin-converting enzyme is mainly a tissue-bound enzyme found on the luminal aspect of vascular endothelial cells (20%-40% of the activity occurs in pulmonary vessels) and catalyzes the conversion of angiotensin I to angiotensin II (8). The main direct physiologic action of angiotensin II is to cause vasoconstriction. This hormone does produce a number of other effects, including central activation of the sympathetic nervous system, the facilitation of peripheral sympathetic transmission, the increase of inward calcium current and force of contraction of heart muscle, direct action on the kidney to produce antidiuresis and antinatriuresis, and direct stimulation of synthesis and secretion of aldosterone. High levels of aldosterone, in turn, produce increased sodium retention and potassium loss and stimulate collagen deposition in the myocardium. Angiotensin II has also been shown to stimulate myocyte hypertrophy independent of any increase in the arterial blood pressure and peripheral vascular resistance (9–11). The use of captopril, an ACE inhibitor, prevents the development of ventricular dilatation and increased ventricular mass in rats following MI induced by coronary artery ligation (12–14). This is further evidence to support the belief that angiotensin II can stimulate ventricular hypertrophy.

The renin–angiotensin system, under normal physiological conditions, is beneficial for counteracting volume depletion and the effects of acute blood loss (15). The response of this system will help to restore blood volume and maintain perfusion pressure. Congestive heart failure is a condition in which there is a perceived decrease in effective blood volume (16), and the renin–angiotensin system may be activated in an attempt to maintain circulatory hemostasis. This compensation in the short term is of benefit, but in the long term, angiotensin II may be detrimental, owing to the increase in myocardial workload (17) and because of potential direct toxicity (18–20). There is also evidence to suggest that the renin–angiotensin system is activated early in patients with LV dysfunction even prior to the development of symptoms (21).

The results of these studies would suggest that inhibition of the renin–angiotensin system should result in an improvement in morbidity and mortality for CHF patients. These studies have provided the rationale for designing clinical trials that examine the effects of ACE inhibitors in patients with symptomatic and asymptomatic LV dysfunction.

CLINICAL TRIALS OF ANGIOTENSIN-CONVERTING ENZYME INHIBITORS IN CONGESTIVE HEART FAILURE PATIENTS

There have been more than 10,000 patients with varying severity of LV dysfunction randomized into trials that have assessed the benefits of ACE inhibitors. As previously stated, the mortality associated with CHF is high, in the range of 20% per year, and the annual hospitalization rates are even greater; therefore, the focus of these trials has been to determine if the pharmacologic therapy results in a reduction of these rates. A therapy that reduces the risk of death by even as little as 10% or 20% could, on a national or international level, have profound public health implications and might, for example, substantially delay several tens of thousands of deaths per year in the United States and Canada alone. Furthermore, a reduction of morbidity in this range would result in fewer hospitalizations and the need for other medical services. Obviously, this could have the potential to reduce health care costs for CHF patients by several millions of dollars per year. Another goal in some of these trials was to determine whether the early institution of therapy could reduce the rate of progression of patients from asymptomatic to symptomatic LV dysfunction. These trials also assessed the effects of ACE inhibitors on functional capacity and quality of life.

Effects on Mortality

The impact of ACE inhibitors has been evaluated in patients with asymptomatic and symptomatic LV dysfunction and following MI. The SOLVD treatment (22), Survival and Ventricular Enlargement (SAVE) (23), first Cooperative North Scandinavian Enalapril Survival Study (CONSENSUS) (7), and Acute Infarction Ramipril Efficacy (AIRE) (24) trials have conclusively demonstrated that ACE inhibitors reduce mortality in patients with heart failure.

Patients with Overt Heart Failure

In the CONSENSUS trial (7), patients who remained in New York Heart Association (NYHA) functional class IV despite 2 weeks of maximum therapy with diuretics, digoxin, and non–ACE inhibitor vasodilators were randomized to either enalapril or a placebo group for an average period of 6 months. The enalapril group had a significant ($p = 0.003$) reduction in mortality, as well as improvements in

NYHA functional class, and reductions in heart size and the need for diuretics. In the SOLVD treatment trial (22), patients included were those mainly in NYHA classes II and III and who were randomized to either placebo or enalapril therapy for an average of 41 months. There was a 16% ($p = 0.0036$) reduction in total mortality risk and a 22% ($p = 0.0045$) reduction in risk attributed to progressive heart failure.

Postmyocardial Infarction with Left Ventricular Dysfunction or Heart Failure

Three to 16 days following an MI, patients with an ejection fraction less than 40%, but without overt heart failure or symptoms of myocardial ischemia, were recruited into the SAVE trial (23) and randomized to receive either captopril or placebo for an average of 42 months. All-cause mortality was reduced by 19% ($p = 0.019$), and cardiovascular mortality was reduced by 21% ($p = 0.014$) in the group taking captopril. Approximately 50% of the patients in the SAVE trial (23) were on diuretics or digoxin at randomization, and the observed significant reduction in cardiovascular mortality was consistent in both subgroups (i.e., those on and not on anti-failure therapy at baseline). This suggests that background anti-failure therapy does not significantly modify the effect of ACE inhibitors. In the recently published AIRE trial (24), patients who had clinical evidence of heart failure were randomized on day 3 to day 10 after the index infarction to either ramipril or placebo for an average of 15 months. There was a 27% ($p = 0.002$) reduction in total mortality in the ramipril group.

In the CONSENSUS II trial (25), in which approximately 6,000 patients with acute MI (no selection based on presence of heart failure or LV dysfunction) were randomized to receive enalapril or placebo, there was no decrease in mortality. This trial was stopped early because of a tendency toward a greater number of deaths in patients receiving enalapril, so that the possibility of demonstrating a significant reduction in mortality was low. This trial had a short follow-up period of 6 months and did not select patients with LV dysfunction or heart failure; these may be reasons why no significant difference was observed for enalapril. Alternatively, neurohormonal adaptations may be important to the acute compensation in the first few hours to days post-MI.

Asymptomatic Left Ventricular Dysfunction

The SOLVD prevention trial (26) randomized asymptomatic patients with ejection fractions of 35% or less to receive either enalapril or placebo for an average of 37 months. There was an 8% ($p = 0.30$) reduction in total mortality and a 12% ($p = 0.12$) reduction in cardiovascular mortality for the enalapril group. During the study, more patients assigned to the placebo than to the enalapril group received digoxin, diuretics, or ACE inhibitors that were not part of the study regimen. This may have accounted for the lack of significant difference between the two groups, as the reduction in mortality with enalapril was due chiefly to a lower incidence of heart failure.

In the trials that included patients with overt heart failure (7,22,24), there was an immediate reduction in mortality with the institution of ACE-inhibitor therapy, with the benefits being sustained for up to 4 years. In patients with asymptomatic LV dysfunction (23,26), benefits were not observed for at least 12 to 18 months; thereafter mortality was reduced during the rest of the long-term treatment in the trial. This indicates that there may be a period during which LV remodeling has to be prevented in asymptomatic LV dysfunction, in order to limit the development of heart failure. This ultimately translates into reduced mortality.

These studies in combination demonstrate that ACE-inhibitor therapy causes a reduction in mortality not only in patients with overt heart failure, but also in those with asymptomatic LV dysfunction. Furthermore, the results demonstrate that ACE-inhibitor therapy may be beneficial in patients who develop asymptomatic or symptomatic LV dysfunction after an MI, whether initiated a few days after the event or deferred for up to 1 year.

Effects on Development of Heart Failure and Hospitalization Rate

In the SOLVD Prevention trial (26), ACE inhibitors reduced the incidence of heart failure by 37%. The prevention of heart failure was observed for various severities and definitions of heart failure, including heart failure diagnosed by the study physician, heart failure requiring the initiation of diuretics or digoxin (43% decrease), heart failure requiring hospitalization (36% decrease), and a trend toward fewer deaths due to heart failure (21% decrease). The SOLVD Treatment trial (22) results demonstrate that in patients with established heart failure, ACE-inhibitor therapy will significantly decrease the risk of one or more hospitalizations in a year. The results from the SAVE trial (23) are consistent with those found in the SOLVD trials: a 37% risk reduction ($p<0.001$) for the development of heart failure and a 22% ($p=0.019$) risk reduction for the development of CHF requiring hospital admission. Finally, the results from the AIRE trial (24) also have demonstrated a significant reduction in the risk of patients developing severe or resistant heart failure. The results from all of these trials were highly significant and collectively indicate that ACE inhibitors prevent clinical deterioration, symptomatic worsening, and hospitalization for heart failure.

Effects on Ischemic Events

In the SOLVD trials, the occurrence of a new MI increased the risk of subsequent death by up to eightfold, and a third of all deaths were preceded by a major ischemic event (27). These data emphasize that reductions in ischemic events should be an integral part of the management of patients with LV dysfunction.

In the SOLVD trials, 25% of patients in the placebo group developed MI or were hospitalized for unstable angina during the 3.5 years of follow-up (27). Treatment with enalapril reduced the incidence of MI by 23% ($p = 0.001$) and hospitalizations for unstable angina by 22% (0.0001). There were reductions in both fatal and nonfatal MIs, although the effects of reducing nonfatal infarction were twice as great as reducing fatal MI. In contrast with the reduction in hospital admission for worsening heart failure with enalapril, which was observed shortly after randomization, the effects on ischemic events were not apparent for at least 6 months. Thereafter the impact increased until a peak effect at about 36 months. This delay in ischemic events resembles the pattern observed in trials of cholesterol lowering (28) and suggests that the mechanism of benefit is not due to acute hemodynamic changes. Instead, the benefits are likely due to structural changes in the vessel wall (29).

The reduction of the risk of recurrent MI by 25% ($p = 0.015$) in the captopril group was also observed in the SAVE trial (23). In the SAVE trial, there was a significant reduction in the need for revascularization procedures but no impact on unstable angina. There were very few MIs diagnosed in the AIRE trial (24), and this trial did not demonstrate an impact on MI rates. The observation that ramipril had a less significant effect on ischemic events than has been found previously may relate to the follow-up time, the high noncompliance rate to treatment allocation by 1 year, and the few cases of MI. Overall, there is still a significant reduction in MI rates with ACE inhibitors by about 20% (29). Collectively, therefore, these data indicate that in patients with low ejection fractions, ACE inhibitors prevent major ischemic events such as MI, unstable angina, and the need for revascularization procedures (Table 1).

The mechanisms responsible for the reduction in ischemic events following the use of ACE inhibitors have not been determined by these trials. The potential mechanisms are reviewed in depth elsewhere (29) but are summarized briefly here and outlined in Table 2. Studies have demonstrated a continuous association between elevations of blood pressure and increased risk of MI even among patients with diastolic blood pressure below 90 mmHg (30). A 5–6-mmHg reduction in diastolic blood pressure has been associated with a 14% reduction in coronary heart disease events (31). In SOLVD a 4-mmHg reduction in diastolic blood pressure was observed; therefore, part of the reduction in mortality may be associated with a decline in blood pressure. Another possibility may be that ACE inhibitors may block some of the direct adverse effects of angiotensin II on the coronary circulation and myocardium. It has been shown that hypertensive patients with high-renin profiles have a higher risk of MI (32). Infusion of angiotensin II into rabbits has been shown to cause myocardial necrosis (33). Furthermore, angiotensin II can adversely affect the balance between cardiac oxygen supply and demand either by a direct coronary vasoconstrictor effect (19) or by increasing the inotropy by raising cytosolic Ca^{2+} concentration in the myocardium (34). Also, angiotensin II regulates protooncogenes that control cell growth and differentiation involved in both the vascular wall and myocardium (34–36). Finally, the prolonged use of ACE inhibitors restores normal endothelial function and vascular dilatation in animal models of heart failure and prevents the proliferative response to vascular injury (34,35). It is therefore likely that reduction in ischemic events may be due to multiple mechanisms.

TABLE 1. *Effect of enalapril on the development of myocardial infarction, hospitalization for worsening angina, and cardiac and total mortality in the SOLVD combined trials*

Outcome	No. of events (%)		Risk reduction (%) (95% C.I.)	Z score	p value
	Placebo	Enalapril			
Myocardial infarction					
Fatal	157(4.6)	139(4.1)	14(−8,32)	1.32	0.19
Nonfatal	230(6.8)	169(5.0)	29(13,41)	3.39	0.001
Either	362(10.6)	288(8.5)	23(11,34)	3.38	0.001
Hospitalization for angina[a]	595(17.5)	499(14.7)	20(9,29)	3.61	0.001
MI or hospitalization for angina	859(25.3)	707(20.8)	22(14,29)	4.89	0.0001
Cardiac deaths, nonfatal MI	918(27.0)	758(22.3)	21(13,28)	4.72	0.0001
Cardiac deaths, nonfatal MI, or hospitalization for angina	1350(39.7)	1117(32.9)	22(16,28)	6.20	0.0001
All deaths, nonfatal MI, or hospitalization for angina	1422(41.8)	1205(35.5)	20(14,26)	5.82	0.0001

[a]The data regarding hospitalization for angina includes both the primary and secondary discharge diagnosis. The numbers of patients hospitalized with a primary diagnosis of worsening angina are: prevention trial (329 placebo vs. 296 enalapril, Z = 1.61); treatment trial (204 placebo vs. 166 enalapril, Z = 2.55); and combined trials (533 placebo vs. 462 enalapril, Z = 2.84).
C.I., confidence interval; MI, myocardial infarction.

Comparison of Angiotensin-Converting Inhibitors with Other Vasodilators

Only one moderately large study, the Vasodilator Heart Failure trial (VHeFT II), has compared the effects of an ACE inhibitor with other vasodilators (37). Patients were randomized to receive either enalapril or the combination of hydralazine plus isosorbide dinitrate. There was a trend toward fewer deaths in the group treated with enalapril. The improvements in ejection fraction and exercise tolerance, however, tended to favor patients receiving the hydralazine plus isosorbide dinitrate. In addition, contrary to the results of the other major trials, the main impact was on ar-

TABLE 2. *Summary of effects of angiotensin-converting enzyme inhibitors in patients with left ventricular dysfunction/heart failure*

Pathophysiologic
  Reduced preload and afterload
  Reduced cardiac dilatation and left ventricular mass
  Reduced levels of angiotensin II, norepinephrine, atrial natriuretic peptide, and aldosterone
  Antiproliferative effects on vascular tissue
Clinical
  Improved functional capacity and reduced symptoms
  Prevention of heart failure
  Prevention of unstable angina and myocardial infarction
  Prevention of hospitalization for heart failure
  Reduced mortality

rhythmic death rather than worsening heart failure. These results may be because both vasodilators may be equally effective in reducing deaths due to pump dysfunction, whereas they may have differing effects on sympathetic activation and on sudden death. For example, hydralazine increases sympathetic activity, whereas ACE inhibitors decrease sympathetic activity.

Vasodilators, as a class, appear to have a beneficial effect on heart failure symptoms. This is an oversimplification, however, as the results of VHeFT I demonstrate that not all vasodilators have the same effect (38). In VHeFT I it was demonstrated that, compared with placebo or the combination of hydralazine plus isosorbide dinitrate, prazosin had no significant effect on heart failure. Furthermore, ACE inhibitors have additional advantages, including inhibition of the renin-angiotensin-aldosterone system, attenuation of the sympathetic nervous system, and blocking the effects of various trophic factors (including angiotensin II) on the myocardium.

Therefore, the results of these studies demonstrate that not all vasodilators are effective for the treatment of heart failure. Another important lesson from these studies is that the impact of treatment on surrogate endpoints, such as exercise tolerance or ejection fraction, may be misleading and may not translate into a clinically worthwhile benefit.

Subgroup Effects

Subgroup analyses of the SOLVD and SAVE trials indicate that treatment was beneficial in a large number of subgroups identified. These included patients of both genders, LV dysfunction of different etiologies, and different background therapies. It appears, however, that the reductions in mortality and hospitalizations for heart failure were greater in patients with more severe degrees of LV dysfunction, and it also appears that by comparing the results in CONSENSUS I, AIRE, the SOLVD treatment trial, and the SOLVD prevention trial, the benefits in terms of both absolute risk reductions and relative risk reductions, especially on mortality, were greater in those with more marked symptoms.

A metaanalysis of all available trials in patients with LV dysfunction and heart failure is required to clarify the effects of ACE inhibitors in a variety of subgroups. With the completion of the TRACE study (Trandolapril Cardiac Evaluation; principal investigators A.J. Camm, J. Carlsen) with trandolapril in 1994, a total of about 14,000 patient data will become available. These data should, therefore, provide more reliable information on subgroup effects than any single trial.

SUMMARY

The results of the trials of ACE-inhibitor therapy overwhelmingly demonstrate their benefits in CHF patients. There is a significant reduction in mortality and morbidity (progression of heart failure or hospitalization) from heart failure. Also

TABLE 3. *Implications of routine use of angiotensin-converting enzyme inhibitors in patients with low ejection fractions (based on the SOLVD trial results)*

	No. of events prevented or delayed by treating 1,000 patients with an angiotensin-converting enzyme inhibitor for 3 years	
	EF≤0.35 + CHF	EF≤0.35 + no CHF
Development of CHF	N/A	90
Hospitalization for CHF	200	65
MI or unstable angina	40	35
Deaths	50	15

EF, ejection fraction; CHF, congestive heart failure; N/A, not applicable.

ACE inhibitors were found to reduce the risk of a heart failure patient having an ischemic event classified as either an MI or unstable angina. This is an important finding because a patient suffering an ischemic event has a much higher mortality risk when compared with other heart failure patients who have not had such an event. Table 3 demonstrates the number of events prevented or delayed by treating 1,000 patients with ACE inhibitors for 3 years. As can be seen, ACE inhibitors have a significant impact on the development of heart failure, hospitalizations, ischemic events, and death in either the group with no heart failure but ejection fraction ≤0.35 or the heart failure group with ejection fraction ≤0.35. These data, therefore suggest that the use of ACE inhibitors could be cost-effective and even lead to a substantial reduction in health care costs in patients with overt heart failure.

Given a tendency toward less benefit in those with better-maintained LV function, as seen in the SOLVD and SAVE trials, it would not be prudent to extrapolate the results of these trials to patients with ejection fractions greater than 40%. Although it appears that the antiischemic effect of ACE inhibitors could potentially be extrapolated to those with relatively preserved LV function, this hypothesis requires direct verification in prospectively designed studies of patients without poor LV function, but who are at high risk of MI. At present, there are at least two large trials looking at the effects of ACE inhibitors in the prevention of ischemic events in high-risk patients without heart failure or LV dysfunction. These include the Quinapril Ischaemic Event Trial (QUIET) study, with quinapril in 1,800 patients, and the Heart Outcomes Prevention and Evaluation (HOPE) study, with ramipril in 8,000 patients. The collective results from these and other smaller trials examining the effects of ACE inhibitors on progression of atherosclerosis should provide useful information regarding both the clinical impact of such therapy in preventing MI and other ischemic events and progression of vascular lesions (Table 4).

The data from these large trials provide a rational basis for the use of ACE inhibitors in patients with asymptomatic or symptomatic LV dysfunction. The currently recommended approach would be to treat these patients as early as possible with ACE-inhibitor therapy.

TABLE 4. *Long-term trials of angiotensin-converting enzyme inhibitors on atherosclerosis or ischemic events in patients without heart failure or low ejection fraction*

Name of trial	ACE inhibitor	Primary outcome	No. of patients	Mean duration of treatment (yr)
HOPE	Ramipril	Myocardial infarction + stroke + death	8,000	3.5
SECURE	Ramipril	B-mode ultrasound	700	3
QUIET	Quinapril	Clinical events; angiographic substudy	1,800	3
SCAT	Enalapril	Angiography	400	3
PART	Ramipril	B-mode ultrasound	600	2

HOPE, Heart Outcomes Prevention and Evaluation Study; SECURE, Study to Evaluate Carotid Ultrasound Changes with Ramipril and Vitamin E; QUIET, Quinapril Ischemic Event Trial; SCAT, Simvastatin/Enalapril Coronary Atherosclerosis Regression Trial; PART, Prevention of Atherosclerosis with Ramipril Therapy.

REFERENCES

1. Yusuf S, Thom T, Abbott RD. Changes in hypertension treatment and in congestive heart failure mortality in the United States. *Hypertension* 1989;13:174–179.
2. McKee PA, Castelli WP, McNamara PM, Kannell WB. The natural history of congestive heart failure: the Framingham Study. *N Engl J Med* 1971;285:1441–1446.
3. Ho KKL, Pinsky JL, Kannel WB, Levy D. The epidemiology of heart failure: the Framingham Study. *J Am Coll Cardiol* 1993;22[Suppl A];6A–13A.
4. Bangdiwala SI, Weiner DH, Bourassa MG, Friesenger GC, Ghali JK, Yusuf S, for the SOLVD Investigators. Studies of Left Ventricular Dysfunction (SOLVD) Registry: rationale, design, methods, and description of baseline characteristics. *Am J Cardiol* 1992;70:347–353.
5. Yusuf S. Overview of the design and key results of the Studies of Left Ventricular Dysfunction (SOLVD). *Heart Failure* 1993;9:28–40.
6. Pfeffer MA, Braunwald E, Moyé LA, et al. Effect of captopril on mortality and morbidity in patients with left ventricular dysfunction after myocardial infarction. *N Engl J Med* 1992;327:669–677.
7. The CONSENSUS Trial Study Group. Effects of enalapril on mortality in severe congestive heart failure. *N Engl J Med* 1987;316:1429–1435.
8. Douglas WW. Polypeptides—angiotensin, plasma kinins, and others. In: Gilman AG, Goodman LS, Rall TW, Murad F, eds. *The pharmacological basis of therapeutics.* 7th ed. Toronto: MacMillan; 1985:639–659.
9. Khairullah PA, Kanabus J. Angiotensin and myocardial protein synthesis. *Perspect Cardiovasc Res* 1983;8:337–347.
10. Aceto JF, Baker KM. [Sar^1] angiotensin II receptor mediated stimulation of protein synthesis of chick heart cells. *Am J Physiol* 1990;258:H806–H813.
11. Morgan HE, Baker KM. Cardiac hypertrophy—mechanical, neural and endocrine dependence. *Circulation* 1991;83:13–25.
12. Pfeffer MA, Pfeffer JM, Steinberg C, Finn P. Survival after an experimental myocardial infarction; beneficial effects of long-term therapy with captopril. *Circulation* 1985;72:406–412.
13. Pfeffer JM, Pfeffer MA. Angiotensin converting enzyme inhibition and ventricular remodelling in heart failure. *Am J Med* 1988;84(3A):37–44.
14. Pfeffer JM, Pfeffer MA, Braunwald E. Influence of chronic captopril therapy on the infarcted left ventricle of the rat. *Circ Res* 1985;57:84–95.
15. Harris P. Evolution and the cardiac patient. *Cardiovasc Res* 1983;17(6):313–319.
16. Schrier RW. Body fluid volume regulation in health and disease: a unifying hypothesis. *Ann Intern Med* 1990;113:155–159.
17. Francis GS, Goldsmith SR, Levine BT, Olivari MT, Cohn JN. The neurohumoral axis in congestive heart failure. *Ann Intern Med* 1984;101:370–377.

18. Tan LB, Jalil JE, Pick R, et al. Cardiac myocyte necrosis induced by angiotensin II. *Circ Res* 1991; 69:1185–1195.
19. Gavras H, Brown JJ, Lever AF, et al. Acute renal failure, tubular necrosis and myocardial infarction induced in the rabbit by intravenous angiotensin II. *Lancet* 1971;2:19–22.
20. Gavras H, Kremer D, Brown JJ, et al. Angiotensin and norepinephrine-induced myocardial lesions: experimental and clinical studies in rabbits and man. *Am Heart J* 1975;89:321–332.
21. Francis GS, Benedict C, Johnstone DE, et al., for the SOLVD Investigators. Comparison of neuro-endocrine activation in patients with left ventricular dysfunction with and without congestive heart failure. A substudy of the Studies of Left Ventricular Dysfunction (SOLVD). *Circulation* 1990; 82:1724–1729.
22. The SOLVD Investigators. Effect of enalapril on survival in patients with reduced left ventricular ejection fractions and congestive heart failure. *N Engl J Med* 1991;325:293–302.
23. Pfeffer MA, Braunwald E, Moyé LA, et al., on behalf of the SAVE Investigators. Effect of captopril on mortality and morbidity in patients with left ventricular dysfunction after myocardial infarction. Results of the Survival and Ventricular Enlargement Trial. *N Engl J Med* 1992;327:669–677.
24. The Acute Infarction Ramipril Efficacy (AIRE) Study Investigators. Effect of ramipril on mortality and morbidity of survivors of acute myocardial infarction with clinical evidence of heart failure. *Lancet* 1993;342:821–828.
25. Swedburg K, Held P, Kjekshus J, et al., on behalf of the CONSENSUS II Study Group. Effects of early administration of enalapril on mortality in patients with acute myocardial infarction. Results of the Cooperative North Scandinavian Enalapril Survival Study II (CONSENSUS II). *N Engl J Med* 1992;327:678–684.
26. The SOLVD Investigators. Effect of enalapril on mortality and the development of heart failure in asymptomatic patients with reduced left ventricular ejection fractions. *N Engl J Med* 1992;327:685–691.
27. Yusuf S, Pepine CJ, Garces C, et al. Effect of enalapril on myocardial infarction and unstable angina in patients with low ejection fractions. *Lancet* 1992;340:1173–1178.
28. Frick MH, Elo O, Haapa K, et al. Helsinki Heart Study: primary prevention trial with gemfibrozil in middle-aged men with dyslipidemia. *N Engl J Med* 1987;317:1237–1245.
29. Lonn EM, Yusuf S, Jha P, et al. Emerging role of angiotensin-converting enzyme inhibitors in cardiac and vascular protection. *Circulation* 1994;90(4):2056–2069.
30. MacMahon S, Peto R, Cutler J, et al. Blood pressure, stroke and coronary heart disease I: prolonged differences in blood pressure: prospective observational studies corrected for the regression dilution bias. *Lancet* 1990;335:765–774.
31. Collins R, Peto R, MacMahon S, et al. Blood pressure, stroke and coronary heart disease II, short-term reductions in blood pressure: overview of randomized drug trials in their epidemiological context. *Lancet* 1990;335:827–838.
32. Alderman MH, Madhavan SH, Ooi WL, Cohen H, Sealey JE, Laragh JH. Association of the renin-sodium profile with the risk of myocardial infarction in patients with hypertension. *N Engl J Med* 1991;324:1098–1104.
33. Gavras I, Gavras GH. The use of ACE-inhibitors in hypertension. In: Kostis JB, DeFelice EA, eds. *Angiotensin converting enzyme inhibitors*. New York: Alan R. Liss; 1987:93–122.
34. Kiowski W, Zuber M, Elsasser S, Erne P, Pfisterer M, Burkart F. Coronary vasodilatation and improved myocardial lactate metabolism after angiotensin converting enzyme inhibition with enalapril in patients with congestive heart failure. *Am Heart J* 1991;122:1382–1388.
35. Ontkean MT, Gay R, Breenberg B. Effects of chronic captopril therapy on endothelium derived relaxing factor activity in heart failure. *J Am Coll Cardiol* 1992;19[Suppl A]:768–774.
36. Katz AM. Angiotensin II: hemodynamic regulator or growth factor? *J Mol Cell Cardiol* 1990;2: 739–747.
37. Cohn JN, Johnson G, Ziesche S, et al. A comparison of enalapril with hydralazine-isosorbide dinitrate in the treatment of chronic congestive heart failure. *N Engl J Med* 1991;325:303–310.
38. Cohn JN, Archibald DG, Ziesche S, et al. Effect of vasodilator therapy on mortality in chronic congestive heart failure: results of a Veterans Administration Cooperative Study. *N Engl J Med* 1986;314:1547–1552.

The Failing Heart, edited by N. S. Dhalla,
R. E. Beamish, N. Takeda, and M. Nagano.
Lippincott-Raven Publishers, Philadelphia © 1995.

23

Biochemistry, Molecular Biology, and Potential Roles of the Cardiac Renin–Angiotensin System

David E. Dostal and Kenneth M. Baker

Weis Center for Research, Geisinger Clinic, Danville, Pennsylvania 17822-2611 United States

The octapeptide angiotensin II (AII), a hormone and neurotransmitter, is the active component of the renin–angiotensin system (RAS). This evolutionarily well-conserved peptide has a major role in the regulation of cardiovascular, renal, and endocrine functions. All of the biological actions of AII are mediated through specific membrane receptors located on or in cells of various organs or tissues, including the vasculature, adrenal, kidney, brain, heart, and liver (1,2). The traditional RAS is a system in which circulating AII is delivered to target organs and cells; however, more recent data support the existence of localized RASs in the brain, adrenal, heart, vasculature, and kidneys. In addition to known biological actions of the hormone, such as regulation of aldosterone biosynthesis and secretion by the adrenal cortex and of vascular smooth muscle contraction, effects of AII on regulation of cell growth and differentiation have recently been demonstrated. The scope of this review will be (a) to provide a discussion of functional characteristics and potential roles of local RASs, with an emphasis on cardiac tissue, and (b) to review the molecular biology and biochemistry of AII-receptor–mediated signal transduction pathways.

BIOCHEMISTRY OF THE RENIN–ANGIOTENSIN SYSTEM

The systemic production of angiotensin peptides in the circulatory system is initiated by the hydrolysis of angiotensinogen by renin to produce the decapeptide angiotensin I (AI; see Fig. 1). Angiotensinogen, the only known substrate for renin, is an α_2-globulin that is synthesized and constitutively secreted by the liver. Renin is an aspartyl protease that is synthesized, stored, and released from the juxtaglomerular cells of the afferent arterioles of the kidney. Angiotensin I is processed by the dipeptidyl peptidase, angiotensin-converting enzyme (ACE), to yield the biolog-

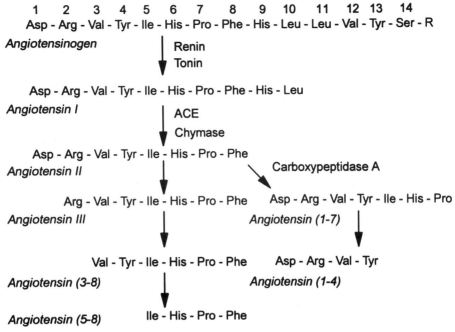

FIG. 1. Biochemistry of the renin–angiotensin system. The enzymes, renin and tonin, cleave angiotensinogen between two leucines in positions 10 and 11 or form the decapeptide, angiotensin I. Angiotensin-converting enzyme and human heart chymase remove residues 9 and 10 (histidine and leucine) to form the octapeptide angiotensin II. Removal of aspartic acid, arginine, and valine from amino acids 1, 2, and 3 by an aminopeptidase forms angiotensin III, angiotensin (3–8), and angiotensin (5–8), respectively. Removal of phenylalanine from position 8 of angiotensin II by carboxypeptidase A yields angiotensin (1–7). Cleavage between tyrosine and isoleucine in positions 4 and 5 by an endopeptidase yields angiotensin (1–4).

ically active AII. Angiotensin-converting enzyme is membrane-bound and anchored in the endothelium of many vascular beds, with highest concentrations found in the lung (3). Angiotensin II can also undergo hydrolysis by an amino- or carboxypeptidase to yield the biologically less active heptapeptides, [2–8] AIII and [1–7] AII, respectively. Cleavage of AIII by aminopeptidase yields the hexapeptide, [1–6] AII. Additional cleavage of these peptides by endo- and carboxypeptidases yields fragments with little activity (2). Although AII is traditionally viewed as a circulating effector hormone, there is substantial evidence to suggest that in the vasculature, adrenal, brain, kidney, and heart there exist local RASs that could contribute to functional responses through autocrine, paracrine, or intracrine pathways (4,5–9). The functional importance of the cardiac RAS may depend on cellular localization of components, the developmental state of the organism, and the metabolic and pathological condition of the heart.

LOCAL CARDIAC RENIN–ANGIOTENSIN SYSTEM COMPONENTS

The interpretation of biochemical and physiological roles for a local RAS in the myocardium is complicated by the presence of multiple cell types such as myocytes or nonmyocytes (fibroblasts, vascular smooth muscle [VSM], pericytes, mesothelial cells) and the spatial arrangement of these cells. It has been documented that rat heart contains all of the RAS components (6–9). Angiotensinogen mRNA and protein have been localized in cultured neonatal rat fibroblasts and cardiomyocytes using reverse transcriptase polymerase chain reaction (RTPCR) and immunohistochemical techniques (8). Immunoreactive angiotensinogen in cultured cardiac myocytes and fibroblasts had a diffuse perinuclear localization, and obvious storage granules were lacking, which was consistent with constitutive secretion. The existence of renin mRNA, detection of the enzyme by renin antibodies, and enzymatic activity indicate that renin is present and may participate in the formation of AI in the heart (8,10,11). Localization of ACE in the adult heart has also been demonstrated by measurements of enzyme activity and quantitative autoradiography (12). Angiotensin-converting enzyme is most abundant in the pulmonary, aortic, mitral, and tricuspid valves, and in the endothelial layers of the coronary arteries. The adventitia of coronary vessels has dense punctate labeling consistent with localization in the vaso vasorum. The right atrium has moderate levels of ACE with lower levels in the left atrium and both ventricles (12). Tissue ACE mRNA levels, however, may not reflect the amount of AII generated by this enzyme, because other proteins may alter the activity of ACE and other proteases can generate AII. Ikemoto et al. (13) have described an endogenous ACE inhibitor in heart tissue and Urata et al. (14), a chymase that converts AI to AII in heart. Thus, perturbations that cause changes in expression of the ACE gene require careful interpretation in terms of physiological function. The biologically active products of the RAS, AI and AII, have been extracted from the hearts of monkeys (15), nephrectomized dogs (16), and cultures of cardiomyocytes and cardiac fibroblasts (9) and have been characterized by high-pressure liquid chromatography and quantified by radioimmunoassay. In the rhesus monkey, AII levels are highest in the right atrium, decreasing in the right ventricle, left atrium, interventricular septum, and left ventricle (15).

Although cardiac tissue contains the primary components and products of the RAS, the functional organization of these components has not been elucidated. It is conceivable that localized production of AII could reach sufficiently high levels in certain areas of the heart to regulate/modulate cardiac function. For functions of the cardiac RAS to be fully understood, the pathways for synthesis, as well as the paracrine and autocrine effects of AII, need to be determined in tissues such as sympathetic and parasympathetic nerves, blood vessels, interstitium, conduction system, and contractile and noncontractile cells. The redistribution of RAS components during development and in heart disease suggests that flexibility exists in this system and that AII is likely to play an important functional role under certain conditions. It remains to be determined whether angiotensin peptides localized in cardiac tissue are produced intra- or extracellularly. Perinuclear localization of renin, angiotensinogen, and ACE in cultured neonatal rat cardiac myocytes and fibroblasts is consistent with constitutive release of these components (8,9). Immunofluorescent staining patterns suggest that AI and AII may be synthesized intracellularly where they could be exported to effect autocrine or paracrine functions or remain and exert intracellular effects. The latter concept is supported by evidence that demonstrated rapid uptake of AII by mitochondria and nuclei of cardiomyocytes and smooth-muscle cells (17). Cytoplasmic (18) and nuclear (19) binding sites for AII have been identified in hepatic tissue; however, their function(s) is (are) unknown. The rapid receptor internalization that occurs following AII binding not only may clear the receptor and degrade the peptide, but also could provide intracellular distribution of AII and/or its metabolites. Cytoplasmic "receptors" may also transport AII to nuclear "receptors" and/or other intracellular locations. The intracellular localization of angiotensins could also be the result of receptor-mediated endocytosis of AI and AII or the production of these peptides within endosomes following co-internalization of angiotensinogen with renin, ACE, or other proteases such as kallikreinin or cathepsins.

Determinants involved in regulation of the RAS probably include locally produced factors, mechanical stimuli (e.g., stretch), neurotransmitters from sympathetic and parasympathetic nerves, and feedback by AII. The distribution of RAS components is altered during development or cardiac hypertrophy or following myocardial infarction, with redistribution primarily to the ventricles (8,20,21). Renin and angiotensinogen are the most likely components of the RAS that may be rate-limiting due to the abundance of ACE activity in the various regions of the heart. Renin has been shown to be the rate-limiting step for AII production in the circulation (7), and when signal strengths of renin and angiotensinogen mRNA are compared in whole hearts from mouse and rat, angiotensinogen mRNA is more abundant, suggesting that renin may also be the rate-limiting component for AII production in the heart. The regulation of ACE gene expression and the role of this enzyme in vivo, in the control of AII production by localized RASs, remains to be elucidated. Tissue-specific inhibition of transgene expression in renin-overexpressing rats and angiotensinogen-overexpressing mice (22,23) may help to clarify the role of a localized versus circulating RAS in the development of heart failure. Cardiac cells from transgenic animals could be studied in culture to determine the effects of altered RAS expression on specific cellular functions. Regulation of RAS expression using a genetic model is attractive because better assessment of cardiac function can be obtained during drug treatment due to the lack of physical constraints imposed by surgical procedures.

CONTRIBUTION OF NON-RENIN–ANGIOTENSIN COMPONENTS TO CARDIAC ANGIOTENSIN SYNTHESIS

The nucleic and amino acid sequences of renin have significant homology with acid proteases and share features of other enzymes in this family, such as pepsin, cathepsin D, tonin, tissue kallikreinin, and chymosin (3,24), which could be involved in AII generation in cardiac tissue. The contribution of non-RAS components to AII synthesis may vary depending on factors such as the metabolic state of the heart. Tissue kallikreinin, a serine protease, has been shown to generate AII directly from angiotensinogen under acidic conditions in vitro (25). It has been demonstrated recently that kallikreinin appears to play a major role in the synthesis of AII in the hearts of bilaterally nephrectomized dogs. When cardiac ischemia was produced by coronary occlusion, a tissue kallikreinin inhibitor blocked AII release into the coronary circulation (16). Under control conditions, however, the majority of AII released into the coronary circulation was due to ACE because the ACE inhibitor, captopril, blocked most release. Alternative pathways for the conversion of AI to AII may also exist, as a chymotrysin-like proteinase (chymase) has been characterized (14,26) and cloned in human heart (27). This heart chymase demonstrated a high degree of catalytic efficiency and substrate specificity for the formation of AII from AI, was unaffected by inhibition of ACE, and was blocked by a soybean–trypsin inhibitor (14). The development of selective heart chymase antagonists will be needed to determine specific roles of the enzyme in vivo.

CARDIAC ANGIOTENSIN RECEPTORS

The presence of AII receptors in heart tissue provides support for a functional cardiac RAS. A high density of AII receptors is present in the atrioventricular node, cells of the intracardiac ganglia, and on parasympathetic nerve bundles in rat heart (28). Fewer receptors have been found associated with atrioventricular bundles and in the atria, ventricles, and media of the aorta; pulmonary arteries; and superior vena cava (28). These locations of receptors are consistent with the local actions of the peptide, which include inotropic and chronotropic effects. The peptide potentiates sympathetic function and inhibits vagal efferent nerve activity (1,2). In blood vessels, AII is a potent vasoconstrictor, the actions of which are mediated by direct effects on VSM and indirectly by facilitating release and inhibition of norepinephrine at sympathetic nerve terminals (1,2).

Evidence for multiple receptor subtypes (plasma membrane, cytosolic, and nuclear) has been derived from biochemical, molecular biological, pharmacological, functional, and radioligand-binding studies. Plasma membrane angiotensin receptors are characterized as AT_1 or AT_2, based on the binding affinity for nonpeptide antagonists, such as losartan (Dup 753) and PD 123177, respectively (29–32). Pharmacological data and ligand-binding studies have indicated that there are additional subtypes of AT_1 (A and B) receptors. The AT_1 class of receptors demonstrates high sensitivity to sulfhydryl reagents, coupling to G proteins, ability to undergo endocytosis, and coupling to increases in Ca^{2+} and phospholipid metabolism, and decreases in adenylyl cyclase. The AT_2 receptor lacks these properties and has not been conclusively linked to a biological response. Recently, AT_1- and AT_2-receptor subtypes have been described in rabbit and rat ventricular myocardium (33,34). In adult rat myocardium, AT_1 and AT_2 receptors each account for 50% of the specific binding (34). High-affinity AT_1 binding sites have been demonstrated on cultured neonatal rat cardiac myocytes (35) and fibroblasts (36). Little is known concerning regulation of angiotensin receptors in the myocardium. Upregulation of AII receptors occurs in myocytes in both ventricles following coronary artery occlusion (37). The enhanced expression of the AT_1 receptor could result in an increase in the transduction of signal production by local or circulating AII, thereby influencing the metabolic and growth properties of surviving cardiomyocytes. In the vasculature, sensitivity to AII varies inversely with circulating AII concentrations, whereas adrenal steroidogenic responsiveness varies directly with AII levels (38). Recent studies using quantitative RTPCR demonstrate that rat vasculature and adrenal have predominately AT_{1A} and AT_{1B} receptors, respectively (39). Angiotensin II decreases the level of AT_{1A}-receptor mRNA and increases AT_{1B}-receptor mRNA in rat (39), suggesting these two receptor subtypes are regulated in opposing fashion by AII.

Utilizing expression cloning strategies to derive cDNAs, the AT_{1A} receptor has been cloned from rat heart (40) and found to be identical to that reported for bovine adrenal zona glomerulosa and rat aortic VSM (41,42). The encoded AT_{1A} receptor consists of 359 amino acid residues with a relative molecular mass of 41,000 Daltons, similar to the deglycosylated form of the AII receptor as determined by sodium dodecyl sulfate-polyacylamide gel electrophoresis (SDS-PAGE). The predicted structure of the protein included seven transmembrane domains that exhibited 20% to 30% sequence homology with other G-protein–coupled receptors. It had only 19% sequence homology with the human *mas* oncogene product, however, which was proposed previously to be an AII receptor (43). Subsequent studies have failed to demonstrate binding to AII or its analogs for the *mas* oncogene product, thus precluding it as an AII receptor gene. Three potential N-glycosylation sites have been identified in the AT_1 receptor: one in the hydrophilic N-terminal extracellular region and two in the third extracellular loop. Serine and threonine residues in the second and C-terminal cytoplasmic domains represent potential sites for regulatory phosphorylation. These regions also contain three tyrosine residues, providing additional possible sites of phosphorylation. Each of the four extracellular loops contains one cysteine residue that is likely to be involved in forming the disulfide bridge conformation required for ligand binding (41,42). Regions of the receptor protein involved in signal transduction, internalization, and desensitization have not been determined. Clarification of the mechanisms of the responses has been confounded by receptor diversity and instability of solubilized receptors. With the cloning of the AT_1 receptor, however, the expression, distribution, functional significance, ligand-binding domains, and regulation can now be further explored using a variety of biochemical and molecular biological techniques.

ANGIOTENSIN TYPE II (AT_2) RECEPTORS IN CARDIAC TISSUE

Despite the presence of AT_2-binding sites in the heart, there is no conclusive evidence for a functional role. Angiotensin II type 2 receptors do not couple to G proteins or undergo ligand-mediated receptor internalization, suggesting that these receptors have a structure different from the AT_1 receptor. The progressive loss of ventricular receptors during the first 10 days after birth in neonatal rat heart suggests that both AT_1 and AT_2 receptors may have an important role in early growth and development (44). Due to the lack of functional data concerning AT_2 receptors, however, it is unclear whether signals generated from this receptor subtype are synergistic or antagonistic with those of the AT_1 receptor. In general, the functional characterization of the AT_2 receptor in tissues containing AT_1 receptors has been hampered by the lack of suitable antagonists, as PD123177 inhibits AT_1 binding at high concentrations and CGP 42112A has partial agonist activity. Several reports have documented AII responses that are selectively blocked by AT_2 antagonists (PD123177 or PD123319) but not by AT_1 antagonists (losartan). These include AII-induced inhibition of trypsin-activated collagenase activity in cultured rat cardiac fibroblasts (45), a stimulated increase in $3',5'$-cyclic monophosphate (cAMP) in cultured neurons from neonatal rat brain (46), and dilatation of rat pial brain arterioles (47). The development of highly selective AT_2 antagonists and antibodies and cloning of this receptor should lead to studies that will provide insight into the physiological function of this receptor.

ATYPICAL ANGIOTENSIN RECEPTORS IN CARDIAC TISSUE

The inability of competitive, nonpeptide AT_1 and AT_2 antagonists (in certain tissues/cells) to totally block AII responses that are inhibited by peptide receptor antagonists suggests there may be AII receptors that cannot be categorized as either AT_1 or AT_2. In some cases, inadequate blocking of the AT_1 receptor using competitive antagonists, such as losartan, could explain these results (36). The use of noncompetitive, nonpeptide AT_1-receptor antagonists (such as Exp 3174) has helped to resolve this issue. The existence of additional receptor subtypes may explain findings such as those in rat liver where saralasin ($Sar^1 Ala^8$ AII) is an antagonist of AII-induced activation of a Ca^{2+}-dependent kinase, but an agonist for inhibition of adenylyl cyclase. Additionally, $Sar^1 Ile^8$ AII is an antagonist for AII-coupled responses in most tissues/organs, but has similar effects as AII on intestinal Na^+ and water transport (48). The heptapeptide [2–8] AIII and [3–8] AII have been shown to be biologically active in a number of tissues and cells, but it is not clear whether the actions of these angiotensin peptides are mediated by an AT_1 receptor or another receptor subtype. A distinct membrane-binding site (AT_4), which specifically binds [3–8] AII saturably, reversibly, and with high affinity, has been described in heart as well as other tissues (49). Pharmacologically, the binding site is distinct from AT_1 and AT_2 because it displays a low affinity ($>10^{-6}$ M) for AII and AIII, and the antagonists $Sar^1 Ile^8$ AII, losartan, and PD123177. Because no function has been determined for the putative AT_4 receptor, it remains to be determined whether this site mediates physiological and/or pathological functions in the myocardium. The high concentration of AT_4 receptors on endothelial cells suggests that this peptide may regulate endothelial cell function, possibly related to the synthesis and release of endogenous substances (e.g., nitric oxide) associated with vasodilation (50).

ANGIOTENSIN II RECEPTOR DESENSITIZATION AND INTERNALIZATION

Angiotensin II receptors in cardiac myocytes, fibroblasts, and VSM rapidly desensitize upon exposure to AII. Desensitization presumably "protects" the tissue against potent effects of the peptide. In view of the high affinity of the receptor for AII, mechanisms other than dissociation of the peptide from the receptor must explain the generally short duration of action of AII in most effector systems. A number of possible mechanisms may explain AT_1-receptor desensitization, including covalent modification of the receptor (2), ligand occupancy, and internalization (51) and inactivation of effectors. In the case of β-adrenergic receptors, phosphorylation of the receptor by cAMP-dependent kinases, PKC, β-adrenergic receptor kinase (52), and tyrosine kinase (53) are responsible for homologous desensitization. Although the AT_1 receptor has potential phosphorylation sites in the cytoplasmic domains, there is no conclusive evidence to indicate that a protein kinase initiates receptor desensitization. However, the presence of receptor kinases for other G protein–coupled receptors such as α-adrenergic and muscarinic, makes it a tenable hypothesis that a specific kinase inactivates the AT_1 receptor. Even though translocation ultimately removes AII receptors from the cell surface and prevents further interactions with exogenous ligand, this mechanism is probably not responsible for the initial rapid desensitization. Receptor internalization and recycling are probably more important for long-term regulation of receptor density on the plasma membrane. Internalization also may influence transcriptional responses related to growth, because a close correlation between AII-receptor sequestration and delayed diacylglycerol (DG) accumulation has been demonstrated in VSM cells following AII stimulation (54), suggesting that internalization may be an initial event for maintaining sustained levels of DG and PKC activity.

ROLE OF THE RENIN–ANGIOTENSIN SYSTEM IN HEART FAILURE

A 1992 multicenter study (55) designed to identify determinants of myocardial infarction found that the frequency of a deletion polymorphism in the gene for ACE was significantly greater in patients with heart failure than in controls, suggesting that this is an important risk factor in heart disease. Angiotensin-converting enzyme inhibitors have also been shown to reduce myocardial infarction size following coronary occlusion (56,57). It is disputed, however, whether the protective effects of ACE inhibitors in heart failure are mediated by decreased synthesis of AII or by a decrease in bradykinin breakdown. In contrast to renin, ACE does not have significant substrate specificity and can metabolize a variety of peptides other than AI, such as bradykinin, enkephalin, neurotensin, and substance P (24). Indirect evidence that supports the role of AII as the primary mediator involved in cardiac remodeling and pathological hypertrophy includes the following: (a) Angiotensin II increases coronary vascular resistance and can induce myocardial necrosis (58). (b) The RAS has been shown to be activated following acute myocardial infarction in humans (59) and experimental animals (56). (c) Cardiac hypertrophy induced by pressure overload in the murine is prevented by administration of an AT_1-receptor antagonist, indicating that AII has a direct effect in mediating cardiac growth in this model (60). (d) Angiotensin-converting enzyme mRNA is increased in myocardium from rats with left ventricular hypertrophy, suggesting that its expression is associated with the hypertrophic response (20). On the other hand, in vivo evidence for the role of ACE in breakdown of bradykinin has recently been demonstrated, in which captopril increased significantly the release of bradykinin ($\sim$ threefold) into the interventricular vein of bilaterally nephrectomized dogs following ischemia induced by coronary artery constriction (16). The function of ACE may depend on where the enzyme is localized as well as the metabolic state of the heart. Recently developed bradykinin and angiotensin-receptor antagonists will be useful in determining the roles of these hormones in various forms of heart failure. Both experimental and clinical studies have documented the efficacy of ACE inhibitors in preventing cardiac hypertrophy and remodeling (61,62), indicating that AII is an important growth factor in the heart. The peptide also contributes to the normal rapid left ventricular growth that occurs in the early neonatal period (63,64). Angiotensin II has positive growth effects in cultured neonatal rat cardiac fibroblasts (36) and myocytes (65,66), and the peptide stimulates collagen and glycoconjugate synthesis in heart and VSM, an effect that may contribute to extracellular matrix remodeling (67).

SIGNAL TRANSDUCTION PATHWAYS MEDIATING ANGIOTENSIN II EFFECTS IN THE HEART

Although it has been documented that the cardiac RAS is activated in heart failure, the primary stimulus for induction is unknown. Increased ventricular wall stress may be an important stimulus for activation of this system because it correlates with myocardial angiotensinogen mRNA levels in the hypertrophying, noninfarcted myocardium during the early postinfarction period (68). The importance of mechanical stretch on cardiac cell growth and activation of the local RAS has been demonstrated by recent in vitro studies. The application of stretch to cultured neonatal rat cardiac myocytes results in activation of mitogen-activated protein kinase (referred to as MAP-kinase or extracellular signal-regulated kinase [ERK]) (69), transcriptional activation of early and intermediate response genes (70,71), followed by the appearance of the hypertrophic phenotype (72). Stretch of primary cardiac nonmyocytes containing a mixture of fibroblasts, smooth-muscle cells, and endothelial cells caused a rapid induction of immediate-early genes followed by hyperplasia rather than hypertrophy (73). When stretched, primary cultures of neonatal rat cardiomyocytes released a humoral factor which acted in an autocrine and/or paracrine fashion to activate *c-fos* (74). Conditioned media from stretched cells, when transferred to nonstretched cardiomyocytes, mimicked the effects of stretch (74). The humoral factor(s) released during stretch remains to be identified; recent evidence, however, suggests that AII may be involved because an ACE inhibitor (captopril) or AT_1-receptor antagonist (losartan) attenuates stretch-induced growth in primary cultures of cardiac myocytes (75).

Angiotensin II can activate intracellular responses in common with conventional peptide growth factors, including calcium mobilization, stimulation of Na^+/H^+ exchange, inositol phosphate metabolism, DG production, PKC activation, Raf-1 hyperphosphorylation, MAP-kinases, ribosomal protein S6-kinase activation, and phosphorylation of nuclear membrane lamins (Fig. 2). Angiotensin II stimulates expression of early (*c-fos, c-jun*) and intermediate response genes (*c-myc, c-myb*), which are important for regulation of cell growth (76–79). The induction of *c-fos* mRNA has been shown to occur by Ca^{2+}- and PKC-dependent pathways, with maximum induction requiring both (80). Antisense oligonucleotides to *c-fos* block the AII-induced stimulation of protein synthesis in VSM (81). AII stimulates hyperphosphorylation of Raf-1 in cultured rat aortic VSM cells within 5 to 10 minutes, a response that is sustained for at least 2 hours (82). The phosphorylation of Raf-1 appears to require PKC activation because downregulation of PKC in VSM cells abolishes AII-induced hyperphosphorylation. Although AII stimulates tyrosine kinase activity (83), the AT_1 receptor does not have intrinsic tyrosine kinase activity, suggesting that nonreceptor tyrosine kinases may be associated with the receptor and transduce the signal in response to ligand binding. This signal may occur through identified components of the signal transduction pathway activated by AII, such as G proteins, PKC, calmodulin-kinase, and/or through unidentified components that interact directly with the receptor. The activation of PLC-γ by tyrosine phosphorylation is probably not required for AII-induced growth, because the AT_1 receptor stimulates intracellular production of inositol triphosphate (IP_3) and DG by activating PLC-β, presumably through G_q or members of the G_{11} subfamily (84).

Phospholipase Cs have been thought to be the only class of signaling enzymes that interact with both G proteins and receptor-regulated tyrosine kinases. Recent evidence suggests that PI-3-kinase may also be regulated by G protein transduction pathways (85), but it remains to be determined whether the PI-3-kinase activity is due to cell-specific expression of a G protein–sensitive form of PI-3-kinase and/or whether transduction proteins other than G_i can activate PI-3-kinase. To date, there is no direct evidence to suggest that the AT_1 receptor activates $p21^{ras}$; however, because $p21^{ras}$ is required for Raf-1 activation (86), and AII activates Raf-1, the AT_1 receptor may activate $p21^{ras}$ through intermediate components. Protein kinase C appears to be involved in $p21^{ras}$ activation in certain cell types (87) because phorbol ester induces an increase in $p21^{ras}$-GAP, although in peripheral blood T lymphocytes phorbol ester does not stimulate $p21^{ras}$-GTP formation. Blockade of tyrosine kinase prevents formation of $p21^{ras}$-GTP by the G protein–coupled CD3 receptor (88). At least two pathways, PKC-dependent and PKC-independent, couple

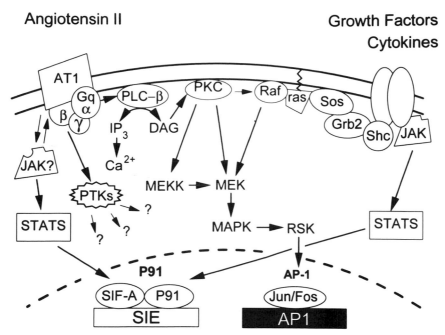

FIG. 2. General scheme by which AII can effect muscle contraction, cell metabolism and growth, and gene expression. Binding of growth factors to their receptors leads to receptor dimerization, activation of intrinsic tyrosine kinases, and autophosphorylation of several sites on the receptor. Cytoplasmic proteins containing SH2 domains, such as Shc and Grb2, bind to the phosphorylated tyrosine residues on the receptor. Shc brings Grb2 and the guanine nucleotide exchange factor, Sos, to the receptor, resulting in sequential activation of p21^{ras} (ras), Raf, a series of protein kinases (mitogen-activated protein kinase, *MAPK*; MAP-kinase kinase, *MEK*; MAP-kinase kinase kinase, *MEKK*), and the transcription factor AP-1. Both MAP-kinase and ribosomal protein kinase (*RSK*) may be translocated to the nucleus to induce gene transcription. Some ligands can induce gene transcription by a more direct pathway involving the cytoplasmic proteins SIF-A and P91 (*STATS*), which are phosphorylated on tyrosine residues by one or more soluble tyrosine kinases, such as Janus kinases (*JAKs*), which have domains that interact with the plasma membrane receptor. The phosphorylated SIF-A and P91 translocate to the nucleus where complexes containing these proteins bind to specific DNA sequences such as the *sis*-inducible element (*SIE*). Binding of angiotensin II to the type-I plasma membrane receptor (*AT$_1$*) stimulates, via a G protein, phospholipase C-β (*PLC-β*), which hydrolyzes phosphatidyl inositol diphosphate (*PIP$_2$*) to form the intracellular messengers inositol trisphosphate (*IP$_3$*) and di-acylglycerol (*DAG*). Similarly, activated growth factor receptors directly interact with PLC-γ, resulting in synthesis of IP$_3$ and DAG. The IP$_3$ releases Ca^{2+} from intracellular stores, which stimulates muscle contraction. Following activation by DAG, protein kinase C (*PKC*) phosphorylates kinases (*Raf, MEK, MEKK*) at various points in the MAPK cascade. Like growth factors and cytokines, AII stimulates phosphorylation of STATS. The kinase(s) responsible for phosphorylation of STATS following AII stimulation is (are) unknown. This activation of STATS may occur through JAK or a similar kinase that directly or indirectly interacts with the AII-receptor complex and/or receptor-associated G-protein subunits (α or βγ). The pathway(s) leading to phosphorylation of soluble protein tyrosine kinases (*PTKs*) is (are) unknown, but may involve the receptor and/or associated G-protein subunits. Even though the targets of PTKs are unknown, these kinases are likely to have a role in activating proximal components of the MAPK cascade.

receptors that lack intrinsic tyrosine kinase activity to $p21^{ras}$. In yeast, $G_{\beta\gamma}$ subunits trigger downstream events (89), with the primary target of $G_{\beta\gamma}$ being Ste20p kinase, which phosphorylates Ste5, a yeast homolog to mammalian $p21^{ras}$ (89). An unidentified mammalian homolog to Ste20p may exist that could link the AT_1 receptor to $p21^{ras}$. There may exist $G_{\beta\gamma}$-regulated kinases in which Ste20p would represent a yeast homolog of such kinases, providing a new mechanism of G protein–mediated transduction, where a protein kinase cascade is activated by $G_{\beta\gamma}$ subunits. The high degree of conservation of G proteins between yeast and humans (90) supports this hypothesis. The muscarinic receptor kinase has been shown to be activated by $G_{\beta\gamma}$ in a reconstituted system (91). A recently identified MAP-kinase kinase kinase (MEKK) in murine, which like Raf-1 activates MAP-kinase kinase, has also been hypothesized to mediate signals originating from G protein–coupled receptors (92).

The MAP-kinase cascade is bidirectional, in which phosphorylation by kinases activates and dephosphorylation inactivates the cascade, although little is known concerning the process of deactivation. The AT_2 receptor has been reported to stimulate protein tyrosine phosphatase activity in PC12W cells (93). Recent experiments (94) show a positive correlation between AT_2-receptor downregulation and PDGF-BB stimulated ^3H-thymidine uptake in VSMC, suggesting that AT_2 may counteract the growth effects of AT_1. Further studies need to be performed to determine whether the AT_2 receptor stimulates significant tyrosine phosphatase activity and if this has a positive or negative effect on cardiac growth.

In contrast to tyrosine kinase receptors, the AT_1 receptor requires 2 to 4 hours of agonist exposure to induce growth in cultured rat cardiomyocytes (95), cardiac fibroblasts (96), and VSM cells (97). This suggests that activation of PKC, MAP-kinases, and early response genes is not sufficient to induce protein (cardiomyocytes and VSM) or DNA synthesis (cardiac fibroblasts). Addition of the AT_1-receptor antagonist EXP 3174 to cardiac fibroblasts, within 90 minutes after AII administration, prevents the AII-induced mitogenic response (96). The mechanisms activated by prolonged stimulation by AII are not apparent, especially because the receptor rapidly desensitizes following agonist binding. Continuous activation of second messenger pathways by the recycling of AT_1 receptors may serve to recruit components required for cell proliferation or hypertrophy. Proximal components recruited may include $p21^{ras}$, Src, or even modified AT_1 receptor. The internalized receptor and/or peptide could also regulate nuclear events related to growth. Determining the need for $p21^{ras}$, Raf-1, or other signaling proteins activated by AII will require the use of dominant interfering protein or neutralizing antibodies. Studies examining the possible delayed and/or multiphasic activation of PLC-γ, $p21^{ras}$ GTPase-activator protein, $p21^{ras}$, PI-3-kinase, and/or $pp60^{src}$ by AII remain to be performed. These studies would provide insight into the sequence of events and factors needed for AII-mediated growth. Angiotensin II induces a biphasic activation of MAP-kinases in cultured neonatal rat cardiac fibroblasts after 5 and 90 minutes of stimulation, whereas carbachol, which is not mitogenic in these cells, produces only an initial rise in MAP-kinase activity (96). It is not clear whether the secondary rise in MAP-kinase activity is required for growth or is coincident with activation of required growth pathways. The secondary rise in MAP-kinase activation could be mediated by recycling of AT_1 receptors and/or indirectly by AII-mediated release of growth factors which act in an autocrine fashion to stimulate tyrosine kinase receptors.

In cardiac fibroblasts, in addition to MAP-kinase, AII stimulates protein tyrosine phosphorylation of p46[Shc], p56[Shc], p125[Fak], and unidentified proteins of 85, 145, and 185 kDa in cardiac fibroblasts (97). It is interesting to note that AII effects in cardiac fibroblasts extend to activation of cytosolic proteins, which are part of the cytokine signal transduction pathway (98). Cytokines have been demonstrated to control proliferation and differentiation and play key roles in the immune and hematopoietic system (99,100). These factors induce activation of a group of cytoplasmic proteins termed *signal transducers and activators of transcription* (STATs) and include the proteins p48, p84, p91, and p113 (99,101). When activated, these STATs form an interferon-stimulated gene factor (ISGF) transcriptional complex that binds to the interferon-stimulated response element (ISRE) and activates transcription (102). Formation of the ISGF complex and its migration to the nucleus requires tyrosine phosphorylation of p84, p91, and p113 (103). This novel gene transcription pathway is shared by all members of the cytokine receptor family. Upon AII stimulation, it has been shown that p91 is phosphorylated in cultured neonatal rat cardiac fibroblasts and in CHO-K1 cells stably expressing the AT_{1A} receptor (98). Through the use of selective nonpeptide receptor antagonists we have established that AII-mediated phosphorylation of these proteins occurs through the AT_1 receptor. This is the first evidence to demonstrate that a G protein–coupled serpentine receptor, such as AT_1, can activate this cytokine pathway. The transducing pathway leading from the activated AT_1 receptor to activation of tyrosine kinase(s) responsible for activation of STATs, however, remains to be defined. Studies involving mutagenesis of cytokine receptors have led to the conclusion that a protein tyrosine kinase physically associates with the cytokine receptor and becomes activated following ligand binding (99). Janus kinases (JAKs), which belong to a family of cytoplasmic protein tyrosine kinases that lack SH2 or SH3 domains, are responsible for activating STATs, following cytokine receptor activation (99,100). It remains to be determined whether activation of a *sis*-inducible element (SIE) by activated AT_1 receptor also occurs through a JAK, and if so, whether the Janus kinase interacts with the AII-receptor complex and/or associated G protein subunits. The activation of cytokine pathways by AII in cardiac tissue suggests that AII may play a significant role in the healing process following cardiac injury such as myocardial infarction or in posttransplantation inflammatory response. The demonstration of angiotensinogen expression by leukocytes (104) suggests that AII may be locally generated by noncardiac cells that migrate to the injured region of the heart.

RELEASE OF GROWTH FACTORS BY ANGIOTENSIN II

A number of studies suggest that AII can modulate growth indirectly by stimulating release of platelet-derived growth factor (PDGF), transforming growth factor beta (TGF-β_1), and basic fibroblast growth factor (bFGF), which in turn could have autocrine and/or paracrine effects. In cultured rat aortic VSM, AII stimulates mRNA for and synthesis of endothelin, TGF-β_1 ,and PDGF (105,106,107). The peptide also stimulates insulin-like growth factor-1 (IGF-I) gene transcription in VSM cells, and AII-stimulated thymidine incorporation is almost completely inhibited in the presence of an anti-IGF-I antibody (108). Angiotensin II also stimulates de novo synthesis and release of endothelin-1 in neonatal rat cardiomyocytes (109). Protein synthesis stimulated by AII in cardiomyocytes was blocked by endothelin-A receptor antagonists and antisense oligonucleotides against prepro endothelin-1 mRNA, suggesting a potential autocrine/paracrine role of endothelin-1 in AII-induced cardiomyocyte growth (109). Angiotensin II–induced release of TGF-β_1 could account for many of the changes that take place upon remodeling, since this factor stimulates synthesis of extracellular matrix, proliferation of VSM cells in coronary arteries, and controls expression of contractile proteins in myocytes (67). Because TGF-β_1 is secreted in a latent form (110), additional mechanisms must be invoked to explain the AII-stimulated increase in active TGF-β_1. Further studies are needed to determine the involvement of autocrine and paracrine factors in mediation of the AII growth response in cardiac cells.

INTEGRATION OF ANGIOTENSIN RECEPTOR SIGNALING WITH TYROSINE KINASE RECEPTORS

The study of potential interactions between G protein–coupled and tyrosine kinase receptors is an important area of research. The AT_1 receptor has mitogenic and other growth-related effects that are of central importance to gene regulation in the heart; however, little is known concerning the acute and chronic interactions between G protein–mediated and tyrosine kinase–activated pathways and how these signaling events apply to developmental and pathological growth. Cross-talk between G protein–coupled and tyrosine-linked receptors has been described at the level of the receptor and G protein (for recent review, see ref. 111). Stimulation of β-adrenergic receptors results in phosphorylation and desensitization of the insulin receptor (112,113). Alternatively, insulin can alter the state of phosphorylation of the β_2-adrenergic receptor by increasing the degree of phosphorylated tyrosine residues while decreasing the level of phosphorylation of phosphothreonine residues (53). Functional cross-regulation between tyrosine kinase and β-adrenergic receptor pathways has been described for G_s, where tyrosine phosphorylation of $G_{s\alpha}$ by pp60[src] increased the activity of G_s (52). It remains to be determined whether pp60[src] phosphorylates G proteins, which couple to phospholipase C and calcium mobilization.

SUMMARY

During the past several decades, we have witnessed the evolution of our understanding of the RAS, with initial identification and synthesis of AII; characterization of the functional responses of angiotensin peptides; identification, characterization, and cloning of angiotensin receptors; and the demonstration of local RASs. The ability to slow the rate of formation of endogenous AII with ACE inhibitors has provided experimental and clinical data demonstrating effectiveness in the treatment of hypertension and congestive heart failure, which supports the involvement of the RAS in these pathological conditions. Although a cardiac RAS may generate AII, the role in normal cellular physiology and contribution to locally mediated biological responses remain to be elucidated. Although the RAS can be pharmacologically interrupted by inhibition of renin and ACE, studies using specific receptor antagonists will be needed to elucidate functional determinants of this system. Future directions using newly developed drugs and molecular biological techniques (e.g., transgenes) should provide a more complete understanding of the molecular mechanisms of angiotensin-induced responses, definition of the various types and functions of AII receptors, and documentation of the biological relevance of a local RAS.

ACKNOWLEDGMENTS

During the writing of this review, our work was supported by grants from the National Institutes of Health (KMB, HL44883, and HL44379), the American Heart Association (KMB 91003030 and 900607; and DED 93008840), the Pennsylvania Affiliate of the American Heart Association (KMB, DED), and the Geisinger Clinic Foundation. Dr. Baker is an Established Investigator of the American Heart Association.

REFERENCES

1. Peach MJ. Renin-angiotensin system: biochemistry and mechanism of action. *Physiol Rev* 1977; 57:313–370.
2. Peach MJ. Pharmacology of angiotensin II. In: Fisher JW, ed. *Kidney hormones*. 1986;3:273–308.
3. Hackenthal E, Paul M, Ganten D, Taugner R. Morphology, physiology, and molecular biology of renin secretion. *Physiol Rev* 1990;70:1067–1116.
4. Dzau VJ. Molecular and physiological aspects of the tissue renin-angiotensin system: emphasis on cardiovascular control. *J Hypertens* 1988;6[Suppl 3]:S7–S12.
5. Phillips MI. Functions of angiotensin in the central nervous system. *Annu Rev Physiol* 1987;49: 413–435.
6. Dostal DE, Baker KM. Evidence for a role of an intracardiac renin-angiotensin system in normal and failing hearts. *Trends Cardiovasc Med* 1993;3:67–74.
7. Lindpaintner K, Ganten D. The cardiac, renin-angiotensin system: an appraisal of experimental and clinical evidence. *Circ Res* 1991;68:905–921.
8. Dostal DE, Rothblum KC, Chernin MI, Cooper GR, Baker KM. Intracardiac detection of angiotensinogen and renin: evidence for a localized renin-angiotensinogen system in neonatal rat heart. *Am J Physiol (Cell Physiol)* 1992;263:C838–C850.
9. Dostal DE, Rothblum KC, Conrad KM, Cooper GR, Baker KM. Detection of angiotensin I and II cultured rat cardiac myocytes and fibroblasts; evidence for local production. *Am J Physiol (Cell Physiol)* 1992;263:C851–C863.
10. Dzau VJ, Ellison KE, Brody T, Ingelfinger J, Pratt RE. A comparative study of the distribution of renin and angiotensinogen messenger ribonucleic acids in rat and mouse tissues. *Endocrinology* 1987;120:2334–2338.

11. Dzau VJ, Re RN. Evidence for the existence of renin in the heart. *Circulation* 1987;75[Suppl I]: I-134–I-136.
12. Yamada H, Fabris B, Allen AM, Jackson B, Johnston CI, Mendelsohn FAO. Localization of angiotensin converting enzyme in rat heart. *Circ Res* 1991;68.141–149.
13. Ikemoto F, Song GB, Tominaga M, Yamamoto K. Endogenous inhibitor of angiotensin converting enzyme in the rat heart. *Biochem Biophys Res Commun* 1989;159:1093–1099.
14. Urata H, Kinoshita A, Misono FM, Bumpus FM, Husain A. Identification of a highly specific chymase as the major angiotensin II–forming enzyme in the human heart. *J Biol Chem* 1990;265: 22348–22357.
15. Lindpaintner K, Wilhelm JJ, Jin M, et al. Tissue renin-angiotensin systems: focus on the heart. *J Hypertens* 1987;5[Suppl 2]:S33–S38.
16. Noda K, Sasaguri M, Ideishi M, Ikeda M, Arakawa K. Role of locally formed angiotensin II and bradykinin in the reduction of myocardial infarct size in dogs. *Circ Res* 1993;27:334–340.
17. Robertson AL, Khairallah PA. Angiotensin II: rapid localization in nuclei of smooth and cardiac muscle. *Science* 1971;172:1138–1139.
18. Kiron MAR, Soffer RL. Purification and properties of a soluble angiotensin II-binding protein from rabbit liver. *J Biol Chem* 1989;264:4138–4142.
19. Booz GW, Conrad KM, Hess AL, Singer HA, Baker KM. Angiotensin II binding sites on hepato-cyte nuclei. *Endocrinology* 1992;130:3641–3649.
20. Shunkert H, Dzau VJ, Tang SS, Hirsch AT, Apstein CS, Lorell BH. Increased rat cardiac angioten-sin converting enzyme activity and mRNA expression in pressure overload left ventricular hyper-trophy: effects on coronary resistance, contractility, and relaxation. *J Clin Invest* 1990;86:1913–1920.
21. Baker KM, Chernin MI, Wixon SK, Aceto JF. Renin-angiotensin system involvement in pressure-overload cardiac hypertrophy in rats. *Am J Physiol* 1990;259:H324–H332.
22. Mullins JJ, Peters J, Ganten D. Fulminant hypertension in transgenic rats harbouring the mouse Ren-2 gene. *Nature* 1990;344:541–544.
23. Kimura S, Mullins JJ, Bunnemann B, et al. High blood pressure in transgenic mice carrying the rat angiotensin gene. *EMBO J* 1992;11:821–827.
24. Erdos EG, Skidgel RA. The unusual substrate and the distribution of human angiotensin I convert-ing enzyme. *Hypertension* 1986;8[Suppl I]:I34–I37.
25. Maruata H, Arakawa K. Confirmation of direct angiotensin formation by kallikrein. *Biochem J* 1983;213:193–200.
26. Kinoshita A, Urata H, Bumpus FM, Husain A. Multiple determinants for the high substrate speci-ficity of an angiotensin II–forming chymase from the human heart. *J Biol Chem* 1991;266:19192–19197.
27. Urata H, Kinoshita A, Perez DM, et al. Cloning of the gene and cDNA for human heart chymase. *J Biol Chem* 1991;266:17173–17179.
28. Allen AM, Yamada H, Mendelsohn FAO. In vitro autoradiographic localization of binding to an-giotensin receptors in the rat heart. *Int J Cardiol* 1990;28:25–33.
29. Wong PC, Hart SD, Zasbel AM, et al. Functional studies of nonpeptide angiotensin II receptor subtype-specific ligands: DuP 753 (AII-I) and PD123177 (AII-2). *J Pharmcol Exp Ther* 1990;255: 584–592.
30. Timmermans PBMWM, Wong PC, Chiu AT, Herblin WF. Nonpeptide angiotensin II receptor an-tagonists. *TIPS* 1991;12:55–62.
31. Bumpus FM, Catt KJ, Chiu AT, et al. Nomenclature of angiotensin receptors. A report of the Nomenclature Committee of the Council for High Blood Pressure Research. *Hypertension* 1991;17:720–721.
32. Catt K, Abbott A. Molecular cloning of angiotensin II receptors may presage further receptor sub-types. *TIPS* 1991;12:279–281.
33. Rogg H, Schmid A, de Gasparo M. Identification and characterization of angiotensin II receptor subtypes in rabbit ventricular myocardium. *Biochem Biophys Res Commun* 1990;173:416–422.
34. Sechi LA, Griffin CA, Grady EF, Kalinyak JE, Schambelan M. Characterization of angiotensin II receptor subtypes in rat heart. *Circ Res* 1992;71:1482–1489.
35. Rogers TB, Gaa ST, Allen IS. Identification and characterization of functional angiotensin II receptors on cultured heart myocytes. *J Pharmacol Exp Ther* 1986;236:438–444.
36. Schorb W, Booz GW, Dostal DE, Conrad KM, Chang KC, Baker KM. Angiotensin II is mitogenic in neonatal rat cardiac fibroblasts. *Circ Res* 1993;72:1245–1254.

37. Meggs LG, Coupet J, Huang H, et al. Regulation of angiotensin II receptors on ventricular myocytes after myocardial infarction in rats. *Circ Res* 1993;72:1149–1162.
38. Douglas JG. Angiotensin receptor subtypes of the kidney cortex. *Am J Physiol* 1987;253:F1–F7.
39. Inagami T, Iwai N, Sasaki K, et al. Angiotensin II receptors: cloning and regulation. *Drug Res* 1993;43:226–228.
40. Thekkumkara TJ, Du J, Dostal DE, Booz GW, Motel TJ, Baker KM. Characterization of permanently transfected AT$_{1A}$ receptors in CHO-K1 cells: desensitization by angiotensin II. *FASEB J* 1993;7:A491.
41. Sasaki K, Yamano Y, Bardhan S, et al. Cloning and expression of a complementary DNA encoding a bovine adrenal angiotensin I type-1 receptor. *Nature* 1991;351:230–233.
42. Murphy TJ, Alexander RW, Griendling KK, Runge MS, Bernstein KE. Isolation of a cDNA encoding the vascular type-1 angiotensin II receptor. *Nature* 1991;351:233–236.
43. Jackson TR, Blair LAC, Marshall J, Goedert M, Hanley MR. The *mas* oncogene encodes an angiotensin receptor. *Nature* 1988;335:437–440.
44. Urata H, Healy B, Stewart RW, Bumpus FM, Husain A. Angiotensin receptors in normal and failing human hearts. *J Clin Endocrinol Metab* 1989;69:54–66.
45. Matsubara L, Brilla CG, Weber KT. Angiotensin II–mediated inhibition of collagenase activity in cultured cardiac fibroblasts. *FASEB J* 1992;6:A941.
46. Sumners C, Tang W, Zelezna B, Raizada MK. Angiotensin II receptor subtypes are coupled with distinct signal transduction mechanisms in neurons and astrocytes from rat brain. *Proc Natl Acad Sci USA* 1991;88:7567–7571.
47. Brix J, Haber RL. The AT$_2$-receptor mediates endothelium-dependent dilation of rat brain arterioles. *FASEB J* 1992;6:A1264.
48. Peach MJ, Dostal DE. The angiotensin II receptor and the actions of angiotensin II. *J Cardiovasc Pharmacol* 1990;16[Suppl 4]:S25–S30.
49. Swanson GN, Hanesworth JM, Sardinia MF, et al. Discovery of a distinct binding site for angiotensin II (3–8), a putative angiotensin IV receptor. *Regul Pept* 1992;40:409–419.
50. Harberl RL, Decker PJ, Einhaupl KM. Angiotensin degradation products mediate endothelium-dependent dilation of rabbit brain arterioles. *Circ Res* 1991;68:1621–1627.
51. Anderson KM, Murahashi T, Dostal DE, Peach MJ. Morphological and biochemical analysis of angiotensin II internalization in cultured rat aortic smooth muscle cells. *Am J Physiol* 1993;274:C179–C188.
52. Hausdorff WP, Pitcher JA, Luttrell DK, et al. Tyrosine phosphorylation of G protein subunits by pp60^{v-src}. *Proc Natl Acad Sci USA* 1992;89:5720–5724.
53. Hadcock JR, Port JD, Gelman MS, Malbon CC. Cross-talk between tyrosine kinase and G-protein-linked receptors: phosphorylation of β$_2$-adrenergic receptors in response to insulin. *J Biol Chem* 1992;267:26017–26022.
54. Griendling KK, Delafontaine P, Rittenhouse SE, Gimbrone MA Jr, Alexander RW. Correlation of receptor sequestration with sustained diacylglycerol accumulation in angiotensin II–stimulated cultured vascular smooth muscle cells. *J Biol Chem* 1987;262:14555–14562.
55. Cambien F, Poirier O, Lecerf L, et al. Deletion polymorphism in the gene for angiotensin-converting enzyme is a potent risk factor for myocardial infarction. *Nature* 1992;359:641–644.
56. Ertl G, Kloner RA, Alexander RW, Braunwald E. Limitation of experimental infarct size by an angiotensin converting enzyme inhibitor. *Circulation* 1982;65:40–48.
57. Hock CE, Ribeiro LGT, Lefer AM. Preservation of ischemic myocardium by a new converting enzyme inhibitor, enalaprilic acid, in acute myocardial infarction. *Am Heart J* 1986;109:222–228.
58. Gavras H, Kremer D, Brown JJ, et al., Angiotensin- and norepinephrine-induced myocardial lesions: experimental and clinical studies in rabbits and man. *Am Heart J* 1975;89:312–331.
59. McAlpine HM, Cobbe SM. Neuroendocrine changes in acute myocardial infarction. *Am J Med* 1988;84[Suppl 3A]:61–66.
60. Wachhorst SP, Rockman HA, Ross J Jr. Inhibition of local angiotensin II action prevents myocardial hypertrophy due to pressure overload in mice. *J Am Coll Cardiol* 1993;21:433A.
61. Lamas GA, Pfeffer MA. Left ventricular remodeling after acute myocardial infarction: clinical course and beneficial effects of angiotensin-converting enzyme inhibition. *Am Heart J* 1991;121:1194–1202.
62. Linz W, Schaper J, Wiemer G, Albus U, Scholkens BA. Ramipril prevents left ventricular hypertrophy with myocardial fibrosis without blood pressure reduction: a one year study in rats. *Br J Pharmacol* 1992;107:970–975.

63. Beinlich CJ, Baker KM, White GJ, Morgan HE. Control of growth in the neonatal pig heart. *Am J Physiol* 1991;261:3–7.
64. Beinlich CJ, White GJ, Baker KM, Morgan ME. Angiotensin II and left ventricular growth in newborn pig heart. *J Mol Cell Cardiol* 1991;23:1031–1038.
65. Katoh Y, Komuro I, Shibasaki Y, Yamaguchi H, Yazaki Y. Angiotensin II induces hypertrophy and oncogene expression in cultured rat heart myocytes. *Circulation* 1989;80:II-A450.
66. Aceto JF, Baker KM. [Sar¹] angiotensin II receptor-mediated stimulation of protein synthesis in chicken heart cells. *Am J Physiol* 1990;258:H806–H813.
67. Scott-Burden T, Hahn AWA, Resink TJ, Bühler FR. Modulation of extracellular matrix by angiotensin II: stimulated glycoconjugate synthesis and growth in vascular smooth mucle cells. *J Cardiovasc Pharmacol* 1990;16[Suppl 4]:S36–S41.
68. Lindpaintner K, Lu W, Niedermajer N, et al. Selective activation of cardiac angiotensinogen gene expression in post-infarction ventricular remodeling in the rat. *J Mol Cell Cardiol* 1993;25:133–143.
69. Yamazaki T, Tobe K, Hoh E, et al. Mechanical loading activates mitogen-activated protein kinase and S6 peptide kinase in cultured rat cardiac myocytes. *J Biol Chem* 1993;268:12069–12076.
70. Komuro I, Kaida T, Shibasaki Y, et al. Stretching cardiac myocytes stimulates protooncogene expression. *J Biol Chem* 1990;265:3595–3598.
71. Sadoshima J, Jahn L, Takahasi T, Kulik TJ, Izumo S. Molecular characterization of the stretch-induced adaptation of cultured cardiac cells: an in vitro model of load-induced cardiac hypertrophy. *J Biol Chem* 1992;267:10551–10560.
72. Komuro I, Katoh Y, Kaida T, et al. Mechanical loading stimulates cell hypertrophy and specific gene expression in cultured rat cardiac myocytes. *J Biol Chem* 1991;266:1265–1268.
73. Sadoshima J, Takahashi T, Jahn L, Izumo S. Roles of mechano-sensitive ion channels, cytoskeleton, and contractile activity in stretch-induced immediate-early gene expression and hypertrophy of cardiac myocytes. *Proc Natl Acad Sci USA* 1992;89:9905–9909.
74. Sadoshima J, Isumo S. Mechanical stretch rapidly activates multiple signal transduction pathways in cardiac myocytes: potential involvement of an autocrine/paracrine mechanism. *EMBO J* 1993;12:1681–1692.
75. Miyata S, Haneda T, Fukuzawa J, et al. Stretch induces hypertrophic growth through renin-angiotensin system in cultured neonatal rat myocytes. In: Yasuda H, Kawaguchi H, eds. *New aspects in the treatment of failing heart*. Tokyo: Springer-Verlag; 1992;223–225.
76. Paquet J-L, Baudouin-Legros M, Brunelle G, Meyer P. Angiotensin II–induced proliferation of aortic myocytes in spontaneously hypertensive rats. *J Hypertens* 1990;8:565–572.
77. Naftilan AJ, Pratt RE, Dzau VJ. Induction of platelet-derived growth factor A-chain and *c-myc* gene expression by angiotensin II in cultured rat vascular smooth muscle cells. *J Clin Invest* 1989;83:1419–1424.
78. Pratt RE, Itoh H, Gibbons GH, Dzau VJ. Role of angiotensin in the control of vascular smooth muscle growth. *J Vasc Med Biol* 1991;3:25–29.
79. Naftilan AJ, Pratt RE, Eldrige CS, Lin HL, Dzau VJ. Angiotensin II induces *c-fos* expression in smooth muscle via transcriptional control. *Hypertension* 1989;13:706–711.
80. Taubman MB, Berk BC, Izumo S, Tsauda T, Alexander RW. Angiotensin II induces *c-fos* mRNA in aortic smooth muscle. Role of Ca^{2+} mobilization and protein kinase C activation. *J Biol Chem* 1989;264:526–530.
81. Rainer RS, Eldrige CS, Gilliland GK, Naftilan AJ. Antisense oligonucleotide to *c-fos* blocks the angiotensin II–induced stimulation of protein synthesis in rat aortic smooth muscle cells. *Hypertension* 1990;16:326.
82. Molloy CJ, Taylor DS, Weber H. Angiotensin II stimulation of rapid protein tyrosine phosphorylation and protein kinase activation in rat aortic smooth muscle cells. *J Biol Chem* 1993;268:7338–7345.
83. Huckel WR, Prokop CA, Dy RC, Herman B, Earp S. Angiotensin II stimulates protein-tyrosine phosphorylation in a calcium-dependent manner. *Mol Cell Biol* 1990;10:6290–6298.
84. Taylor SJ, Chae HZ, Rhee SG, Exton JH. Activation of the β1 isozyme of phospholipase C by a subunit of the G_q class of G proteins. *Nature* 1991;350:516–518.
85. Stephens L, Eguinoa A, Corey S, Jackson T, Hawkins PT. Receptor stimulated accumulation of phosphatidylinositol (3,4,5)-trisphosphate by G-protein mediated pathways in human myeloid derived cells. *EMBO J* 1993;12:2265–2273.
86. Williams NG, Roberts TM, Li P. Both $p21^{ras}$ and $pp60^{v-src}$ are required, but neither alone is sufficient to activate the Raf-1 kinase. *Proc Natl Acad Sci USA* 1992;89:2922–2926.

87. Nakafuku M, Satoh T, Kaziro Y. Differentiation factors, including nerve growth factor, fibroblast growth factor, and interleukin-6, induce an accumulation of an active Ras-GTP complex in rat pheochromocytoma PC12 cells. *J Biol Chem* 1992;267:19448–19454.
88. Izquierdo M, Downward J, Graves JD, Cantrell DA. Role of protein kinase C in T-cell antigen receptor regulation of p21^{ras}: evidence that two p21^{ras} regulatory pathways coexist in T cells. *Mol Cell Biol* 1992;12:3305–3312.
89. Leberer E, Dignard D, Hougan L, Thomas DY, Whiteway M. Dominant-negative mutants of a yeast G-protein β subunit identify two functional regions involved in pheromone signalling. *EMBO J* 1992;11:4805–4813.
90. Whiteway M, Hougan L, Dignard D, et al. The STE4 and STE18 genes of yeast encode potential β and γ subunits of the mating factor receptor-coupled G protein. *Cell* 1989;56:467–477.
91. Haga K, Haga T. Activation by G protein βγ subunits of agonist- or light-dependent phosphorylation of muscarinic acetylcholine receptors and rhodopsin. *J Biol Chem* 1992;267:2222–2227.
92. Lange-Carter CA, Pleiman CM, Gardner AM, Blumer KJ, Johnson GL. A divergence in the MAP kinase regulatory network defined by MEK kinase and raf. *Science* 1993;260:315–319.
93. Bottari SP, King IN, Reichlin S, Dahlstroem I, Lydon N, de Gasparo M. The angiotensin AT$_2$ receptor stimulates protein tyrosine phosphatase activity and mediates inhibition of particulate guanylate cyclase. *Biochem Biophys Res Commun* 1992;183:206–211.
94. Kambayashi Y, Bardhan S, Inagami T. Peptide growth factors markedly decrease the ligand binding of angiotensin II type 2 receptor in cultured vascular smooth muscle cells. *Biochem Biophys Res Commun* 1993;194:478–482.
95. Baker KM, Aceto JF. Angiotensin II stimulation of protein synthesis and cell growth in chick heart cells. *Am J Physiol* 1990;259:H610–H618.
96. Schorb W, Singer HA, Dostal DE, Baker KM. Angiotensin II is a potent simulator of MAP-kinase activity in neonatal rat cardiac fibroblasts. *J Mol Cell Cardiol* 1994 (In press).
97. Schorb W, Peeler TC, Madigan NN, Conrad KM, Baker KM. Angiotensin II–induced protein tyrosine phosphorylation in neonatal rat cardiac fibroblasts. *J Biol Chem* 1994;269:19626–19632.
98. Bhat GJ, Thekkumkara TJ, Thomas WG, Conrad KM, Baker KM. Angiotensin II stimulates *sis*-inducing factor-like DNA binding activity: Evidence that the AT$_{1A}$ receptor activates transcription factor-Stat91 and/or a related protein. *J Biol Chem* 1994;269:31443–31449.
99. Ihle JN, Witthuhn BA, Quelle FW, et al. Signaling by the cytokine receptor superfamily: JAKs and STATs. *TIPS* 1994;19:222–227.
100. Wilks AF, Harpur AG. Cytokine signal transduction and the JAK family of protein tyrosine kinases. *Bioessays* 1994;16:313–320.
101. Fu XF, Kessler DS, Veals SA, Levy DE, Darnell JE Jr. IGF3, the transcriptional activator induced by interferon α, consists of multiple interacting polypeptide chains. *Proc Natl Acad Sci USA* 1992; 87:8555–8559.
102. Schindler C, Fu XY, Improta T, Aebersold R, Darnel JE Jr. Proteins of transcription factor ISGF-3: one gene encodes the 91- and 84-kDa ISGF-3 proteins that are activated by interferon α. *Proc Natl Acad Sci USA* 1992;89:7836–7839.
103. Shuai K, Ziemiecki A, Wilks AF, et al. Polypeptide signalling to the nucleus through tyrosine phosphorylation of Jak and Stat proteins. *Nature* 1993;366:580–583.
104. Gomez RA, Norling LL, Wilfong N, et al. Leukocytes synthesize angiotensinogen. *Hypertension* 1993;21:470–475.
105. Geisterfer AA, Peach MJ, Owens GK. Angiotensin II induces hypertrophy, not hyperplasia, of cultured rat aortic smooth muscle cells. *Circ Res* 1988;62:749–756.
106. Stouffer GA, Owens GK. Angiotensin II–induced mitogenesis of spontaneously hypertensinve rat-derived cultured smooth muscle cells is dependent on autocrine production of transforming growth factor-beta. *Circ Res* 1992;70:820–828.
107. Hahn AW, Resink TJ, Scott-Burden T, Powell J, Dohi Y, Bühler FR. Stimulation of endothelin mRNA and secretion in rat vascular smooth muscle cells: a novel autocrine function. *Cell Reg* 1990;1:649–659.
108. Delafontaine P, Lou H. Angiotensin II regulates insulin-like growth factor I gene expression in vascular smooth muscle cells. *J Biol Chem* 1993;268:16866–16870.
109. Ito H, Hirata Y, Adachi S, et al. Endothelin-1 is an autocrine/paracrine factor in the mechanism of angiotensin II-induced hypertrophy in cultured rat cardiomyocytes. *J Clin Invest* 1993;92:398–403.
110. Sporn MB, Roberts AB, Wakefield LM, Assoian RK. Transforming growth factor-beta: biological function and chemical structure. *Science* 1986;233:532–534.

111. Port JD, Malbon CC. Integration of transmembrane signaling: cross-talk among G-protein linked receptors and other signal transduction pathways. *Trends Cardiovasc Med* 1993;3:85–92.
112. Arner P, Hellmer J, Ewerth S, Ostman J. Effect of glucose on beta-adrenergic induced down-regulation of insulin receptor binding in human fat cells. *Biochem Biophys Res Commun* 1984;122: 97–102.
113. Liu CY, Mills SE. Decreased insulin binding to porcine adipocytes in vitro by beta-adrenergic agonists. *J Anim Sci* 1990;68:1603–1608.

The Failing Heart, edited by N. S. Dhalla,
R. E. Beamish, N. Takeda, and M. Nagano.
Lippincott-Raven Publishers, Philadelphia © 1995.

24

The Functional Role of Angiotensin and Endothelin in Failing and Nonfailing Human Myocardium

Christian Holubarsch, Burkert Pieske, Bodo Kretschmann,
Stephan Schmidt-Schweda, Markus Meyer, Klaus Schlotthauer,
Thorsten Ruf, Gerd Hasenfuss, and Hanjörg Just

*Department of Cardiology and Angiology, University of Freiburg,
79106 Freiburg, Germany*

The two polypeptides angiotensin and endothelin have several activities in common: (a) Concentrations of both naturally occurring substances are increased in heart failure (1–7). (b) Both substances exhibit considerable vasoconstrictive activities (8–12). (c) Both substances induce cardiac hypertrophy in isolated cardiac myocytes of animals (13–15). (d) On the basis of animal experiments with angiotensin II (16–19) and endothelin (20,21), it is believed that both substances have positive inotropic effects also in human myocardium, although no or limited data are available (22). We therefore studied extensively the functional role of angiotensin and endothelin in isolated right atrial as well as left ventricular myocardium of human failing and nonfailing hearts using experimental physiological conditions (37°C and 60 beats per minute).

METHODS

Source of Human Cardiac Tissue

Experiments were performed in a variety of different human myocardial preparations: (a) Long, thin trabeculae were prepared from human right atria. The tissues were obtained from patients undergoing routine aortocoronary bypass surgery. They did not suffer from heart failure symptoms; their left ventricular ejection fraction was mostly normal (23,24). (b) Muscle strip preparations were cut from left ventricular papillary muscles which were obtained from patients suffering from mitral valve stenosis or mitral valve regurgitation. (c) A number of preparations could be

295

obtained from normal left human ventricles which could not be used for transplantation for technical reasons. (d) Muscle strips were also prepared from the left ventricular free wall of explanted hearts of patients with dilated cardiomyopathy at the end stage of heart failure (23,34). (e) Right ventricular myocardium was obtained from four infants that had to undergo reconstructive heart surgery for tetralogy of Fallot (23,24).

Handling of Cardiac Tissue, Preparation Procedure, and Experimental Conditions

In all cases, transportation and preparation of cardiac tissues were performed in Krebs-Ringer solution containing 30 mM 2,3-butanedione monoxime (25). This cardioprotective solution also contained insulin and was used to minimize cutting injury (25). Time between excision of the tissues and start of measurements was between 30 minutes and 6 hours. More details about preparation procedure and experimental details are given elsewhere (23), but it is important to note that the experimental temperature was 37°C, and the stimulation rate was 60 beats per minute.

Aequorin Light Measurements

During the equilibration period, the atrial or ventricular preparation was kept at l_{max}, the optimal muscle length at which maximum systolic force is developed. The experimental temperature was 37°C, and the preparation was stimulated at 60 beats per minute. Then, the electrical stimulus was switched off and the calcium-regulated bioluminescent photoprotein aequorin was macroinjected into the resting muscle (26). The aequorin light signal was detected by a photomultiplier tube (XP 2803, Philipps, Hamburg, Germany). To optimize the efficiency of the system, an ellipsoidal mirror was used to reflect photons to the phototube (Scientific Instruments, Heidelberg, Germany).

Experimental Protocol

After mechanical stabilization, angiotensin I, angiotensin II, or endothelin (Sigma-Aldrich Chemical Co., Diesenhofen, Germany) was added to the bathing solution at increasing concentrations, from 10^{-10} to 10^{-6} M (angiotensin) and from 10^{-9} to 10^{-5} M (endothelin). Additionally, the following substances were used: saralasin (10^{-5} M), propranolol (10^{-6} M), prazosin (10^{-5} M), enalaprilate (10^{-5} M), and the new angiotensin receptor antagonist ICI D 8731 (26).

Statistical Analysis

Average values are given as mean $\pm$ SEM in figures. The paired t-test was applied using the Bonferroni–Holmes procedure.

RESULTS

Angiotensin II: Mechanical Experiments

Both angiotensin I and II exert positive inotropic effects in preparations of human right atrial trabeculae (Fig. 1A). This concentration-dependent effect is maximum at 10^{-7} M angiotensin II and at 10^{-6} M angiotensin I. We have shown earlier (23) that the effect of angiotensin I can be completely blocked by preincubation in 10^{-5} M enalaprilate. In contrast, preincubation in 10^{-6} M propranolol and 10^{-5} M prazosin has no influence on the positive inotropic effects of angiotensin II, whereas saralasin—a peptide-angiotensin receptor antagonist—blocks the positive inotropic effects of angiotensin I and II (23,24).

We also tested angiotensin I and II in preparations of human left ventricles with a variety of diseases (idiopathic dilated cardiomyopathy, mitral valve stenosis, mitral valve incompetence) and in donor hearts (23,24). In none of these preparations was any increase in peak developed force observed (Fig. 1B). Because it is known that the number of angiotensin II receptors is greater in the myocardium from infants, we also studied right ventricular preparations obtained from infants suffering from tetralogy of Fallot. Again, no positive inotropic effect could be observed in any of the ten preparations studied (Fig. 1C).

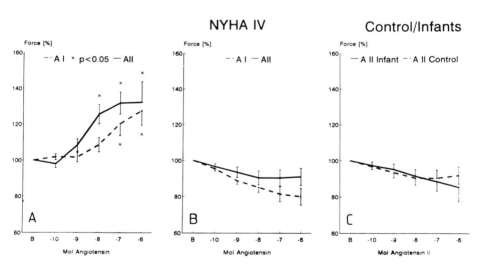

FIG. 1. Influence of angiotensin I and II on isometric peak force of human nonfailing right atrial trabeculae (**A**). By increasing the angiotensin concentrations, peak developed force is concentration dependently increased. The maximum increase in force is about 30% at 10^{-7} M angiotensin II and at 10^{-6} M angiotensin I. Influence of angiotensin II on isometric force development of human left ventricular myocardium from nonfailing (donor heart, mitral valve stenosis, mitral valve regurgitation) and from failing hearts (dilative cardiomyopathy NYHA III–IV) (**B**). Right ventricular preparations from infants suffering from tetralogy of Fallot were also exposed to angiotensin II. In none of these preparations could any positive inotropic effect be detected (**C**).

Angiotensin: Aequorin Light Measurements

To gain more insight into molecular mechanisms by which the positive inotropic effect of angiotensin is brought about in human atrial tissue, aequorin experiments were performed. As can be seen from Fig. 2, there is a parallel increase in the aequorin light signal and the peak developed force, both of which are angiotensin concentration–dependent. This information indicates that angiotensin II increases force development by increasing the number of activated crossbridges, a mechanism that is very similar to an experimental increase in extracellular calcium concentration (26,27). Figure 2 also indicates that the selective angiotensin II–receptor

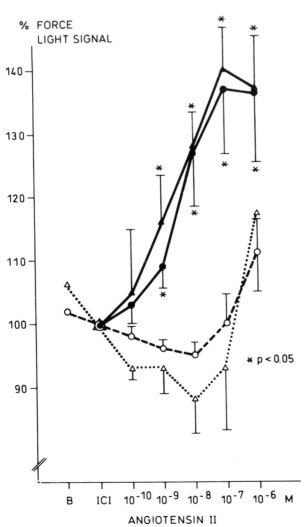

FIG. 2. Dose-response curves for angiotensin II in human atrial preparations: Peak developed force as well as calcium transients (peak aequorin light signals) are illustrated. When preparations were pretreated by ICI D-8731 (10^{-6} M), the effects of angiotensin II on both light signal and peak developed force are blocked.

antagonist ICI D 8731 (10^{-6} M) completely blocks the effect of angiotensin on both the calcium transient and force development.

DISCUSSION

Positive Inotropic Effects of Angiotensin

Reports in the literature have shown that the positive inotropic response of the mammalian myocardium to angiotensin depends on the chosen species on the one hand and on the used experimental conditions on the other. Consistent positive inotropic effects are demonstrated in hamster (22,23), cat (16), and rabbit (18,28) myocardium, whereas no positive inotropic effect could be observed in guinea pig (29), dog (19), and ferret (28) myocardium. Even negative inotropic effects were reported in cultured neonatal rat cardiomyocytes (30). On the other hand, the quantity of the positive inotropic response of a preparation to angiotensin is considerably dependent on temperature, stimulation rate, and calcium concentration (31). We therefore attempted to simulate physiological conditions in our experiments with isolated human cardiac tissue by (a) setting the experimental temperature to 37°C, (b) choosing a stimulation rate of 60 beats per minute, and (c) using a calcium concentration of 2.5 mM.

When using this approach, a very consistent positive inotropic effect of angiotensin was observed in atrial preparations (Fig. 1A). On the average, the increase in peak developed force was $33\% \pm 6\%$. In contrast, no effect was measured in human left ventricular myocardium, neither in preparations from human hearts without left ventricular dysfunction (donor hearts, mitral valve stenosis) nor in those from hearts with left ventricular dysfunction (mitral valve incompetence, idiopathic dilated cardiomyopathy). Even in preparations from right ventricles of infants, no response of the myocardium to angiotensin was elicited (Figs. 1B,C) (23).

The fact that angiotensin has no effect on myocardial mechanical function in right and left ventricular myocardium can be interpreted in three different ways: (a) Angiotensin II receptors may be absent in human ventricular myocardium. (b) Angiotensin II receptor subtype modulation may be responsible for uneffectivness of angiotensin II in ventricular human myocardium. (c) Signal transduction within the cell may be different between atrial and ventricular human myocardium. Currently, we favor the third hypothesis for a variety of reasons: The existence of angiotensin II receptors have clearly been demonstrated in human failing and nonfailing myocardium (32). Although the angiotensin-receptor subtype populations may be different between atrial and ventricular human myocardium, a complete switch from effective receptor subtypes in atrial tissue to uneffective receptor subtypes in left ventricular myocardium is unlikely (33). Therefore, differences in signal transduction between atrial and ventricular myocardium in men have to be discussed (see later).

Positive Inotropic Effects of Endothelin

Endothelin exerts significant positive inotropic effects in right atrial preparations from nonfailing human hearts (35) as well as in left ventricular preparations from failing human hearts (36). This finding is consistent with several animal studies. Positive inotropic responses to endothelin have been reported in isolated rat cardiomyocytes (20,21) and in papillary muscle preparations of rat, guinea pig, and rabbit (28). Although we have not yet studied the existence of endothelin receptor subtypes by using specific antagonists, it is very likely that the positive inotropic effect is mediated by the ET_A-subtype receptor (28).

Signal Transduction Mechanisms

In right atrial human myocardium, we have shown that angiotensin II and endothelin increase peak developed force in association with a similar increase in the calcium transient (26,27,35). Both substances have been shown to increase intracellular inositol (1,4,5)-triphosphate ($InsP_3$), which in turn binds to intracellular $InsP_3$ receptors (34) and facilitates calcium release, probably from the sarcoplasmic reticulum (Fig. 3). The situation is totally different in left ventricular human myocardium: (a) Angiotensin II has neither positive inotropic effects in adult human left ventricular myocardium nor in infant right ventricular myocardium. (b) Endothelin exerts a positive inotropic effect in left ventricular human myocardium. We have currently demonstrated, however, that this increase in contractile force is not associated with any significant change in the calcium transient (36). Therefore, the positive inotropic effect of endothelin is calcium-independent, and a different mechanism of positive inotropy of endothelin has to be postulated. The most likely

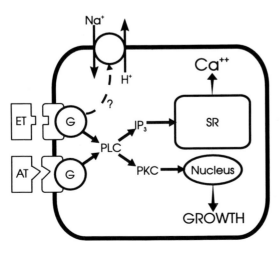

FIG. 3. Schematic illustration of angiotensin and endothelin receptors, signal transduction, and second messengers. The hypothesis is that the sarcoplasmic reticulum of human atrial myocardium exhibits IP3 receptors, allowing calcium release, whereas that of ventricular human myocardium does not (see text). AT, angiotensin II; ET, endothelin; PLC, phospholipase C; G, G protein; IP3, inositol (1,4,5)-triphosphate; PKC, proteine kinase C; SR, sarcoplasmatic reticulum; Na^+-H^+, sodium–hydrogen exchanger.

explanation for the different functional responses between atrial and ventricular myocardium in men would be that $InsP_3$ receptors exist only in the sarcoplasmic reticulum of atria but are absent in that of ventricular human myocardium (Fig. 3). This hypothesis is supported by the fact that the distribution of $InsP_3$ and ryanodine receptors, which both regulate intracellular calcium release from the sarcoplasmic reticulum, vary considerably between different cells. Some cells have either ryanodine-sensitive stores exclusively like skeletal muscle or $InsP_3$-sensitive stores like oocytes, whereas others contain both types of receptors (vascular smooth muscle, neurons) (34). It might well be that the sarcoplasmic reticulum of atrial muscle has both $InsP_3$ receptors and ryanodine receptors, whereas that of ventricular myocardium processes only ryanodine receptors. This hypothesis would easily explain why angiotensin II has no effect on isometric contractile force and endothelin has no effect on intracellular calcium transients. Furthermore, this hypothesis would be consistent with the observation that both angiotensin II and endothelin can induce cardiac hypertrophy in isolated cardiomyocytes via activation of protein kinase C (see Fig. 3) (13–15). Further studies are necessary to prove this concept for adult human ventricular myocardium.

How is the positive inotropic effect of endothelin in human left ventricular myocardium brought about? The answer comes from a study of Krämer et al. (21). These authors were able to demonstrate that endothelin increases contractility in isolated rat myocytes by activation of the sodium–hydrogen exchanger (21). Such an activation may increase intracellular pH and thereby lead to a leftward shift of the force-pCa curve of the contractile proteins. Then, at a given calcium concentration, more force is developed by the contractile machinery (37,38). This mechanism of action, however, has not yet been proven for human left ventricular myocardium (Fig. 3). It is also unclear which molecular coupling may exist between the endothelin receptor system and the sodium–hydrogen exchanger (Fig. 3).

Clinical Aspects

Angiotensin and endothelin play an important role in the genesis and progression of congestive heart failure syndrome. The use of angiotensin-converting enzyme (ACE) inhibitor has been clearly demonstrated to be of benefit for patients with heart failure symptoms as well as those with left ventricular dysfunction. The fact that angiotensin II exerts significant positive inotropic effects in atrial but not in ventricular human myocardium is of clinical importance for two reasons: (a) Even though the renin–angiotensin system may be maximally activated in patients with heart failure, ACE inhibitors will not exert negative inotropic effects on the left ventricle as known, for example, with β-blocker therapy. (b) The negative inotropic effect of ACE inhibition in atrial muscle may positively contribute to a reduction of left ventricular end-diastolic pressure and thereby to the prevention of progressive left ventricular dilatation (24).

Because of the beneficial effects of a therapeutic blockade of the renin–angiotensin system, one might speculate that endothelin-receptor antagonists may also be useful in the treatment of heart failure for three different reasons: (a) The vaso-contrictive effect of endothelin might be abolished. (b) The positive inotropic effect in the atrial cardiac muscle of endothelin may be blocked, thereby decreasing left ventricular filling pressure as postulated for ACE inhibitors (discussed earlier). (c) Because endothelin seems to have the same influence on cardiac growth (15) and left ventricular dilatation as angiotensin (13,14), progression of left ventricular dys-function may be stopped or slowed. By blocking the positive inotropic effect of endothelin in human left ventricular myocardium, however, cardiac contractility may be reduced in a situation where inotropic support of the heart is necessary. Therefore, when using endothelin antagonists in patients with severe heart failure, potential negative inotropic effects have been taken into consideration. Further-more, it is necessary to study the interaction between angiotensin and endothelin because one polypeptide might be able to trigger release of the other from en-dothelium or myocytes and—because of common signal transduction pathways (see Fig. 3)—their simultaneous actions may potentiate their effects in an unex-pected way.

SUMMARY

Both polypeptides angiotensin and endothelin play important roles in a variety of cardiovascular disorders, including arterial hypertension, cardiac hypertrophy, and congestive heart failure. Little has been known, however, about the functional ef-fects of both polypeptides in human failing and nonfailing myocardium. We there-fore studied the mechanical effects of angiotensin I and II and endothelin in a large number of isolated human cardiac tissues contracting under physiological condi-tions (37°C, 60 beats/minute). Whereas angiotensin I and II exhibited positive ino-tropic effects in human atrial preparations, no effects could be found in human right and left venrticular preparations from failing and nonfailing hearts. In contrast, endothelin increased peak-developed tension both in atrial and left ventricular hu-man preparations. These differential effects of angiotensin and endothelin are ex-plained on the basis of different signal transduction pathways, for endothelin and angiotensin on the one hand and between atrial and ventricular human myocardium on the other.

ACKNOWLEDGMENT

This work was supported by the Deutsche Forschungsgemeinschaft (HO 915/4-1 and HA 1233/3-1).

REFERENCES

1. Francis GS, Benedict C, Johnsstone DE, et al. Comparison of neuro-endocrine activation in patients with left ventricular dysfunction with or without heart failure. *Circulation* 1990;82:1724–1729.

2. Swedberg K, Eneroth P, Kjekshus J, Snapinn S. Effects of enalapril and neuroendocrine activation on prognosis in severe congestive heart failure. *Am J Cardiol* 1990;66:40D–45D.
3. Margulies KB, Hildebrand FL, Lerman A, Perrella M, Burnett JC. Increased endothelin in experimental heart failure. *Circulation* 1990;82:2226–2230.
4. Cody RJ, Haas GJ, Binkley PF, Capers Q, Kelley R. Plasma endothelin correlates with the extent of pulmonary hypertension in patients with chronic congestive heart failure. *Circulation* 1992;85:504–509.
5. Lerman A, Kubo SH, Tschumperlin LK, Burnett JC. Plasma endothelin concentrations in humans with end-stage heart failure and after heart transplantation. *J Am Coll Cardiol* 1992;20:849–853.
6. McMurray JJ, Ray SG, Abdullah I, Dargie HJ, Morton JJ. Plasma endothelin in chronic heart failure. *Circulation* 1992;85:1374–1379.
7. Wei C-M, Lerman A, Rodeheffer RJ, et al. Endothelin in human congestive heart failure. *Circulation* 1994,89:1580–1586.
8. Lindpaintner K, Ganten D. The cardiac renin-angiotensin system: an appraisal of present experimental and clinical evidence. *Circ Res* 1991;68:905–921.
9. Hill WHP, Andrus EC. The cardiac factor in the "pressor" effects of renin and angiotensin. *J Exp Med* 1941;74:91–103.
10. Yanagisawa M, Kurihara H, Kimura S, et al. A novel potent vasoconstrictor peptide produced by vascular endothelial cells. *Nature* 1988;332:411–415.
11. Miller WL, Redfield MM, Burnett JC. Integrated cardiac, renal, and endocrine actions of endothelin. *J Clin Invest* 1989;83:317–320.
12. Lerman A, Hildebrand FL, Aarkus LL, Burnett JC. Endothelin has biological actions at pathophysiological concentrations. *Circulation* 1991;83:1808–1814.
13. Sadoshima J, Izumo S. Molecular characterization of angiotensin II–induced hypertrophy of cardiac myocytes and hyperplasia of cardiac fibroblasts: critical role of the AT_1-receptor subtype. *Circ Res* 1993;73:413–423.
14. Sadoshima J, Izumo S. Signal transduction pathways of angiotensin II–induced C-fos gene expression in cardiac myocytes in vivo. *Circ Res* 1993;73:424–438.
15. Ito H, Hirata Y, Hiroe M, et al. Endothelin-1 induces hypertrophy with enhanced expression of muscle-specific genes in cultured neonatal rat cardiomyocytes. *Circ Res* 1991;69:209–215.
16. Koch-Weser J. Myocardial action of angiotensin. *Circ Res* 1964,14:337–343.
17. Dempsey PJ, McCallum ZT, Kent KM, Cooper T. Direct myocardial effects of angiotensin II. *Am J Physiol* 1971;220:477–481.
18. Bonnardeaux JL, Park WK, Regoli D. Effects of angiotensin and catecholamines on the transmembrane potential and isometric force of rabbit isolated atria. *Arch Int Pharmacodyn Ther* 1977;229:83–94.
19. Kobaiashi M, Furukawa Y, Chiba S. Positive chronotropic and inotropic effects of angiotensin II in the dog heart. *Eur J Pharmacol* 1978;501:17–25.
20. Kelly RA, Eid H, Krüger BK, et al. Endothelin enhances the contractile responsiveness of adult rat ventricular myocytes to calcium by a pertussis toxin-sensitive pathway. *J Clin Invest* 1990;86: 1164–1171.
21. Krämer BK, Smith TW, Kelly RA. Endothelin and increased contractility in adult rat ventricular myocytes. *Circ Res* 1991;68:269–279.
22. Moravec CS, Schlüchter MD, Paranandi L, et al. Inotropic effects of angiotensin II on human cardiac muscle in vivo. *Circulation* 1990;82:P1973–P1984.
23. Holubarsch Ch, Hasenfuss G, Schmidt-Schweda S, et al. Angiotensin I and II exert inotropic effects in atrial but not in ventricular human myocardium. *Circulation* 1993;88:1228–1237.
24. Holubarsch Ch, Schmidt-Schweda S, Knorr A, et al. Functional significance of angiotensin receptors in human myocardium. *Eur Heart J* 1994;15[Suppl D]:88–91.
25. Mulieri LA, Hasenfuss G, Ittleman F, Blanchard EM, Alpert NR. Protection of human left ventricular myocardium from cutting injury with 2,3-butanedione monoxime. *Circ Res* 1989;65:1441–1444.
26. Pieske B, Holubarsch Ch, Schmidt-Schweda S, Kretschmann B, Schranz D, Hasenfuss G. Inotropic effects of angiotensin I and II in human auricular and ventricular myocardium. *Circulation* 1992; 86[Suppl I]:3052.
27. Pieske B, Kretschmann B, Schmidt-Schweda S, et al. Influence of angiotensin II on force of contraction and intracellular Ca^{2+} transients in human atrial myocardium. *J Heart Failure* 1993;1 [Suppl]:75.
28. Endo M. Cardiac endothelin and angiotensin receptors and signal transduction. Report on occasion of the Japanese-German Joint Seminar on Physiologic and Pathophysiologic Regulation on Cardio-

vascular Receptors, Ion Channels and Intracellular Signal Transduction. Osaka, Japan, October 1994.

29. Baker KM, Singer JA. Identification and characterization of guinea pig angiotensin II ventricular and atrial receptors: coupling to inositol phosphate production. *Circ Res* 1988;62:896–904.
30. Allen IS, Cohen NM, Dhallan RS, Gaa ST, Lederer WJ, Rogers TB. Angiotensin II increases spontaneous contractile frequency and stimulates calcium current in cultured neonatal rat heart myocytes: insights into the underlying biochemical mechanisms. *Circ Res* 1988;62:524–534.
31. Koch-Weser J. Nature of the inotropic action of angiotensin on ventricular myocardium. *Circ Res* 1965;16:230–237.
32. Urata H, Healy B, Steward RW, Bumpus FM, Husain A. Angiotensin II receptors in normal and failing human hearts. *J Clin Endocrinol Metab* 1989;69:54–66.
33. Regitz-Zagrasek V, Auch-Schwelck W, Neuss M, Fleck E. Regulation of the angiotensin receptor subtypes in cell cultures, animal models and human diseases. *Eur Heart J* 1994;15[Suppl D]:92–97.
34. Berridge MJ. Inositol triphosphate and calcium signalling. *Nature* 1993;361:315–325.
35. Meyer M, Lehnart S, Holubarsch Ch, Hasenfuss G, Just H. Wirkmechanismen von Endothelin-1 am menschlichen Vorhofmyokard. *German J Cardiol* 1994;83[Suppl I]:494.
36. Pieske B, Kretschmann B, Burmeister Ch, et al. Influence of isoproterenol and endothelin on intracellular Ca^{2+}-transients and isometric force in isolated human ventricular myocardium. *Circulation* 1993;88[Suppl]:3065.
37. Allen DG, Orchard CH. The effects of changes of pH on intracellular calcium transients in mammalian cardiac muscle. *J Physiol* 1983;335:555–567.
38. Solaro RJ, Lee JA, Kentish JC, Allen DG. Effects of acidosis on ventricular muscle from adult and neonatal rats. *Circ Res* 1988;63:779–787.

The Failing Heart, edited by N. S. Dhalla,
R. E. Beamish, N. Takeda, and M. Nagano.
Lippincott-Raven Publishers, Philadelphia © 1995.

25

Renin–Angiotensin System and Volume Overload–Induced Cardiac Remodeling

Marcel Ruzicka and Frans H.H. Leenen

Hypertension Unit, University of Ottawa Heart Institute,
Ottawa, Ontario, K1Y 4E9 Canada

Cardiac hypertrophy induced by cardiac volume or pressure overload has for a long time been considered a physiological adaptation to increase in cardiac load. It also represents, however, a major independent risk factor for cardiovascular morbidity and mortality. Morphological and functional changes associated with pressure or volume overload–induced cardiac hypertrophic growth increase risk for fatal arrhythmias, myocardial ischemia, and heart failure. Besides hemodynamic stimuli, humoral factors, in particular the renin–angiotensin system, have recently been implicated as either direct cardiac trophic stimuli or as factors mediating the hypertrophic response of the heart to cardiac pressure or volume load. In this chapter, we deal with methodological aspects of cardiac volume overload in rats, associated changes in hemodynamics and renin–angiotensin system, and their relevance for cardiac remodeling and progression into heart failure.

MODELS OF VOLUME OVERLOAD–INDUCED CARDIAC HYPERTROPHY IN RATS

To address the pathophysiological mechanisms of volume overload–induced cardiac remodeling, several experimental models of cardiac volume overload have been established. Besides surgical techniques used to produce cardiac volume overload, iron- and/or copper-deficient diet-induced anemia, as well as arterial vasodilators (such as minoxidil or hydralazine), cause cardiac volume overload. We will discuss several methodological aspects, in particular the predictability of the level of cardiac volume overload and the extent of hypertrophic response, and problems/difficulties related to the induction of volume overload, which determine the suitability of different models of cardiac volume overload for studies on mechanisms of development and maintenance of cardiac hypertrophy.

Surgical Models of Cardiac Volume Overload–Induced Cardiac Hypertrophy

Cardiac Volume Overload by an Aortocaval Shunt

The microsurgical technique described by Flaim et al. (1) and Stumpe et al. (2) was used until recently to produce an aortocaval shunt in rats. Briefly, after a midline incision in the abdominal wall, the abdominal aorta and vena cava are exposed and isolated for a distance of about 20 mm. Under a dissecting microscope, a segment of aorta and vena cava is isolated by placement of two bulldog clamps across the main vessels below the left renal artery and above the aortic bifurcation. Openings of approximately equal size (about 1–1.5 mm) are made through the medial walls at the midpoint of the isolated segments of aorta and vena cava. The opposing edges of the two openings are attached using microsurgical sutures. Clamps are then removed and the patency of the shunt is confirmed visually by the presence of mixing arterial blood in the vena cava (1). Alternatively, an end-to-side anastomosis is produced between the distal end of the left iliolumbar vein and the side of the aorta (3). This approach leaves the opportunity to easily close the shunt by a single ligature around the iliolumbar vein. These surgical procedures (including closing of abdominal incision) take about 40 minutes to complete. It is obvious that these techniques are demanding and require personnel trained in microvascular surgery. Because the size of the incision can only approximately be determined, the size of the shunt varies substantially from rat to rat, as reflected in the large variability in shunt flow (1), cardiac output (3), and heart weight (3,4). The poor control over the size of the shunt during surgery results in a large fistula in some rats and contributes to a high mortality rate from acute heart failure during the first 24 hours after shunt surgery. For example, Flaim et al. (1) reported a long-term survival rate (2 months) of only 23% with acute heart failure within 24 hours after surgery as causing the majority of deaths. Similarly, Liu et al. (3) reported a survival rate of 47%, with the majority of deaths due to heart failure within 24 hours after the shunt. In addition to death from acute heart failure, abdominal bleeding may contribute to high surgical mortality rate.

Overall, the poor control over the size of the fistula and the high surgical mortality rate make this labor-intensive technique less suitable for the induction of aortocaval shunt as a model of cardiac volume overload as compared with the recently described "needle technique."

Recently, Garcia and Diebold (5) introduced a simple, rapid, and effective method of producing an aortocaval shunt in rats. Briefly, in anesthetized rats, the vena cava and abdominal aorta are exposed by opening the abdominal cavity via a midline incision. The aorta is then clamped below the left renal artery and subsequently punctured with a disposable needle caudal two-thirds of the distance between the left renal artery and the aortic bifurcation. The needle is advanced into the aorta, perforating the adjacent wall and penetrating the vena cava. The needle is then removed and the aorta puncture-point is sealed by a drop of cyanoacrylate glue. This surgical procedure does not require microsurgical equipment. In our hands

(6,7), the procedure is substantially faster (the whole procedure, including closing of abdominal cavity, takes about 20 minutes) than the microsurgical techniques described previously and has minimal surgical mortality (less than 5%). Last, but not least, there is an excellent control over the size of the shunt, which is determined by the external diameter of the needle used to puncture the aorta and vena cava. Depending on the gauge of the needle used, the size of the shunt and, in turn, the degree of volume overload–induced cardiac hypertrophy can be modified from small to fairly large (Fig. 1).

Opening of an aortocaval shunt results in hypertrophy of both right ventricle (RV) and left ventricle (LV). Most of the hypertrophic response to cardiac volume overload by aortocaval shunt occurs within 4 to 5 weeks after surgery (Fig. 1). For example, aortocaval shunt by an 18-gauge needle increases LV weight by about 24% and 45% at 1 and 4 weeks after surgery, respectively, with only minimal further changes at 10 weeks (6,7). Right ventricular weight increased by about 40% and 78% at the same time points, respectively, with no further increase at 10 weeks (6,7). Similar results were reported by others (4,8,9). For example, Hatt et al. (8) reported an increase in heart weight by about 42% 1 month after aortocaval shunt with no further increase at up to 6 months of follow-up. The more marked hypertrophic response of the RV versus LV (6,7,9,10) to the aortocaval shunt may be related to substantially more (diastolic wall) stress per cardiomyocyte in RV versus LV because of the smaller number of cardiomyocytes and thinner wall of the RV (11,12). Alternatively, differences in hemodynamics in LV and RV after the shunt (see discussion that follows) may explain the more pronounced RV hypertrophy.

Left ventricular eccentric hypertrophy with a more pronounced increase in LV internal diameter as compared to LV wall thickness develops in response to aor-

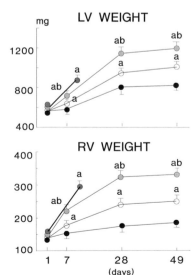

FIG. 1. Time course of increases in left ventricular (LV) and right ventricular (RV) weights in response to different size of the aortocaval shunt. Values are mean ± SEM (n = 6–10/group/time point). a, $p < 0.05$ vs. control; b, $p < 0.05$ vs. aortocaval shunt by 21-gauge needle; ●, control; ○, aortocaval shunt by 21-gauge needle; ◙, aortocaval shunt by 18-gauge needle; ◐, aortocaval shunt by 16-gauge needle. Part of the data is derived from Ruzicka et al. (6,7), with permission of the American Heart Association.

LV INTERNAL DIAMETER

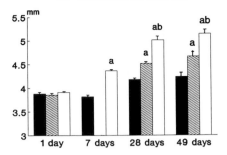

LV WALL THICKNESS

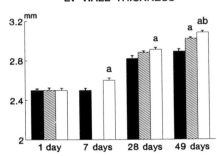

FIG. 2. Time course of changes in left ventricular (LV) internal diameter and LV wall thickness in response to different size of the aortocaval shunt. Bars represent mean ± SEM (n = 6–10/group/time point). a, p <0.05 vs. control; b, p <0.05 vs. aortocaval shunt by 21-gauge needle; ■, control; ▨, aortocaval shunt by 21-gauge needle; □, aortocaval shunt by 18-gauge needle. Data from Ruzicka et al. (6), with permission of the American Heart Association.

tocaval shunt (Fig. 2). For example, aortocaval shunt by an 18-gauge needle increases LV internal diameter by about 20% at 4 weeks after surgery, while LV wall thickness increases by only 3% (6) (Fig. 2). Again, only minimal further changes in LV geometry were observed at 10 weeks after aortocaval shunt (7). Whether the age of animals used to open an aortocaval shunt affects the extent of the hypertrophic response of the heart (as it does in volume-overload aortic insufficiency; see next section) has not yet been assessed.

In conclusion, the model of volume overload–induced cardiac hypertrophy by aortocaval shunt induced by the "needle technique" (5) is clearly suitable (based on high reproducibility, easy-to-modulate extent of volume overload, and low surgical mortality) for studies on mechanisms in development and maintenance of cardiac hypertrophy.

Cardiac Volume Overload by Aortic Insufficiency

Uematsu et al. (13) described a simple method for producing graded aortic insufficiency in rats and subsequent development of volume overload–induced cardiac hypertrophy. In anesthetized animals, the peripheral portion of the right common carotid artery is ligated and a slightly curved polyethylene rod (0.8 mm outside diameter) is inserted retrogradely into the artery. The visible curvature of the rod is used as a guide as the rod is moved forward to touch the right cusp of the aortic valve. The rod is further forwarded to perforate the cusp and then is slightly moved backward and rotated by about 120°, and the left valve cusp is perforated in the same way. The perforation of each of the valve cusps can be verified by the stepwise increase in pulse pressure (13). Uematsu et al. (13) reported a stepwise increase in right common carotid artery pulse pressure by 47% and 87% after perforation of the right and both right and left cusps of the aortic valve. The disruption of only the right cusp of the aortic valve increased heart weight by about 20% and 35% as compared with control rats at 2 and 4 weeks after surgery (13). An increase in (combined LV and RV) cardiac weight by 47% and 68% was reported in rats with aortic insufficiency due to the disruption of both cusps of the aortic valve at the same time points (13). Regarding changes in LV versus RV weights, at 2 months after disrupting both cusps of the aortic valve, LV weight had increased by 43% and RV weight by about 60% (14). Similar results were reported by Isoyama et al. (15). In contrast, at 28 days after disruption of both cusps of the aortic valve, Roberston et al. (16) reported an increase in LV weight by about 40%, but only a minimal increase in RV weight. In this model, the development of RV hypertrophy likely reflects a failing LV and the transmission of high LV filling pressure into the RV. Minimal changes in RV weight in the latter study (16) may therefore suggest less aortic insufficiency (and less increase in LV end-diastolic pressure [LVEDP]), as compared with previously mentioned studies (14,15). Data on LVEDP or pulse pressure, however, were not reported by Robertson et al. (16).

Isoyama et al. (15) showed that the age of the animals at the time of induction of aortic insufficiency affects the degree of cardiac hypertrophy. A similar degree of aortic insufficiency (as assessed from the similar increase in LVEDP) increased LV weight by about 42% at 4 weeks in adult (9-months-old) rats with aortic insufficiency, but by only 22% in old (18- to 22-months-old) rats ($p < 0.05$). In contrast, RV weight showed a more pronounced increase ($p < 0.05$) in old (52%) as compared with young (39%) rats. This difference may relate to the development of more marked LV failure in old rats as compared with young rats (see next section).

Altogether, this method does not require expensive technical equipment, it gives the possibility to induce graded volume overload, and it has virtually no mortality related to the surgical procedure (13). At present it is difficult to assess its reproducibility, because there are only a few studies showing data on both cardiac hemodynamics and morphology.

Anemia-induced Cardiac Volume Overload

An iron- and copper-deficient diet in young growing rats causes anemia and consequently cardiac volume overload. For example, Olivetti et al. (12) reported the effects of a standard diet with 240 mg of iron/kg and 35 mg of copper/kg and an iron- and copper-deficient diet (10 mg of iron/kg and 2 mg of copper/kg) for

7 weeks. The iron- and copper-deficient diet significantly decreased hemoglobin concentration (51 ± 10 g/l vs. 127 ± 6 g/l), and hematocrit (18 ± 3 vs. 41 ± 3) and caused somewhat lower body weight (by about 10%). Cardiac hypertrophy developed in the anemic rats; LV and RV weight increased by 49% and 70%, respectively, as compared with the rats on a standard diet. Dilation of both RV and LV in response to anemia (as assessed from the increase in ventricular wall area) was substantially more pronounced than the increases in RV and LV wall thickness. Diets deficient in only copper or iron cause similar results (17,18). For example, rats (initial body weight 50 to 60 g) on a copper-deficient diet (0.2 mg of copper/kg) for 7 weeks developed anemia (as assessed from the decrease in hematocrit, 24 ± 3 vs. 44 ± 1, and hemoglobin, 69 ± 18 g/l vs. 125 ± 8 g/l, compared with age-matched control rats on a standard diet) and cardiac hypertrophy (increase in LV weight by about 58% after 7 weeks [17]). Similarly, in rats (3 weeks old) given an iron-deficient diet for 4 weeks hematocrit decreased (17 vs. 45) and cardiac weight increased by about 55% (18). Anemia represents an easy-to-reproduce model of volume overload–induced cardiac hypertrophy with virtually no mortality related to the experimental procedure. Surprisingly, there are no reports on graded anemia and its effect on the heart (in particular, the threshold of anemia causing cardiac effects). Similarly, the effect of reversal of anemia on anemia-induced cardiac changes has not yet been evaluated. In contrast to the surgical models of volume overload–induced cardiac hypertrophy with a rapid increase in cardiac volume load and fast development of cardiac hypertrophy (mostly during the first week after surgery), anemia and the cardiac hypertrophy develop gradually over a period of weeks (19,20).

The possible effect of age on the cardiac hypertrophic response to anemia has not yet been properly addressed. Neffgen and Korecky (19) reported similar increases in heart weight (by about 60%) in young (weaning period) and young adult (10 weeks) rats for a period of 4 to 10 weeks on an iron-deficient diet, resulting in a decrease in hemoglobin from about 110 g/l to about 40 g/l. However, whether the cardiac hypertrophic response to anemia-induced volume overload is blunted in old rats (of similar age, as employed by Isoyama et al. [15], about 18 months old) remains to be assessed.

Pharmacologically Induced Cardiac Volume Overload

When different antihypertensive drugs were assessed for their potential to regress LV hypertrophy for a given decrease in blood pressure, arterial vasodilators were found to actually potentiate LV hypertrophy (21). In addition, minoxidil and hydralazine change the geometry of pressure overload–induced concentric LV hypertrophy into an eccentric one, and also cause RV hypertrophy (21,22). These results indicate that cardiac volume overload by arterial vasodilators maintains/aggravates LV hypertrophy despite decreased blood pressure. Indeed, both hydralazine and minoxidil cause an increase in cardiac volume load and in cardiac weight in normotensive rats (23–28). Consistent with previous studies from this lab (23,24,27), and with data reported by others (25), we repeatedly found (7,28) a gradual increase in LV (by about 20%) and RV (by about 40%) over a period of 5 weeks in normotensive rats on minoxidil treatment (120 mg/l in drinking water [Fig. 3]) with no further changes at 10 weeks of treatment. The more pronounced RV hypertrophy than LV hypertrophy in this model may be explained by more diastolic wall stress per cardiomyocyte in RV (at a given level of volume overload because of fewer cardiomyocytes in RV [11,12]) or may point to a combination of both diastolic wall stress and systolic wall stress (possibly as the result of pulmonary hypertension by minoxidil [26]). Similarly, as in other models of volume overload, LV eccentric hypertrophy develops, associated with an increase in LV internal diameter (by about 11% at 5 weeks) and only minimal (n.s.) changes in LV wall thickness. This is the only model in which the time course of spontaneous regression of changes after withdrawal of minoxidil has been evaluated (7). As shown in Fig. 3, minoxidil-induced cardiac hypertrophy nearly completely disappears within 2 to 5 weeks after discontinuation of minoxidil.

In summary, minoxidil-induced cardiac hypertrophy is easy to produce; the time course of development as well as the degree of RV and LV hypertrophy is consistent. In addition, this model has virtually no mortality. Thus, minoxidil-induced

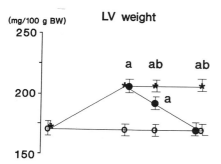

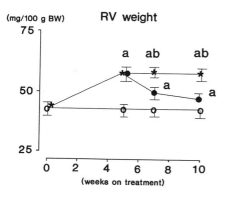

FIG. 3. Changes in left ventricular (LV) and right ventricular (RV) weight during administration of minoxidil and in response to its discontinuation after 5 weeks of treatment. Values are mean ± SEM (n = 6–8/group/time point). a, p <0.05 vs. control; b, p <0.05 vs. discontinued minoxidil; ○, control; *, continuous minoxidil treatment; ●, minoxidil discontinued at 5 weeks. From Ruzicka et al. (7), with permission of the American Heart Association.

cardiac hypertrophy clearly represents an experimental model suitable for studies on prevention/regression of volume overload–induced cardiac hypertrophy.

CHANGES IN CARDIAC HEMODYNAMICS BY DIFFERENT MODELS OF CARDIAC VOLUME OVERLOAD

Cardiac Volume Overload by an Aortocaval Shunt

Opening of an aortocaval shunt results in a rapid increase in cardiac volume load (as assessed from the increase in end-diastolic pressure in RV and LV). Both LV and RV end-diastolic pressures peak shortly after opening of an aortocaval shunt (3,6,29). As mentioned earlier, the technique by Garcia and Diebold (5) allows modification of the size of the aortocaval shunt and therefore the level of cardiac volume overload. For example, one day of aortocaval shunt by a 21-, 18-, and 16-gauge needle increased LVEDP to 6.3 ± 0.5, 10.5 ± 0.6, and 14.7 ± 0.8 mmHg, respectively, as compared with 1.4 ± 0.3 mmHg in sham-operated rats (Fig. 4). Thereafter, LVEDP gradually (over a period of 4–5 weeks) decreases, likely as the result of the increase in chamber size, and then remains relatively stable (Fig. 4) (3,4,6,7,10). For example, in rats with shunt by 21- and 18-gauge needles, LVEDP decreased from (aforementioned) peak values to 4.0 ± 0.5 and 6.8 ± 0.5 mmHg, respectively, after 4 weeks and then remained at this level up to 10 weeks after the shunt (Fig. 4) (6,7). Stroke volume increases immediately after the shunt (29) and then further increases from 1 to 4 weeks after the surgery (3). Cardiac output increases, mainly by the increase in stroke volume (1,3,4,6,7,10), by 20% to 50% depending on the size of the needle used to create the aortocaval shunt (6,7) and does not deteriorate for up to 10 weeks after the shunt (7).

Whereas the aortocaval shunt increases the LVEDP, LV peak systolic pressure (LVPSP) and blood pressure (systolic and diastolic) decrease shortly after opening of the aortocaval shunt (3,6). Systolic and diastolic blood pressure and LVPSP gradually (over a period of 4 weeks) return toward normal in rats with small and

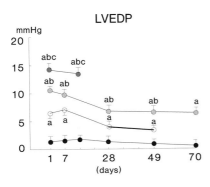

FIG. 4. Time course of changes in left ventricular end-diastolic pressure (LVEDP) in response to different sizes of the aortocaval shunt. Values are mean $\pm$ SEM (n = 6–10/group/time point). a, p <0.05 vs. control; b, p <0.05 vs. aortocaval shunt by 21-gauge needle; c, p <0.05 vs. aortocaval shunt by 18-gauge needle; ●, control; ○, aortocaval shunt by 21-gauge needle; ⊘, aortocaval shunt by 18-gauge needle; ◑, aortocaval shunt by 16-gauge needle. Part of the data is derived from Ruzicka et al. (6,7) with permission of the American Heart Association.

medium size of the shunt (3,4,6,7). In contrast, LVPSP and blood pressure may remain decreased in rats with large aortocaval fistulas (e.g., by 16-gauge needle [Ruzicka and Leenen, *unpublished observations*]). A decrease in total peripheral resistance (1,3,6) clearly contributes to this decrease in LVPSP and blood pressure. However, whereas total peripheral resistance shows only small changes from acute to chronic shunt (3,4,6,7), LVPSP and blood pressure return toward normal (3,6). The increased LVEDP and decreased LVPSP and blood pressure shortly after the shunt may point to a (temporarily) depressed LV function. Indeed, LV dP/dt$_{max}$ is depressed during the first week after the shunt (3), but returns toward normal within 4 to 5 weeks after the shunt surgery (3), and stroke volume further increases from 1 to 4 weeks after the shunt surgery (3). The increase in LVPSP and blood pressure toward normal levels in parallel with the increase in LV dP/dt$_{max}$, stroke volume, and the development of LV hypertrophy and dilation suggest that LV pumping ability after opening the aortocaval shunt initially does not compensate for the decrease in total peripheral resistance caused by the shunt.

Similarly, as in the LV, RV end-diastolic pressure increases shortly after the aortocaval shunt (3). In contrast to LV, however, RV peak systolic pressure also increases acutely (likely as the result of increased venous return with minimal change in pulmonary vascular resistance) (3,29). For example, in rats with an aortocaval shunt of 1-week duration, RV end-diastolic pressure and systolic pressure increased to 8.4 ± 0.9 and 45 ± 2 mmHg, as compared with 2.5 ± 0.5 and 34 ± 1 mmHg in sham-operated controls (3). While RV systolic pressure remained at this level for up to 5 months (4), RV end-diastolic pressure decreased (4.8 ± 0.5 mmHg at 5 months after surgery) (4).

Cardiac Volume Overload by Aortic Insufficiency

Similar to the previous model, LVEDP increases rapidly after disruption of one or two cusps of the aortic valve and then gradually decreases (14,15). For example, Isoyama et al. (15) reported an increase in LVEDP from 4.8 ± 0.6 to 12.0 ± 1.5 mmHg immediately after surgery and then a gradual decrease over a period of 4 weeks to 8.5 ± 0.9 mmHg (Fig. 5). Whereas aortic systolic pressure shows only small decreases, aortic diastolic pressure decreases significantly, resulting in a rise in pulse pressure immediately after surgery (e.g., from 29 ± 2 to 41 ± 2 mmHg with no major changes after up to 4 weeks of follow-up) (Fig. 5). Similar to the previous model, an increase in stroke volume accounts for the increase in cardiac output, because no changes in heart rate were reported (14–16,30).

Isoyama et al. (15) showed that the age of the animal used determines the time course of changes in hemodynamics (Fig. 5). As described earlier, LVEDP showed a rapid increase immediately after surgery and then a gradual decrease in adult rats (9 months; Fig. 5). In contrast, in old (18–22 months) rats, aortic insufficiency caused a similar immediate increase in LVEDP to 11.0 ± 0.7 mmHg, but LVEDP further increased to 16.9 ± 3.1 mmHg at 2 weeks, with no further major changes at

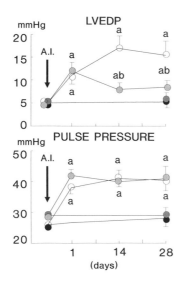

FIG. 5. Effects of age of the rats on time course of changes in left ventricular end-diastolic pressure (LVEDP) and pulse pressure after aortic insufficiency. Values are mean ± SEM (n = 8–10/group/time point). a, p <0.05 vs. control (of the same age); b, p <0.05 vs. aortic insufficiency in 18–22-month-old rats; ◔, control: 9 months old; ●, control: 18–22 months old; ⊘, aortic insufficiency: 9 months old; ○, aortic insufficiency: 18–22 months old. Data derived from Isoyama et al. (15), with permission of the American Society for Clinical Investigation, Inc.

4 weeks after surgery (Fig. 5). As described in the previous section, these old rats developed less cardiac hypertrophy, which appears not to compensate for the increased cardiac volume load resulting in persistent elevation of LVEDP (and diastolic wall stress) (15). The further increase in LVEDP may reflect deterioration in LV systolic/diastolic function.

There are no reports on changes in RV hemodynamics after aortic insufficiency in rats. Thus, one may only speculate that the development of RV hypertrophy (14,15) after experimental aortic insufficiency in rats points to increased pulmonary artery pressure caused by high LVEDP and left atrial pressure.

Cardiac Volume Overload by Minoxidil

The acute effects of minoxidil on LVEDP in rats have not yet been assessed. One may assume, however, that cardiac volume overload by minoxidil develops more gradually (presumably over a period of hours/days), as compared with surgical models. After 1 week on minoxidil, LVEDP follows a similar time course of changes as described in aforementioned models of volume overload (i.e., as LV eccentric hypertrophy develops, LVEDP decreases somewhat, and then remains stable over 5–10 weeks) (28). For example, Tsoporis et al. (23) showed an increase in LVEDP to about 7 mmHg after 1 week on minoxidil-treated rats. Left ventricular end-diastolic pressure decreases to about 4 mmHg at 5 weeks on treatment (vs. about 2 mmHg in control rats) and remains at this level for up to 10 weeks of treatment (28). Because the initial increase in LVEDP precedes the volume expansion (23), and cannot be prevented by diuretics (24), it appears that a shift of blood from the peripheral to the central compartment (26) mostly contributes to the initial (1–2 weeks) increase in LVEDP (23,24). Chronically, an increase in blood volume appears to account for the persistent increase in LVEDP (23), as suggested from the normalization of LVEDP at this stage by diuretics (24). Left ventricular peak systolic pressure shows only small (n.s.) decreases over a period of 10 weeks with minoxidil. The increase in cardiac output in minoxidil-treated rats relates to an increase in stroke volume, with no significant changes in heart rate over a period of 10 weeks (23,24,27,28).

Right ventricular pressures have not yet been assessed in rats treated with arterial vasodilators such as hydralazine or minoxidil. However, persistent increases in right atrial pressure (RAP) for up to 10 weeks on minoxidil treatment, as well as development of RV hypertrophy, point to an increase in RV pressures (23,24).

Cardiac Volume Overload by Anemia

There are no reports on changes in LVEDP, LVPSP, and RV pressures during diet-induced anemia in normotensive rats. In spontaneously hypertensive rats (SHR), anemia (a decrease in hemoglobin from 16.7 g/l to 6.9 g/l) induced by a diet deficient in iron and copper decreased LVPSP and blood pressure, increased LVEDP and heart rate, and had no effect on RV pressures (31). Spontaneously hypertensive rats, anemic for 12 weeks, showed an LVEDP of 8.6 ± 1.6 mmHg, as compared with 3.0 ± 1.4 and 4.4 ± 2.3 mmHg in Wistar Kyoto rats (WKY) and SHR of the same age but on a normal diet (31). At the same time point, heart rate was increased to about 500 beat/min as compared to about 400 beats/min in both groups on regular diets, and LVPSP was decreased to 112 ± 11 mmHg, as compared with 180 ± 17 and 130 ± 8 mmHg in control SHR and WKY (31).

CHANGES IN CIRCULATORY VERSUS CARDIAC RENIN–ANGIOTENSIN SYSTEM IN DIFFERENT MODELS OF CARDIAC VOLUME OVERLOAD

There are no reports on changes in the circulatory and cardiac renin–angiotensin system (RAS) in rats with cardiac volume overload by aortic insufficiency or by anemia. Thus, the following discussion deals with volume overload by aortocaval shunt or minoxidil treatment.

Aortocaval Shunt

Opening of the aortocaval shunt results in a rapid increase in plasma renin activity (PRA) (Fig. 6). This response is part of the initial stimulation of neurohumoral systems after aortocaval shunt and appears to be a function of the size of the aortocaval shunt and consequently the inability of the heart to keep the blood pressure

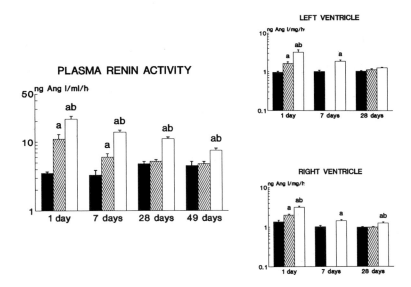

FIG. 6. Effects of aortocaval shunt on plasma and left ventricular (LV) and right ventricular (RV) renin activity. a, p <0.05 vs. control; b, p <0.05 vs. aortocaval shunt by 21-gauge needle; ■, control; ▨, aortocaval shunt by 21-gauge needle; ☐, aortocaval shunt by 18-gauge needle. Figures derived from Ruzicka et al. (6), with permission of the American Heart Association.

within normal range (6). In the long term, PRA returns toward normal in rats with a small (by 21-gauge needle) shunt, but may persist significantly increased in rats with a big shunt (Fig. 6). There are no reports on plasma angiotensinogen, angioten-sin-converting enzyme (ACE), and angiotensin (Ang) II after aortocaval shunt in rats.

In both LV and RV, renin activity increases to about 3.2 ng Ang I/mg/h (com-pared with 1.0–1.3 ng Ang I/mg/h) at 1 day after shunt surgery (Fig. 6). Renin activity then gradually decreased and was no longer different from that of sham-operated rats at 4 weeks after shunt surgery. Most of the increase in cardiac renin activity at 1 day after the shunt is plasma-derived because no increase in renin activity occurs in either ventricle when bilateral nephrectomy precedes aortocaval shunt surgery (Fig. 7). In agreement with this, there is no parallel increase in LV renin mRNA at 1 day after the shunt (32). The increase in LV and RV renin activity at 1 week after surgery (6), however, is accompanied by an increase in renin mRNA (32), which may suggest that renin of cardiac origin contributes to the increase at 7 days after surgery. Angiotensinogen has not been assessed in the heart after aor-tocaval shunt, but LV angiotensinogen mRNA does not increase at 1 and 7 days after surgery, as compared with control rats (32). Angiotensin-converting enzyme activity and ACE mRNA, as well as AT_1 and AT_2 receptors and their mRNAs, have not yet been evaluated. Similarly, the effect of aortocaval shunt on actual cardiac Ang II levels remains to be assessed.

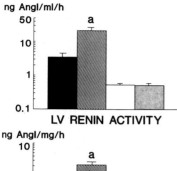

FIG. 7. Effect of bilateral nephrectomy preceding the opening of the aortocaval shunt on plasma and left ventricular (LV) renin activity at 1 day after shunt surgery. Bars are mean ± SEM (n = 6–7/group). a, *p* <0.05 vs. control; ■, control; □, bilateral nephrectomy; ▨, aortocaval shunt by 18-gauge needle; ▩, bilateral nephrectomy and aortocaval shunt by 18-gauge needle.

Minoxidil Treatment

Plasma renin activity increases within the first few days after minoxidil treatment (21,23,24) and remains significantly increased up to 10 weeks after treatment (Table 1). For example, Ruzicka and Leenen (28) showed that PRA increased to about 10 ng Ang I/ml/h at 2 weeks on minoxidil, and then remained at this level up to 10 weeks on treatment. In contrast to aortocaval shunt, the increase in LV and RV renin activity is delayed, as compared with the increase in PRA (Table 1). For example, while PRA is already increased at 2 weeks on minoxidil, LV and RV renin activity remain within control values at that time point (Table 1). Subsequently, LV

TABLE 1. *Changes in plasma and cardiac tissue renin activity during development of minoxidil-induced cardiac hypertrophy*

	2 weeks	5 weeks	10 weeks
PRA (ng Ang I/ml/h)			
Control	2.1 ± 0.1	3.4 ± 0.2	2.6 ± 0.2
Minoxidil	9.3 ± 0.6[a]	10.7 ± 0.7[a]	8.0 ± 0.5[a]
LV-renin activity (ng Ang I/mg/h)			
Control	0.99 ± 0.06	1.07 ± 0.04	1.14 ± 0.03
Minoxidil	1.04 ± 0.03	2.10 ± 0.05[a]	2.18 ± 0.09[a]
RV-renin activity (ng Ang I/mg/h)			
Control	1.01 ± 0.05	1.00 ± 0.02	1.07 ± 0.03
Minoxidil	1.03 ± 0.04	2.27 ± 0.06[a]	2.22 ± 0.05[a]

Data from Ruzicka and Leenen (28), with permission of the American Physiological Society.
Values are mean ± SEM (n = 6–7/group).
[a]*p*<0.05 vs. controls.
PRA, plasma renin activity; LV, left ventricle; RV, right ventricle.

and RV renin activity increase at 5 weeks on minoxidil and remain increased up to 10 weeks (Table 1). Based on these data, one cannot determine whether the increase in cardiac renin activity reflects an active uptake from the circulation (33) or whether renin is produced locally. Effects of chronic minoxidil treatment on other components (i.e., angiotensinogen, ACE, Ang II, AT_1 and AT_2 receptors) of the RAS and their cardiac mRNAs have not yet been evaluated.

RELEVANCE OF CHANGES IN HEMODYNAMICS AND RENIN–ANGIOTENSIN SYSTEM FOR DEVELOPMENT/MAINTENANCE OF VOLUME OVERLOAD–INDUCED CARDIAC HYPERTROPHY

An increase in ventricular diastolic wall stress (and thus an increase in stretch of cardiomyocytes) as the result of cardiac volume overload results in activation of protein synthesis in the myocyte and the rapid production of new contractile proteins (34–37). The cardiac response is aimed at compensating for the increase in hemodynamic stress, and an increase in diastolic wall stress (by cardiac volume overload) results in series sarcomere replication (35). Prolongation of each cardiac myocyte and resulting increase in chamber size ("without" LV wall thickening) reduces diastolic wall stress (and LVEDP) and permits the ventricle to pump an increased stroke volume (35). An increase in chamber radius at the end of systole, however, then results in increased systolic wall stress (35). For complete and full compensation to volume overload, the wall thickness should therefore increase as well (35).

Whereas an increase in cardiac volume load may be the primary hypertrophic stimulus, nonhemodynamic trophic factors may directly stimulate cardiomyocytes in parallel with the physical stress or may translate physical stress into growth response. For example, Sadoshima et al. (38) and Sadoshima and Izumo (39,40) showed that in vitro stretched cardiomyocytes release Ang II, which in turn stimulates cardiomyocytes' growth. This trophic effect of Ang II is likely mediated via a membrane AT_1 receptor, as suggested from the blockade of this effect by the AT_1-receptor blocker losartan (38). In vivo, cardiac volume load increases LVEDP, which determines diastolic wall stress (stress = pressure × radius/2 × thickness). If the increase in LVEDP (and wall stress) is the primary and only stimulus for the cardiac hypertrophic response, then plotting LV weight against LVEDP should show a similar relation in different models (assuming similar levels of cardiac afterload). Indeed, as expected, LVEDP and LV weight show highly significant correlations in aortocaval shunt- and minoxidil treatment–induced cardiac hypertrophy (Fig. 8) (7). Significantly more hypertrophy for a given increase in LVEDP, however, is present in the aortocaval shunt model of volume overload, as compared with the minoxidil model (Fig. 8) (7). Considering that systolic pressure and cardiac afterload appear to decrease similarly in both models, additional nonhemodynamic factor(s) may potentiate/attenuate the hypertrophic response to a different extent in the two models. In addition, if LVEDP is the only trophic stimulus in these models of

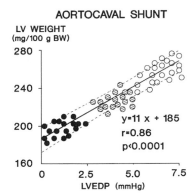

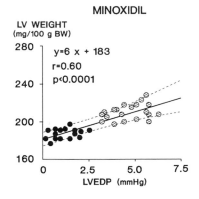

FIG. 8. Relation between left ventricular end-diastolic pressure (LVEDP) and left ventricular (LV) weight in rats with chronic aortocaval shunt or chronic minoxidil treatment. Regression line for aortocaval shunt: n = 51, combined data of control rats and rats with chronic aortocaval shunt. Broken lines represent 95% confidence interval. Regression line for minoxidil: n = 90, combined data of control rats and rats on chronic minoxidil. Broken lines represent 95% confidence interval. ●, control; ◐, aortocaval shunt by 21-gauge needle; ○, aortocaval shunt by 18-gauge needle; ⊘, minoxidil., Data derived from Ruzicka et al. (6,7,28), with permission of the American Heart Association and the American Physiological Society.

cardiac hypertrophy, one may expect prevention/regression of LV hypertrophy in proportion to the prevention in rise/decrease in LVEDP by treatment. If not, other trophic factors are involved primarily or secondarily (i.e., initiated by treatment). In the following section, we discuss the evidence for the role of the RAS as a trophic stimulus in the development and maintenance of volume overload–induced cardiac hypertrophy.

Aortocaval Shunt

As described previously, opening of an aortocaval shunt results in a rapid increase in LVEDP. The bigger the shunt, the higher the LVEDP (6). Moreover, the higher the LVEDP, the more RV and LV hypertrophy (Fig. 8). To assess whether the RAS is involved in the hypertrophic response, we employed two different types of blockers of the RAS (i.e., the ACE inhibitors, enalapril and quinapril, and the Ang II–receptor blocker, losartan). All blockers to a similar extent prevented the rise in LVEDP, but only losartan and quinapril prevented/attenuated RV hypertrophy and LV hypertrophy and LV dilation relative to their hemodynamic effects (Table 2)

TABLE 2. *Prevention of increases in left ventricular end-diastolic pressure and in left ventricular and right ventricular weights induced by an aortocaval shunt with treatment by enalapril, quinapril, and losartan*

	LVEDP (mmHg)	LV weight (mg/100 g bw)	RV weight (mg/100 g bw)
Control	1.1 ± 0.5	193 ± 3	56 ± 3
Control + enalapril	1.0 ± 0.4	179 ± 3	54 ± 3
Shunt	8.0 ± 0.8^a	250 ± 7^a	80 ± 3^a
Shunt + enalapril	$3.8 \pm 0.7^{a,b}$	243 ± 5^a	76 ± 2^a
Control	1.1 ± 0.5	193 ± 3	56 ± 3
Control + quinapril	2.0 ± 0.8	183 ± 3	54 ± 2
Shunt	8.0 ± 0.8^a	250 ± 7^a	80 ± 3^a
Shunt + quinapril	$4.0 \pm 0.5^{a,b}$	$214 \pm 6^{a,b}$	$61 \pm 2^{a,b}$
Control	0.0 ± 1.2	201 ± 2	44 ± 2
Control + losartan	-1.0 ± 0.5	185 ± 3	43 ± 2
Shunt	7.8 ± 2.0^a	245 ± 5^a	59 ± 3^a
Shunt + losartan	$2.6 \pm 1.5^{a,b}$	$205 \pm 9^{a,b}$	$50 \pm 3^{a,b}$

Data derived from Ruzicka et al. (6) and Ruzicka and Leenen (41), with permission of the American Heart Association.
Values are $\pm$ SEM (n = 6–9/group).
[a]$p < 0.05$ vs. control.
[b]$p < 0.05$ for enalapril-, quinapril-, and losartan-treated shunt vs. untreated shunt.
LV, left ventricular; RV, right ventricular; LVEDP, LV end-diastolic pressure.

(6,41). In contrast, enalapril did not even attenuate the hypertrophic response of the heart after aortocaval shunt, despite preventing the rise in LVEDP (6,41). Enalapril and quinapril similarly decreased LVEDP and similarly blocked the pressor effect of intravenous Ang I, indicating a similar degree of blockade of the circulatory ACE by the two ACE inhibitors (41–43). Their contrasting effects on prevention of cardiac hypertrophy may therefore point to different affinities for cardiac ACE between enalapril (low) and quinapril (high) (42,43). If so, these data suggest that an increase in stretch of the cardiomyocytes by LVEDP is translated into a hypertrophic response via Ang II released by stretched cardiomyocytes (38–40). At present, there are no data on the relation between the amount of stretch on the cardiomyocyte and the amount of the Ang II generated/released. One may speculate that enalapril actually increased the amount of Ang II generated in the heart for a given level of LVEDP (and stretch), possibly by (enhanced passive) uptake from increased circulatory renin and Ang I.

Minoxidil

As described, minoxidil causes cardiac volume overload, increases plasma and cardiac renin activity, and results in LV eccentric hypertrophy and RV hypertrophy. Losartan combined with minoxidil treatment only minimally affected LVEDP but prevented RV and LV hypertrophy and LV dilation (28). In contrast, enalapril prevented most of the rise in the LVEDP by minoxidil, but failed to prevent the cardiac hypertrophic response (28). Prevention of cardiac hypertrophy by losartan, despite only small effects on LVEDP, may suggest that Ang II is released by cardiomyocytes in response to stretch and mediates growth of cardiomyocytes (38–40). One cannot exclude the possibility that minoxidil per se enhanced cardiac Ang II generation, resulting in the hypertrophic response of the cardiomyocytes. Similarly, as described for the aortocaval shunt, the failure of enalapril to prevent cardiac hypertrophy despite decreasing LVEDP, may point to the low affinity of enalapril for cardiac tissue ACE (42,43), and even enhanced cardiac Ang II generation for a given level of LVEDP by (enhanced passive) uptake from high-plasma renin and Ang I.

MAINTENANCE OF VOLUME OVERLOAD–INDUCED CARDIAC HYPERTROPHY AND/OR PROGRESSION TO HEART FAILURE

In all models of cardiac volume overload studied (i.e., aortocaval shunt, aortic insufficiency, or minoxidil), treatment with ACE inhibitors such as enalapril, perindopril, captopril, or the Ang II–receptor blocker losartan reverses LV hypertrophy and dilation in parallel with their effects on LVEDP (7,14,28,44,45). For example, in rats with an aortocaval shunt by an 18-gauge needle, enalapril or losartan added from 5 to 10 weeks after shunt decreased LVEDP from 6.4 ± 1.2 to 3.0 ± 0.6 and 2.0 ± 0.5 mmHg and reduced LV weight and dilation in parallel with their effects on LVEDP (Fig. 9). In rats on minoxidil, when treatment is discontinued after 5 weeks, LVEDP decreases back to normal and LV hypertrophy and LV dilation disappear (see Fig. 3). Similarly, enalapril and losartan added to minoxidil from 5 to 10 weeks normalize LVEDP and reduce RV and LV hypertrophy and LV dilation to an extent similar to that which occurs after withdrawal of minoxidil (Table 3). The

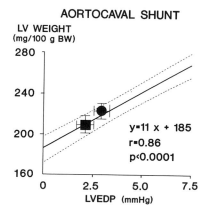

AORTOCAVAL SHUNT

LV WEIGHT
(mg/100 g BW)

$y = 11 x + 185$
$r = 0.86$
$p < 0.0001$

LVEDP (mmHg)

FIG. 9. Effect of enalapril and losartan on left ventricular (LV) weight in relation to their effect on left ventricular end-diastolic pressure (LVEDP) from 5 to 10 weeks of aortocaval shunt. For regression line, see Fig. 8. Broken lines represent 95% confidence interval. Values are mean ± SEM (n = 6–8/group). ■, aortocaval shunt plus losartan; ●, aortocaval shunt plus enalapril. Figure derived from Ruzicka et al. (7) with permission of the American Heart Association.

TABLE 3. *Effects of enalapril versus losartan on LVEDP and LV weight during the maintenance phase of cardiac hypertrophy induced by minoxidil*

	LVEDP (mmHg)	LV weight (mg/100 g bw)
Control	0.0 ± 0.2	176 ± 4
Control + enalapril	0.5 ± 0.3	160 ± 3[a]
Control + losartan	0.2 ± 0.2	157 ± 7[a]
Minoxidil	4.5 ± 0.8[a]	215 ± 4[a]
Minoxidil + enalapril	1.2 ± 0.6[b]	171 ± 2 + [b]
Minoxidil + losartan	1.0 ± 0.4[b]	179 ± 3 + [b]

Data derived from Ruzicka et al. (7), with permission of the American Heart Association.
Values are mean ± SEM (n = 12–16/group).
[a]$p < 0.05$ vs. control.
[b]$p < 0.05$ for minoxidil or shunt + treatment vs. minoxidil or shunt untreated.
LV, left ventricular; RV, right ventricular; LVEDP, LV end-diastolic pressure.

decrease in LVEDP by blockers of the RAS is likely caused by a decrease in cardiac afterload and by improvement in LV systolic and diastolic performance (46), as suggested from a persistent increase in cardiac output at lower filling pressures. In all three models of cardiac volume overload (i.e., aortocaval shunt, aortic insufficiency, and minoxidil), hemodynamic effects of the RAS appear, therefore, to continue to play a role in determining filling pressures of the heart and thereby the maintenance of cardiac hypertrophy. In contrast to the development phase, however, the RAS no longer appears to directly stimulate cardiomyocytes' growth during maintenance of aortocaval shunt- and minoxidil-induced cardiac hypertrophy.

SUMMARY

Large aortocaval fistulas may never be compensated (as suggested from persistent decreases in LVPSP and increases in LVEDP), and heart failure develops within a few days to weeks after shunt surgery. Cardiac hypertrophy, however, compensates for moderate cardiac volume overload and only slowly progresses into the heart failure, as suggested from a close-to-normal LV ejection fraction (60 ± 2% vs. 73 ± 2%) at 3 months after aortocaval shunt by an 18-gauge needle (47). Whereas the RAS appears to directly stimulate cardiomyocytes' growth in response to cardiac volume overload by an aortocaval shunt or minoxidil during the development of the cardiac hypertrophy, the RAS appears no longer to do so during chronic cardiac volume overload. On the other hand, the RAS appears to contribute to the maintenance of the cardiac hypertrophy by maintaining high filling pressures. Because the progression of compensated cardiac volume overload into congestive heart failure in rats has not yet been assessed, we cannot at present assess whether the RAS is involved in such progression. Similarly, whether treatment with blockers of the RAS and resulting attenuation of development/reduction of cardiac hypertrophy would prevent/slow the progression of chronic volume overload into congestive heart failure remains to be evaluated.

ACKNOWLEDGMENTS

Research by the authors described in this review was supported by operating grants from the Heart and Stroke Foundation of Ontario. Dr. Ruzicka was supported by a research fellowship from the Heart and Stroke Foundation of Canada. Dr. Leenen was supported by a career investigatorship from the Heart and Stroke Foundation of Ontario.

REFERENCES

1. Flaim SF, Minteer WJ, Nellis SH, Clark DP. Chronic arteriovenous shunt: evaluation of a model for heart failure. *Am J Physiol* 1979;236:H698–H704.
2. Stumpe KO, Solle H, Klein H, Fruck F. Mechanism of sodium and water retention in rats with experimental heart failure. *Kidney Int* 1973;4:309–317.
3. Liu Z, Hilbeling DR, Crockett WB, Gerdes AM. Regional changes in hemodynamics and cardiac myocyte size in rats with aortocaval fistulas: 1. Developing and established hypertrophy. *Circ Res* 1991;69:52–58.
4. Liu Z, Hilbeling DR, Gerdes AM. Regional changes in hemodynamics and cardiac myocyte size in rats with aortocaval fistulas: 2. Long-term effects. *Circ Res* 1991;69:59–65.
5. Garcia R, Diebold S. Simple, rapid, and effective method of producing aortocaval shunts in the rat. *Cardiovasc Res* 1990;24:430–432.
6. Ruzicka M, Yuan B, Harmsen E, Leenen FHH. The renin-angiotensin system and volume overload-induced cardiac hypertrophy in rats. Effects of angiotensin converting enzyme inhibitor versus angiotensin II receptor blocker. *Circulation* 1993;87:921–930.
7. Ruzicka M, Yuan B, Leenen FHH. Effects of enalapril versus losartan on regression of volume overload-induced cardiac hypertrophy in rats. *Circulation* 1994;90:484–491.
8. Hatt P-Y, Rakusan K, Gastineau P, Laplace M. Morphometry and ultrastructure of heart hypertrophy induced by chronic volume overload (aorto-caval fistula in the rat). *J. Mol Cell Cardiol* 1979; 11:989–998.
9. Brown LA, Nunez DRJ, Wilkins MR. Differential regulation of natriuretic peptide receptor messenger RNAs during the development of cardiac hypertrophy in the rat. *J Clin Invest* 1993;92:2702–2712.
10. Huang M, Hester RL, Guyton AC. Hemodynamic changes in rats after opening an arteriovenous fistula. *Am J Physiol* 1992;262:H846–H851.
11. Anversa P, Ricci R, Olivetti G. Quantitative structural analysis of the myocardium during physiologic growth and induced cardiac hypertrophy: a review. *J Am Coll Cardiol* 1986;7:1140–1149.
12. Olivetti G, Lagrasta C, Quaini F, et al. Capillary growth in anemia-induced ventricular wall remodeling in the rat. *Circ Res* 1989;65:1182–1192.
13. Uematsu T, Yamazaki T, Matsuno H, Hayashi Y, Nakashima M. A simple method for producing graded aortic insufficiencies in rats and subsequent development of cardiac hypertrophy. *J Pharmacol Methods* 1989;22:249–257.
14. Gay RG. Captopril reduces left ventricular enlargement induced by chronic volume overload. *Am J Physiol* 1990;259:H796–H803.
15. Isoyama S, Grossman W, Wei JY. Effect of age on myocardial adaptation to volume overload in the rat. *J Clin Invest* 1988;81:1850–1857.
16. Robertson E, Hof RP, Zierhut W. Effect of hypertrophy induced by pressure overload or volume overload on reperfusion induced arrhythmias in anaesthetised rats. *Cardiovasc Res* 1993;27:515–519.

17. Farquharson C, Duncan A, Robins SP. The effects of copper deficiency on the pyridinium crosslinks of mature collagen in the rat skeleton and cardiovascular system. *PSEBM* 1989;192:166–171.
18. Beard J. Feed efficiency and norepinephrine turnover in iron deficiency. *PSEBM* 1987;184:337–344.
19. Neffgen JF, Korecky B. Cellular hyperplasia and hypertrophy in cardiomegalies induced by anemia in young and adult rats. *Circ Res* 1972;30:104–113.
20. Datta BN, Silver MD. Cardiomegaly in chronic anemia in rats. An experimental study including ultrastructural, histometric and stereologic observations. *Lab Invest* 1975;32:503–514.
21. Sen S. Regression of cardiac hypertrophy. Experimental animal model. *Am J Med* 1983;86:87–93.
22. Tsoporis J, Leenen FHH. Effects of arterial vasodilators on cardiac hypertrophy and sympathetic activity in rats. *Hypertension* 1988;11:376–386.
23. Tsoporis J, Yuan B, Leenen FHH. Arterial vasodilators, cardiac volume load, and cardiac hypertrophy in normotensive rats. *Am J Physiol* 1989;256:H876–H880.
24. Tsoporis J, Fields N, Lee RMKW, Leenen FHH. Arterial vasodilation and cardiovascular changes in normotensive rats. *Am J Physiol* 1991;260:H1944–H1952.
25. Sen S, Tarazi RC, Bumpus FM. Cardiac hypertrophy and antihypertensive therapy. *Cardiovasc Res* 1977;11:427–433.
26. Tarazi RC, Dustan HP, Bravo EL, Niarchos AP. Vasodilating drugs: contrasting hemodynamic effects. *Clin Sci Mol Med* 1976;51:575S–578S.
27. Fields N, Tsoporis J, Leenen FHH. Differential effects of the calcium antagoinist, nisoldipine, versus the arterial vasodilator, minoxidil, on ventricular anatomy, intravascular volume, and sympathetic activity in rats. *J Cardiovasc Pharmacol* 1989;14:826–835.
28. Ruzicka M, Leenen FHH. Renin-angiotensin system and minoxidil-induced cardiac hypertrophy in rats. *Am J Physiol* 1993;265:H1551–H1556.
29. Flaim SF, Minteer WJ, Zelis R. Acute effects of arterio-venous shunt on cardiovascular hemodynamics in rat. *Pflugers Arch* 1980;385:203–209.
30. Umemura K, Zierhut W, Rudin M, et al. Effect of spirapril on left ventricular hypertrophy due to volume overload in rats. *J Cardiovasc Pharmacol* 1992;19:375–381.
31. Olivetti G, Quaini F, Lagrasta C, et al. Effects of genetic hypertension and nutritional anaemia on ventricular remodelling and myocardial damage in rats. *Cardiovasc Res* 1993;27:1316–1325.
32. Boer PH, Ruzicka M, Lear W, Harmsen E, Rosenthal J, Leenen FHH. Stretch-mediated activation of cardiac renin gene. *Am J Physiol* 1994;268:H1630–H1636.
33. Danser AHJ, van Kats JP, Admiraal PJJ, et al. Cardiac renin and angiotensins. Uptake from plasma versus in situ synthesis. *Hypertension* 1994;24:37–48.
34. van Bilsen M, Chien KR. Growth and hypertrophy of the heart: towards an understanding of cardiac specific and inducible gene expression. *Cardiovasc Res* 1993;27:1140–1149.
35. Grossman W, Lorell BH. Hemodynamic aspects of left ventricular remodeling after myocardial infarction. *Circulation* 1993;87[Suppl VII]:VII-28–VII-30.
36. Geenen DL, Malhotra A, Scheuer J. Angiotensin II increases cardiac protein synthesis in adult rat heart. *Am J Physiol* 1993;265:H238–H243.
37. Aceto JF, Baker KM. [Sar[1]]angiotensin II receptor–mediated stimulation of protein synthesis in chick heart cells. *Am J Physiol* 1990;258:H806–H813.
38. Sadoshima J, Xu Y, Slayter HS, Izumo S. Autocrine release of angiotensin II mediates stretch-induced hypertrophy of cardiac muscle in vitro. *Cell* 1993;75:977–984.
39. Sadoshima J, Izumo S. Molecular characterization of angiotensin II–induced hypertrophy of cardiac myocytes and hyperplasia of cardiac fibroblasts. Critical role of the AT_1 receptor subtype. *Circ Res* 1993;73:414–423.
40. Sadoshima J, Izumo S. Signal transduction pathways of angiotensin II–induced c-*fos* gene expression in cardiac myocytes in vitro. *Circ Res* 1993;73:424–438.
41. Ruzicka M, Leenen FHH. Relevance of blockade of cardiac and circulatory angiotensin converting enzyme for the prevention of volume overload-induced cardiac hypertrophy. *Circulation* 1995;91:16–19.
42. Cushman DW, Wang FL, Fung WC, Harvey CM, DeForrest JM. Differentiation of angiotensin-converting enzyme (ACE) inhibitors by their selective inhibition of ACE in physiologically important target organs. *Am J Hypertens* 1989;2:294–306.
43. Nakajima T, Yamada T, Setoguchi M. Prolonged inhibition of local angiotensin-converting enzyme after single or repeated treatment with quinapril in spontaneously hypertensive rats. *J Cardiovasc Pharmacol* 1992;19:102–107.

44. Arnal JF, Philippe M, Laboulandine I, Michel JB. Effect of perindopril in rat cardiac volume overload. *Am Heart J* 1993;126:776–782.
45. Qing G, Garcia R. Chronic captopril and losartan (DuP 753) administration in rats with high-output heart failure. *Am J Physiol* 1992;263:H833–H840.
46. Schunkert H, Dzau VJ, Tang SS, Hirsch AT, Apstein CS, Lorell BH. Increased rat cardiac angiotensin converting enzyme activity and mRNA expression in pressure overload left ventricular hypertrophy: effect on coronary resistance, contractility, and relaxation. *J Clin Invest* 1990;86:1913–1920.
47. Yang XP, Sabbah HN, Liu YH, et al. Ventriculographic evaluation in three rat models of cardiac dysfunction. *Am J Physiol* 1993;265:H1946–H1952.

The Failing Heart, edited by N. S. Dhalla,
R. E. Beamish, N. Takeda, and M. Nagano.
Lippincott-Raven Publishers, Philadelphia © 1995.

26

Role of Angiotensin Receptors in the Regulation of Vascular Growth

Peter Zahradka, Laura Saward, and Lorraine Yau

Department of Physiology, Division of Cardiovascular Sciences, Faculty of Medicine, University of Manitoba, St. Boniface General Hospital Research Centre, Winnipeg, Manitoba, R2H 2A6 Canada

Atherosclerosis and hypertension are vascular diseases that contribute to the development of ischemic heart disease and its eventual progression to congestive heart failure (1,2). One of the principal characteristics of both atherosclerosis and hypertension is the narrowing of vessel diameter due to growth of the smooth-muscle cells present in the medial or intimal layers. For this reason, the factors that stimulate smooth-muscle cell growth are important components in the processes that determine whether there is a significant risk of developing cardiovascular disease (Fig. 1).

CELL PROLIFERATION OR CELL HYPERTROPHY

Cell growth is an essential feature in the development of multicellular organisms; uncontrolled cell growth, however, is generally deleterious to long-term survival. Although such events are associated usually with disorders such as cancer, they also contribute to the development of many cardiovascular diseases. Maladaptive cardiac hypertrophy, atherosclerosis, and some forms of hypertension, in particular, may originate from defects in those systems that regulate cell growth. An understanding of the mechanisms that govern the growth and proliferation of cardiac and vascular tissues can therefore provide useful information applicable to the treatment and control of these specific illnesses.

Cell proliferation can be viewed as the end result of a process that requires successful completion of at least three distinct events (Fig. 2). The primary characteristic of growing cells is the duplication of the genetic information, and this event can be measured by incorporation of radiolabeled thymidine during DNA synthesis (3). The progression to S phase, however, must be preceded by the synthesis of numerous RNA molecules. For example, the stimulation of proto-oncogenes such as

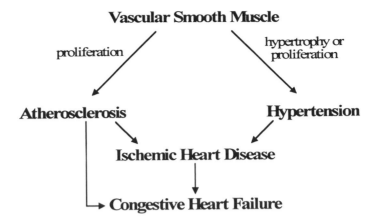

FIG. 1. Changes in smooth-muscle growth status contribute to the development of cardiovascular disease.

c-*fos*, c-*myc*, and c-*jun* has been used as an indicator that cells have departed the quiescent state (4). It must also be noted, however, that the bulk (>80%) of the cellular RNA is found in the ribosomal fraction rather than as mRNA. Therefore, simple assays that monitor uridine incorporation into a cell are actually a measure of ribosomal RNA synthesis (5,6) and, for this reason, can also serve as a marker for cell growth. Finally, the mitotic index, the percentage of cells undergoing mitosis, is the truest measure of cell proliferation because it distinguishes growth in cell number from hypertrophic growth. In a proliferating cell population, this value typically approaches 5%, but reaches more than 80% in one that is synchronously progressing through the cell cycle (3). A complete evaluation of cell growth thus requires the measurement of all of these events because a distinction between cell proliferation (growth with cell division) and hypertrophy (growth without cell division) cannot be made by using a single indicator.

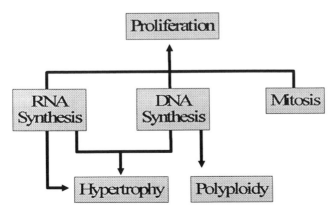

FIG. 2. Macromolecular synthesis and cell division can signify distinct patterns of cell growth.

RIBOSOME BIOGENESIS

Cell growth involves an ordered series of events that begins with the binding of a mitogen to its receptor and is followed by activation of a second messenger system(s), induction of immediate early gene expression, and the eventual stimulation of genes required for mobilizing the cellular machinery needed for DNA replication and mitosis. In parallel with these events, the cellular content of ribosomes is increased to ensure that sufficient amounts of ribosomal subunits are available for translation of the newly synthesized mRNAs (7). To achieve this objective, the cell must provide four species of ribosomal RNA (rRNA) and more than 80 distinct ribosomal proteins (r-proteins) through the actions of three different RNA polymerases. In addition, the sites of synthesis include the nucleus (5S rRNA and r-protein mRNA), nucleolus (18S, 28S, and 5.8S rRNAs plus subunit assembly) and the cytoplasm (r-proteins). The complexity of this process necessitates the existence of an efficient mechanism to coordinate all of the separate events in order to minimize the wasting of valuable resources.

The synthesis of the ribosomal components and their assembly into functional subunits can be viewed as three separate processes (7). Gene activation represents one aspect that has been considered in some detail in a variety of systems. The transition from quiescence following growth factor stimulation as well as entry into the terminally differentiated state have undergone the greatest scrutiny. The most common model for regulation of ribosome biogenesis involves direct control of 45S rRNA gene transcription, while expression of both r-protein and 5S rRNA genes remains unaltered (7,8). Changes in the occupancy of the 45S rRNA gene promoter by RNA polymerase I is governed through a distinct transcription factor, TFIC or TIF-IA (depending on the laboratory nomenclature), that is tightly coupled to the polymerase (9,10). This factor mediates the interaction of specific promoter-bound transcription factors with RNA polymerase and in this manner determines whether the transcription initiation complex is completed. The mechanism by which TFIC/TIF-IA accomplishes this function has yet to be identified, although both de novo synthesis of the protein or its modification by phosphorylation have been postulated.

Within the context of these events, additional regulation can occur at several of the later stages, and this becomes evident even in those situations where rRNA gene transcription is the primary site for control. In particular, the processing of the 45S rRNA transcript into the individual rRNA molecules concurrent with ribosome assembly can play an important role (11). As well, this coupled assembly/processing scheme imparts a useful means of controlling cellular levels of the other ribosomal components (7). For example, both the r-proteins and 5S rRNA will be degraded if they are in excess over the 45S rRNA, because protection from the degradation activities is achieved only after incorporation into subunits. Alternatively, feedback inhibition can decrease the transcription of the r-protein genes, although this mechanism has been found to be more prevalent in yeast than in mammalian systems. Therefore, based on these observations, any control of cell growth must involve ribosome biogenesis and, in particular, rRNA gene transcription.

The question that remains then involves how ribosome biogenesis contributes to cell proliferation beyond its role in providing the necessary components for protein production. It has been established that rRNA synthesis is rapidly induced upon addition of growth factors. This effect is not inhibited directly by cycloheximide, although this agent will eventually repress rRNA synthesis following passage of a defined lag period (12). These data not only suggest that stimulation of rRNA gene expression is an immediate early event, but that sustained transcription requires production of a factor with a short half-life. This close connection between growth and rRNA synthesis indicates that certain mechanisms exist to couple rRNA synthesis to cell growth. A paper by Rakowicz-Szulczynska and Koprowski, for example, showed that inhibition of rRNA synthesis blocked platelet-derived growth factor (PDGF) -dependent cell proliferation (13). Therefore, the modulation of rRNA synthesis is sufficient for controlling cell growth without necessarily affecting induction of other immediate early genes such as c-*fos*.

GROWTH STIMULATORY EFFECTS OF ANGIOTENSIN II

Vascular smooth-muscle cells have retained the ability to migrate and grow in response to specific external stimuli. These characteristics are essential for the efficient repair and maintenance of the vasculature. For instance, smooth-muscle cell hypertrophy is an important component of the adaptive process associated with chronic hypertension. In this case, increased cell growth reinforces those portions of the vascular wall that are under stress. The same processes that are involved in the beneficial and adaptive growth of smooth-muscle cells, however, also contribute to the development and pathology of vascular diseases such as hypertension and atherosclerosis (14,15). A key event in all of these processes is the conversion of differentiated smooth-muscle cells to a growing population, an event that encompasses a switch from an adult, contractile phenotype to a less contractile (i.e., synthetic) fetal phenotype (16,17). Of the many growth factors capable of inducing these changes, angiotensin II is physiologically relevant because its synthesis via an autocrine mechanism has been shown to occur in smooth-muscle cells (18,19). Angiotensin II has been established as a stimulator of smooth-muscle cell growth that increases RNA and protein synthesis (20,21) and induces protooncogene expression (22,23). In a number of cases, DNA synthesis also occurs, suggesting that exposure to angiotensin II can trigger cell proliferation (24–26).

Our laboratory has been using two smooth-muscle cell models to further define angiotensin II's influence on various cell growth processes. A10 smooth-muscle cells, originally derived from rat thoracic aorta (27), are a homogeneous cell population capable of alternating between a proliferative and differentiated phenotype in response to changes in serum content. Two features were demonstrated by these cells: (a) Differentiated cells are quiescent (do not synthesize DNA), and (b) they express the appropriate muscle-specific markers (desmin, smooth-muscle α-actin, creatine kinase, acetylcholine receptor) as measured by both Northern blot analysis and immunofluorescent microscopy. In addition to this model, primary smooth-muscle cells from adult porcine coronary artery have been prepared by an explant method. These cells are also capable of a reversible transition between proliferating and contractile phenotypes based on similar criteria. In this way, it has been possible to demonstrate that these cell populations are appropriate representatives of vascular smooth-muscle cells.

The treatment of smooth-muscle cells with angiotensin II triggers a complex series of events that eventually leads to cell growth (22,25). First, there is an induction of c-*fos* and c-*myc* expression that follows the immediate early pattern characteristic of cells that are traversing the G_0 to G_1 boundary. In addition, there is an increase in RNA and protein synthesis. These responses have been used as indicators that the cells have initiated growth. In both A10 and porcine coronary artery models, similar events were triggered by angiotensin II (28). On examining the effect on DNA synthesis, however, it was observed that replication occurred only in the coronary artery cells. Thus these cells have distinct reactions to stimulation by angiotensin II. Although it is not possible at this time to indicate what might account for these different responses, it is nevertheless possible to show that A10 smooth-muscle cells do not reach S phase in the presence of angiotensin II, while primary cultures of porcine coronary artery progress further in the cell cycle. Given these distinct models for the action of angiotensin II, it has been possible to determine some of the cellular events associated with the two currently known angiotensin II receptors.

ANGIOTENSIN II RECEPTOR FUNCTION IN SMOOTH MUSCLE

The cellular actions of angiotensin II are mediated by specific cell surface receptors that are coupled to distinct signaling systems and cellular responses. To date, at least two receptor subtypes have been identified according to their pharmacological properties (29). The AT_1 receptor is highly abundant in adult vascular smooth muscle. It functions, in part, by stimulating Ca^{2+} mobilization from intracellular stores and for this reason is responsible for the contractile actions associated with angiotensin II. In addition, it has been linked to proto-oncogene expression (22,23) and the activation of processes that result in DNA synthesis (24,25). This receptor is characterized primarily through its interaction with the nonpeptide antagonist losartan (DuP753). The AT_2 receptor, in contrast, is not abundant on adult vascular smooth muscle, accounting for less than 5% of the total angiotensin II binding activity (30). It has only been recently cloned and found to share limited homology (34%) with the AT_1 receptor (31,32). No specific function has yet been identified for this receptor. Nevertheless, its greater abundance in fetal and developing tissues, as well as its tight regulation by growth factors, suggests the AT_2 receptor has a growth-related function (30,33). Binding of angiotensin II to this receptor is prevented by the nonpeptide antagonist, PD123319. The current list of angiotensin II receptors is rapidly expanding, with several new receptor subtypes reported as recently as 1992 (34,35). Their relationship to the two classes already described, however, has yet to be determined. A functional understanding of their importance must wait until their basic properties have been delineated and specific antagonists have been synthesized.

As previously described, the cellular actions of angiotensin II are mediated primarily by the AT_1 receptor (36). For this reason, there is substantial clinical interest in losartan, the AT_1 receptor antagonist, as a therapeutic agent for hypertension, atherosclerosis, and other cardiovascular complications associated with excessive cell growth. One potential disadvantage with this agent, however, is its interference with other critical processes that are not coupled to growth. For instance, stimulation of extracellular matrix production or smooth-muscle cell contraction, which is inhibited by losartan (37,38), may be beneficial under certain conditions. Therefore, the availability of another agent that does not interfere with these processes may be useful.

The evidence collected in our studies has indicated that RNA synthesis, and more specifically ribosomal RNA gene transcription, is stimulated by angiotensin II. To determine which receptor subtype is responsible for this effect, both A10 and coronary artery smooth-muscle cells were treated with angiotensin II in the presence of either losartan or PD123319. No change in the rate of RNA synthesis was observed after stimulation of A10 cells with angiotensin II in the presence of losartan; PD123319, however, effectively inhibited this process (28). A direct link between the AT_2 receptor and RNA synthesis is therefore indicated. With the coronary artery cells, the angiotensin II–mediated increase in RNA synthesis was prevented by both antagonists, suggesting that activation of both receptors was necessary (Saward and Zahradka, *in preparation*). Although the underlying cause for this difference in receptor subtype contribution cannot be determined on the basis of these data, it is possible that either the tissue source (fetal thoracic aorta versus adult coronary artery), the culture conditions (cell line versus primary culture), or the species (rat versus pig) could contribute. Alternatively, this difference may represent a distinction between cells that will undergo hypertrophy as opposed to proliferation. In either case, the ability of PD123319 to block RNA synthesis may represent an alternative possibility for controlling certain diseases that involve activation of the renin–angiotensin system.

Current information regarding the contributions of the AT_1 and AT_2 receptors to cell growth suggests the presence of distinct systems responsible for rRNA synthesis and cell cycle progression. This concept is not a novel finding, considering that numerous reports have already indicated that, although growth and DNA replication are coordinated in proliferating cells, the cell cycle and ribosome biogenesis can actually be uncoupled (39–41). In particular, it has been proposed that separate systems must be activated for each process (40). According to this logic, a growth factor must therefore stimulate one pathway that leads to cell growth and another that leads to DNA synthesis in order to induce proliferation. In contrast, stimulation of only one pathway would lead to either hypertrophy or polyploidy (see Fig. 2). Given the lack of an AT_1-mediated response in A10 smooth-muscle cells, this culture system would be ideal for studies of the signaling systems associated with the AT_2 receptor.

INTRACELLULAR MEDIATORS OF ANGIOTENSIN II RECEPTOR SIGNALS

Extracellular agents can trigger the transition from G_0 into G_1 through specific cell surface receptors that stimulate the production of second messenger molecules within the cell. Angiotensin II has been shown to operate through specific G-protein–coupled cascades (42). The cloning of the AT_1 and AT_2 receptors indicated that both proteins have the seven transmembrane domains characteristic of G-protein–linked receptors (31,32). The unique feature of the AT_2 receptor is its possible connection to an uncharacterized pertussis toxin-sensitive G protein that mediates the inhibition of tyrosine phosphatase activity (32,43). This function has not been previously noted, and it further supports the view that not all of the cardiovascular effects of angiotensin II are directed by the AT_1 receptor.

Various signaling systems have been linked to angiotensin II, with Ca^{2+} mobilization, protein kinase C activation, and phosphoinositol pathways being the best established (36). Although these cascades are usually associated with changes in contractility, they also have a distinct impact on cell growth properties. Other intracellular signaling molecules, such as prostaglandins, have also been linked to angiotensin II function (44,45). It has been clearly established that prostaglandins mediate vascular tone, a function that complements the effects of angiotensin II (46). Any connection between prostaglandins and angiotensin II in the regulation of cell growth remains tenuous, however, largely due to the difficulty in clearly identifying the lipid species that are synthesized following angiotensin II treatment. In order to approach this problem without the necessity of dealing with a specific prostaglandin, indomethacin was added to cultures of A10 smooth muscle simultaneously with angiotensin II. The presence of this cyclooxygenase inhibitor blocked the expected increase in RNA synthesis (28). Because this response is controlled solely by the AT_2 receptor, it would appear that prostaglandins may be an important component of the AT_2 signaling system. A similar result was obtained with the coronary artery smooth-muscle cells, indicating that prostaglandins function similarly in both cell models.

The observation that prostaglandins regulate rRNA synthesis is a novel finding, because little is known of the mechanisms that couple cell growth with ribosome biogenesis. To evaluate this potential connection in more detail, coronary artery smooth-muscle cells were treated directly with purified prostaglandins, and their effect on RNA synthesis was measured. Both PGE_2 and $PGF_{2\alpha}$, but not PGI_2, increased RNA synthesis in a dose-dependent manner (Yau and Zahradka, *in preparation*). These results clearly demonstrate that prostaglandins are important mediators of rRNA production. Nevertheless, until a comprehensive evaluation of the prostaglandin species produced in response to angiotensin II is completed, it will be impossible to tell whether PGE_2 or $PGF2_\alpha$ serves as a mediator for angiotensin II or if the results described here indicate there is a separate pathway for control of cell growth by exogenously produced prostaglandins.

In the mid-1980s there was an increased awareness that cell proliferation was actually a coordinated process involving both cell growth and progression through the cell cycle as exemplified by duplication of the genome and eventual production of two daughter cells. The work of Baserga, Zetterberg, and Adam clearly demonstrated that these individual processes could be uncoupled (39–41). For this reason, it was proposed that the ribosome cycle was regulated via processes distinct from those that controlled cell cycle progression. Recent evidence for such a scheme has been obtained from yeast as well as other higher organisms (47). The evidence provided by experiments obtained from this laboratory suggests that the AT_2 receptor makes an important contribution to smooth-muscle cell growth. This conclusion is especially evident in A10 smooth-muscle cells, because their response to angiotensin II (which involves increasing the rate of rRNA synthesis) occurs only through an AT_2 receptor–dependent mechanism. Most significantly, this cellular response is completely insensitive to the AT_1 receptor antagonist losartan. Although both AT_1 and AT_2 receptors are necessary for stimulating RNA synthesis in coronary artery smooth-muscle cells, the realization that the AT_2 receptor mediates certain aspects of cell growth provides an added dimension for controlling those conditions associated with excessive cell growth. More specifically, given that the AT_1 receptor regulates the contractile as well as various growth-related responses of angiotensin II, AT_2 receptor antagonists may provide an alternative approach for managing cardiovascular diseases such as atherosclerosis and restenosis that are not primarily associated with changes in vascular tone.

SUMMARY

The growth and proliferation of vascular smooth-muscle cells is an important element in hypertension and atherosclerosis. Many of the factors that stimulate smooth-muscle cell growth are produced within the vasculature through local autocrine and paracrine systems. One of the most important agents is angiotensin II, because treatment with converting-enzyme inhibitors has proved efficacious in preventing both atherosclerosis and hypertension. This therapy, however, also causes an elevation in bradykinin levels, which can lead to certain undesirable side effects. As an alternative strategy, specific antagonists of the angiotensin II receptor subtypes are being investigated as possible successors to ACE inhibitors for controlling vascular disease. To date, considerable attention has been focused on the AT_1 receptor, because it has been found to mediate the majority of actions ascribed to angiotensin II. In contrast, the biological function of the AT_2 receptor remains undefined. Our laboratory has been evaluating the cellular events involved in angiotensin II–stimulated growth of vascular smooth-muscle cells. Using both the A10 smooth-muscle cell line and primary cultures of coronary smooth-muscle cells, we have established that the stimulation of ribosomal RNA by angiotensin II is an early event that is distinct from the pathways leading to DNA synthesis. Evidence supporting a role for the AT_2 receptor in mediating rRNA synthesis through prostaglandins has also been obtained. These data indicate that the AT_2 receptor must be considered in any model for the cellular actions of angiotensin II and may provide an additional approach for managing vascular disease.

ACKNOWLEDGMENTS

Studies from this laboratory have been supported by grants from the Medical Research Council Group in Experimental Cardiology, Juvenile Diabetes Foundation International, and by MRC studentships to L. S. and L. Y.

REFERENCES

1. Stokes J, Kannel WB, Wolf PA, D'Agostino RB, Cupples LA. Blood pressure as a risk factor for cardiovascular disease. *Hypertension* 1989;13[Suppl I]:I13–I18.
2. Ross R. The pathogenesis of atherosclerosis: a perspective for the 1990s. *Nature* 1993;362:801–809.
3. Baserga R. Measuring parameters of growth. In: Baserga R, ed. *Cell growth and division*. Oxford: IRL Press; 1989:1–16.
4. Leutz A, Graf T. Relationships between oncogenes and growth control. In: Sporn MB, Roberts AB, eds. *Peptide growth factors and their receptors II*. New York: Springer-Verlag; 1991:655–703.
5. Zahradka P, Yau L. ADP-ribosylation and gene expression. *Mol Cell Biochem* 1994;138:91–98.
6. Mauck JC, Green H. Regulation of RNA synthesis in fibroblasts during transition from resting to growing state. *Proc Natl Acad Sci USA* 1973;70:2819–2822.
7. Larson DE, Zahradka P, Sells BH. Control points in eucaryotic ribosome biogenesis. *Biochem Cell Biol* 1991;69:5–22.
8. Zahradka P, Larson DE, Sells BH. Regulation of ribosome biogenesis in differentiated rat myotubes. *Mol Cell Biochem* 1991;104:189–194.
9. Schnapp A, Pfleiderer C, Rosenbauer H, Grummt I. A growth-dependent transcription initiation factor (TIF-IA) interacting with RNA polymerase I regulates mouse ribosomal RNA synthesis. *EMBO J* 1990;9:2857–2863.
10. Mahajan PB, Thompson EA Jr. Hormonal regulation of transcription of rRNA. Purification and characterization of the hormone-regulated transcription factor IC. *J Biol Chem* 1990;265:16255–16233.
11. Hadjiolov AA. Biogenesis of ribosomes in eukaryotes. *Subcell Biochem* 1980;7:1–80.
12. Gokal PK, Cavanaugh AH, Thompson EA Jr. The effects of cycloheximide upon transcription of rRNA, 5S RNA and tRNA genes. *J Biol Chem* 1986;261:2536–2541.
13. Rakowicz-Szulczynska EM, Koprowski H. Antagonistic effect of PDGF and NGF on transcription of ribosomal DNA and tumor cell proliferation. *Biochem Biophys Res Commun* 1989;163:649–656.
14. Schwartz SM, Campbell GR, Campbell JH. Replication of smooth muscle cells in vascular disease. *Circ Res* 1986;58:427–444.
15. Herrman JR, Hermans WRM, Vos J, Serruys PW. Pharmacological approaches to the prevention of restenosis following angioplasty. The search for the Holy Grail? (Part I). *Drugs* 1993;46:18–52.
16. Thyberg J, Hedin U, Sjolund M, Palmberg L, Bottger BA. Regulation of differentiated properties and proliferation of arterial smooth muscle cells. *Arteriosclerosis* 1990;10:966–990.
17. Pauletto P, Chiavegato A, Giuriato L, et al. Hyperplastic growth of smooth muscle cells in renovascular hypertensive rabbits is characterized by the expansion of an immature cell phenotype. *Circ Res* 1994;74:774–788.
18. Naftilan AJ, Zuo WM, Ingelfinger J, Ryan TJ, Pratt RE, Dzau VJ. Localization and differential regulation of angiotensinogen mRNA expression in the vessel wall. *J Clin Invest* 1991;87:1300–1311.
19. Rakugi H, Jacob HJ, Krieger JE, Ingelfinger JR, Pratt RE. Vascular injury induces angiotensinogen gene expression in the media and neointima. *Circulation* 1993;87:283–290.
20. Andrawis NS, Abernathy DR. Verapamil blocks basal and angiotensin II–induced RNA synthesis of rat aortic vascular smooth muscle cells. *Biochem Biophys Res Comm* 1992;183:767–773.

21. Berk BC, Vershtein V, Gordon HM, Tsuda T. Angiotensin II–stimulated protein synthesis in cultured vascular smooth muscle cells. *Hypertension* 1989;13:305–314.
22. Naftilan AJ. The role of angiotensin II in vascular smooth muscle growth. *J Cardiovasc Pharmacol* 1992;20[Suppl 1]:S37–S40.
23. Millet D, Desgranges C, Campan M, Gadeau A-P, Costerousse O. Effects of angiotensins on cellular hypertrophy and c-*fos* expression in cultured arterial smooth muscle cells. *Eur J Biochem* 1992; 206:367–372.
24. Weber H, Taylor DS, Molloy CJ. Angiotensin II induces delayed mitogenesis and cellular proliferation in rat aortic smooth muscle cells. *J Clin Invest* 1994;93:788–798.
25. Deaman MJAP, Lombardi DM, Bosman FT, Schwartz SM. Angiotensin II induces smooth muscle cell proliferation in the normal and injured rat arterial wall. *Circ Res* 1991;68:450–456.
26. Huckle WR, Earp HS. Regulation of cell proliferation and growth by angiotensin II. *Prog Growth Factor Res* 1995;5:177–194.
27. Kimes BW, Brandt BL. Characterization of two putative smooth muscle cell lines from rat thoracic aorta. *J Cell Physiol* 1983;98:349–366.
28. Saward L, Zahradka P. The angiotensin type 2 receptor mediates RNA synthesis in A10 vascular smooth-muscle cells. 1995 [submitted].
29. Steinberg MI, Wiest SA, Palkowitz AD. Non-peptide angiotensin II antagonists. *Cardiovasc Drug Rev* 1993;11:312–358.
30. Viswanathan M, Tsutsumi K, Correa FMA, Saavedra JM. Changes in expression of angiotensin receptor subtypes in the rat aorta during development. *Biochem Biophys Res Commun* 1991;179: 1361–1367.
31. Mukoyama M, Nakajima M, Horiuchi M, Sasamura H, Pratt RE, Dzau VJ. Expression cloning of type 2 angiotensin II receptor reveals a unique class of seven-membrane receptors. *J Biol Chem* 1993;268:24539–24542.
32. Kambayashi Y, Bardhan S, Takahashi K, et al. Molecular cloning of a novel angiotensin II receptor isoform involved in phosphotyrosine phosphatase inhibition. *J Biol Chem* 1993;268:24543–24546.
33. Feuillan PP, Millan MA, Auguilera G. Angiotensin II binding sites in the rat fetus: characterization of receptor subtypes and interaction with guanyl nucleotides. *Regul Pept* 1993;44:159–169.
34. Swanson GN, Henesworth JM, Sardinia MF, et al. Discovery of a distinct binding site for angiotensin (3–8), a putative angiotensin IV receptor. *Regul Pept* 1992;40:409–419.
35. Sandberg K, Ji H, Clark AJL, Shapira H, Catt KJ. Cloning and expression of a novel angiotensin II receptor subtype. *J Biol Chem* 1992;267:9455–9458.
36. Chiu AT, Roscoe WA, McCall DE, Timmermans BMWM. Angiotensin II-1 receptors mediate both vasoconstrictor and hypertrophic responses in rat aortic smooth muscle cells. *Receptor* 1991;1:133–140.
37. Crawford DC, Chobanian AV, Brecher P. Angiotensin II induces fibronectin expression associated with cardiac fibrosis in the rat. *Circ Res* 1994;74:727–739.
38. Weinen W, Mauz ABM, Van Meel JCA, Entzeroth M. Different types of receptor interaction of peptide and nonpeptide angiotensin II antagonists revealed by receptor binding and functional studies. *Mol Pharmacol* 1992;41:1081–1088.
39. Seuwen K, Adam G. Only one of the two signals required for initiation of the cell cycle is associated with cellular accumulation of ribosomal RNA. *Biochem Biophys Res Commun* 1983;117:223–230.
40. Baserga R. Growth in size and cell DNA replication. *Exp Cell Res* 1984;151:1–5.
41. Zetterberg A, Larsson O. Coordination between cell growth and cell cycle transit in animal cells. *Cold Spring Harbor Symp Quant Biol* 1991;56:137–147.
42. Anand-Srivastava MB. Angiotensin II receptors negatively coupled to adenylate cyclase in rat myocardial sarcolemma. *Biochem Pharmacol* 1989;38:489–496.
43. Takahasi K, Bardhan S, Kambayashi Y, Shirai H, Inagami T. Protein tyrosine phosphatase inhibition by angiotensin II in rat pheochromocytoma cells through type 2 receptor, AT2. *Biochem Biophys Res Commun* 1994;198:60–66.
44. Leung KH, Chang RSL, Lotti VJ, et al. AT1 receptors mediate the release of prostaglandins in porcine smooth muscle cells and rat astrocytes. *Am J Hypertens* 1992;5:648–656.
45. Jaiswal N, Tallant EA, Diz DI, Khosla MC, Ferrario CM. Subtype 2 angiotensin receptors mediate prostaglandin synthesis in human astrocytes. *Hypertension* 1991;17:1115–1120.
46. Dorn GW, Becker MW, Davis MG. Dissociation of the contractile and hypertrophic effects of vasoconstrictor prostanoids in vascular smooth muscle. *J Biol Chem* 1992;267:24987–24905.
47. Murray A, Hunt T. *The cell cycle*. New York: Freeman and Company, 1993.

The Failing Heart, edited by N. S. Dhalla,
R. E. Beamish, N. Takeda, and M. Nagano.
Lippincott-Raven Publishers, Philadelphia © 1995.

27

Treatment of Symptomatic Heart Failure

Kanu Chatterjee and Teresa DeMarco

*Division of Cardiology, Moffitt-Long Hospital, University of California at
San Francisco, San Francisco, California 94143*

The objectives of therapeutic interventions in patients with chronic heart failure due to left ventricular systolic dysfunction are to alleviate symptoms and improve quality of life and prognosis. Congestive symptoms and fatigue, tiredness, and poor exercise tolerance are the major symptoms experienced by most patients with chronic heart failure. Although the mechanisms of congestive symptoms, such as exertional dyspnea, are not entirely clear, the congestive symptoms are frequently relieved with a decrease in intracardiac volumes and systemic and pulmonary venous pressures. Pathogenesis of impaired exercise tolerance, fatigue, and tiredness in chronic heart failure is also not clear. Decreased skeletal muscle blood flow and various abnormalities of structural and metabolic function of the skeletal muscles have been thought to be contributory (1). Neuroendocrine activation has also been regarded as an important pathogenic mechanism for symptomatology and progression of heart failure (2). In patients with symptomatic heart failure due to left ventricular systolic dysfunction, plasma renin activity, angiotensin II, and aldosterone levels are significantly increased (3). There is also evidence for increased tissue angiotensin activity, particularly in renal vascular, endothelial, and myocardial tissues (4). This increased circulating and tissue angiotensin activity contributes to altered renal, peripheral, and central hemodynamics. Angiotensin II–mediated increased release of aldosterone from the adrenal glands is associated with sodium and fluid retention and increased intravascular and intracardiac volumes, which is a major mechanism for the congestive symptoms. Aldosterone, in addition, may exert a direct deleterious effect on the extracellular matrix and increase collagenosis and fibrosis (5). An activated renin–angiotensin system also appears to be important in ventricular remodeling associated with increased left ventricular mass and systolic and end-diastolic volume, and reduced ejection fraction (6). Ventricular remodeling following initial myocardial insult is an essential mechanism for progressive ventricular dysfunction and worsening heart failure. Abnormal coronary hemodynamics and myocardial energetics and perfusion may also contribute to deteriorating ventricular function and progression of heart failure (7). In patients with ischemic or nonischemic dilated cardiomyopathy associated with clinical heart failure, myocar-

337

dial oxygen consumption is significantly increased, probably due to an increase in myocardial oxygen demand primarily resulting from increased left ventricular wall stress. Myocardial perfusion may be impaired, not only in patients with ischemic cardiomyopathy, but also in patients with nonischemic cardiomyopathy without atherosclerotic obstructive coronary artery disease. Endothelium-dependent coronary vasodilatation appears to be impaired in patients with dilated cardiomyopathy (8). Reduced coronary vasodilatory reserve and a concomitant increase in myocardial oxygen requirements may induce myocardial ischemia, even in the absence of coronary artery disease, and may be a contributing factor for the progression of heart failure. Enhanced renin–angiotensin and adrenergic activity may be contributory to abnormal coronary hemodynamics and myocardial energetics. Increased systemic and cardiac adrenergic activity, which is frequently observed in patients with symptomatic heart failure due to left ventricular systolic dysfunction, may also produce deleterious effects on peripheral and central hemodynamics as well as myocardial mechanical and metabolic function. Increased cardiac adrenergic activity may be associated with myocardial beta-adrenergic receptor dysfunction and impaired myocardial contractile response, contributing to impaired cardiac performance in patients with chronic heart failure (9). Furthermore, neuroendocrine abnormalities have been associated with a worse prognosis and increased plasma renin activity, and norepinephrine levels have been reported to influence the prognosis adversely (10,11). Thus, correction of an abnormal neuroendocrine profile has emerged as an additional objective for treatment of chronic heart failure (Fig. 1).

INITIAL THERAPY IN SYMPTOMATIC HEART FAILURE

Diuretics

Diuretic therapy (12) is essential for the relief of congestive symptoms of patients with chronic heart failure. Patients with symptoms and signs of volume overload should be considered for diuretic therapy (Table 1). The major hemodynamic effects during diuretic therapy are reduction of right atrial and pulmonary capillary wedge pressure (PCWP) with little or no change in cardiac output. The reduction in systemic and pulmonary venous pressures results partly from diuresis and a decrease in intravascular volume, but also from peripheral venodilatation, which also decreases intracardiac volumes. It has been postulated that venodilatation may be a direct effect of furosemide or it may be prostaglandin-mediated. Diuretic therapy may also improve pulmonary compliance and decrease airway resistance, which is associated with improved efficiency of respiratory work.

In some patients with severe, chronic congestive heart failure, intravenous administration of relatively large doses of furosemide may cause a transient deterioration in hemodynamics and left ventricular performance. Cardiac output may transiently decrease along with an increase in PCWP, and this deterioration of cardiac performance has been related to an increase in systemic vascular resistance resulting

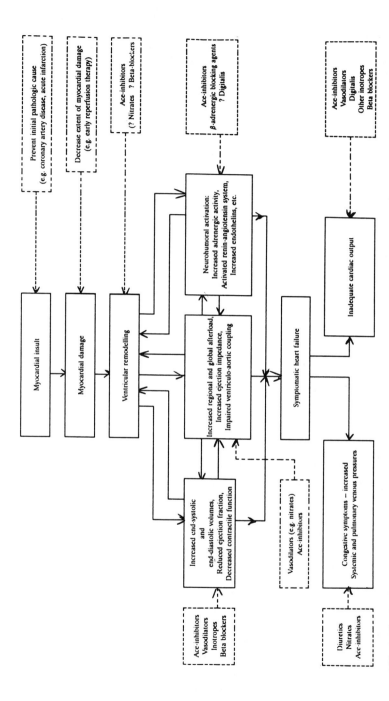

FIG. 1. The pathophysiologic mechanisms of development of heart failure following initial myocardial insult. Significant impairment of systolic function results when the extent of myocardial damage reaches a threshold level and ventricular remodeling occurs. Progressive impairment of cardiac function, peripheral hemodynamics, and neurohumoral activation establish a vicious cycle resulting in progressive heart failure. Potential therapeutic interventions to prevent the development of this vicious cycle of chronic heart failure are indicated.

TABLE 1. *Treatment strategies in symptomatic heart failure*

Mild-to-moderate heart failure
 Diuretics, ACE inhibitors, and preferably digoxin, even in patients with sinus rhythm.
  Intolerance or contraindication to ACE inhibitors → hydralazine, isosorbide dinitrate,
  diuretics, and digoxin.
 Absence of congestive symptoms; diuretics may be withheld.
Severe heart failure
 Diuretics (usually loop diuretics), larger doses than in patients with mild-to-moderate heart
  failure, digoxin, and ACE inhibitors. ACE inhibitors are started at a low dose, with the dose
  increased slowly to maximal tolerable dose. In hypotensive patients and in patients
  intolerant of ACE inhibitors, hydralazine/isosorbide dinitrate, in addition to digoxin and
  diuretics.
Refractory heart failure
 Correction of complicating factors.
 Increased dose of loop diuretics; addition of metolazone.
 Combination of ACE inhibitors and hydralazine/isosorbide dinitrate in addition to digoxin and
  diuretics in selected patients.
 Combination of loop diuretics and spironolactone and lower doses of ACE inhibitors and
  digoxin in selected patients.
 Beta-blockers in addition to digoxin, diuretics, and ACE inhibitors or hydralazine/isosorbide
  dinitrate in selected patients.
 Low-dose amiodarone in addition to diuretics and ACE inhibitors or hydralazine/isosorbide
  dinitrate. Digoxin should be withdrawn or dose should be reduced.
 Dual-chamber pacing in addition to pharmacotherapy in selected patients.
 "Tailored" therapy with intravenous vasodilators and inotropic agents followed by
  nonparenteral vasodilators, ACE inhibitors, and digoxin to maintain similar improved
  hemodynamics in selected patients.
 Intermittent intravenous inotropic therapy in selected patients.
 Ultrafiltration and hemodialysis in selected patients.
 "Experimental" nonglycosidic inodilators, along with amiodarone, vasodilators, or ACE
  inhibitors in selected patients.

from increased plasma renin activity and increased vasopressin and norepinephrine release. This deterioration of cardiac performance, however, particularly elevation of PCWP following intravenous administration of furosemide, is usually very transient, and for clinical purposes, these potentially adverse effects should not be regarded as contraindications for the use of intravenous furosemide when it is indicated. Chronic long-term diuretic therapy alone, however, may cause a reduction in cardiac output and hypotension, despite a persistent reduction in systemic and pulmonary venous pressure. Left ventricular filling pressure may decrease to a very low level during chronic diuretic therapy, partly explaining the mechanism of decreased stroke volume and cardiac output. Chronic aggressive diuretic therapy, however, is also associated with an increase in plasma renin activity and increased angiotensin II and norepinephrine levels. Enhanced renin–angiotensin and adrenergic activity can increase left ventricular outflow resistance by increasing peripheral vascular tone, which may in turn impair left ventricular pump performance. Furthermore, aggressive diuretic therapy alone may induce electrolyte imbalance as well as deterioration of renal function. The neurohumoral abnormalities in response to diuretic therapy may also modify the diuretic response (12). Angiotensin II increases salt and water reabsorption directly into the proximal convoluted tubule and attenuates the diuretic response. Angiotensin II stimulates aldosterone production, which will diminish the natriuresis of the diuretic agents by increasing sodium transport in the collecting tubule. Metabolic alkalosis, hyperuricemia, hyperglycemia, and hyperlipidemia are established complications of chronic diuretic therapy. A clinical problem of diuretic therapy in congestive heart failure is the development of diuretic resistance. Noncompliance and excessive salt intake are important resistance factors. Decreased renal perfusion due to hypotension, low cardiac output, or both, and a reduction of glomerular filtration rate may decrease solute delivery to the site of diuretic action and cause an inadequate diuretic response. The concomitant use of the nonsteroidal antiinflammatory agents can cause blunting of the diuretic response of the loop diuretics, probably due to nonsteroidal-induced inhibition of prostaglandin secretion and counteraction of their tubular action. Loop diuretics cause vasodilation of the afferent renal arterioles secondary to the release of prostaglandins. Nonsteroidal agents block the vascular effects of the loop diuretics. It is apparent that although diuretics can relieve congestive symptoms, diuretic therapy alone is not indicated because of potential adverse effects on cardiac performance, neuroendocrine profile, and renal function and electrolyte balance.

Digitalis

Maintenance chronic digitalis therapy is indicated for the management of symptomatic patients with chronic heart failure due to left ventricular systolic dysfunction. The beneficial hemodynamic effects of chronic digitalis therapy have been documented in patients with chronic congestive heart failure in sinus rhythm (13). Cardiac output increases along with a reduction in pulmonary and systemic venous pressures. In the majority of patients, arterial pressure remains unchanged, although systemic vascular resistance and heart rate tend to decline. Although improvement in left ventricular function results, at least partly, from enhanced contractile function, due to its positive inotropic effect, improvement in ventricular performance and systemic hemodynamics appears to result also from improved peripheral hemodynamics. Digitalis therapy in chronic heart failure is associated with decreased forearm vascular resistance and increased forearm blood flow (14). This reduction in peripheral vascular resistance appears to be mediated primarily by reduction in systemic adrenergic activity, as it has been documented that following digitalis therapy, muscle sympathetic nerve activity declines. The mechanism of decreased adrenergic activity appears to be unrelated to its positive inotropic effect, as the use of more potent positive inotropic agents does not usually decrease muscle sympathetic nerve activity, although the magnitude of increase in cardiac output with these agents may be greater than that with digitalis. Digitalis may also decrease plasma renin activity in patients with chronic heart failure. Aldosterone concentration may also decrease along with decreased plasma renin activity. The mechanisms for these beneficial neuroendocrine changes with digitalis in chronic heart failure are not entirely clear. Orthostatic stress, which unloads mechanosensitive cardiopulmonary baroreceptors, showed that digitalis potentiated the baroreflex-mediated afferent inhibitory modulation of sympathetic neural responses. These findings suggest that digitalis causes a selective improvement in abnormal baroreceptor responsiveness and decreases sympathetic outflow, which may be the principle mechanism for digitalis-induced peripheral vasodilatation. Whatever the mechanisms, the peripheral vascular effects of digitalis and sympatho-inhibition appear to contribute significantly in improving central hemodynamics in chronic heart failure. Large-scale prospective randomized clinical trials have also demonstrated the efficacy of digitalis therapy in the management of patients with chronic heart failure due to left ventricular systolic dysfunction. The Captopril Digoxin Multicenter Trial (15) compared the effects of captopril or digoxin with placebo in patients with mild-to-moderate chronic congestive heart failure with left ventricular ejection fraction of 40% or less. During the study, 84% of patients were maintained on diuretics. Compared with placebo, digoxin increased ejection fraction significantly. Lack of digoxin was associated with a higher frequency of worsening heart failure and a need for hospitalization for the treatment of heart failure. In the Milrinone Digoxin Multicenter Trial (16), patients with more severe heart failure (New York Heart Association class III–IV) with left ventricular ejection fractions of 35% or less were randomized to placebo, digoxin, or milrinone. All patients were taking diuretics, and about half of these patients were also on vasodilator therapy. Digoxin therapy caused a significant increase in exercise capacity and left ventricular ejection fraction compared with placebo, and the incidence of worsening heart failure was greater without digoxin. The Prospective Randomized Study of Ventricular Failure and the Efficacy of Digoxin (PROVD) (17) has also reported that withdrawal of digoxin in patients with stable chronic heart failure with left ventricular ejection fraction of 35% or less, and not treated with angiotensin-converting enzyme (ACE) inhibitors, is associated with clinical and hemodynamic deterioration. To assess the role of digoxin therapy in patients receiving converting-enzyme inhibitors, a digoxin withdrawal study was performed (Randomized Assessment of Digoxin on Inhibitors of the Angiotensin-Converting Enzyme, RADIANCE) in patients with mild-to-moderate heart failure (New York Heart Association class II–III) with reduced left ventricular ejection fraction (18). Withdrawal of digoxin was associated with worsening heart failure, decreased functional class and exercise tolerance, and worsening quality of life. Left ventricular ejection fractions also deteriorated after withdrawal of digoxin. A meta-analysis of double-blind randomized control trials also suggests that digoxin reduces the risk of clinical deterioration (19). Thus, presently, maintenance digitalis therapy is indicated for treatment of symptomatic patients with chronic heart failure. It is not known at the moment, however, whether digitalis therapy alone can improve the prognosis of patients with chronic heart failure. Because the addition of certain vasodilators or ACE inhibitors to digitalis and diuretic therapy can potentially improve the prognosis of patients with chronic heart failure, digitalis and diuretic therapy alone should not be considered for long-term management of patients with systolic ventricular failure.

Vasodilators and Angiotensin-Converting Enzyme Inhibitors

That vasodilator therapy can improve left ventricular systolic function and systemic hemodynamics in patients with heart failure has been amply demonstrated (20). In patients with chronic heart failure, however, a poor correlation exists between initial improvement in systemic hemodynamics and subsequent changes in symptoms and prognosis during vasodilator therapy. Furthermore, many vasodilators do not influence long-term clinical status or prognosis, despite causing substantial improvement in hemodynamics and left ventricular function initially. Alpha-adrenergic blocking agents, such as prazosin, have been shown to improve systemic hemodynamics during short-term therapy (21); the symptomatic status and prognosis of patients treated with alpha-adrenergic blocking agents, however, remain unchanged compared with conventional treatment with digitalis and diuretics (22). Similarly, first-generation calcium entry blocking agents, such as nifedipine and diltiazem, can improve hemodynamics in patients with chronic heart failure, but do not influence the clinical status or prognosis (23). With the dihydropyridine class of calcium channel blockers, such as nifedipine, worsened heart failure and increased frequency of hospital admission for treatment of heart failure have been reported (24). Diltiazem has been reported to increase the risk of adverse cardiac events, including mortality, in patients with pulmonary congestion and reduced left ventricular ejection fraction following myocardial infarction (25). Intravenous prostacyclin, another potent peripheral vasodilator, can also influence adversely the prognosis of patients with severe refractory heart failure. Thus, for vasodilator therapy of chronic heart failure, alpha-adrenergic blocking agents or first-generation calcium entry blocking agents are not the drugs of choice and are generally contraindicated.

In the Veterans Administration (VA) Heart Failure Trial I, a hydralazine/isosorbide dinitrate combination was found to improve the prognosis of patients with mild to moderately severe chronic heart failure (22). There was a 28% reduction in the risk of mortality at 1 year in patients treated with hydralazine/isosorbide dinitrate in addition to conventional treatment with digitalis and diuretics. The mortality benefit persisted during the duration of follow-up. The incidence of intolerance to hydralazine/isosorbide dinitrate due to side effects, however, was also considerable. In a number of prospective randomized controlled studies, ACE inhibitors have also been shown to improve the prognosis of patients with mild to moderately severe chronic heart failure. In the Studies of Left Ventricular Dysfunction (SOLVD) Treatment Trial, patients with reduced left ventricular ejection fraction (35% or less), with mild-to-moderate clinical heart failure, were randomized to conventional treatment; that is, digitalis and diuretics, or enalapril, were added (23). The addition of enalapril to conventional therapy substantially decreased mortality and rate of hospitalization for treatment of heart failure. It is of interest that the incidence of acute coronary events, including unstable angina, reinfarction, and death from coronary events, was also substantially reduced with treatment with enalapril. In the Cooperative North Scandinavian Enalapril Survival Study (CONSENSUS) Trial, patients with severe heart failure (New York Heart Association class IV) were randomized to conventional treatment or to enalapril (24). Treatment with enalapril was associated with a substantial reduction in mortality at 6 months (40%) and at 1 year (31%). These controlled studies therefore suggest that the addition of either hydralazine/isosorbide dinitrate or ACE inhibitors to conventional treatment has the potential to improve prognosis in patients with chronic heart failure, in addition to improving in symptomatic status as well as quality of life.

One of the practical clinical issues is about the choice between the hydralazine/isosorbide dinitrate combination or ACE inhibitors for vasodilator therapy of chronic heart failure. Angiotensin-converting enzyme inhibitors provide some advantages over the direct-acting vasodilators for long-term management of patients with chronic heart failure. Angiotensin-converting enzyme inhibitors, in general, improve the abnormal neuroendocrine profile of patients with chronic heart failure (25). There is usually a decrease in adrenergic activity, as reflected by a decrease in norepinephrine levels. Circulating angiotensin II levels also decrease, and there is evidence that tissue angiotensin II activity is decreased. Because the converting enzyme is the same as kininase II, which is required for the breakdown of bradykinin, converting-enzyme inhibitors increase the bradykinins that contribute to vasodilatation. Furthermore, bradykinin-mediated prostacyclin release is increased, which may also be contributory to vasodilatation with ACE inhibitors. Occasionally, however, angiotensin II activity and aldosterone levels increase despite adequate treatment with ACE inhibitors. It has been suggested that this breakthrough phenomenon may be due to formation of angiotensin II by the activation of a nonconverting enzyme pathway. An enzyme called angiotensin convertase, which is homologous to mast cell chymase, can potentially form angiotensin II and increase both circulating and tissue angiotensins (26). Angiotensin II–mediated aldosterone release may also, therefore, increase. The clinical relevance of this breakthrough phenomenon during converting-enzyme inhibitor therapy remains unclear. Angiotensin-converting enzyme inhibitors can also produce sustained beneficial systemic and coronary hemodynamic effects. Angiotensin-converting enzyme inhibitors, in general, increase coronary blood flow by primary coronary vasodilatation. Coronary vasodilatation with ACE inhibitors is partly mediated by bradykinin because bradykinin antagonists attenuate coronary vasodilatation (27). Angiotensin-converting enzyme inhibitors, in general, decrease myocardial oxygen requirements and oxygen consumption by decreasing arterial pressure, heart rate, and ventricular volume (28). Angiotensin II exerts a positive inotropic effect, and therefore ACE inhibitors potentially can reduce the contractile function. The clinical significance of this negative inotropic effect of ACE inhibitors remains unclear; it might be contributory, however, to a decrease in myocardial oxygen consumption.

Converting-enzyme inhibitors can prevent ventricular remodeling following acute ischemic or nonischemic myocardial injury. In patients with postinfarction left ventricular systolic dysfunction, ACE inhibitor therapy is associated with decreased end-systolic volume, an increase in ejection fraction, and significant attenuation of an increase in left ventricular end-diastolic volume (29). Lack of increase, or even a decrease in left ventricular mass, has also been observed during converting-enzyme inhibitor therapy. Even in patients with established, moderately severe heart failure, ACE inhibitor therapy can increase left ventricular ejection fraction and decrease ventricular dilatation (30). In the Survival and Ventricular Enlargement Trial (31), patients with depressed left ventricular ejection fraction (40% or less) following myocardial infarction were randomized to conventional treatment or to captopril, an ACE inhibitor. Treatment with ACE inhibitors was associated with a substantial reduction in cardiovascular mortality and development of congestive heart failure. Furthermore, there was a decrease in the incidence of acute coronary events, including re-infarction and unstable angina. In the SOLVD Prevention Trial (32), patients with asymptomatic left ventricular systolic dysfunction with ejection fractions of 35% or less were randomized to conventional treatment or to enalapril, another converting-enzyme inhibitor. Treatment with enalapril also decreased the incidence of mortality and hospitalization for treatment of heart failure. There was also a reduction in the acute coronary events. These studies demonstrate, therefore, that ACE inhibitors may be of benefit in preventing the development of heart failure, even in patients with asymptomatic left ventricular systolic dysfunction. In the VA Heart Failure Trial II (33), patients with mild-to-moderate heart failure were ranomized either to receive enalapril or hydralazine/isosorbide dinitrate combination in addition to conventional treatment with digitalis and diuretics. The magnitude of the decrease in mortality with enalapril was greater than that with hydralazine/isosorbide dinitrate. Thus, ACE inhibitors are preferable to the hydralazine/isosorbide dinitrate combination for the initial treatment of patients with symptomatic heart failure. Those patients who cannot tolerate ACE inhibitors or develop unacceptable side effects should be considered for treatment with hydralazine/isosorbide dinitrate.

REFRACTORY HEART FAILURE

Clinicians are likely to encounter patients who remain symptomatic or develop recurrence of congestive heart failure despite adequate treatment with vasodilators or ACE inhibitors and digitalis and diuretics. The therapeutic options for these patients with refractory heart failure are limited (see Table 1). Cardiac transplantation should be considered for the appropriate patients. It cannot be offered to the vast majority of patients with refractory heart failure, however. Several pharmacologic and nonpharmacologic therapeutic maneuvers have been proposed for the treatment of such patients. In patients with apparently refractory heart failure, the potential complicating factors that can diminish the response to therapy should be recognized and corrected. Unexplained anemia, thyrotoxicosis, overt or silent myocardial ischemia, worsening mitral regurgitation, and uncontrolled hypertension are a few complicating factors that can produce refractory heart failure. With increasing severity of heart failure or persistence of congestive state, the doses of loop diuretics should be increased until the systemic venous pressure falls to normal levels and the body weight has stabilized. The doses of furosemide can be titrated to as high as 240 mg twice daily. It is desirable, however, to add thiazide diuretics, particularly metolozone, 2.5 to 10 mg initially, one to three times weekly, and then, if required, once daily. The addition of potassium-sparing diuretics is also helpful, not only to promote diuresis, but also to prevent severe hypokalemia, which tends to occur more frequently when loop and thiazide diuretics are combined. Natriuresis by furosemide is also sometimes potentiated by the addition of ultra-low doses of captopril (1 mg), but not the usual dose of captopril (34). The addition of low-dose dopamine (1–2 mg/kg/min) or dopexamine may sometimes enhance the response of the diuretic drugs. In the presence of markedly reduced cardiac output, an increase in the cardiac output with the use of inotropic, vasodilator, or inodilator drugs may restore the response of the diuretic drugs. In patients with marked persistent elevation of systemic venous pressure, the response of loop diuretics is better when given intravenously rather than orally (35). Constant infusion of furosemide after the loading dose has been found to be better than intermittent intravenous administration in patients with severe heart failure (36). The more severe the heart failure, the more likely the use of multiple diuretic drugs with different mechanisms of action will be required for so-called sequential nephron blockade.

In persistently volume-overloaded states with intractable peripheral edema, elevated venous pressure, and impaired renal function, ultrafiltration or hemodialysis may be considered, provided the blood pressure remains adequate (37,38). Ultrafiltration or hemodialysis can sometimes be performed in hypotensive patients by maintaining adequate blood pressure with the use of a vasopressor, such as dopamine, norepinephrine, or neosynephrine. Ultrafiltration has been reported to produce sustained hemodynamic and beneficial neuroendocrine effects in some patients with severe heart failure. A sustained reduction in plasma norepinephrine level, plasma renin activity, and aldosterone level may occur in some patients. Ultrafiltration, as expected, decreases PCWP and right atrial pressure, with some reduction in arterial pressure. Cardiac output also tends to decrease initially but returns to baseline level within a few days. Systemic vascular resistance also initially increases but returns to baseline. Although ultrafiltration can produce beneficial hemodynamic and neuroendocrine effects in some patients with severe heart failure, their prognoses are not necessarily improved. Thus, ultrafiltration should be considered only in selected patients with persistent volume overload and congestive symptoms and in those who are unresponsive to diuretic therapy.

In some patients with refractory heart failure, aggressive vasodilator and inotropic therapy is necessary, with hemodynamic monitoring to assess response to therapy. Initially, intravenous vasodilators or inotropic agents are used to optimize hemodynamic improvement. In patients with low cardiac output, elevated PCWP, and systemic vascular resistance, but with adequate arterial pressure, intravenous sodium nitroprusside often improves the hemodynamics. In the presence of persistently elevated PCWP despite aggressive diuretic therapy, intravenous nitroglycerin can be added to sodium nitroprusside for further reduction in PCWP. When the increase in cardiac output with intravenous vasodilator therapy is inadequate, the addition of adrenergic agonists, such as dobutamine, or phosphodiesterase inhibitors, such as amrinone or milrinone, may be associated with a further increase in cardiac output. When the optimal hemodynamic improvements are achieved with the use of intravenous vasodilator and inotropic drugs, attempts are made to maintain the same hemodynamic improvement with nonparenteral vasodilator drugs and diuretics. Combination of hydralazine/isosorbide dinitrate and ACE inhibitors occasionally can maintain hemodynamic improvement. The addition of alpha-adrenergic blocking agents, such as prazosin or doxazosin, to ACE inhibitors may also be of benefit in maintaining adequate hemodynamic improvement. A combination of vasodilators with ACE inhibitors, however, not infrequently induces hypotension and renal failure. These patients require frequent and close supervision and follow-up evaluations, including assessment of changes in renal function and adjustment and re-adjustment of diuretic and vasodilator therapy. Intermittent intravenous inotropic therapy with dobutamine, dopamine, amrinone, or milrinone is sometimes necessary to maintain clinical improvement. Although continuous low-dose dobutamine infusion at home has been successful in some selected patients, such therapy may be associated with an increase in mortality (39). Presently, intravenous inotropic therapy in patients with refractory heart failure should be performed under supervision, if feasible.

Although acute and short-term inotropic therapy with the use of adrenergic agents or phosphodiesterase inhibitors produces beneficial hemodynamic and clinical effects, long-term therapy with these agents is associated with increased mortality. In the xamoterol, a partial beta$_1$ agonist trial, patients with moderately severe and severe heart failure were randomized to receive conventional treatment or to receive xamoterol (40). Treatment with xamoterol was associated with an increase in cardiovascular mortality. Similarly, in the Prospective Randomized Milrinone Survival Evaluation (PROMISE) trial patients already treated with digitalis, diuretics, and ACE were randomized to receive either placebo or milrinone, a phosphodiesterase inhibitor (41). Milrinone treatment increased all-cause mortality, and cardiovascular mortality increased by more than 50% in patients with severe heart failure. In the Prospective Randomized Flosequinan Longevity Evaluation (PROFILE) Trial, patients with moderately severe chronic heart failure were randomized to receive either placebo or flosequinan, a directly acting vasodilator agent with significant positive inotropic effect at high doses. The majority of these patients were receiving ACE inhibitors along with digitalis and diuretics before randomization. After initial hemodynamic and clinical improvement with flosequinan, the clinical status of the patients receiving the active drug deteriorated and a higher mortality was observed in patients receiving flosequinan (41a). Thus, long-term therapy with nonglycosidic positive inotropic agents does not appear to be beneficial.

Recently, a new inotropic agent, vesnarinone, has been reported to improve the prognosis of patients with moderately severe chronic heart failure due to impaired left ventricular systolic function (42). The mechanism of action of vesnarinone is different from those of adrenergic inotropic agents and phosphodiesterase inhibitors. It appears to decrease transmembrane potassium current and increases intracellular sodium and also action potential duration (43). Its phosphodiesterase-inhibiting effect is relatively minor. In a prospective randomized trial, the addition of low-dose vesnarinone (60 mg/daily) to conventional treatment (digitalis, diuretics, and ACE inhibitors) was associated with a substantial reduction in mortality (44). The use of a larger dose of vesnarinone, however, caused a marked increase in mortality. Thus, the role of vesnarinone treatment for the management of patients with refractory heart failure remains unresolved.

Beta-blocker therapy has been shown to improve clinical status, exercise tolerance, and left ventricular systolic function in some patients with chronic left ventricular failure. The rationale for the beta-blocker therapy is to attenuate the adverse effects of enhanced systemic and cardiac adrenergic activity. Despite the potential deleterious effects on cardiac function due to their negative inotropic effects, beta-adrenergic receptor antagonists have been shown to improve left ventricular function and symptoms in patients with chronic heart failure due to dilated cardiomyopathy (45). Left ventricular ejection fraction tends to improve, and the increase in total stroke volume results from a decrease in end-systolic volume, as end-diastolic dimensions and volumes usually remain unchanged (46). In patients who tolerate chronic beta-blocker therapy, cardiac output tends to increase along with a decrease in left ventricular end-diastolic pressure, PCWP, and systemic vascular resistance (47). In addition to improved hemodynamics and left ventricular function, symptomatic improvement also occurs along with an increase in exercise tolerance. In most studies, metoprolol, a cardioselective beta-adrenergic antagonist, has been used; other beta adrenergic antagonists, however, have also been shown to produce similar beneficial hemodynamic and clinical effects (48). Bucindolol, a nonselective beta-adrenergic blocking drug with direct vasodilatory effects (48); labetalol, a combined alpha- and beta-adrenergic blocking agent (49); carvidolol, an alpha- and beta-adrenoreceptor antagonist (50); and nevivolol and celiprolol, beta-adrenergic blocking agents with vasodilating properties (51,52) have also been shown to improve left ventricular systolic function and symptomatic status in patients with heart failure.

Beta-adrenergic blocking drugs, however, do not always improve cardiac function and symptoms or exercise tolerance in patients with chronic heart failure (53). During the introduction of beta-adrenergic blocking therapy, a rapid hemodynamic and clinical deterioration can occur. Administration of full beta-blocking doses may decrease cardiac output and blood pressure and increase left ventricular filling pressure, along with an increase in plasma catecholamine levels. Patients who are clinically unstable or who are obviously symptomatic at rest may not tolerate even lower doses of beta-blocking drugs. As many as 20% of patients may be intolerant to even lower doses of metoprolol during the initiation of therapy.

The beneficial effects of chronic beta-blocker therapy on the prognosis of patients with chronic heart failure have not been established. Initial uncontrolled studies reported an improved prognosis in patients with nonischemic cardiomyopathy (54). Controlled prospective randomized studies have failed to demonstrate any survival benefit in patients with moderately severe heart failure (New York Heart Association classes II and III) (55). A reduction in the need for and delay of cardiac transplantation, however, has been observed with chronic beta-blocker therapy (55). The mechanism for improvement in ventricular systolic function and symptomatic status of patients with chronic heart failure using beta-blocker therapy has not been clarified. Upregulation of the beta-adrenoreceptors, increased myocardial contractile response, improved substrate utilization and myocardial energetics, and improvement in left ventricular diastolic function may all be contributory (56,57). The selection of patients appropriate for beta-blocker therapy is difficult in clinical practice. Patients with overt heart failure with depressed left ventricular systolic function, but who are clinically stable, may be the most appropriate candidates for beta-blocker therapy. It needs to be emphasized that beta-blocker therapy alone is unlikely to be of benefit, and all patients selected for beta-blocker therapy should also be treated with diuretics, digitalis, and ACE inhibitors, if feasible.

Amiodarone is a type III antiarrhythmic drug that also possesses a weak, negative inotropic effect. It also has direct vasodilatory and nonspecific antiadrenergic properties. It exerts beneficial effects on coronary hemodynamic and myocardial energetics and can potentially relieve myocardial ischemia. Acute intravenous administration of amiodarone or the use of large doses of oral amiodarone can transiently depress left ventricular systolic function (58). Oral long-term low-dose administration of amiodarone, however, is not usually associated with any significant deterioration of hemodynamics and left ventricular function at rest or during exercise. Indeed, a significant increase in left ventricular ejection fraction can occur in some patients with chronic low-dose amiodarone therapy (59). Uncontrolled studies have reported a beneficial effect of amiodarone therapy on survival of patients with chronic heart failure due to left ventricular systolic dysfunction (60). The results of the prospective studies, however, have been inconclusive. Some studies have reported a decrease in mortality with amiodarone therapy, and others have reported no survival benefit (61–63). The effect of amiodarone therapy in patients with refractory heart failure, however, has not been evaluated. In selected patients with severe refractory heart failure that is unresponsive to digitalis, diuretic, and vasodilator or ACE inhibitor therapy, amiodarone has been reported to improve left ventricular systolic function and survival (64). The beneficial effects of amiodarone are not observed before 4 to 6 weeks of chronic maintenance therapy. This is probably related to the pharmacodynamic and pharmacokinetic features of amiodarone. Amiodarone may be of particular benefit in patients who require long-term nonglycosidic inotropic therapy. It might be of benefit in patients who are in atrial fibrillation with a rapid ventricular response.

Patients suitable for amiodarone therapy are difficult to determine in clinical practice. Those patients who are in atrial fibrillation with a rapid ventricular response, despite adequate digitalis therapy, may be appropriate candidates for long-term amiodarone treatment. Patients who cannot tolerate beta-blocker therapy may also be candidates for long-term amiodarone treatment. Long-term amiodarone treatment, however, may produce serious side effects, such as pulmonary fibrosis, hypo- and hyperthyroidism, hepatic dysfunction, and polyneuropathy. Skin discoloration and corneal deposits are frequent but are not contraindications for amiodarone therapy. Extreme sinus bradycardia or atrioventricular dissociation may occur, particularly with concomitant digoxin therapy.

Dual-chamber pacing (65,66) has been reported to improve hemodynamics and symptoms in patients with severe heart failure due to dilated cardiomyopathy. The clinical experience with such therapy, however, is extremely limited, and preliminary experience suggests that only patients with prolonged PR interval and diastolic mitral regurgitation are likely to benefit from dual-chamber pacing with appropriate and effectively timed atrial contraction. Doppler echocardiographic evaluation is necessary for the selection of patients likely to benefit from dual-chamber pacing.

SUMMARY

All symptomatic patients with chronic heart failure due to left ventricular systolic dysfunction should be treated initially with digitalis, diuretics, and ACE inhibitors. Those patients who cannot tolerate ACE inhibitors should be considered for hydralazine/isosorbide dinitrate combination therapy. Patients who become refractory to triple therapy may benefit from beta-blocker or amiodarone therapy. Whenever feasible, however, ACE inhibitor therapy should be continued with beta-blockers or amiodarone. Some patients require combination vasodilator therapy for symptomatic and hemodynamic improvement. The impact of such therapy on the prognosis of patients needs to be emphasized.

REFERENCES

1. Minotti JR, Dudley G. Pathophysiology of exercise intolerance and the role of exercise training in congestive heart failure. *Curr Opinion Cardiol* 1993;8:397.
2. Packer M. The neurohormonal hypothesis: a theory to explain the mechanism of disease progression in heart failure. *J Am Coll Cardiol* 1992;20:248.
3. Chatterjee K, Viquerat CE, Daly P. Neurohumoral abnormalities in heart failure. *Heart Failure* 1985;1:69.
4. Motwanti JG, McAlpine H, Kennedy N, et al. Plasma brain natriuretic peptide as an indicator for angiotensin-converting enzyme inhibition after myocardial infarction. *Lancet* 1993;341:1109.
5. Weber KT, Brilla CG. Pathologic hypertrophy and cardiac interstitium. Fibrosis and renin–angiotensin aldosterone system. *Circulation* 1991;83:1849.
6. Lamas GA, Pfeffer MA. Left ventricular remodeling after acute myocardial infarction: clinical course and beneficial effects of angiotensin-converting enzyme inhibition. *Am Heart J* 1991;121: 1194.
7. DeMarco T, Chatterjee K, Rouleau JL, et al. Abnormal coronary hemodynamics and myocardial energetics in patients with chronic heart failure caused by ischemic heart disease and dilated cardiomyopathy. *Am Heart J* 1988;115:809.
8. Treasure CB, Vita JA, Cox DA, et al. Endothelium-dependent dilation of the coronary microvasculature is impaired in dilated cardiomyopathy. *Circulation* 1990;81:772.
9. Bristow MR, Ginsberg R, Minobe W, et al. Decreased catecholamine sensitivity and beta adrenergic receptor density in failing human hearts. *N Engl J Med* 1982;307:205.
10. Cohn JN, Levine TB, Olivari MT, et al. Plasma norepinephrine as a guide to prognosis in patients with chronic congestive heart failure. *N Engl J Med* 1984;311:819.

11. Rockman HA, Juneau C, Chatterjee K, et al. Long-term predictors of sudden and low output death in chronic congestive heart failure secondary to coronary artery disease. *Am J Cardiol* 1989;64: 1344.
12. Mujais SK, Nora NA, Levin ML. Principles and clinical uses of diuretic therapy. *Prog Cardiovasc Dis* 1992;35:221.
13. Gheorghiade M, Hall V, Lakier J, et al. Comparative hemodynamic and neurohormonal effects of intravenous captopril and digoxin and their combinations in patients with severe heart failure. *J Am Coll Cardiol* 1989;13:134.
14. Ferguson DW, Berg WJ, Sanders JS, et al. Sympathoinhibitory responses to digitalis glycosides in heart failure patients: direct evidence from sympathetic neural recordings. *Circulation* 1989;80:65.
15. The Captopril–Digoxin Multicenter Research Group. Comparative effects of therapy with captopril and digoxin in patients with mild to moderate heart failure. *JAMA* 1988;259:539.
16. DiBianco R, Shabetai R, Kostuk W, et al. A comparison of oral milrinone, digoxin and their combination in the treatment of patients with chronic heart failure. *N Engl J Med* 1989;320:677.
17. Uretsky BF, Young JB, Shahidi FE, et al. Randomized study assessing the effect of digoxin withdrawal in patients with mild to moderate congestive heart failure: results of the PROVED Trial. *J Am Coll Cardiol* 1993;22:955.
18. Packer M, Gheorghiade M, Young JB, et al. Withdrawal of digoxin from patients with chronic heart failure treated with angiotensin-converting-enzyme inhibitors. *N Engl J Med* 1993;312:1.
19. Jaeschke R, Oxman AD, Guyatt GH. To what extent do congestive heart failure patients in sinus rhythm benefit from digoxin therapy? A systemic overview and meta-analysis. *Am J Med* 1990; 88:279.
20. Chatterjee K, Parmley WW. The role of vasodilator therapy in heart failure. *Prog Cardiovasc Dis* 1992;35:221.
21. Packer M, Meller J, Gorlin R, et al. Hemodynamic and clinical tachyphylaxis to prazosin-mediated afterload reduction in severe chronic congestive heart failure. *Circulation* 1979;59:531.
22. Cohn JN, Archibald D, Ziesche G, et al. Effect of vasodilator therapy on mortality in chronic congestive heart failure: results of a Veterans Administration Cooperative Study (V-HEFT). *N Engl J Med* 1986;314:1547.
23. The SOLVD Investigators. Effect of enalapril on survival in patients with reduced left ventricular ejection fractions and congestive heart failure. *N Engl J Med* 1991;325:293.
24. Elkayam U, Amin J, Mehra A, et al. A prospective, randomized, double-blind cross-over study to compare the efficacy and safety of chronic nifedipine therapy with that of isosorbide dinitrate and their combination in the treatment of chronic congestive heart failure. *Circulation* 1990;82:1954.
25. Goldstein RE, Boccuzzi SJ, Cruess D, et al. Diltiazem increases late onset congestive heart failure in post-infarction patients with early reduction in ejection fraction. *Circulation* 1991;83:52.
26. Dzau VJ, Packer M, Swartz SL, et al. Prostaglandins in relationship to renin–angiotensin system and hyponatremia. *N Engl J Med* 1984;310:347.
27. Ruocco NA Jr, Yu TK, Bergelson BA, et al. Augmentation of coronary blood flow by ACE inhibition enhanced by endogenous bradykinin but not by angiotensin II receptor blockade. *Circulation* 1992;86[Suppl I]:640.
28. Craeger MA, Halperin JL, Bernard DB, et al. Acute regional circulatory and renal hemodynamic effects of converting enzyme inhibition in patients with congestive heart failure. *Circulation* 1981; 64:483.
29. Sharpe N, Smith H, Murphy J, et al. Early prevention of left ventricular dysfunction after myocardial infarction with angiotensin-converting enzyme inhibition. *Lancet* 1991;337:872.
30. Kris-Etherton PM, Kisloff L, Kassouf RA, et al. Teaching principles and cost of sodium-restricted diets. *J Am Diet Assoc* 1982;80:55.
31. Pfeffer MA, Braunwald E, Moye LA, et al. Effect of captopril on mortality and morbidity in patients with left ventricular dysfunction after myocardial infarction: results of the survival and ventricular enlargement trial. *N Engl J Med* 1992;327:669.
32. The SOLVD Investigators. Effect of enalapril on mortality and the development of heart failure in asymptomatic patients with reduced left ventricular ejection fractions. *N Engl J Med* 1992;327:682.
33. Cohn JN, Johnson G, Zeische S, et al. A comparison of enalapril with hydralazine-isosorbide dinitrate in the treatment of chronic congestive heart failure. *N Engl J Med* 1991;325:303.
34. Motwani JG, Fenwick MK, Morton JJ, et al. Furosemide-induced natriuresis is augmented by ultra low dose captopril but not by standard doses of captopril in chronic heart failure. *Circulation* 1992;86:439.

35. Vasko MR, Brown-Cartwright D, Knochel PA, et al. Furosemide absorption altered in decompensated congestive heart failure. *Ann Intern Med* 1985;102:314.
36. Lahav M, Regev A, Ra'Anani P, et al. Intermittent administration of furosemide vs. continuous infusion preceded by a loading dose for congestive heart failure. *Chest* 1992;102:725.
37. Simpson IA, Rae AP, Gribben J, et al. Ultrafiltration in the management of refractory congestive heart failure. *Br Heart J* 1986;55:334.
38. Akiba T, Taniguchi K, Marumo F, et al. Clinical significance of renal hemodynamics in severe congestive heart failure: responsiveness to ultrafiltration therapies. *Jpn Circ J* 1989;53:191.
39. Dies F, Krell MJ, Whitlow P, et al. Intermittent dobutamine in ambulatory out-patients with chronic cardiac failure. *Circulation* 1986;74[Suppl II]:II-39.
40. The Xamoterol in Severe Heart Failure Study Group: Xamoterol in severe heart failure. *Lancet* 1990;336:1.
41. Packer M, Carver JR, Rodeheffer RJ, et al. Effect of oral milrinone on mortality in severe chronic heart failure. *N Engl J Med* 1991;325:1468.
41a. Packer M, Rouleau J, Swedberg K, et al. Effect of flosequinan on survival in chronic heart failure: preliminary results of the profile study. *Circulation* 1993;I-301:88.
42. Feldman AM, Bristow MR, Parmley WW, et al. Results of a multi-center study of OPC-8212 in chronic congestive heart failure. *Circulation* 1992;86:I-374.
43. Feldman AM, Baughman KL, Lee WK, et al. Usefulness of OPC-8212, a quinoline derivative for chronic congestive heart failure in patients with ischemic heart disease or idiopathic dilated cardiomyopathy. *Am J Cardiol* 1991;68:1203.
44. Feldman AM, Bristow MR, Parmley WW, et al. Effects of vesnarinone on morbidity and mortality in patients with heart failure. *N Engl J Med* 1993;329:149.
45. Fowler MB. Beta blockers in cardiac failure. *Curr Opinion Cardiol* 1991;6:368.
46. Engelmeier RS, O'Connell JB, Walsh R, et al. Improvement in symptoms and exercise tolerance by metoprolol in patients with dilated cardiomyopathy. A double-blind, randomized placebo-controlled trial. *Circulation* 1985;72:536.
47. Waagstein F, Caidahl K, Wallentin I, et al. Long-term B-blockade in dilated cardiomyopathy: effects of short- and long-term metoprolol treatment followed by withdrawal and readministration of metoprolol. *Circulation* 1989;80:551.
48. Gilbert EM, Anderson JL, Deitchman D, et al. Long-term beta blocker vasodilator therapy improves cardiac function in idiopathic dilated cardiomyopathy. A double-blind, randomized study of bucindolol versus placebo. *Am J Med* 1990;88:223.
49. Leung WH, Lau CP, Wong CK, et al. Improvement in exercise performance and hemodynamics by labetalol in patients with idiopathic dilated cardiomyopathy. *Am Heart J* 1990;199:884.
50. Dasgupta P, Broadhurst P, Raftery EB, et al. Value of carvedilol in congestive heart failure secondary to coronary artery disease. *Am J Cardiol* 1990;66:1118.
51. Wisenbaugh T, Katz I, Davis J, et al. Long-term (3 month) effects of nebivolol on cardiac performance in patients with dilated cardiomyopathy. *Circulation* 1992;86[Suppl I]I-645.
52. Chatterjee K. Potential use of third-general B-blockers in heart failure. *J Cardiovasc Pharmacol* 1989;14[Suppl 7]:S22.
53. Currie PF, Kelly MJ, McKenzie A, et al. Oral beta-adrenergic blockade with metoprolol in chronic severe dilated cardiomyopathy. *J Am Coll Cardiol* 1984;3:203.
54. Swedberg K, Hjalmarson A, Waagstein F, et al. Prolongation of survival in congestive cardiomyopathy by receptor blockade. *Lancet* 1979;1:1374.
55. Waagstein F, Bristow MR, Swedberg K, et al. Beneficial effects of metoprolol in idiopathic dilated cardiomyopathy. *Lancet* 1993;342:1441.
56. Eichhorn EJ, Bedotto J, Mallow CR, et al. Effect of B-adrenergic blockade on myocardial function and energetics in congestive heart failure: improvements in hemodynamic, contractile, and diastolic performance with bucindolol. *Circulation* 1989;82:473.
57. Fowler MB, Bristow MR, Laser JA, et al. Beta blocker therapy in severe heart failure: improvement related to beta, adrenergic receptor up regulation? *Circulation* 1984;70[Suppl 2]:112.
58. Schwartz A, Shen E, Morady F, et al. Hemodynamic effects of intravenous amiodarone in patients with depressed left ventricular function and recurrent ventricular tachycardia. *Am Heart J* 1983;106: 848.
59. Hamer AW, Arkles LB, Johns JA. Beneficial effects of low dose amiodarone in patients with congestive heart failure: a placebo controlled trial. *J Am Coll Cardiol* 1989;14:1768.

60. Dargie HJ, Cleland JGF, Leckie BJ, et al. Relation of arrhythmias and electrolyte abnormalities to survival in patients with severe chronic heart failure. *Circulation* 1987;76[Suppl IV]:IV-98.
61. Nicklas JM, McKenna WH, Stewart RA, et al. Prospective double-blind placebo-controlled trial of low-dose amiodarone in patients with severe heart failure and asymptomatic frequent ventricular ectopy. *Am Heart J* 1991;122:1016.
62. Teo K, Yusuf S, Furberg C. Overview of randomized trials of low-dose amiodarone on mortality in cardiac patients. *Circulation* 1992;86[Suppl I]:I-534.
63. Nul DR, Doval H, Grancelli H, et al. Amiodarone reduces mortality in severe heart failure. *Circulation* 1993;88:I-603(abst).
64. Galli FC, DeMarco T, Chatterjee K. Does amiodarone improve survival of patients with refractory heart failure due to dilated cardiomyopathy? *Clin Res* 1993;42(1):38A.
65. Hochleitner M, Hortnagl H, Ng KC, et al. Usefulness of physiologic dual-chamber pacing in drug resistant idiopathic dilated cardiomyopathy. *Am J Cardiol* 1990;66:198.
66. Brecker SJD, Ziao HB, Sparrow J, et al. Effects of dual-chamber pacing with short atrioventricular delay in dilated cardiomyopathy. *Lancet* 1992;340:1308.

The Failing Heart, edited by N. S. Dhalla,
R. E. Beamish, N. Takeda, and M. Nagano.
Lippincott-Raven Publishers, Philadelphia © 1995.

28

Clinical Implications of Inotropic Agents in Heart Failure

Marrick L. Kukin

*Heart Failure Program, Coronary Care Unit, Mount Sinai Medical Center,
New York, New York 10029-6574*

The consequences of impaired left ventricular function lead to the clinical syndrome of congestive heart failure. With decreased left ventricular contractility, there is a subsequent decrease in cardiac output and stroke volume. Among the many pathophysiologic responses following these events are both neurohormonal activation and decreased renal perfusion. The acute effect of neurohormonal activation is to increase systemic vascular resistance and thereby maintain blood pressure. This acute response to preserve blood pressure, however, when unchecked, can lead to long-term adverse consequences by increasing afterload and causing further left ventricular dysfunction. Similarly, decreases in stroke volume cause decreased renal perfusion and subsequent salt and water retention as an attempt to maintain blood volume. Whereas these responses may acutely benefit stroke volume, the long-term consequence of sodium and fluid retention is peripheral edema.

Treatments for heart failure have been targeted to counteract these pathophysiologic consequences of impaired left ventricular function. The angiotensin-converting enzyme (ACE) inhibitors block the renin–angiotensin system and have proven beneficial in reducing the morbidity and mortality of heart failure. Diuretics counteract the renal response of salt and water retention. However, neither of these pharmacologic approaches directly affects the underlying problem of impaired left ventricular function.

The goal of inotropic therapy has been to address the impairment of left ventricular function and thereby both improve cardiac performance and reduce the symptoms of heart failure. Congestive heart failure, however, is not purely a problem with the left ventricle but rather is a syndrome of complex interactions between the heart, the peripheral vasculature, the kidneys, neurohormonal alterations, and the baroreceptors. This complex grouping of abnormalities may explain the problems that have been seen thus far with inotropic therapy in clinical trials in the treatment of congestive heart failure.

Although inotropic agents have shown benefit in small hemodynamic and exercise trials, they have not shown consistent benefits when tested in mortality trials. Inotropic agents can improve contractility. This "benefit," however, appears to be at the expense of energy depletion (1), proarrhythmia, and increased mortality.

In this chapter we review studies looking at β-agonists, phosphodiesterase inhibitors, and two compounds with vasodilating and inotropic properties—flosequinan and vesnarinone—to illustrate the risks and benefits of inotropic therapy in heart failure.

THE β-AGONIST DOBUTAMINE

Continuous and intermittent therapy with dobutamine has been shown to improve cardiac output and to lower pulmonary wedge pressure and systemic vascular resistance (2–4). Dobutamine, however, is proarrhythmic, which is true of most inotropic agents. One study, by Dies et al. (5), enrolled 60 outpatients with class III and IV heart failure to receive intermittent dobutamine or placebo as a continuous infusion for 2 days a week in a 24-week randomized, double-blind trial. By an intention-to-treat analysis, 20 patients died in this study: 5 patients on placebo, 13 on dobutamine, and 2 who crossed from placebo to dobutamine ($p = 0.147$). In an actual treatment analysis, 5 of 30 patients on placebo and 15 of 38 patients on dobutamine died ($p = 0.08$). This adverse effect on mortality caused this trial to be terminated prematurely.

The parenteral route of administration and the proarrthymic effect of dobutamine have relegated its use primarily to intensive care and monitored units for acute exacerbations of congestive heart failure.

PHOSPHODIESTERASE INHIBITORS

The use of phosphodiesterase inhibitors as inotropic agents has shown benefits when endpoints such as exercise and hemodynamics have been evaluated (6–11). The phosphodiesterase inhibitors, however, also have been shown to be arrhythmogenic, and therefore, their potential adverse effect on mortality was questioned.

The Prospective Randomized Milrinone Survival Evaluation (PROMISE) trial (12) is illustrative of this problem with phosphodiesterase inhibitors. In this trial, 1,088 patients with class III and IV heart failure on background therapy of digoxin, diuretics, and ACE inhibitors were randomized to receive milrinone (10 mg po qid) or placebo. This trial was prematurely terminated by the Data and Safety Monitoring Board (DSMB) due to a 28% increase in all-cause mortality ($p = 0.038$) and a 34% increase in cardiovascular mortality ($p = 0.016$). This effect was most marked in the class IV patients, with a 53% increase in mortality ($p = 0.006$).

In this study, Holter monitors were obtained at baseline and after 1 week, 1 month, and 6 months of therapy. Three proarrhythmia criteria were prespecified (13) in this study: (a) increase of ventricular premature beats, (b) increased runs of ventricular tachycardia (VT), and (c) the increased length of VT, defined as a doubling of the length of the longest baseline VT event. All three of these criteria occurred more frequently with milrinone compared with placebo ($p<0.05$). Milrinone increased the risk of sudden death by 69% ($p<0.005$). Thus, there was a significant association between the worsening of asymptomatic arrhythmias and mortality. This study showed that milrinone increased mortality, primarily via a proarrhythmic effect.

FLOSEQUINAN

Flosequinan is a novel vasodilator that has shown significant hemodynamic effects (14–16). Its mechanism of action appears to involve the inosityl triphosphate (IP3 pathway) and protein kinase C, which caused vasodilatation by its effect on the endothelium and endothelial-derived relaxation factors (17).

The drug was also shown in acute intravenous studies to be a positive inotropic agent (18). Pressure volume loops in 14 of 15 patients showed a shift upward and to the left after administration of intravenous flosequinan at a dose demonstrating increased contractility. Given the adverse mortality effects seen with other inotropes, the effects of this drug with both vasodilating and inotropic properties were questioned.

An international trial, the Prospective Randomized Flosequinan Longevity Evaluation Study, (19) was undertaken to evaluate the effect of this drug on mortality. In this trial, 2,345 patients were randomized to receive flosequinan (100 mg/d) or matching placebo. All patients were on a background therapy of digoxin, diuretic, and ACE inhibitors. For those patients who could not tolerate the 100-mg dose of flosequinan, there was a fallback dose of 75 mg (which 20% of the patients received). The initial evaluation period of tolerability was single-blind for 1 month, and then patients were double-blind randomized to flosequinan or placebo. The trial was prematurely terminated in April 1993 when the DSMB found a 40% excess in mortality in patients receiving the 100-mg dose of the medication compared with placebo ($p=0.0004$). Holter monitors were not obtained in this trial, and the final relationship of sudden death and drug therapy has not yet been reported. There was, however, a clear increase in mortality with the active therapy.

VESNARINONE

Although the mechanism of vesnarinone is not precisely defined, it appears to have some minimal effect on phosphodiesterase inhibition, with some blockade of the sodium and potassium channels and blocking effects on the cytokine system (20). The mortality trial with vesnarinone, published by Feldman et al. (21), showed significantly different effects with high and low dosages of the medication. This trial was initially structured with three arms—placebo, 60 mg, and 120 mg. After 253 patients were randomized to the three groups, the 120-mg treatment group was terminated due to a significant excess in mortality in those patients on this high dose. The trial continued to randomize patients to 60 mg versus placebo, however, until a total of 477 patients were randomized to either 60 mg of vesnarinone or placebo.

When the placebo versus 60-mg arms were analyzed, there was a 62% reduction in the risk of dying from all-cause mortality ($p = 0.003$). The significant dose-response differences seen in the vesnarinone trial, where 120 mg caused excess mortality and 60 mg decreased mortality, compared with placebo raises as many questions as it answers. For this and other reasons, the Food and Drug Administration has asked for further placebo-controlled data before approving this drug for heart failure use.

SUMMARY

These four categories of drugs illustrate the potential benefits and significant problems associated with pharmacologic attempts to increase inotropic forces. The increase achieved in contractility has a significant "cost"—energy depletion, proarrthymia, and increased mortality.

The examples given here also illustrate another problem encountered in new drug development—Do acute dose-response relationships persist when a drug is used chronically? Acutely higher dosages of pharmacologic substances appear to increase both the hemodynamic and the inotropic effects of these agents. Whether the same relationship holds in the chronic setting is unproven. Furthermore, the acute safety of drugs may be quite different from potential toxicities that may develop with chronic dosing. This raises several difficult problems in evaluating a drug: (a) Are there different mechanisms of action at different dosages? (b) are there active metabolites of a single agent? and (c) is there significant tissue accumulation of the compound?

In conclusion, whereas the attempt to improve heart failure by directly improving contractility may be theoretically appealing, there have been numerous and consistent adverse effects. This is especially true when assessing the ultimate endpoint of mortality. Whether the safety and efficacy of a new inotropic agent can be evaluated without a costly and time-consuming mortality trial remains a significant scientific and regulatory dilemma. Research continues to develop drugs that can improve contractility and thereby improve the symptoms of heart failure without the adverse consequences of increasing mortality. Given the described examples and the potential energy costs associated with augmenting intropy in a failing heart, however, this remains an elusive goal for any drug that is mechanistically a "pure" inotrope. Perhaps there will be greater yield in drug development for heart failure if the focus is not solely on the problem of contractility but rather encompasses the broader interactions of the heart, the peripheral vasculature, the kidney, neurohormones (including cytokines), and baroreceptors. Only when we view congestive heart failure as a complex syndrome of multiple interactions arising from an initial insult to the myocardium can we hope to gain insight into the pathophysiology of the disease and thereby make significant progress in our therapeutic approaches.

REFERENCES

1. Katz AM. Cardiomyopathy of overload: a major determinant of prognosis in congestive heart failure. *N Engl J Med* 1990;322:100–110.
2. Krell MJ, Kline EM, Bates ER, et al. Intermittent, ambulatory dobutamine infusions in patients with severe congestive heart failure. *Am Heart J* 1984;112:787–791.
3. Applefeld MM, Newman KA, Grove WR, et al. Intermittent, continuous outpatient dobutamine infusion in the management of congestive heart failure. *Congest Heart Failure* 1983;51:455–458.
4. Leier CV, Huss P, Lewis RP, Unverferth DV. Drug-induced conditioning in congestive heart failure. *Circulation* 1982;65:1382–1387.
5. Dies F, Krell MJ, Whitlow P, et al. Intermittent dobutamine in ambulatory outpatients with chronic cardiac failure. *Circulation* 1986;74[Supp II]:II-38–II-152.
6. Dibianco R, Shabetai R, Silverman BD, Leier CV, Benotti JR. Oral amrinone for the treatment of chronic congestive heart failure: results of a multicenter randomized double-blind and placebo-controlled withdrawal study. *J Am Coll Cardiol* 1984;4:855–866.
7. Massie B, Bourassa M, Dibianco R, et al. Long-term oral administration of amrinone for congestive heart failure: lack of efficacy in a multicenter controlled trial. *Circulation* 1985;71:963–971.
8. Simonton CA, Chatterjee K, Cody RJ, et al. Milrinone in congestive heart failure: acute and chronic hemodynamic and clinical evaluation. *J Am Coll Cardiol* 1985;6:453–459.
9. LeJemtel TH, Maskin CS, Mancini D, Sinoway L, Feld H, Chadwick B. Systemic and regional hemodynamic effects of captopril and milrinone administered alone and concomitantly in patients with heart failure. *Circulation* 1985;72:364–369.
10. Uretsky BF, Jessup M, Konstam MA, et al. Multicenter trial of oral enoximone in patients with moderate to moderately severe congestive heart failure. *Circulation* 1990;82:774–780.
11. Swan HJC. Enoximone in chronic heart failure. *Circulation* 1990;82:1049–1050.
12. Packer M, Carver JR, Rodenheffer RJ, et al. Effects of oral milrinone on mortality in severe chronic heart failure. *N Engl J Med* 1991;325:1468–1475.
13. Massie BM, Podrid PJ, Hendrix GH, et al. Does asymptomatic worsening of arrhythmia predict sudden death in heart failure? Evidence for clinically significant proarrhythmia during milrinone therapy. *J Am Coll Cardiol* 1992;19:78A.
14. Falotico R, Haertlein BJ, Lakas-Weiss CS, et al. Positive inotropic and hemodynamic properties of flosequinan, a new vasodilator, and a sulfone metabolite. *J Cardiovasc Pharmacol* 1989;14:412–418.
15. Corin WJ, Monrad ES, Strom JA, et al. Flosequinan: a vasodilator with positive inotropic activity. *Am Heart J* 1991;121:537–540.
16. Kessler PD, Packer M. Hemodynamic effects of BTS 494665, a new long-acting systemic vasodilator drug, in patients with severe congestive heart failure. *Am Heart J* 1987;113:137.
17. Lang D, Lewis MJ. The effects of flosequinan on endothelin-1 induced changes in inositol 1,4,5-triphosphate levels and protein kinase C activity in rat aorta. *Eur J Pharmacol* 1992;226:259–264.
18. Burstein S, Semigran MJ, Dec GW, Boucher CA, Fifer MA. Positive inotropic and lusitropic effects of intravenous flosequinan in patients with heart failure. *J Am Coll Cardiol* 1992;20:822–829.
19. Swedburg K, Packer M, Rouleau J. Oral presentations on PROFILE study (Prospective Randomized Flosequinan Longevity Evaluation Study) American College of Cardiology Scientific Session. March 14, 1994, Altanta, Georgia.
20. Matsumori A, Shioi T, Yamada T, Matsui S, Sasayama S. Vesnarinone, an inotropic agent, inhibits cytokine production by stimulated human blood from patients with heart failure. *Circulation* 1994;89:955–958.
21. Feldman AM, Bristow MR, Parmley WW, et al. Effects of vesnarinone on morbidity and mortality in patients with heart failure. *N Engl J Med* 1993;329:149–155.

The Failing Heart, edited by N. S. Dhalla,
R. E. Beamish, N. Takeda, and M. Nagano.
Lippincott-Raven Publishers, Philadelphia © 1995.

29

Subcellular Mechanism of Action of a Novel Cardiotonic Quinolinone Derivative OPC-18790 in Mammalian Cardiac Muscle: Selective Inhibition of Isozymes of Phosphodiesterase and Contractile Regulation

Masao Endoh, Yumi Katano, and Youichi Kawabata

*Department of Pharmacology, Yamagata University School of Medicine,
Yamagata 990-23 Japan*

Adenosine $3',5'$-monophosphate (cyclic AMP) plays a crucial role in regulation of cardiac contractile function induced by β-adrenoceptor agonists and certain cardiotonic agents including cyclic AMP phosphodiesterase (PDE) inhibitors. Cyclic AMP PDE, the enzyme that hydrolyzes cyclic AMP to inactive $5'$-AMP, has been shown to be composed of several isozymes in myocardial cells (1–3). These isozymes may share differential physiological roles in regulation of the contractile function in intact myocardial cells (4–6). Selective inhibition of PDE isozymes is responsible for the functional modulation, and a number of newly developed cardiotonic agents such as amrinone, milrinone, enoximone, and piroximone selectively inhibit PDE III (7–13). It has been demonstrated that the distribution of soluble and particulate PDE III shows a wide range of species-dependent variation in mammalian myocardial cells and that rat cardiac muscle lacks particulate PDE III (11). In rat ventricular myocardium, Ro 20-1724 and rolipram—selective PDE IV inhibitors—are extremely effective in enhancing the cyclic AMP accumulation and positive inotropic effect induced by isoproterenol (14).

In the present study, the inotropic profile of a new cardiotonic quinolinone derivative OPC-18790 [(±)-6-(3-[3,4-dimethoxybenzylamino]-2-hydroxypropoxy)-2 (1H)-quinolinone] (Fig. 1, upper panel) was investigated in rat and rabbit ventricular muscle in comparison with selective PDE inhibitors: milrinone, rolipram, Ro 20-1724, another quinolinone derivative Y-20487 [6-(3,6-dihydro-2-oxo-2H-1,3,4-thiadiazin-5-y1)-3,4-dihydro-2(1H)-quinolinone] (Fig. 1, lower panel) (15), and a nonselective inhibitor 3-isobutyl-1-methylxanthine (IBMX). In previous studies, a quinolinone cardiotonic vesnarinone (OPC-8212) that elicits the positive inotropic

FIG. 1. Chemical structures of OPC-18790 and Y-20487.

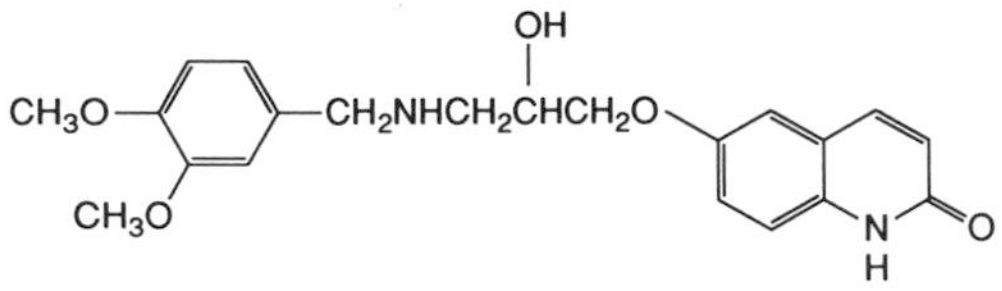

effect by selective inhibition of PDE III (16,17) has been demonstrated to be an effective agent for the treatment of patients with congestive heart failure (18,19). Vesnarinone, however, is water-insoluble, and therefore only oral preparation is available. OPC-18790 has been developed as a water-soluble quinolinone cardiotonic (20,21).

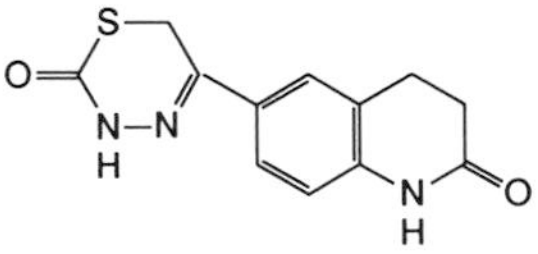

MATERIALS AND METHODS

Three preparations were used to investigate the action and interaction of the compounds on the cyclic AMP level and force of contraction: isolated rat cardiac myocytes, rat right ventricular papillary muscles, and the isolated right ventricular papillary muscle of the rabbit.

Determination of Cyclic AMP in Isolated Rat Ventricular Cardiomyocytes

Male Wistar rats (190–240 g) were lightly anesthetized with ether and heparinized (500 U i.p.). Hearts were quickly removed, and retrograde perfusion was performed through the aorta with Krebs-Henseleit solution containing collagenase (70 U/ml) and 0.1% bovine serum albumin (BSA) in the presence of 50 µM Ca^{2+} according to the method of Powell and Twist (22), with a slight modification. The constituent of the solution (mM) was Na^+ 142.9; K^+ 5.9; Mg^{2+} 1.2; Ca^{2+} 1.25; $H_2PO_4^-$ 1.2; HCO_3^- 24.9; SO_4^{2-} 1.2; Cl^- 127.8; glucose 5.0; and pyruvic acid 2.0; pH was 7.4 when bubbled with 95% O_2 and 5% CO_2. The viability of the freshly prepared cells was about 90%. Incubation of cardiac myocytes and extraction of cyclic AMP from the cells were performed according to the method described by Katada and Ui (23), with a slight modification. Briefly, each incubation tube contained 100 μl of cells (5×10^5 cells/ml) suspended with Krebs-Henseleit solution containing 2% BSA and 100 μl of physiological saline with drugs. Incubation was carried out at 37°C. At the end of incubation, 200 μl of 0.2 N HCl was quickly added and the tube immersed in boiling water for 3 minutes to extract cyclic AMP. After centrifugation at $600 \times g$ for 10 minutes, cyclic AMP was assayed in duplicate by the sensitive radioimmunoassay method (Yamasa Shoyu Co., Choshi, Japan). Cyclic AMP levels were determined 2 minutes after the administration of various concentrations of the PDE inhibitors, or 2 minutes after administration of isoproterenol. In the experiments in which the influence of the PDE inhibitors on the isoproterenol-induced accumulation of cyclic AMP were studied, the PDE inhibitors at a concentration of 10^{-5} M were allowed to act for 5 minutes prior to administration of various concentrations of isoproterenol.

Isolated Rat and Rabbit Right Papillary Muscle

Papillary muscles isolated from rat and rabbit right ventricles were used. The experimental procedures have been described previously for rat (14) and rabbit (24), but briefly, male Wistar rats (300–400 g) or albino rabbits (1.6–2.1 kg) were lightly anesthetized with ether, and right ventricular papillary muscles were isolated and mounted in 20-ml organ baths containing Krebs-Henseleit solution bubbled with 95% O_2 and 5% CO_2 at a temperature of $37 \pm 0.5°C$ (pH 7.4). Muscles were electrically stimulated by square-wave pulses of 5-ms duration and a voltage of about 20% above the threshold at 1 Hz. Force of isometric contractions was recorded on a thermal pen–writing oscillograph (Recti-Horiz-8K, NEC-San-ei Instruments Co., Tokyo, Japan) by means of strain-gauge transducers (UL-10GR, Shinkoh Communication Industry Co., Tokyo, Japan). After an equilibration period of 1 hour, the experiments were started. The PDE inhibitors and isoproterenol were administered in a cumulative manner. The positive inotropic effect of PDE inhibitors was expressed as the percentage of the maximal response to isoproterenol (10^{-6}–10^{-5} M) determined at the end of each experiment. The influence of the various PDE inhibitors at a concentration of 10^{-5} M on the concentration-response curve for the positive inotropic effect of isoproterenol was compared.

Statistical Analysis

Experimental values were presented as means ± SEM. Statistical significance of drug-induced changes was estimated by Student's t test. For multiple comparisons (comparison of the concentration-response curves for isoproterenol in the absence [control] and presence of PDE inhibitors), analysis of variance, including Scheffe's test for variables, was applied. Differences between two groups were considered to be significant when the F value from the analysis of variance indicated a significant difference among groups at a level of $p < 0.05$.

Drugs and Chemicals Used

The drugs used were obtained from the following sources: 3-isobutyl-1-methylxanthine (IBMX, Aldrich Chemical Co., Milwalkee, Wisconsin, USA); rolipram (Schering AG, Berlin, Germany); milrinone (Starling-Winthrop Research Institute, Rensselaer, NY, USA); OPC-18790 [($\pm$)-6-(3-[3,4-dimethoxybenzylamino]-2-hydroxypropoxy)-2(1H)-quinolinone] (Otsuka Pharmaceutical Co., Tokushima, Japan); Y-20487 [6-(3,6-dihydro-2-oxo-2H-1,3,4-thiadiazin-5-yl)-3,4-dihydro-2(1H)-quinolinone] (Yoshitomi Pharmaceutical Industries, Osaka, Japan); (-)-isoproterenol hydrochloride (Sigma Chemical Co., St. Louis, Missouri, USA); and cyclic AMP assay kit (Yamasa Shoyu Co., Choshi, Japan). IBMX was dissolved in 50% N,N-dimethylformamide at 4×10^{-2} M and diluted to the desired concentration with physiological saline solution; milrinone in 0.5 N lactic acid at 4×10^{-2} M; rolipram in dimethyl sulfoxide (DMSO) at 4×10^{-2} M; Ro 20-1724 in 95% ethanol at 4×10^{-2} M; OPC-18790 in 0.9% NaCl at 4×10^{-2} M; and Y-20487 in DMSO at 4×10^{-2} M. Milrinone and rolipram were diluted with 0.9% NaCl, and Y-20487 was diluted with 70% DMSO (7×10^{-5} M) and then with 0.9% NaCl to the desired concentration.

RESULTS

Direct Inotropic and Cyclic AHP Accumulating Effects on the Rat Ventricular Muscle

The concentration-response curves for the inotropic effect of OPC-18790, Y-20487, milrinone, rolipram, Ro 20-1724, and IBMX in the isolated rat papillary muscle are shown in Fig. 2. IBMX elicited a highest positive inotropic effect with the EC_{50} of approximately 3×10^{-5} M. Milrinone ($> 10^{-5}$ M) elicited a significant positive inotropic effect, but the effect was much less than that of IBMX. Rolipram and Y-20487 up to a concentration of 3×10^{-4} M did not affect the force of contraction. While Ro 20-1724 and OPC-18790 significantly decreased the force of contraction, the OPC-18790 at 3×10^{-4} M elevated the force to a level equivalent to the baseline.

Figure 3 shows the concentration-response curves for cyclic AMP accumulation induced by the PDE inhibitors in rat ventricular cardiomyocytes. IBMX elicited a concentration-dependent cyclic AMP accumulation. The maximal response was not achieved by the highest concentration of IBMX examined (5×10^{-4} M). Milrinone

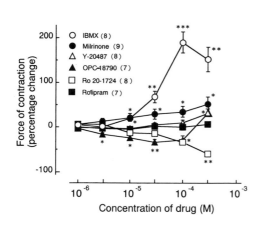

FIG. 2. The concentration-response curves for the inotropic effect of IBMX, milrinone, Y-20487, OPC-18790, Ro 20-1724, and rolipram in the isolated rat papillary muscle. *Ordinate*, force of contraction expressed as a percentage change; *abscissa*, molar concentration of the compounds. Numbers in parentheses are numbers of experiments. Basal force of contraction and the maximal response to isoproterenol in individual experimental groups: 0.69 ± 0.14 and 4.57 ± 1.39 mN (IBMX), 0.84 ± 0.28 and 3.28 ± 0.30 mN (milrinone), 1.90 ± 0.44 and 5.66 ± 0.59 mN (Y-20487), 1.20 ± 0.28 and 4.50 ± 1.10 mN (OPC-18790), 0.84 ± 0.11 and 3.28 ± 0.30 mN (Ro 20-1724), and 1.03 ± 0.24 and 3.75 ± 0.6 mN (rolipram).

and Y-20487 ($>10^{-4}$ M) also caused a significant cyclic AMP accumulation. Rolipram, Ro 20-1724, and OPC-18790 did not significantly affect the cyclic AMP level up to 5×10^{-4} M.

Influence of Phosphodiesterase Inhibitors on the Isoproterenol-induced Effect in the Rat Ventricular Muscle

The influence of IBMX, milrinone, Y-20487, OPC-18790, Ro 20-1724, and rolipram (10^{-5} M each) on the concentration-response curves for the positive inotropic effect of isoproterenol is shown in Fig. 4. IBMX, Y-20487, and OPC-18790

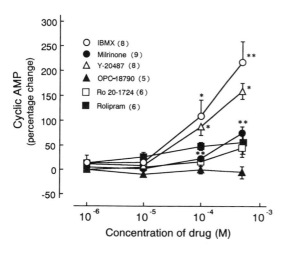

FIG. 3. The concentration-response curves for the cyclic AMP accumulation induced by IBMX, milrinone, Y-20487, OPC-18790, Ro 20-1724, and rolipram in the isolated rat ventricular cardiomyocytes. The cyclic AMP level was determined 2 minutes after the administration of individual compounds. *Ordinate*, cyclic AMP level expressed as a percentage of the basal content; *abscissa*, molar concentration of the compounds. Numbers in parentheses are numbers of determinations. Control cyclic AMP level in the absence of drug administration (pmol/10^5 cells): 1.06 ± 0.08 (IBMX), 1.16 ± 0.20 (milrinone), 0.96 ± 0.10 (Y-20487), 0.80 ± 0.13 (OPC-18790), 1.26 ± 0.12 (Ro 20-1724), and 1.02 ± 0.14 (rolipram).

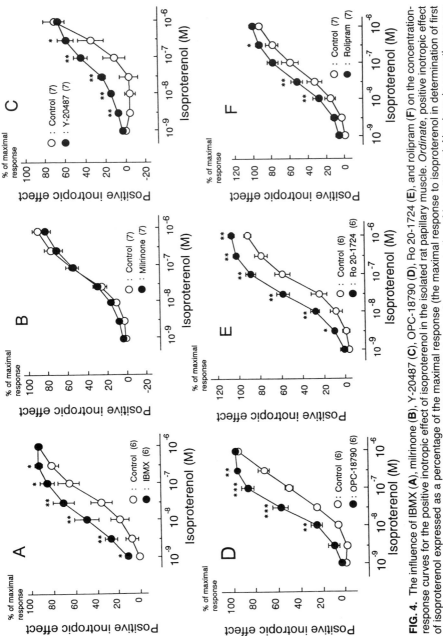

FIG. 4. The influence of IBMX (**A**), milrinone (**B**), Y-20487 (**C**), OPC-18790 (**D**), Ro 20-1724 (**E**), and rolipram (**F**) on the concentration-response curves for the positive inotropic effect of isoproterenol in the isolated rat papillary muscle. *Ordinate*, positive inotropic effect of isoproterenol expressed as a percentage of the maximal response (the maximal response to isoproterenol in determination of first concentration-response curve was defined as 100%); *abscissa*, molar concentration of isoproterenol. Numbers in parentheses are numbers of experiments. Basal force of contraction and the maximal response to isoproterenol in individual experimental groups: 1.34 ± 0.25 and 5.58 ± 0.62 mN (IBMX), 1.05 ± 0.25 and 5.92 ± 0.17 mN (milrinone), 0.81 ± 0.10 and 4.23 ± 0.99 (Y-20487), 1.20 ± 0.19 and 5.77 ± 0.81 mN (OPC-18790), 1.40 ± 0.27 and 5.37 ± 0.66 (Ro 20-1724), and 0.97 ± 0.34 and 4.35 ± 0.64 mN (rolipram), respectively.

TABLE 1. *Extent of the shift of the concentration-response curve for the positive inotropic effect of isoproterenol to the left exerted by isozyme-selective and non-selective phosphodiesterase inhibitors expressed as pD_2 value*

Compounds	ΔpD_2 value	
	Rat	Rabbit
IBMX	0.70 ± 0.16 (6)[a]	0.67 ± 0.05 (5)[b]
Milrinone	0.17 ± 0.05 (7)	0.42 ± 0.05 (5)[a]
Y-20487	0.85 ± 0.23 (7)[a]	0.84 ± 0.23 (7)[a]
OPC-18790	0.76 ± 0.14 (5)[a]	0.91 ± 0.14 (6)[a]
Ro 20-1724	0.49 ± 0.09 (6)[c]	0.11 ± 0.03 (5)
Rolipram	0.42 ± 0.05 (7)[c]	0.07 ± 0.07 (7)

Values presented are means $\pm$ SEM of ΔpD_2 values; numbers in parentheses are numbers of experiments. ΔpD_2 value = pD_2 value (with PDE inhibitors) $- pD_2$ value (control).
[a]$p < 0.01$.
[b]$p < 0.001$.
[c]$p < 0.05$.

shifted the concentration-response curves for isoproterenol to the left approximately to a similar extent. Ro 20-1724 and rolipram produced a significant shift of the curve for isoproterenol to the left and upward, while milrinone did not. The extent of the shift by these PDE inhibitors of the concentration-response curves for isoproterenol to the left is presented as pD_2 values (difference in $-\log EC_{50}$) in Table 1. The extent of the shift by Y-20487 (0.85) and OPC-18790 (0.76) was comparable to that by IBMX (0.70). Ro 20-1724 (0.49) and rolipram (0.42) caused a comparable shift of a lesser extent, but these compounds produced an upward shift of the curve for isoproterenol (Fig. 4).

Influence of the PDE inhibitors on the concentration-response curve for the isoproterenol-induced cyclic AMP accumulation is shown in Fig. 5. Milrinone did not significantly enhance the isoproterenol-induced cyclic AMP accumulation (Fig. 5A). While OPC-18790 and Y-20487 enhanced significantly the response to isoproterenol at 10^{-7} M (OPC-18790) and 10^{-6} M (Y-20487), respectively, the extent was much less than that produced by IBMX (Fig. 5A). Rolipram and Ro 20-1724 were much more effective than IBMX in enhancing the isoproterenol-induced cyclic AMP accumulation (Fig. 5B).

Effects of Phosphodiesterase Inhibitors on the Rabbit Papillary Muscle

The direct positive inotropic effects of the compounds on the isolated rabbit papillary muscle are shown in Fig. 6. OPC-18790 elicited a more pronounced positive inotropic effect than IBMX in the rabbit. Milrinone and Y-20487 were less effective than IBMX. Rolipram and Ro 20-1724 did not increase the force of contraction in the rabbit.

The influence of the PDE inhibitors on the positive inotropic effect of isoprotere-

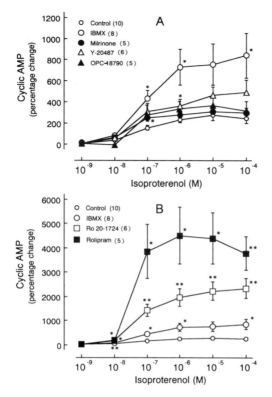

FIG. 5. Influence of IBMX, milrinone, Y-20487, and OPC-18790 (**A**), and IBMX, Ro 20-1724, and rolipram (**B**) on the concentration-response curve for the isoproterenol-induced cyclic AMP accumulation in the isolated rat ventricular cardiomyocytes. Influence of IBMX was presented in both A and B for comparison. Phosphodiesterase inhibitors were allowed to act for 5 minutes before the administration of isoproterenol. The cyclic AMP level was determined 2 minutes after the administration of isoproterenol. *Ordinate,* cyclic AMP level expressed as a percentage of the basal content; *abscissa,* molar concentration of isoproterenol. Numbers in parentheses are numbers of determinations. Control cyclic AMP levels in the absence of drug administration (pmol/10^5 cells): 1.36 ± 0.12 (control), 1.90 ± 0.32 (IBMX), 1.26 ± 0.20 (milrinone), 0.94 ± 0.14 (Y-20487), 0.81 ± 0.22 (OPC-18790), 1.50 ± 0.20 (Ro 20-1724), and 1.10 ± 0.14 (rolipram).

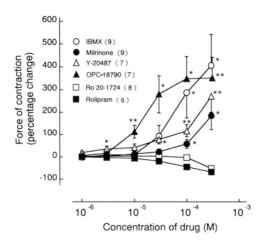

FIG. 6. The concentration-response curves for the positive inotropic effect of IBMX, milrinone, Y-20487, OPC-18790, Ro 20-1724, and rolipram in the isolated rabbit papillary muscle. *Ordinate,* force of contraction expressed as a percentage change; *abscissa,* molar concentration of the compounds. Numbers in parentheses are numbers of experiments. Basal force of contraction and the maximal response to isoproterenol in individual experimental groups: 1.83 ± 0.46 and 13.90 ± 2.95 mN (IBMX), 1.78 ± 0.35 and 12.04 ± 2.01 mN (milrinone), 2.18 ± 0.56 and 9.88 ± 2.08 mN (Y-20487), 2.08 ± 0.78 and 8.86 ± 2.94 mN (OPC-18790), 2.57 ± 0.44 and 8.96 ± 0.65 mN (Ro 20-1724), and 1.38 ± 0.18 and 10.38 ± 3.19 (rolipram), respectively.

nol in the rabbit is shown in Fig. 6 and Table 1. OPC-18790 and IBMX shifted the concentration-response curve for the isoproterenol-induced positive inotropic effect to the left to an identical extent. IBMX, Y-20487, and OPC-18790 shifted the concentration-response curve for the positive inotropic effect of isoproterenol to the left to an identical extent. Milrinone shifted the curve for isoproterenol to the left to a lesser extent, whereas rolipram and Ro 20-1724 did not affect the curve for isoproterenol (Fig. 7, Table 1).

DISCUSSION

The present findings with selective PDE isozyme inhibitors indicate (a) that the types of isozymes responsible for the regulation of cyclic AMP metabolism and contractile function show a species-dependent variation in mammalian ventricular muscle; and (b) that the different types of PDE isozymes may play differential roles in the regulation of cyclic AMP metabolism and contractile function in myocardial cells. Namely, different types of isozymes are responsible for the direct positive inotropic effect of PDE inhibitors and for the activity of PDE inhibitors to enhance the β-adrenoceptor–mediated action.

Species-dependent Variation of Phosphodiesterase Isozymes Involved in Contractile Regulation

It is evident that cyclic AMP metabolism by different types of PDE isozymes shows a wide range of species-dependent variation (14,15,25,26). In the rabbit ventricular muscle, milrinone was effective in inducing the positive inotropic effect and enhancing the positive inotropic action of isoproterenol, while rolipram and Ro 20-1724 were ineffective, an indication that PDE III but not PDE IV is of functional relevance in the rabbit, as is the case in most other mammalian species (4). By contrast, it is considered that in the rat cardiac muscle, PDE IV plays an important role in the hydrolysis of cyclic AMP accumulated in response to β-adrenoceptor stimulation, because rolipram and Ro 20-1724 were extremely effective in enhancing the cyclic AMP accumulation induced by β-adrenoceptor stimulation (13,14).

Direct Positive Inotropic Effect and Enhancing Effect on β-Adrenoceptor–Mediated Action

It is intriguing that in the rat ventricular muscle, rolipram and Ro 20-1724 enhanced the β-mediated action, but they did not produce any direct stimulatory action on the contractile force and cyclic AMP accumulation in the absence of β-stimulation. On the other hand, milrinone induced a weak but significant direct positive inotropic action, but it did not enhance the β-mediated response. These findings imply that different types of PDE isozymes are involved in the direct positive ino-

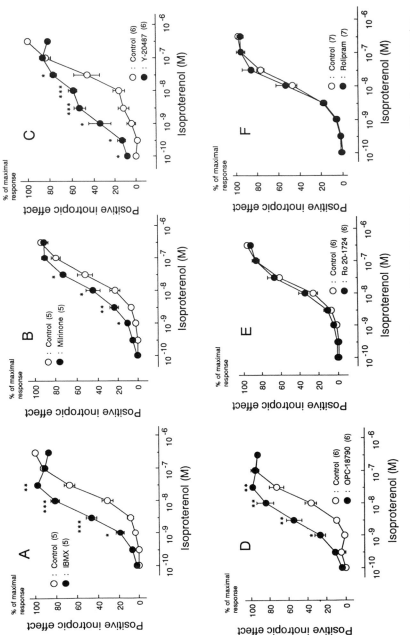

FIG. 7. The influence of IBMX (**A**), milrinone (**B**), Y-20487 (**C**), OPC-18790 (**D**), Ro 20-1724 (**E**), and rolipram (**F**) on the concentration-response curves for the positive inotropic effect of isoproterenol in the isolated rabbit papillary muscle. *Ordinate,* positive inotropic effect of isoproterenol expressed as the percentage of the maximal response (the maximal response to isoproterenol in determination of first concentration-response curve was defined as 100%); *abscissa,* molar concentration of isoproterenol. Numbers in parentheses are numbers of experiments. Two curves were significantly different from each other for OPC-18790, milrinone, and IBMX (analysis of variance). Basal force of contraction and the maximal response to isoproterenol in individual experimental groups: 3.20 ± 1.12 and 13.69 ± 2.16 mN (IBMX), 3.83 ± 0.81 and 16.9 ± 1.48 mN (milrinone), 5.24 ± 1.47 and 17.60 ± 2.53 mN (Y-20487), 1.94 ± 0.33 and 8.61 ± 0.90 mN (OPC-18790), 5.12 ± 1.11 and 17.59 ± 2.05 mN (Ro 20-1724), and 2.90 ± 0.59 and 15.1 ± 1.88 (rolipram), respectively.

tropic effect and the effect to enhance the β-adrenoceptor–mediated response in the rat.

Because IBMX, a nonselective PDE inhibitor (4,27,28), was more effective than other agents in inducing a direct cyclic AMP–accumulating and positive inotropic action in the rat, it is considered that in addition to selective inhibition of PDE III and/or IV, inhibition of other types of isozymes may also contribute to the direct effect of PDE inhibitors. Alternatively, IBMX may have induced the activation of adenylate cyclase by disinhibition of Gi protein–mediated inhibitory action (29). In the rabbit, OPC-18790 was more potent than IBMX and equi-effective to IBMX in inducing the positive inotropic effect, indicating that the combined inhibition of PDE III and IV may be sufficient to maximally activate the cyclic AMP-mediated regulatory mechanism.

Cellular Cyclic Adenosine Monophosphate Accumulation and Contractile Regulation

In the rat ventricular myocytes, the selective inhibition of PDE IV by rolipram and Ro 20-1724 enhanced the isoproterenol-induced cyclic AMP accumulation more effectively than IBMX: The accumulation of cyclic AMP in a tremendous amount was induced by the concomitant presence of isoproterenol and these PDE IV inhibitors. These observations imply that there may be PDE isozymes that are inhibited by PDE IV inhibitors, but not by IBMX. Because the IBMX-insensitive PDE isozyme has been found (30), it is probable that such an isozyme may play a role in rat myocardial cells. Alternatively, it is probable that the inhibition of PDE V induced by IBMX may have resulted in cyclic GMP accumulation (31) that in turn stimulated PDE II (5,6,32) to lead to lowering of the cyclic AMP accumulation. Such a regulation induced by cyclic GMP has been demonstrated in cardiac muscle (33).

The cyclic AMP accumulation induced by isoproterenol and PDE IV inhibitors in the rat is not directly related to the functional regulation: IBMX was more effective than the selective PDE IV inhibitor in enhancing the positive inotropic effect of isoproterenol. While the cyclic AMP accumulation induced by PDE IV inhibition may be functionally less relevant than the accumulation caused by IBMX, this accumulation may have been responsible for the potentiation of the maximal response to isoproterenol in the rat heart.

Effects of OPC-18790

OPC-18790 and Y-20487, which enhanced the positive inotropic effect of isoproterenol in the rat, exerted an effect similar to that of IBMX in the rabbit papillary muscle. These findings imply that OPC-18790 and Y-20487 may exert an inhibitory action on both types of isozymes PDE III and PDE IV, and thereby exhibit a characteristic action on the cyclic AMP-related signal transduction process.

In the present study, the contractile response was dissociated from cellular cyclic AMP accumulation under various experimental conditions: (a) OPC-18790 enhanced the isoproterenol-induced positive inotropic effect to the same extent as IBMX, whereas it produced much less cyclic AMP accumulation as compared with IBMX; (b) selective PDE IV inhibitors rolipram and Ro 20-1724 markedly enhanced the isoproterenol-induced cyclic AMP accumulation, while it shifted the concentration-response curve for the inotropic response to isoproterenol to a lesser degree than did OPC-18790 and IBMX. Although it has to be taken into consideration that the inotropic and cyclic AMP responses were assessed in different preparations, the differential actions of these PDE isozyme selective inhibitors and their interaction with isoproterenol on contractile and cyclic AMP responses strongly suggest the existence of complex compartmentalized cyclic AMP accumulation in intact rat myocardial cells.

These results are essentially in line with the previous observations that the inotropic effect of selective PDE isozyme inhibitors varies widely among mammalian species (14,15,25). It has been established in most mammalian species that newly developed cardiotonic agents, including amrinone and milrinone, are selective inhibitors of PDE III isozyme and thereby induce functional modulation in association with cyclic AMP accumulation that is less than that elicited by nonselective PDE inhibitors such as IBMX and theophylline (7,8). These newly developed cardiotonic agents have been shown to be less effective in the rat cardiac muscle compared with other species (11,25).

From the foregoing discussion, it is evident that PDE IV may play an important role in the cyclic AMP metabolism under stimulation of β-adrenoceptors in rat cardiac myocytes, while inhibition of other types of PDE isozyme, including PDE III, may be responsible for the direct cardiostimulatory action of PDE inhibitors. New cardiotonic agents, OPC-18790 and Y-20487, show unique characteristics due to concomitant inhibitory action on PDE III and PDE IV isozymes. Although the clinical relevance of the new type of PDE isozyme inhibitor is unknown at the moment, it became evident that the specific isozyme is involved in the interaction with β-stimulation, and that the inhibition of another type of isozyme may result in cyclic AMP accumulation in functionally relevant compartments in myocardial cells. It is, therefore, worthwhile to evaluate clinically the PDE inhibitor with combined isozyme selectivity in the treatment of heart failure.

SUMMARY

The inotropic effects of a new cardiotonic agent OPC-18790 [($\pm$)-6-(3-[3,4-dimethoxybenzylamino]-2-hydroxypropoxy)-2(1H)-quinolinone] was investigated in rat and rabbit ventricular muscle in comparison with selective PDE isozyme inhibitors, milrinone (PDE III–selective), rolipram and Ro 20-1724 (PDE IV-selective), another quinolinone derivative Y-20487 [6-(3,6-dihydro-2-oxo-2H-1,3,4-thiadiazin-5-yl)-3,4-dihydro-2(1H)-quinolinone], and a nonselective inhibitor 3-isobutyl-1-methylxanthine (IBMX). In the rat, milrinone elicited a significant accumulation of adenosine 3′,5′-monophosphate (cyclic AMP) and induced a positive inotropic effect, but the effect was much less than that of IBMX. Milrinone scarcely affected the β-adrenoceptor–mediated effects induced by isoproterenol. Whereas rolipram and Ro 20-1724 did not elicit accumulation of cyclic AMP and positive inotropic effect by themselves, they enhanced markedly accumulation of cyclic AMP and positive inotropic effect induced by isoproterenol. In the rat, OPC-18790 and Y-20487 did not change the cyclic AMP level, and OPC-18790 caused a slight negative inotropic effect. Although OPC-18790 and Y-20487 enhanced the positive inotropic effect of isoproterenol to the same extent as IBMX, they enhanced the isoproterenol-induced cyclic AMP accumulation much less than IBMX. In the rabbit, milrinone elicited a positive inotropic effect by itself and enhanced the isoproterenol-induced positive inotropic effect, while rolipram and Ro 20-1724 were ineffective. OPC-18790 was more effective than IBMX to produce the positive inotropic effect in the rabbit, and OPC-18790 and Y-20487 were equi-effective to IBMX to enhance the isoproterenol-induced positive inotropic effect. These results indicate that in the rat ventricular myocardium, PDE IV plays a crucial role in the breakdown of cyclic AMP generated by β-adrenoceptor stimulation, whereas other types of isozymes, including PDE III, may be responsible for the cyclic AMP accumulation and direct positive inotropic effect induced by PDE inhibitors. In the rabbit ventricular muscle, on the other hand, PDE III, but not PDE IV, may be involved in the regulation. The present findings imply that (a) different PDE isozymes are involved in regulation of cyclic AMP metabolism and cardiac contractile function in rat and rabbit; (b) the direct inotropic effect of PDE inhibitors and the effect of PDE inhibitors to enhance the positive inotropic effect of β-adrenoceptor stimulation can be exerted by different isozymes of PDE; (c) the relation between cellular accumulation of cyclic AMP and the positive inotropic effect is different, depending on individual PDE inhibitors, during their interaction with β-stimulation. OPC-18790 and Y-20487 exert characteristic inotropic action different from other agents, probably through inhibition of PDE III and PDE IV isozymes.

ACKNOWLEDGMENTS

This work was partly supported by Grant-in-Aid for Scientific Research on Priority Areas (No. 62624004, 63641002, and 01641003) from the Ministry of Education, Science, and Culture, Japan. We are grateful to Otsuka Pharmaceutical Co. (Tokushima, Japan) for the generous supply of OPC-18790 [(±)-6-(3-[3,4-dimethoxybenzylamino]-2-hydroxypropoxy)-2(1H)-quinolinone] and to Yoshitomi Pharmaceutical Industries (Osaka, Japan) for Y-20487 [6-(3,6-dihydro-2-oxo-2H-1,3,4-thiadiazin-5-yl)-3,4-dihydro-2(1H)-quinolinone].

REFERENCES

1. Hidaka H, Yamaki T, Ochiai Y, Asano T, Yamabe H. Cyclic 3′:5′-nucleotide phosphodiesterase determined in various human tissues by DEAE-cellulose chromatography. *Biochim Biophys Acta* 1977;484:398–407.

2. Thompson WJ, Terasaki WL, Epstein PM, Strada SJ. Assay of cyclic nucleotide phosphodiesterase and resolution of multiple molecular forms of the enzyme. *Adv Cyclic Nucleotide Res* 1979;10:69–92.

3. Beavo JA. Multiple isozymes of cyclic nucleotide phosphodiesterase. *Adv Second Messenger Phosphoprotein Res* 1988;22:1–38.

4. Weishaar RE, Cain MH, Bristol JA. A new generation of phosphodiesterase inhibitors: multiple molecular forms of phosphodiesterase and the potential for drug selectivity. *J Med Chem* 1985;28:537–545.

5. Reeves ML, Leigh BK, England PJ. The identification of a new cyclic nucleotide phosphodiesterase activity in human and guinea-pig cardiac ventricle. Implications for the mechanism of action of selective phosphodiesterase inhibitors. *Biochem J* 1987;241:535–541.

6. Silver PJ. Biochemical aspects of inhibition of cardiovascular low (K_m) cyclic adenosine monophosphate phosphodiesterase. *Am J Cardiol* 1989;63:2A–8A.

7. Kariya T, Willie LJ, Dage RC. Biochemical studies on the mechanism of cardiotonic activity of MDL 17,043. *J Cardiovasc Pharmacol* 1982;4:509–514.

8. Endoh M, Yamashita S, Taira N. Positive inotropic effect of amrinone in relation to cyclic nucleotide metabolism in the canine ventricular muscle. *J Pharmacol Exp Ther* 1982;221:775–783.

9. Bristol JA, Sircar I, Moos WH. Cardiotonic agents I. 4,5-Dihydro-6-[4(1H-imidazol-l-yl)phenyl]-3 (2H)-pyridazinones. Novel positive inotropic agents for the treatment of congestive heart failure. *J Med Chem* 1984;27:1099–1101.

10. Harrison SA, Reifsnyder DH, Gallis B, Cadd GG, Beavo JA. Isolation and characterization of bovine cardiac muscle cGMP-inhibited phosphodiesterase: a receptor for new cardiotonic drugs. *Mol Pharmacol* 1986;29:506–514.

11. Weishaar RE, Kobylarz-Singer DC, Steffen RP, Kaplan HR. Subclasses of cyclic AMP–specific phosphodiesterase in left ventricular muscle and their involvement in regulating myocardial contractility. *Circ Res* 1987;61:539–547.

12. Kitas PA, Artman M, Thompson WJ, Strada SJ. Subcellular distribution of high-affinity type IV cyclic AMP phosphodiesterase activity in rabbit ventricular myocardium: relations to the effects of cardiotonic drugs. *Circ Res* 1988;62:782–789.

13. Kauffman RF, Utterback BG, Robertson DW. Characterization and pharmacological relevance of high affinity binding sites for [^{3}H]LY186126, a cardiotonic phosphodiesterase inhibitor, in canine cardiac membranes. *Circ Res* 1989;65:154–163.

14. Katano Y, Endoh M. Differential effects of Ro 20-1724 and isobutylmethylxanthine on the basal force of contraction and β-adrenoceptor-mediated response in the rat ventricular myocardium. *Biochem Biophys Res Commun* 1990;167:123–129.

15. Katano Y, Endoh M. Effects of a cardiotonic quinolinone derivative, Y-20487 on the isoproterenol-induced positive inotropic action and cyclic AMP accumulation in rat ventricular myocardium: comparison with rolipram, Ro 20-1724, milrinone, and isobutylmethylxanthine. *J Cardiovasc Pharmacol* 1992;20:715–722.

16. Taira N, Endoh M, Iijima T, et al. Mode and mechanism of action 3,4-dihydro-6-[4-(3,4-dimethoxybenzoyl)-1-piperazinyl]-2(1H)-quinolinone (OPC-8212), a novel positive inotropic drug, on the dog heart. *Arzneim Forsch/Drug Res* 1984;34[Suppl I]:347–355.

17. Yanagisawa T, Endoh M, Taira N. Involvement of cyclic AMP in the positive inotropic effect of OPC-8212, a new cardiotonic agent, on the canine ventricular muscle. *Jpn J Pharmacol* 1984;36:379–388.

18. OPC-8212 Multicenter Research Group. A placebo-controlled, randomized, double-blind study of OPC-8212 in patients with mild chronic heart failure. *Cardiovasc Drugs Ther* 1990;4:419–425.

19. Feldman AM, Bristow MR, Parmley WW, et al., for the Vesnarinone Study Group. Effects of vesnarinone on morbidity and mortality in patients with heart failure. *N Engl J Med* 1993;329:149–155.

20. Hosokawa T, Mori T, Fujiki H, et al. Cardiovascular actions of OPC-18790: a novel positive inotropic agent with little chronotropic action. *Heart Vessels* 1992;7:66–75.

21. Endoh M, Kawabata Y, Katrano Y, Norota I. Effects of a novel cardiotonic agent (±)-6-[3-(3,4-dimethoxybenzylamino)-2-hydroxypropoxy]-2(1H)-quinolonone (OPC-18790) on contractile force, cyclic AMP level, and aequorin light transients in dog ventricular myocardium. *J Cardiovasc Pharmacol* 1994;23:723–730.

22. Powell, T, Twist VW. A rapid technique for the isolation and purification of adult cardiac muscle cells having respiratory control and a tolerance to calcium. *Biochem Biophys Res Commun* 1976;72:327–333.

23. Katada T, Ui M. Islet activating protein: enhanced insulin secretion and cyclic AMP accumulation in pancreatic islets due to activation of native calcium ionophores. *J Biol Chem* 1979;254:469–479.
24. Kushida H, Hiramoto T, Endoh M. The preferential inhibition of α_1- over β-adrenoceptor–mediated positive inotropic effect by organic calcium antagonists in the rabbit papillary muscle. *Naunyn Schmiedebergs Arch Pharmacol* 1990;341:206–214.
25. Nicolson CD, Challiss RAJ, Shahid M. Differential modulation of tissue function and therapeutic potential of selective inhibitors of cyclic nucleotide phosphodiesterase isoenzymes. *Trends Pharmacol Sci* 1991;12:19–27.
26. Shahid M, Wilson M, Nicholson CD, Marshall RJ. Species-dependent differences in the properties of particulate cyclic nucleotide phosphodieterase from rat and rabbit ventricular myocardium. *J Pharm Pharmacol* 1990;42:283–284.
27. Chasin M, Harris DN. Inhibitors and activators of cyclic nucleotide phosphodiesterase. *Adv Cyclic Nucleotide Res* 1976;7:225–264.
28. Korth M. Effects of several phosphodiesterase-inhibitors on guinea-pig myocardium. *Naunyn Schmiedebergs Arch Pharmacol* 1978;302:77–86.
29. Parsons WJ, Ramkumar V, Stiles GL. Isobutylmethylxanthine stimulates adenylate cyclase by blocking the inhibitory regulatory protein, G_i. *Mol Pharmacol* 1988;34:37–41.
30. Lavan BE, Lakey T, Houslay MD Resolution of soluble cyclic nucleotide phosphodiesterase isoenzymes, from liver and hepatocytes, identifies a novel IBMX-insensitive form. *Biochem Pharmacol* 1989;38:4123–4136.
31. Davis CW, Kuo JF. Differential effects of cyclic nucleotides and their analogs and various agents on cyclic GMP–specific and cyclic GMP–specific phosphodiesterases purified from guinea pig lung. *Biochem Pharmacol* 1978;27:89–95.
32. Komas N, Le Bec A, Stoclet JC, Lugnier C. Cardiac cGMP-stimulated cyclic nucleotides phosphodiesterase: effects of cGMP analogues and drugs. *Eur J Pharmacol* 1991;206:5–13.
33. Hartzell C, Fischmeister R. Opposite effects of cyclic GMP and cyclic AMP on Ca^{2+} current in single heart cells. *Nature* 1986;323:273–275.

The Failing Heart, edited by N. S. Dhalla,
R. E. Beamish, N. Takeda, and M. Nagano.
Lippincott-Raven Publishers, Philadelphia © 1995.

30

A New Adjunctive Treatment of Chronic Heart Failure Employing a Calcium Sensitizer

Tohru Izumi, Haruhiko Kuwano, Satoru Hirono, Hiroyuki Hosono, Haruo Hanawa, Makoto Kodama, and Takashi Tsuda

First Department of Internal Medicine, Niigata University School of Medicine, Niigata 951 Japan

REFRACTORY PATIENTS WITH CHRONIC HEART FAILURE

How to treat patients with chronic heart failure is a worldwide task among internal cardiologists (1). Due to the increase of the elder population, the number of patients with chronic heart failure has increased in developed countries (2). The present advances in diagnosis and treatment of the failing heart are able to relieve most patients from a serious state in a relatively short period of time. Inevitably, however, several patients fall into a refractory state, and they do not respond to any medical agents. For these people, unfortunately, we have failed to offer an effective therapy. Especially in Japan, where cardiac transplantation has not yet been established as a standard protocol, the task becomes more urgent in comparison with other countries.

Figure 1 represents the difficulties of treatment in such refractory cases when using only conventional therapies. This patient had a diagnosis of cardiomyopathy at 40 years of age. Until that time, he had been an excellent public servant. At age 40, however, he was suddenly attacked by acute pulmonary edema without any apparent triggers. Using diuretics and digitalis, he was able to return to his ordinary business. Despite such fundamental therapies, however, his disease gradually worsened. As an outpatient, he was obliged to receive advanced therapy in combination with the administration of captopril and denopamine. At 43 years of age, he had to be hospitalized once more due to the repetitive occurrence of orthopnea. In our hospital, his pump function was barely kept at a steady state using a maximal dosage of furosemide and captopril. His daily activity was extremely limited; he spent entire days at home. Two years later, after the sudden onset of atrial fibrillation, his deterioration accelerated. After that, his physical state became very fragile. For example, drug-induced anemia exacerbated his pump failure to a critical point. In the terminal stage, he had to repeat hospitalization, but at much shorter intervals

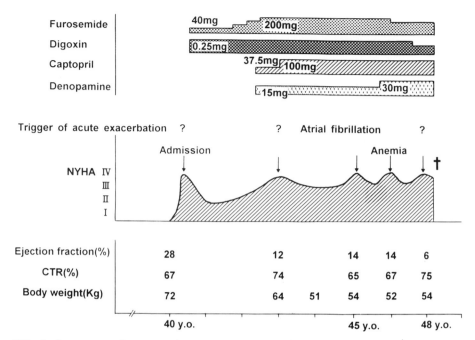

FIG. 1. A representative case refractory to any conventional therapies. Despite the maximal dosage of furosemide and captopril, the patient's circulatory state worsened. In the terminal stage, he was always listed as New York Heart Association (NYHA) function class 4, and was bedridden during the entire time.

than previously (i.e., every 4 months). In the final stage, he was constantly listed as New York Heart Association (NYHA) function class 4, and was bedridden for long periods. Finally, he died suddenly.

As can be seen clearly by his clinical course indicating ejection fraction in echography, cardiac thoracic ratio in chest X-rays, and body weight, despite every effort in combination with fundamental and advanced therapies, his cardiac state was refractory to any agents. These difficulties might be more emphasized in Japan than in other countries, because cardiac transplantation has not been introduced here. Even if this protocol were accepted, however, it would still have been difficult to offer a well-matched donor heart for him, because available hearts could be supplied only in extremely limited numbers. To maintain patients with such refractory chronic heart failure as good candidates for transplantation, and also to positively offer a strong alternative therapy in which these patients can be relieved from suffering, a new effective adjunctive therapy is desperately needed.

Through recent large-scale trials to investigate new drugs, the longevity of patients with refractory chronic heart failure has been clarified epidemiologically. By a survival curve obtained from the Prospective Randomized Milrinone Survival Evaluation (PROMISE), performed in 1991 (3), half of the survivors remained alive

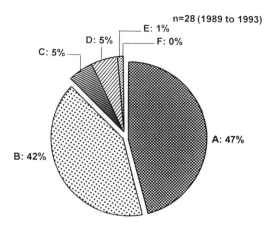

FIG. 2. Proportion of NYHA class 4 patients who were admitted to the Niigata University hospital during a 5-year period. A, valvular heart disease (MR and/or AR); B, dilated cardiomyopathy; C, infective endocarditis; D, primary pulmonary hypertension; E, congenial anomaly; F, coronary heart disease.

only up to 6 months. Eighteen months later, most of the patients had died. The data corresponds completely with those obtained from the Cooperative North Scandinavian Enalapril Survival Study (CONSENSUS), reported in 1987 (4). In Japan, the composition of refractory cases is quite different from that in the United States and European countries (1,5). Figure 2 shows our data for the previous 5 years on the proportion of NYHA class 4 patients. Inoperable valvular regurgitation, including either mitral and/or aortic valves (also the tricuspidal valve, in part), still ranks at the top of five underlying cardiovascular diseases: 47%. Half occupied the postoperative stage of either rheumatic or nonrheumatic valvular dysfunction. If patients with infective endocarditis were added to it, the proportion would reach 52%. Dilated cardiomyopathy ranks second at 42%. In contrast with U.S. and European surveys (1,5), where coronary heart disease is extremely rare, here it was nonexistent.

INODILATORS

Currently, several adjunctive drugs have been introduced to treat patients with chronic heart failure. Among these, angiotensin-converting enzyme (ACE) inhibitors (4,6,7) and beta blockades (8) have succeeded in gaining a definitive position in clinical medicine. In contrast to these, since the PROMISE trial, new cardiac inotropic agents are not being accepted (9). Although these agents can relieve patients in the short term, they fail to enhance the longevity of the patients. Presently, the use of inotropic agents has become challenging even when employing a relatively low dosage (10).

As McCall and O'Rourke have well indicated (11), in the refractory phase of the failing heart, two hemodynamical vicious cycles, namely an overincrease of afterload and preload, are functioning. These two cycles are deleteriously accelerated by humoral factors such as renin, angiotensin II, aldosterone, and vasopressin. Under this condition, physicians are forced to simultaneously resolve these difficult disorders. Clinically, patients associated with such vicious cycles are characterized with systemic hypotension and congestion. When only the conventional agents must be employed, it is extremely difficult to overcome the disorders and shift from the vicious-cycle state. Even the additional use of an ACE inhibitor might reduce blood pressure and worsen organ circulation to a critical level. The addition of a beta blockade might deteriorate the vicious cycle further, even when given in a small dosage. From these points of view, distinguished specialists, when considering energy kinetics in the failing heart (12), look for an agent that functions as a vasodilator (e.g., an ACE inhibitor) and also works as an inotropic drug to maintain the organ circulation. This agent was named *inodilator* by Opie et al. in 1986 (13). Of these agents, pimobendan (i.e., benzimidazole pyridazinone), has emerged as an important candidate (14). This new medication inhibits phosphodiesterase (PDE) activity and also increases calcium sensitizing to the contractile proteins, so it is now called a calcium sensitizer (15). In vitro and in vivo, beneficial vasodilative and inotropic effects are recognized (14,16).

Another type of calcium sensitizer, MCI-154, has been investigated (17). Its calcium-sensitizing effect is more powerful in comparison with pimobendan's. This drug has no effect as a PDE inhibitor. Vesnarinone and its derivatives have been nominated as other types of inodilators (18), but they do not belong to the category of calcium sensitizers.

PIMOBENDAN

In a national pimobendan trial held with the permission of the Japanese Health and Welfare Ministry (19), we met a valuable patient (20,21): a 55-year-old male taxi driver who was diagnosed as having dilated cardiomyopathy 3 years prior. He had a long and tremendous struggle, and he had to be hospitalized four times. Finally, he was bedridden for more than 6 months in a state of NYHA function class 4. Only with the oral use of 5.0 mg pimobendan per day could he recover from this serious state. His body weight decreased from 58 to 53 kg in 2 weeks, and his pulmonary congestion and plural effusion improved dramatically. He regained his activity day by day. In a short while, he could tolerate 6 METS of exercise. Two months later, he was well enough to be discharged from our hospital and resume his normal routine. Just prior to discharge, we tested whether his circulatory state was dependent on this new medicine. With his permission, a pimobendan washout test was performed. Using bedside Swan-Ganz catheterization, his hemodynamics were monitored during a 48-hour period. The hemodynamics were checked on the first day of pimobendan use, and also checked at the same time on the second day without the administration of pimobendan. The check times were selected at 12:00 and 2:00 PM. In comparison with daily oral administration of 5.0 mg of pimobendan, his hemodynamics obviously worsened after the abstinence. The withdrawal effect was especially clearly demonstrated in cardiac index (1.15 to 0.99 l/min/m^2 at 12:00 PM and 1.34 to 0.88 l/min/m^2 at 2:00 PM), AV-O$_2$ difference (10.2 to 11.8 vol% at

12:00 and 8.7 to 13.2 vol% at 2:00), total pulmonary vascular resistance (1,136 to 1,787 dyne/sec/cm^{-5} at 12:00 and 1,107 to 1,694 dyne/sec/cm^{-5} at 2:00), and systemic vascular resistance (3,002 to 3,619 dyne/sec/cm^{-5} at 12:00 and 2,595 to 3,811 dyne/sec/cm^{-5} at 2:00). Comparing cardiac status before and after pimobendan use, his daily life was highly activated from orthopnea at midnight by normal walking, and the exercise capacity was enhanced: peak VO^2 changed from 12.5 to 17.5 ml/kg/min. His systemic blood pressure did not change after use and was well maintained, ranging from 100/70 to 80/50 mmHg. In correspondence with the improvement, cardiac chamber size was minimized from 73% to 64% in cardiothoracic ratio, and the cardiac wall was more active than it was the previous day. With radioisotope (RI) angiography, ejection fraction increased from 15% to 26%.

Further investigation was warranted from this experience. Of patients with chronic heart failure, symptomatic and hospitalized patients were enrolled in a national trial and examined further. Patients had to satisfy three criteria: cardiomegaly—more than 55% cardiothoracic ratio in chest X-ray; increased left ventricular enddiastolic diameter—more than 6.0 cm; and reduced left ventricular fractional shortening in echocardiogram—less than 0.30. Consequently, the subjects were concentrated in two disease categories: dilated cardiomyopathy (12 cases) and volume-overloaded hearts (8 cases). The patients with valvular regurgitation were judged to be inoperable because of reasons such as high risk by operation. Total cases comprised 6 women and 14 men. The average age was 57 ± 11 years. Fractional shortening was 0.19 on average. NYHA function ranged from classes 2 to 4. For evaluation, Swan-Ganz bedside monitoring was employed. For these patients, after administration of 2.5 mg of pimobendan, their hemodynamics were checked hourly at stages of up to 6 hours later. The hemodynamics after bolus administration of pimobendan is summarized in Fig. 3. The beneficial effect was better documented in the volume-overloaded hearts than in the cardiomyopathic hearts. The favorable effects were significantly revealing in the filling pressure (mean right atrial pressure and diastolic pulmonary artery pressure) and total vascular resistance, both in the pulmonary and systemic circulation. In the volume-overloaded heart, mean right atrial pressure decreased from 5 to 2 mmHg, and diastolic pulmonary pressure decreased from 13 to 11 mmHg 6 hours later. Corresponding with the reduction, total pulmonary resistance was reduced from 445 to 337 dyne/sec/m^{-5}, and total systemic resistance was reduced from 1,227 to 1,186 dyne/sec/m^{-5}. On the other hand, the cardiomyopathic hearts did not change as remarkably as the volume-overloaded hearts. In other words, a correlation between stroke volume index and filling pressure was plotted on the pulmonary circulation and systemic circulation, respectively. The favorable function could be more clearly recognized in the volume-overloaded hearts than in the cardiomyopathic hearts (Fig. 4).

Next, the pimobendan effect was compared with that of captopril in the same patient (22). The test was performed in ten of the patients. When using pimobendan, the heart rate increased rapidly after bolus administration. Change in the stroke volume and the AV-O$_2$ difference was not significant in either drug. Concerning the filling pressure, mean right atrial pressure reduced remarkably after the use of pimo-

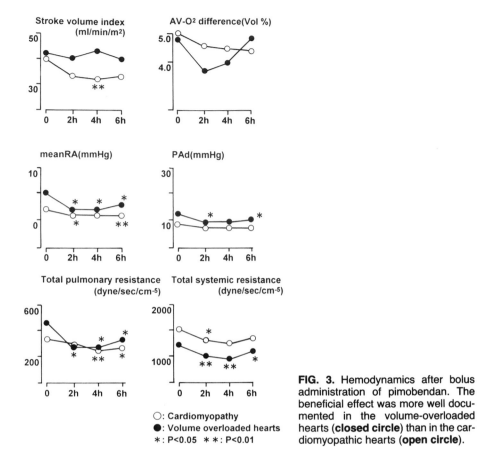

FIG. 3. Hemodynamics after bolus administration of pimobendan. The beneficial effect was more well documented in the volume-overloaded hearts (**closed circle**) than in the cardiomyopathic hearts (**open circle**).

○: Cardiomyopathy
●: Volume overloaded hearts
*: P<0.05 **: P<0.01

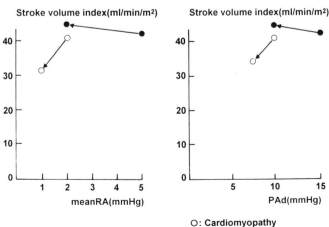

FIG. 4. A correlation between stroke volume indices and filling pressure was plotted in the pulmonary circulation (**left panel**) and systemic circulation (**right panel**), respectively. The favorable function could be recognized in the volume overloaded hearts (**closed circle**).

○: Cardiomyopathy
●: Volume overloaded hearts

bendan, and the effect was maintained over 6 hours. Both drugs reduced mean aortic blood pressure to a similar level. Concerning the vascular resistance, in comparison with captopril, pimobendan reduced systemic and pulmonary resistance to a much greater extent (Fig. 5). This vasodilator action was maintained longer when using pimobendan compared with captopril.

Considering the individual hemodynamic benefits and symptomatic improvement, nine patients were selected from the enrolled patients who wanted to take the medicine. All of them agreed to enter a long-term trial to document the results (23). The trial comprised five patients with dilated cardiomyopathy and four with volume-overloaded hearts. The NYHA function in dilated cardiomyopathy ranged from class 3 to 4 despite fundamental therapies. On the other hand, volume-overloaded hearts functioned from Class 2 to 3. They were given a daily oral administration of 5 mg pimobendan and were followed biweekly as outpatients. Their status was assessed through physical examination and echographic study. After 6 months of pimobendan use, all of them responded well to this adjunctive therapy. Despite the use of pimobendan, their systemic blood pressures were maintained within the

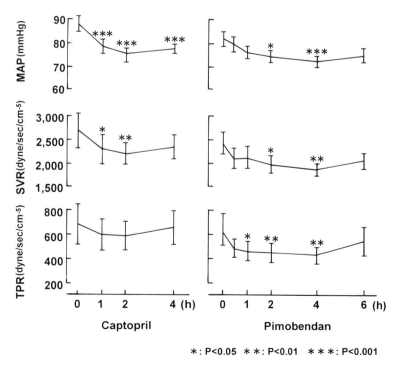

∗ : P<0.05   ∗ ∗ : P<0.01   ∗ ∗ ∗ : P<0.001

FIG. 5. The effect of pimobendan (**right panel**) was compared with that of captopril (**left panel**) in the same patient. In regard to vascular resistance, pimobendan lowered systemic and pulmonary resistance to a much greater degree than did captopril. MAP, mean aortic pressure; SVR, total systemic vascular resistance; TPR, total pulmonary resistance.

normal range. At this point, they were examined via the washout test, to determine whether their hemodynamics were dependent on this medicine. Their hemodynamics were monitored in the afternoon by using a bedside Swan-Ganz catheterization, and changes were checked hourly after abstinence for 2 days. The data were compared between fundamental therapy plus pimobendan on the first day and that without pimobendan on the second day. Noticeably, the withdrawal effect also was confirmed, even after 6 months of use, as shown in Fig. 6. The AV-O_2 difference worsened significantly after abstinence: from 5.5 to 6.6 vol% at 4 hours and from 5.4 to 7.0 vol% at 6 hours. Mean right atrial and diastolic pulmonary artery pressures increased: from 3 to 5 mmHg at 4 hours and from 2 to 5 mmHg at 6 hours, and from 12 to 15 mmHg at 4 hours and from 11 to 14 mmHg at 6 hours, respectively. Vascular resistance also increased in both the systemic and pulmonary circulation: from 1,683 to 1,891 dyne/sec/cm^{-5} at 4 hours and from 1,657 to 2,077 dyne/

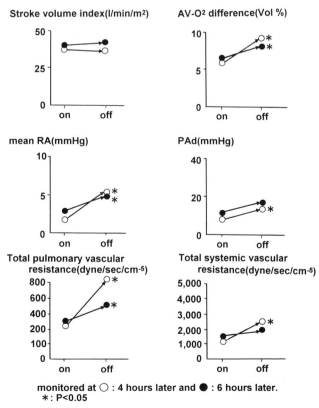

monitored at ○ : 4 hours later and ● : 6 hours later.
*: P<0.05

FIG. 6. After 6 months of use, patients' hemodynamics were tested to determine degree of dependency on pimobendan; bedside Swan-Ganz catheterization was used. Noticeably, the withdrawal effect was also confirmed in the washout, and was especially shown in the AV-O_2 difference, filling ventricular pressures, and vascular resistances.

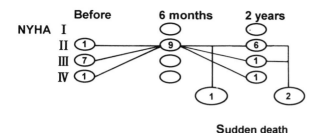

FIG. 7. Two-year follow-up results using NYHA function. During the trial, unexpected sudden cardiac death occurred in three cases.

sec/cm^{-5} at 6 hours, and from 444 to 670 dyne/sec/cm^{-5} at 4 hours and from 438 to 1,222 dyne/sec/cm^{-5} at 6 hours, respectively.

Figure 7 indicates 2 year follow-up results. After 6 months of use, all patients resumed normal daily activities, and six of them have maintained this favorable effect even after 2 years. During the trial, however, unexpected sudden cardiac death occurred in three patients, but these events were limited to patients with cardiomyopathic hearts. In two cases, death occurred after 2 years. Except for one case, patients with volume-overloaded hearts could maintain their enhanced daily activities even after 2 years. During the interval, however, cardiac size and cardiac wall motion did not improve obviously. Out of nine patients, some symptomatic complaints were raised: cold sweating in three cases, hand edema in two cases, and palpitation in two cases.

MCI-154

In Japan, another new type of calcium sensitizer, MCI-154, has already been used to investigate its clinical effects. We also met a dramatic patient (Fig. 8), a 36-year-old Japanese male businessman. He was diagnosed as having dilated cardiomyopathy 8 years prior. Four months after entering our care, he was listed as NYHA class 4, and his life could only be barely maintained with intermittent dobutamine infusion therapy. Although an adjunctive therapy using milrinone was tried, he failed to graduate from the infusion therapy. In this patient, MCI-154 was administered orally as an open trial. After use, his symptoms improved dramatically, and he was able to resume his daily activities. Structurally, the cardiac size decreased abruptly. The cardiac thoracic ratio from chest X-rays decreased dramatically from 60% to 48% in only 1 month. After 6 months, the left atrial chamber decreased from 5.2 to 2.8 cm, and the end-diastolic diameter of the left ventricular chamber decreased from 7.0 to 5.5 cm. Accordingly, cardiac wall motion improved remarkably from 9% to 34% in ejection fraction. Hemodynamically, the effect was confirmed. Mean pulmonary artery pressure decreased from 35 to 14 mmHg, and mean right atrial pressure decreased from 12 to 1 mmHg. The cardiac index improved from 1.8 to 3.4 l/min/m^2.

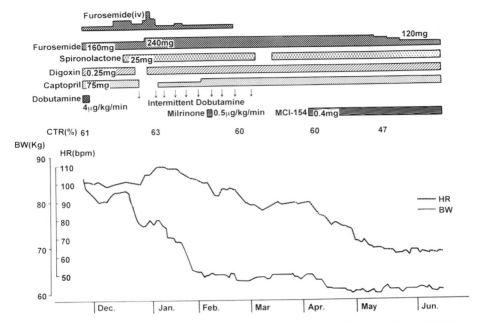

FIG. 8. A patient responded dramatically to another new type of calcium sensitizer, MCI-154.

IMPLICATIONS AND TASKS

The findings of our experience with these calcium sensitizers on a small number of patients are summarized as follows. First, among patients with chronic heart failure, there are some patients that are dramatically responsive to these calcium sensitizers, as described in Fig. 8. At the present time, however, how to differentiate the responder remains uncertain. This response to calcium sensitizers was seen in patients with dilated cardiomyopathy and volume-overloaded hearts. Little was known about its effect on ischemic hearts. Second, in patients who are sufficiently responsive to the agent, not only in the short term but also the long term, the withdrawal effect of this medicine can be detected. Among vasodilators, there is frequently a tolerance developed to the agent over long-term use (24). From our data, at least through 6 months, the calcium sensitizer was found to maintain the inodilator function. Third, the favorable effect is more exaggerated in patients with valvular regurgitation than in those with idiopathic cardiomyopathy. Although the exact mechanism is unclear, the inodilator action must be beneficial to support the pump function in regurgitation. This beneficial action must be evaluated in detail. Fourth, calcium sensitizers are more effective in the pulmonary circulation than in the systemic circulation. As clearly indicated in comparison with captopril, this action is unique. As an arteriovasodilator, this medicine is similar in action to ACE inhibitors. Noticeably, despite long use, it did not reduce the systemic blood pressure.

The venovasodilator effect is also very powerful and continues for a long period. It is a noticeable additional action, but, if this medicine is used in combination with ACE inhibitors, the pharmacological interaction remains unresolved. Whether this agent can be used in combination with ACE inhibitors, even in the patients with hypotension, must be examined. Fifth, from the results of a long follow-up study, the problem of unexpected sudden death was closed up. At the present time, it does not seem to be linked directly with the pimobendan administration in all cases. It is probably related to the underlying disease, but, there is also no proof to refute the interaction. Further large-scale studies are required to investigate the safety of this agent. Sixth, whether this adjunctive therapy can improve the humoral factors has not yet been determined (25).

Finally, it is emphasized that, among inodilators, this calcium sensitizer will be an important adjunctive agent that can relieve patients from refractory chronic heart failure. To devise a definite role for this treatment, further clinical and experimental investigations must be facilitated, and, during a given trial, the heterogeneity of patients with chronic heart failure must be considered.

SUMMARY

We reviewed our clinical experience of a new adjunctive therapy for patients with refractory chronic heart failure. In this therapy, two new agents (pimobendan and MCI-154), which are categorized as calcium sensitizers, are employed. Among refractory patients, there are some who are dramatically responsive to calcium sensitizers. Their vasodilative and inotropic effects seem to respond not only in the short term but also in the long term after administration. This favorable response is more exaggerated in patients with valvular regurgitation than in those with dilated cardiomyopathy. Pimobendan and MCI-154 may improve both pulmonary and systemic circulation in the failing heart. It is recommended that unexpected adverse effects be investigated before general use.

ACKNOWLEDGMENT

These investigations were supported in part by a grant from the Ministry of Health and Welfare of Japan to the Research Committee for Epidemiology and Etiology of Idiopathic Cardiomyopathy.

REFERENCES

1. Armstrong PW, Moe GW. Medical advances in the treatment of congestive heart failure. *Circulation* 1994;88:2941–2952.
2. Kannel WB, Balanger AJ. Epidemiology in heart failure. *Am Heart J* 1991;121:951–957.
3. Packer M, Carver JR, Rodeheffer RJ, et al., for the PROMISE Study Research Group. Effect of oral milrinone on mortality in severe chronic heart failure. *N Engl J Med* 1991;325:1468–1475.

4. The CONSENSUS Trial Study Group. Effect of enalapril on mortality in severe congestive heart failure. Result of the Cooperative North Scandinavian Enalapril Survival Study (CONSENSUS). *N Engl Med* 1987;316:1429–1435.
5. Anderson B, Waagstein F. Spectrum and outcome of congestive heart failure in a hospitalized population. *Am Heart J* 1993;126:632–640.
6. The SOLVD Investigators. Effect of enalapril on survival in patients with reduced left ventricular ejection fractions and congestive heart failure. *N Engl J Med* 1991;325:293–302.
7. Pfeffer MA, Braunwald E, Moyer LA, et al., on behalf of the SAVE Investigators. Effect of captopril on mortality and morbidity in patients with left ventricular dysfunction after myocardial infarction. *N Engl J Med* 1992;327:669–677.
8. Waagstein F, Caidahl K, Wallentin I, et al. Long-term beta-blockade in dilated cardiomyopathy: effects of short-and long-term metoprolol treatment followed by withdrawal and readministration of metoprolol. *Circulation* 1989;80:551–563.
9. Katz AM. Potential deleterious effects of inotropic agents in the therapy of chronic heart failure. *Circulation* 1986;73[Supp 3]:184–190.
10. Packer M. The search for the ideal positive inotropic agent. *N Engl J Med* 1993;329:201–202.
11. McCall D, O'Rourke R. Congestive heart failure. *Mod Conc Cardiol Dis* 1985;52:55–60.
12. Hasenfuss G, Holubarsch C, Heiss HW, et al. Influence of the calcium sensitizer UDCG-115 on hemodynamics and myocardial energetics in patients with idiopathic dilated cardiomyopathy. Comparison with nitroprusside. *Basic Res Cardiol* 1989;84[Suppl 1]:225–233.
13. Opie LH. "Inodilators." *Lancet* 1986;1:1336.
14. Kubo SH, Goullub S, Rahko P, et al., for the Pimobendan Multicenter Research Group. Beneficial effects of pimobendan on exercise tolerance and quality of life in patients with heart failure. *Circulation* 1992;85:942–949.
15. Lee JA, Allen DG. Calcium sensitizer. A new approach to increasing the strength of the heart. *Br Med J* 1990;300:551–552.
16. Fujino K, Sperlakis N, Solaro RJ, et al. Sensitization of dog and guinea pig heart myofilaments to Ca^{2+} activation and the inotropic effect of pimobendan: comparison with milrinone. *Circ Res* 1988;63:911–922.
17. Abe Y, Kitada Y, Narimatsu A. Beneficial effect of MCI-154, a cardiotonic agent, on ischemic contractile failure and myocardial acidosis of dog hearts: comparison with dobutamine, milrinone and pimobendan. *J Pharmacol Exp Ther* 1992;261:1087–1095.
18. Feldman AM, Bristow MR, Parmley WW, et al., for the Vesnarinone Study Group. Effect of vesnarinone on morbidity and mortality in patients with heart failure. *N Engl J Med* 1993;329:149–155.
19. Kato K, Yasuda J, Taniguchi K, et al. Pimobendan therapy on chronic heart failure—open multicenter trial. *Rinsho Kenkyu* 1991;68:3539–3531 [in Japanese].
20. Nonaka R, Tsuda T, Izumi T, et al. A case with refractory chronic heart failure dramatically responsive to pimobendan. *Shinyaku Rinsho* 1991;40:1661–1668 [in Japanese].
21. Fujita T, Tsuda T, Izumi T, et al. A case of dilated cardiomyopathy with intractable heart failure treated with adjunctive therapy of pimobendan and denopamine. *Nippon Naika Gakkai Zasshi* 1992;81:1108–1110 [in Japanese].
22. Tsuda T, Izumi T, Kodama M, et al. Acute hemodynamics of pimobendan in chronic heart failure. A comparative crossover study of captopril and pimobendan. *Jpn Heart J* 1992;33:193–203.
23. Kato K, Ito H, Izumi T, et al. Pimobendan therapy on chronic heart failure—long term multicenter trial. *Rinsho Kenkyu* 1992;69:2275–2297 [in Japanese].
24. Elkayama U. Tolerance to organic nitrates: evidence, mechanism, clinical relevance, and strategies for prevention. *Ann Intern Med* 1991;114:667–677.
25. Erlemeier HH, Kupper W, Bleifeld W. Comparison of hormonal and hemodynamic changes after long-term oral therapy with pimobendan or enalapril—a double-blind randomized study. *Eur Heart J* 1991;12:889–899.

The Failing Heart, edited by N. S. Dhalla,
R. E. Beamish, N. Takeda, and M. Nagano.
Lippincott-Raven Publishers, Philadelphia © 1995.

31

Effects of an Endogenous Inotropic Factor in Low-Flow Ischemia

*†Jagdish C. Khatter, *Moses Agbanyo, and †Francis Darkwa

*Departments of *Medicine (Cardiology) and †Pharmacology and Therapeutics,
University of Manitoba, Health Sciences Centre,
Winnipeg, Manitoba R3E 0Z3 Canada*

Endogenous inhibitors of the sodium pump have been investigated for some time. In the late 1960s Dahl et al. (1) and later Haddy and Overbeck (2) suggested that a low molecular weight digitalis-like inhibitor of the Na^+/K^+ pump may exist in circulation. Much effort has since been made to demonstrate the existence of endogenous digitalis-like substances in animals as well as humans. Gruber et al. (3,4) were first to show digoxin-like immunoreactive material in the plasma of volume-expanded dogs. Subsequently, this material was also demonstrated in the serum of 54 patients with renal impairment (5). Haupert and Sancho (6) described the existence of an inhibitor of the sodium pump in the hypothalamus. There are no reports so far that it circulates in blood plasma. Further studies showed (7) that hypothalamic factor shows inotropy on beating rat heart myocytes that exceeds those where ouabain shows toxic effects. The hypothalamic factor, however, also leads to contractions of vascular smooth-muscle rings of rat aorta (8).

Digitalis-like inotropic factor has also been isolated and purified in our laboratory from left ventricle tissue of porcine (9) and human heart (10). It is acid-resistant, unaffected by proteases, and shows charged ionic properties (11). The factor lacks digitalis-like cardiotoxicity, namely, an increase in resting tension and arrhythmia in large enough doses (12). In canine and guinea pig trabeculae, the endogenous inotropic factor (EIF) was shown to depress the postrest potentiation in the contractility. We concluded that the EIF may prevent the increase in the accumulation of calcium in sarcoplasmic reticulum generally observed with digitalis (12). More recently, the EIF was demonstrated to cause relaxation of rat aortic smooth muscle precontracted with phenylepinephrine (13). The smooth-muscle relaxation effect of EIF was further shown to be endothelium-dependent and may be associated with the release of nitric oxide (13). These characteristics of EIF indicate a high potential in its use for the therapy of heart failure. In this study, we investigated the effects of EIF in Langendorff-perfused isolated guinea pig heart with low-flow ischemia.

METHODS

Isolation of Endogenous Inotropic Factor–Containing Extract

Endogenous inotropic factor–containing extract was isolated from porcine left ventricular tissue, as described by us earlier (9). Briefly, 150 g of left ventricular tissue was extracted using acetone/HCl, delipidated and then submitted to gel permeation and ion exchange chromatographies. The final extract was freeze-dried and dissolved in 100 ml Krebs-Henseleit buffer for isolated heart perfusions.

Isolated Heart Perfusions

Isolated guinea pig hearts of either sex (200–300 g) were perfused retrograde using Krebs-Henseleit bicarbonate buffer solution (pH 7.4) gassed with 95% O_2/5% CO_2. The hearts were paced at 3 Hz at a voltage setting of 10% above the threshold. Isometric contractile force was measured with a Grass FT03 force transducer, and a 2-g tension was applied. After 20 minutes of equilibration at 32°C, at a flow rate of 8 ml/min, the flow rate was altered to 2 ml/min to induce low-flow ischemia. Five minutes after the ischemia, 100 ml of Krebs solution containing either EIF or 1 μM ouabain was used to perfuse the hearts in a recirculating manner at a flow rate of 2 ml/min. Control experiments were treated in the same manner, except that EIF or ouabain was omitted in the perfusion medium.

RESULTS

Inotropic Effect of Endogenous Inotropic Factor

Because EIF inhibits membrane Na^+/K^+-ATPase, we investigated its inotropic effect in retrograde Langendorff-perfused isolated guinea pig heart and compared with ouabain. Extracted from 150 g of left ventricle tissue of porcine heart and dissolved in 100 ml of Krebs-Henseleit buffer, EIF caused a 20% to 25% increase in contractile force within 2 to 5 minutes of retrograde perfusion in a recirculating manner. The increase in the contractile force could be seen even after 40 minutes of continued perfusion (Fig. 1). Ouabain (1 μM) caused a slower increase of up to 10% in contractile force and required 8 to 10 minutes for maximum inotropy. The positive inotropy was followed by a negative inotropic effect, a manifestation of cardiotoxicity, such that after 40 minutes of perfusion, the contractile force had declined by 80% below the basal force.

Effects of Endogenous Inotropic Factor on Contractile Force in Ischemic Heart

In low-flow ischemia, induced by reduction in perfusion to 2 ml/min, the contractile force declined by 50% to 55% (data not shown) within 5 minutes of perfusion.

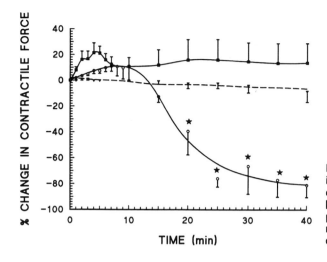

FIG. 1. Time-course % change in contractile force for 1 μM ouabain (○ --- ○), EIF (■ --- ■), and control (▼ --- ▼) heart perfused at 8 ml/min. *Significantly different from both control and EIF (*p*<0.05).

When either EIF or ouabain were added to the perfusion medium after 5 minutes of ischemic flow, ouabain caused a continued negative inotropic effect such that after 40 to 45 minutes of perfusion, there was a further reduction of 60% to 70% in contractile force (Fig. 2). In the presence of EIF, however, there was no significant decline in contractile force, even after 40 to 45 minutes of continued perfusion.

Effects of Endogenous Inotropic Factor on the Resting Tension in Normal and Ischemic Heart

In a normal perfused heart, ouabain (1 μM) perfusion caused an increase in resting tension such that after 40 minutes of perfusion, the resting tension had in-

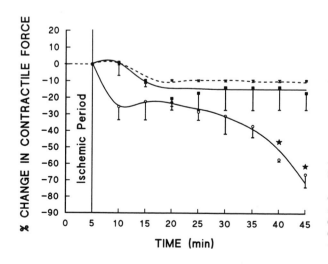

FIG. 2. Time-course % change in contractile force for 1 μM ouabain (○ --- ○), EIF (■ --- ■), and control (▼ --- ▼) hearts perfused at 2 ml/min; % changes were calculated 5 minutes after induction of ischemia. *Significantly different from both control and EIF (*p*<0.05).

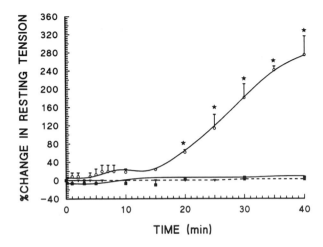

FIG. 3. Time-course % change in resting tension for 1 μM ouabain (○ --- ○), EIF (■ --- ■), and control (▼ --- ▼) hearts perfused at 8 ml/min. *Significantly different from both control and EIF (p<0.05).

creased by as much as 280% (Fig. 3). No such increases in resting tension were observed in the presence of EIF perfusion. In ischemic heart (low-flow for 5 minutes), ouabain perfusion caused a further increase in the resting tension such that 45 minutes of continued perfusion caused an increase in the resting tension by as much as 65% (Fig. 4). Perfusion of EIF in ischemic heart caused no such increase in the resting tension, even after 45 minutes of continued perfusion.

DISCUSSION

Digitalis has been long in use to treat atrial fibrillation and heart insufficiency, especially in congestive heart failure. All of the present information in the literature

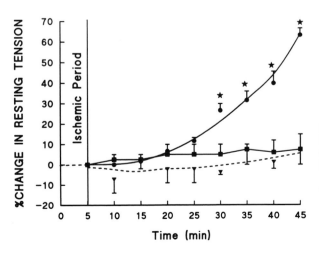

FIG. 4. Time-course % change in resting tension for 1 μM ouabain (● --- ●), EIF (■ --- ■), and control (▼ --- ▼) heart perfused at 2 ml/min; % changes were calculated 5 minutes after induction of ischemia. *Significantly different from both control and EIF (p< 0.05).

favors the concept that digitalis-like compounds can be synthesized endogenously in mammals (14–16). More recently, the endogenous factor was characterized to be pharmacologically and immunoreactively identical to ouabain (14). H'NMR analysis of EIF, however, indicates the presence of no such steroid molecule (data not shown). This would clearly demonstrate that EIF isolated from the porcine heart tissue is a unique compound and is unlike any other Na^+/K^+-ATPase inhibitor reported in the literature. Its unique characteristics of inotropy without digitalis-like toxicity and its relaxation effect on vascular smooth muscle support this concept. Na^+/K^+-ATPase inhibitor isolated from the hypothalamus was also recently shown to have inotropic property (8), but as opposed to EIF, causes a vasoconstriction of the vascular smooth muscle. The data obtained in this study further demonstrate that EIF is a safe inotropic agent, even in ischemic heart condition. Clearly, the study demonstrated that, unlike digitalis, EIF had no deleterious effects, such as negative inotropy or increase in resting tension during continuous perfusion of ischemic heart. This may be due partially to its relaxation effect on vascular smooth muscle (13) and consequent increased perfusion of the heart muscle as opposed to ouabain, which caused vasoconstriction. Endogenous inotropic factor, however, showed no protective effect, either when perfused during the induction of ischemia (data not shown) or after the induction of ischemia.

SUMMARY

This study was undertaken to examine the effects of an EIF on isolated perfused guinea pig heart under ischemic conditions induced by low flow (2 ml/min). Isolated hearts were perfused using a recirculating system and the drugs in Kreb's solution were delivered to the heart via a three-way valve. Ouabain perfused (1 μM) hearts under normal flow conditions (8 ml/min) demonstrated a 10% increase in developed tension within 8 to 10 minutes, which was followed by a negative inotropic effect such that after 40 to 45 minutes of perfusion, the contractile force had declined by 80% below the basal force and the resting tension had increased by over 280%. Endogenous inotropic factor–perfused hearts (normal flow) showed a 20% to 25% increase in the developed tension within 2 to 5 minutes, which was maintained for more than 45 minutes without any change in the resting tension. In low-flow ischemia (2 ml/min), the contractile force declined by 50% to 55% within 5 minutes of perfusion. Ouabain perfusion at this point caused a continued negative inotropic effect such that after 40 to 45 minutes there was a further reduction of 60% to 67% in contractile force and as much as a 65% increase in the resting tension. In perfusion with EIF, however, there was no significant decline in the contractile force or increase in the resting tension, even after 45 minutes of continued perfusion. These data demonstrate that EIF is a safe inotropic agent, even in ischemic heart conditions.

ACKNOWLEDGMENTS

This work was supported by a grant from the Medical Research Council of Canada. Francis Darkwa received a studentship from the Department of Pharmacology and Therapeutics, Faculty of Medicine, University of Manitoba.

REFERENCES

1. Dahl LK, Knudsen KD, Iwai J. Humoral transmission of hypertension: evidence from parabiosis. *Circ Res* 1969;25/26[Suppl I]:121–133.
2. Haddy FJ, Overbeck HS. The role of humoral agents in volume expanded hypertension. *Life Sci* 1976;19:935–948.
3. Gruber KA, Whitaker JM, Buckalew VM Jr. Endogenous digitalis-like substance in plasma of volume expanded dogs. *Nature* 1980;287:743–745.
4. Gruber KA, Rudel LL, Bullock BC. Increased circulating levels of an endogenous digoxin-like factor in hypertensive monkeys. *Hypertension* 1982;4:348–354.
5. Graves SW, Brown B, Valdes R. An endogenous digoxin-like substance in patients with renal impairment. *Ann Intern Med* 1983;99:604–608.
6. Haupert GT, Sancho JM. Sodium transport inhibitor from bovine hypothalamus. *Proc Natl Acad Sci USA* 1979;76:4658–4660.
7. Hallaq HA, Haupert GT. Positive inotropic effect of the endogenous Na^+/K^+-ATPase inhibitor from the hypothalamus. *Proc Natl Acad Sci* 1989;86:10080–10084.
8. Haupert GT, Kachories C, Hallaq HA. Physiological regulation of the Na^+/K^+-ATPase; positive inotropic and vasoconstrictive effects of the hypothalamic Na^+/K^+-ATPase inhibitor. In: *Proceedings of the IUPHAR Satellite Meeting*, "Endogenous digitalis-like factors-purification, properties, physiological functions." Giessen, 1990:35(abst).
9. Khatter JC, Agbanyo M, Hoeschen RJ. Isolation and characterization of an endogenous digitalis-like substance from left ventricle tissue of porcine heart. *Life Sci* 1986;39(25):2483–2492.
10. Khatter JC, Agbanyo M, Zhang M, et al. Pharmacological characterization of an endogenous inotrope from human heart. *Proceedings of the 95th meeting of the American Society for Clinical Pharmacology and Therapeutics*. 1994:152, OI-A-4(abst).
11. Khatter JC, Agbanyo M, Navaratnam S. An endogenous inotropic substance from heart tissue has digitalis-like properties. *Life Sci* 1991;48(5):387–396.
12. Navaratnam S, Bose D, Agbanyo M, Khatter JC. Positive inotropic effect of porcine left ventricular extract on canine ventricular muscle. *Br J Pharmacol* 1990;101:370–374.
13. Chao H, Khatter JC. An endogenous inotropic factor induces relaxation of vascular smooth muscle. *J Pharmacol Exp Ther* 1995 [*submitted*].
14. Hamlyn JM, Blaustein MP, Bova S, et al. Identification and characterization of a ouabain-like compound from human plasma. *Proc Natl Acad Sci USA* 1991;88:6259–6263.
15. Shaikh JM, Lau BWC, Siegfried BA, Valdes R Jr. Isolation of digitalis-like immunoreactive factors from mammalian adrenal cortex. *J Biol Chem* 1991;266:13672–13678.
16. Goto A, Yamada K, Ishii M, et al. Existence of a polar digitalis-like factor in mammalian hypothalamus. *Biochem Biophys Res Commun* 1989;161:953–958.

The Failing Heart, edited by N. S. Dhalla,
R. E. Beamish, N. Takeda, and M. Nagano.
Lippincott-Raven Publishers, Philadelphia © 1995.

32

Cholesterol-Lowering Therapy for Reduction of Myocardial Infarction and Prevention of Heart Failure

Mark E. McGovern

*Department of Cardiovascular Clinical Research and Development, Bristol-Myers Squibb Co.,
Pharmaceutical Research Institute, Princeton, New Jersey 08540 United States*

Atherosclerosis remains the leading cause of death in most developed countries. In the United States, approximately 1.5 million people suffer a myocardial infarction (MI) each year, and almost 6 million people are estimated to be living with some manifestation of coronary heart disease (CHD) (1,2), including heart failure. Based on data from the National Health and Nutrition Examination Survey (NHANES I) (3) of 14,407 adult outpatients 25 to 74 years of age, the prevalence of heart failure has been estimated to be between 1% and 2% of the United States population, with 10- and 15-year mortality rates in the 40% to 55% range, respectively (3). Death rates were greater in those ≥ 55 years of age, and higher in men than in women, especially for men in the 65- to 74-year age group where 10-year mortality from heart failure was over 70% (3). Furthermore, ischemic heart disease now accounts for the majority of cases of heart failure, according to registry data from the Studies of Left Ventricular Dysfunction (SOLVD) trial (4). This trial was conducted in an outpatient office practice setting, and therefore, the patients should be broadly representative of the general population of subjects with heart failure. Among the 6,273 patients in the registry database, ischemic heart disease was the etiology of heart failure in 68.5% of cases. A history of angina and previous MI were reported in 60% and 63.4% of patients, respectively (4).

While the value of vasodilator therapy, digitalis, and diuretics in the treatment of patients with left ventricular dysfunction is widely acknowledged, less attention has been given to the use of lipid-lowering interventions for prevention of heart failure among patients at risk for MI. Among the recognized risk factors for atherosclerosis, the strongest independent predictor of risk of death from CHD is elevated blood cholesterol (5,6); the low-density lipoprotein cholesterol (LDL-C) fraction is the main contributor to this relationship (7). Substantial evidence from clinical trials supports the value of cholesterol-lowering interventions to reduce progression of coronary atherosclerotic plaque and associated cardiovascular clinical sequelae in patients with hypercholesterolemia (8–13). The majority of these data, however, derives from clinical trials of patients with marked hyperlipidemia (e.g., LDL-C> 190 mg/dl [4.9 mmol/l]), and until recently clinical trial evidence for a benefit of lipid-lowering therapies for patients with moderately elevated blood cholesterol typical of the majority of subjects with manifest coronary artery disease (CAD) (14,15) was less definitive.

Results have now been reported from two clinical trials of lipid-lowering intervention that evaluated cardiovascular clinical outcomes in patients with CAD and moderate hypercholesterolemia: Pravastatin Limitation of Atherosclerosis in the Coronary Arteries (PLAC I) and Pravastatin, Lipids, and Atherosclerosis in the Carotid Arteries (PLAC II). These trials were randomized, double-blind, placebo-controlled, 3-year trials of pravastatin, a 3-hydroxy-3-methylglutaryl coenzyme A (HMG CoA) reductase inhibitor, administered as a monotherapy regimen. Prior to randomization, all patients were instructed in a fat- and cholesterol-restricted diet (American Heart Association Phase I or equivalent) (16). PLAC I was a multicenter study in 408 patients (mean age 57 years; 77% were men) with established CAD (at least one 50% stenosis in a major coronary artery) and LDL-C≥130 mg/dl (3.4 mmol/l) and <190 mg/dl (4.9 mmol/l). Progression of coronary atherosclerosis was evaluated using quantitative coronary arteriography (15). PLAC II was a single-center study of 151 patients (mean age 63 years; 85% were men) with LDL-C≥60th< 90th percentiles for the United States population (approximately 146 mg/dl [3.8 mmol/l] − 192 mg/dl [5.0 mmol/l] for the age and sex of the patient population enrolled); documented CAD (remote MI or coronary angiography showing one or more 50% stenoses); and early carotid atherosclerosis. Presence of carotid atherosclerosis was defined as a focal thickening of the combined arterial intima plus media of ≥1.3 mm in either the distal common carotid artery, bifurcation region, or proximal internal carotid. Progression of carotid atherosclerosis was assessed using quantitative B-mode ultrasound (17). In both studies the mean baseline LDL-C was approximately 164 mg/dl (4.2 mmol/l); between 40% (PLAC I) and 60% (PLAC II) of patients had previous MI (15,17).

The results of these two trials showed that pravastatin therapy significantly reduced atherosclerosis progression in the coronary (PLAC I) (18) and carotid (PLAC II) (19) arteries. In PLAC I the major effect was on progression in coronary artery segments with a stenosis <50% at baseline and development of new lesions (defined as an increase of at least 16% diameter stenosis in any segment with a stenosis <16% at baseline) (18). In PLAC II the principal treatment effect was a reduction in the rate of progression of intimal-medial thickening in the distal common carotid artery segment (19). More importantly, cardiovascular clinical event rates, in particular MIs, were significantly reduced in each study among the patients treated with pravastatin. In a pooled event analysis between PLAC I and PLAC II, for the combined endpoint of nonfatal MI or CHD death there were 14 events in the pravastatin group and 27 in the placebo group ($p = 0.014$; Kaplan-Meier lifetable analysis), a 52% reduction in the event rate. Of particular interest was the observation that effects on clinical events in each trial began to emerge relatively rapidly (i.e., within 9 months to 1 year of initiating treatment) (19). These findings are supported by the results of another recently reported study with pravastatin in 1,062 patients (mean age 55 years; 77% were men) with hypercholesterolemia (serum total cholesterol levels from 5.2 mmol/l [200 mg/dl] to 7.8 mmol/l [300 mg/dl]; mean baseline LDL-C was 4.6 mmol/l [181 mg/dl]) plus two additional atherosclerotic risk factors (20). In the latter study, in the initial 26-week, double-blind, placebo-controlled treatment period, there were significantly more serious cardiovascular adverse events in the placebo group (13 events, 2.4%) than in the pravastatin group (one event, 0.2%) ($p<0.001$). Six MIs, five hospitalizations for unstable angina, and one sudden cardiac death occurred in the placebo group, compared with none of these events in the pravastatin group (20). These findings of a rapid emergence of an effect on clinical outcomes contrast with the generally held view that lipid-lowering interventions begin to affect cardiovascular clinical events only after several years of therapy, as seen in the Coronary Primary Prevention Trial (8), the Helsinki Heart Study (9), and the Program on the Surgical Control of the Hyperlipidemias (10). Furthermore, the reduction in clinical event rates within a relatively short time frame suggests that mechanisms other than regression of atherosclerotic plaque may have been involved. Among the various hypotheses advanced to explain the rapid reduction in cardiovascular events are restoration of normal endothelial-dependent vasorelaxation, which is abnormal in the presence of hypercholesterolemia and/or established atherosclerosis (21), effects on platelets or other components of the coagulation system (20,22), and plaque stabilization (23).

The data from PLAC I and PLAC II are also in accord with previous trials in patients with marked hypercholesterolemia (8–13) and extend the benefits of lipid-lowering therapy to the large number of patients with CAD and only moderately elevated blood cholesterol. The results show that cholesterol-lowering intervention with pravastatin reduced the incidence of acute MI by more than 50%. It also may be assumed that the clinical complications of MI, such as heart failure, were thereby avoided or prevented in a certain number of patients at risk in the pravastatin treatment group. Data from the Framingham study estimate the probability of developing heart failure as 1.8% per year in patients diagnosed with first nonfatal MI (24). In this context, the results of PLAC I and PLAC II, extrapolated to the general population of patients at risk for an acute ischemic event, suggest that the incidence of heart failure may be reduced significantly by lipid-lowering therapy and may have significant implications from a public health perspective.

In conclusion, the demonstrated effects of lipid-lowering interventions in reducing MI incidence can be predicted to significantly impact the subsequent development of clinical complications such as heart failure. Cholesterol-lowering therapies should be added to the currently recognized class of anti–heart failure agents.

SUMMARY

Atherosclerotic CHD, in particular MI, is now the leading cause of heart failure in the United States. It therefore stands to reason that treatments aimed at preventing

MI should have a significant impact on the subsequent incidence of heart failure in patient populations at risk. An elevated blood cholesterol level, especially the LDL-C fraction, is the strongest independent risk factor for CHD. Data supporting the value of lowering markedly elevated blood cholesterol levels (e.g., LDL-C>190 mg/dl [4.9 mmol/l]) in preventing acute ischemic syndromes are available from several reported clinical trials. The collective results of these studies have shown that cholesterol lowering retards progression of coronary atherosclerotic plaque and improves cardiovascular morbidity. Results have recently been reported from two regression clinical trials in patients with only moderately elevated cholesterol levels and CAD: PLAC I and PLAC II. Each study was a randomized, double-blind, placebo-controlled, 3-year evaluation using the HMG CoA reductase inhibitor, pravastatin, as a monotherapy regimen for 3 years. Efficacy assessments included atherosclerosis progression (PLAC I: coronary, N = 408; PLAC II: carotid, N = 151) and clinical events. The results show that in each study, both progression of atherosclerosis and cardiovascular clinical event rates were reduced in the patients treated with pravastatin. Between PLAC I and PLAC II, treatment with pravastatin resulted in a 52% reduction in the event rate for the combined endpoint of nonfatal MI or CHD death. These results are in accord with previous trials in patients with marked hypercholesterolemia and extend the benefit to patients with CAD and moderately elevated cholesterol levels. More importantly, the benefits of lipid-lowering therapy in reducing the overall incidence of MI should have an impact on the subsequent development of clinical complications such as heart failure.

ACKNOWLEDGMENT

These studies were supported by research grants from the Bristol-Myers Squibb Pharmaceutical Research Institute, Princeton, New Jersey.

REFERENCES

1. Destefano F, Merritt RK, Anda RF, Casper ML, Eaker ED. Trends in nonfatal heart disease in the United States, 1980 through 1989. *Arch Intern Med* 1993;153:2489–2494.
2. AHA Special Report. The cholesterol facts: a summary of the evidence relating dietary fats, serum cholesterol, and coronary heart disease. *Circulation* 1990;81:1721–1733.
3. Schocken DD, Arrieta MI, Leaverton PE, Ross EA. Prevalence and mortality rate of congestive heart failure in the United States. *J Am Coll Cardiol* 1992;20:301–306.
4. Bourassa MG, Gurne O, Bangdiwala SI, et al. Natural history and patterns of current practice in heart failure. The Studies of Left Ventricular Dysfunction (SOLVD) Investigators. *J Am Coll Cardiol* 1993;22[4 Suppl A]:14A–19A.
5. Kannel WB, Castelli WP, Gordon T, McNamara PM. Serum cholesterol, lipoproteins, and the risk of coronary heart disease: the Framingham Study. *Ann Intern Med* 1971;74:1–12.
6. Martin MT, Hulley SB, Browner WS, Buller LH, Wentworth D. Serum cholesterol, blood pressure, and mortality: implications from a cohort of 361,662 men. *Lancet* 1986;2:933–936.
7. Stamler J. Population studies. In: Levy RI, Rifkind BM, Dennis BH, et al., eds. *Nutrition, lipids, and coronary heart disease*. New York: Raven Press; 1979:25–88.
8. Lipid Research Clinics Program. The Lipid Research Clinics coronary primary prevention trial results. I. Reduction in incidence of coronary heart disease. *JAMA* 1984;251:351–364.

9. Frick MH, Elo O, Haapa K, et al. Helsinki Heart Study: primary-prevention trial with gemfibrozil in middle-aged men with dyslipidemia. Safety of treatment, changes in risk factors, and incidence of coronary heart disease. *N Engl J Med* 1987;317:1237–1245.
10. Buchwald H, Varco RL, Matts JP, et al. Effect of partial ileal bypass surgery on mortality and morbidity from coronary heart disease in patients with hypercholesterolemia. *N Engl J Med* 1990;323: 946–955.
11. Brensike JF, Levy RI, Epstein SE, et al. Effects of therapy with cholestyramine on progression of coronary arteriosclerosis: results of the NHLBI type II coronary intervention study. *Circulation* 1984;69:313–324.
12. Brown BG, Albers JJ, Fisher LD, et al. Regression of coronary artery disease as a result of intensive lipid-lowering therapy in men with high levels of apolipoprotein B. *N Engl J Med* 1990;323:1289–1298.
13. Watts GF, Lewis B, Brunt JNH, et al. Effects on coronary artery disease of lipid-lowering diet, or diet plus cholestyramine, in the St. Thomas' Atherosclerosis Regression Study (STARS). *Lancet* 1992;339:563–569.
14. Romm PA, Green CE, Reagan K, Rackley CE. Relation of serum lipoprotein cholesterol levels to presence and severity of angiographic coronary artery disease. *Am J Cardiol* 1991;67:479–483.
15. Pitt B, Ellis SG, Mancini GBJ, Rosman S, McGovern ME. Design and recruitment in the United States of a multicenter quantitative angiographic trial of pravastatin to limit atherosclerosis in the coronary arteries (PLAC I). *Am J Cardiol* 1993;72:31–35.
16. Nutrition Committee, American Heart Association. Dietary guidelines for healthy American adults. A statement for physicians and health professionals by the Nutrition Committee, American Heart Association. *Circulation* 1986;74:1465A–1468A.
17. Crouse JR, Byington RP, Bond MG, et al. Pravastatin, lipids, and atherosclerosis in the carotid arteries: design features of a clinical trial with carotid atherosclerosis outcome. *Controlled Clin Trials* 1992;13:495–506.
18. Pitt B, Mancini GBJ, Ellis G, Rosman S, McGovern ME. Pravastatin Limitation of Atherosclerosis in the Coronary Arteries (PLAC I). *J Am Coll Cardiol* 1994;131A.
19. Furberg CD, Byington RP, Crouse JR, Espeland MA. Pravastatin, lipids, and major coronary events. *Am J Cardiol* 1994;73:1133–1134.
20. The Pravastatin Multinational Study Group for Cardiac Risk Patients. Effects of pravastatin in patients with serum total cholesterol levels from 5.2 to 7.8 mmol/liter (200 to 300 mg/dl) plus two additional atherosclerotic risk factors. *Am J Cardiol* 1993;721:1031–1037.
21. Creager MA, Cooke JP, Mendelsohn ME, et al. Impaired vasodilation of forearm resistance vessels in hypercholesterolemic humans. *J Clin Invest* 1990;86:228–234.
22. Jay RH, Rampling MW, Betteridge DJ. Abnormalities of blood rheology in familial hypercholesterolemia: effects of treatment. *Atherosclerosis* 1990;85:249–256.
23. Brown GB, Zhao XQ, Sacco DE, Albers JJ. Arteriographic view of treatment to achieve regression of coronary atherosclerosis and to prevent plaque disruption and clinical cardiovascular events. *Br Heart J* 1993;69:S48–S53.
24. The Framingham Study, Section 35. Survival following initial cardiovascular events and subsequent events as a function of previous event; Department of Health and Human Services, National Institutes of Health publication #88-2969. 1988.

The Failing Heart, edited by N. S. Dhalla,
R. E. Beamish, N. Takeda, and M. Nagano.
Lippincott-Raven Publishers, Philadelphia © 1995.

33

Effect of Propionyl-L-Carnitine on Heart and Skeletal Muscle Metabolism During Congestive Heart Failure

Federica de Giuli, Anna Cargnoni, Evasio Pasini, *Anna Mazzoletti,
*Roberta Confortini, and †Roberto Ferrari

*Fondazione Clinica del Lavoro, Centro di Fisiopatologia Cardiovascolare "S. Maugeri,"
25064 Gussago, Brescia, Italy; *Cattedra di Cardiologia, Spedali Civili di Brescia,
25123 Brescia, Italy; and †Department of Cardiology, Universitá degli Studi di Brescia,
25123 Brescia, Italy*

Carnitine is an essential cofactor in the intermediary metabolism of fatty acids. Most of the endogenous carnitine is located in the muscle, both cardiac and skeletal (1). Because oxidized fatty acids are the primary substrate for the cardiac muscle, carnitine deficiency can impair myocardial energy fluxes and, therefore, heart function (2).

Carnitine prevents fatty acid accumulation and lactic acid production and hence helps muscle function (3–5). It has been found to increase exercise tolerance in patients with ischemic heart and peripheral vascular diseases (6–9). Systemic carnitine deficiency produces a reversible form of cardiomyopathy (10,11). Low levels of carnitine have been found in adults with mild or moderate heart failure (12,13) and in the explanted heart of patients affected by dilated (14) or ischemic (15) cardiomyopathy. Therapy with L-carnitine, the active isomer of carnitine, has also been found to be beneficial in dipptheritic- (16) and anthracycline- (17) induced myocarditis. The role of carnitine for the treatment of heart failure, however, remains unknown. In this article, we review the literature and our own data (18–23) on the effects of propionyl-L-carnitine in heart failure.

Propionyl-L-carnitine is a naturally occurring component of the carnitine pool which exists endogenously and is maintained in a homeostatic balance. The empirical formula is $C_{10}H_{20}O_4NCI$, and the molecular weight is 253.7. Propionyl-L-carnitine is formed by means of carnitine acetyltransferase from propionyl-CoA, a product of methionine, threonine, valine, and isoleucine as well as of odd-chain fatty acids.

Pharmacokinetic studies have demonstrated that, in humans, the plasma concentration of propionyl-L-carnitine increases following intravenous administration and then decreases to baseline values within 6 to 24 hours (24). This time span varies with dosage. The plasma concentrations of L-carnitine follow a similar pattern, but in a more sustained fashion. Urinary excretion of all these compounds increases after the intravenous dose of propionyl-L-carnitine and the excretion rates reach their highest values during the first 24 hours following administration.

Propionyl-L-carnitine has several advantages over L-carnitine. First of all, as just mentioned, it increases plasma and cellular carnitine content, thus enhancing free fatty acid (FFA) oxidation in carnitine-deficient states as well as increasing glucose oxidation rates (25). Second, muscular carnitine transferases have higher affinity for propionyl-L-carnitine than for L-carnitine or its other derivatives. Therefore, propionyl-L-carnitine is highly specific for both skeletal and cardiac muscle (26). Third, while having a mechanism of action similar to carnitine, it carries the propionyl group, and enhances the uptake of this agent by myocardial cell (27). This is particularly important, as propionate can be used by mitochondria as an anaplerotic substrate, thus providing energy in the absence of oxygen consumption (28). Interestingly, propionate alone cannot be administered due to its toxicity (29). Finally, due to the particular structure of the molecule with a long lateral tail, propionyl-L-carnitine has specific pharmacological action independent of its effect on muscle metabolism, resulting in peripheral dilatation and positive inotropism (19,30).

RATIONALE FOR THE USE OF PROPIONYL-L-CARNITINE IN HEART FAILURE AT EXPERIMENTAL LEVEL

The rationale for using propionyl-L-carnitine for the treatment of heart failure relies on its effects on both cardiac and skeletal muscle. The effects of propionyl-L-carnitine on the normal aerobic myocardium have been tested in several different experimental preparations and in patients with coronary artery disease but normal left ventricular function.

When given acutely to isolated and perfused heart preparation, propionyl-L-carnitine does not modify left ventricular pressure (18). When given intravenously through in vivo preparation, propionyl-L-carnitine causes a dose-dependent, short-lasting enhancement of cardiac output, both in dogs studied under open- and closed-chest conditions (24,25). In these preparations, arterial blood pressure, heart rate, and contractility varied slightly and unpredictably. Propionyl-L-carnitine does not elicit electrocardiographic effects. These responses are not modified by alpha- or beta-adrenergic blockade, nor by administration of calcium antagonists. They are, however, abolished by the combination of all of these interventions. Mesenteric iliac and renal blood flows are also increased. In addition, propionyl-L-carnitine causes coronary vasodilation with reduced oxygen extraction; this effect lasts longer than the general hemodynamic effects and is not seen with L-carnitine alone. All of these cardiovascular actions of propionyl-L-carnitine can be attributed to its pharmacologic properties, rather than to its role as a metabolic intermediate.

The hemodynamic effect of propionyl-L-carnitine has been evaluated in ten patients with coronary artery disease but with normal left ventricular function (26,27). The drug was administered intravenously at a dose of 15 mg/kg. Propionyl-L-carnitine improves the stroke volume and reduces the ejection impedence as a result of a decrease in systemic and pulmonary resistance and of an increase in arterial compliance. Total external heart power improves with a proportionally smaller increase in the energy requirement, suggesting that propionyl-L-carnitine has a positive inotropic property.

Interestingly, when administered chronically to the animals several days before the isolation of the heart, propionyl-L-carnitine increases the performance of the aerobic myocardium independently from changes of peripheral hemodynamics or coronary flow (18,28).

To investigate whether the chronic effect is specific for propionyl-L-carnitine or is due to L-carnitine or propionic acid, we have designed experiments in which rabbits were treated for 10 days with either saline, L-carnitine (1 mmol/kg), propionic acid (1 mmol/kg), or propionyl-L-carnitine (1 mmol/kg) (19). Propionic acid resulted in 98% mortality after 10 days. No death could be detected after propionyl-L-carnitine or L-carnitine treatment. Treatment with L-carnitine failed to modify the volume-pressure curves of the isolated left ventricle. On the contrary, treatment with propionyl-L-carnitine prevented the decrease of the optimum developed pressure and the rise in end-diastolic pressure, which remained constant even after overstretching.

In our previous studies (18,19), we postulated the hypothesis that the rise in end-diastolic pressure enhances the mechanical performance of the heart by improving its metabolism. It is known that pyruvate increases heart contractility allowing a more efficient energy utilization (29). Administration of pyruvate leads to a higher cytosolic phosphorylation potential, which in conjuction with a reduced inorganic phosphate (Pi) concentration translates into an increased contraction.

We investigated whether a similar mechanism is at the basis of the propionyl-L-carnitine effects. Energy metabolism does not seem to be involved, because high-energy phosphates, Pi, and mitochondrial function remain unchanged after chronic propionyl-L-carnitine administration (19). These findings, however, lead to some important implications. Usually, typical inotropic agents such as digitalis, calcium, and adrenergic compounds stimulate contractility by increasing myofibrillar energy utilization at the expense of energy supply. Consequently, these agents cause a decline in PCr/Pi ratio, suggesting that they place the heart in a supply/demand imbalance (29). This was not the case for propionyl-L-carnitine. Energy metabolism remained unchanged despite the increase in myocardial performance.

Finally, we investigated whether the mechanical effects of prolonged treatment with propionyl-L-carnitine are related to electrophysiological changes. It is known that acute administration of propionyl-L-carnitine does not influence the action potential parameters (30). On the contrary, chronic treatment causes a prolongation of the action potential duration in the plateau phase (19). This action appears to be a specific effect for propionyl-L-carnitine, as prolonged treatment with L-carnitine does not cause any electrophysiological change (19). During the repolarization phase, which is modified by propionyl-L-carnitine, important events occur that are able to influence contractility (31). It is attractive to correlate the effect on papillary muscle action potential duration with that on cardiac mechanical performance, because propionyl-L-carnitine, but not L-carnitine, affects both of them. In addition, the electrophysiological and mechanical effects of propionyl-L-carnitine are not dependent on the extracellular calcium concentration. The improvement in mechanical performance, however, is observed not only in the spontaneously beating heart, but also at driving rates at which the effect on action potential duration is completely lost. Consequently, the relationship between the two events remains uncertain and the intrinsic difference between the two experimental preparations does not allow one to draw a definitive link.

In addition, research conducted with ischemic myocardium by Broderick et al. (32) on isolated rat hearts and global no-flow ischemia showed that during the reperfusion of previously ischemic hearts, propionyl-L-carnitine stimulated glucose oxidation and significantly improved the functional recovery, as measured by heart rate and peak systolic pressure. This work supports the theory that carnitine's beneficial effects on ischemic myocardium is a result of its ability to overcome the inhibition of glucose oxidation induced by increased levels of fatty acids. Other work also suggests an intracellular mechanism of action and implies that better protection is provided if the agent is administered prior to the ischemic insult (33). Paulson et al. (34) studied isolated rat hearts subjected to global, low-flow ischemia. During reperfusion, the propionyl-L-carnitine group exhibited a significantly greater recovery of all hemodynamic variables. Interestingly, a concentration of 1 mM of propionyl-L-carnitine had no significant protective effect, while concentrations of 5.5 mM and 11 mM significantly improved recovery of cardiac output. This beneficial effect was determined to be greater than that of L-acetylcarnitine or L-carnitine on a molar basis. Equally, propionyl-L-carnitine has been found to directly improve postischemic stunning (34).

Specific experimental studies have been conducted on the efficacy of this agent with respect to congestive heart failure (33–40). In particular, treatment with propionyl-L-carnitine (50 mg/kg, intra-arterially) for 4 days significantly improves the hemodynamic of pressure-overloaded (by constriction of the abdominal aorta) conscious rats (40). The beneficial effects were more significant for the rats with the higher cardiac hypertrophy and the greater carnitine deficiency (40). In another study, papillary muscles were isolated from rats that had been treated with 180 mg/kg propionyl-L-carnitine for 8 weeks, starting from weaning (35). Aortic constriction was performed at 8 weeks of age and lasted 4 weeks. The papillary muscles of untreated animals showed increased time-to-peak tension and reduced peak rate of tension rise and delay. Propionyl-L-carnitine normalized all of these parameters (35). The effects of propionyl-L-carnitine has also been tested on isolated myocytes obtained by pressure-overloaded rats. Compared with normal cells, myocytes from untreated animals subjected to aortic clamping showed depressed palmitate oxidation and reduced adenosine triphosphate/adenosine diphosphate (ATP/ADP) ratio. propionyl-L-carnitine corrected this defect in the energy-producing system of the hypertrophied cells. This in turn results in preservation of α/β myosin heavy chain.

In an infarct model of heart failure, chronic administration of propionyl-L-carnitine (60 mg/kg per os given for 5 months) positively influenced ventricular remodeling, being equi-effective to enalapril (1 mg/kg per os) in limiting the magnitude of left ventricular dilatation estimated by pressure-volume curves (36). Propionyl-L-carnitine limited the alterations in ventricular chamber stiffness induced by infarction both at low and at high filling pressure (36). In isolated myocytes obtained from infarcted rats, propionyl-L-carnitine increased peak systolic Ca^{2+}, peak shortening (17%), and the velocity of cell shortening to a greater extent than in normal cells (38).

We investigated the effects of propionyl-L-carnitine (250 mg/kg intraperitoneally for 2 months) on the perfused heart obtained from rabbits with streptozotocin-induced diabetes (37). Cardiac performance was determined under basal conditions and during a stepwise increase in volume of a saline-filled balloon inserted into the left ventricle. Propionyl-L-carnitine prevented the decrease in developed pressure and the increase in diastolic pressure due to progressive filling of the left ventricular balloon. The same treatment also prevented the depression in the function of the sarcoplasmic reticulum observed in untreated rats. Ca^{2+}-stimulated ATPase activity, Ca^{2+} uptake, and Mg^{2+} ATPase activity were similar to those of the nondiabetic heart. On the contrary, treatment with propionyl-L-carnitine failed to reserve the diabetes-induced changes in the sarcolemmal Ca^{2+} ATPase (39).

Thus propionyl-L-carnitine displayed a therapeutic effect in a number of models of chronic heart failure, namely pressure overload, infarction, and diabetic cardiomyopathies. In several occasions the effect of propionyl-L-carnitine was apparent under conditions of high energy demand, induced by an increase in work load. It seems therefore likely that propionyl-L-carnitine is able to correct some metabolic steps of the process that leads to heart failure. In addition, propionyl-L-carnitine could be helpful in heart failure for a specific action on peripheral heart muscle.

In general, a patient with heart failure complains of fatigue and shortness of breath. Usually these symptoms are alleviated by the administration of diuretic, digoxin, and vasodilator therapy, and the majority of patients experience resolution of symptoms at rest. Unhappily, however, many patients continue to experience exertional symptoms and frequently report that they are unable to perform regular activities of daily life. During maximal exercise testing, patients with heart failure terminate exercise earlier than normal subjects of comparable weight and gender.

Traditionally, fatigue and shortness of breath have been related to a low cardiac output and increased end-diastolic pressure. Although there may be some validity to this claim, recent studies have demonstrated that the origin of symptoms in heart failure is much more complex (41,42). In chronic heart failure, unlike acute heart failure, shortness of breath is not related simply to end-diastolic pressure either at rest or at peak exercise (42). Many subtle changes do take place in the lungs, such as an increased ventilation for a given carbon dioxide production and weakness of the diaphragm. Equally, exertional fatigue is not simply the result of skeletal muscle underperfusion (43–45).

We measured leg flow responses to a low-work-load bicycle exercise mimicking the small amount of activity encountered in daily life by using a femoral venous thermodilution catheter in a group of patients with heart failure. We found a significant decrease in flow responses to exercise in the majority of patients, although in some the flow response was within the normal limits (46). The inability of muscle blood flow to increase normally during exercise in patients with heart failure is due primarily to an abnormality of arterial vasodilation, as evidenced by a failure of leg vascular resistances to decrease normally during exercise (44,46). This, in turn, could be due to (a) compression of capillaries and intrinsic vascular changes due to fluid and sodium retention (47); (b) increase in sympathetic activation and angiotensin II, impairing dilatation (48); and (c) abnormality of vascular endothelium and vascular remodeling (49).

While abnormalities of the peripheral circulation in chronic heart failure patients have been frequently described as a major determinant of exercise limitation, Wiener et al. have found no relationship between plethysmographic measurements of exercising forearm blood flow and muscle metabolism measured by phosphorus nuclear magnetic resonance (NMR) spectroscopy (50). These researchers suggest that other mechanisms, such as alterations in mitochondrial population or substrate utilization, may be responsible for the depressed exercise performance.

Perhaps the best evidence that muscle deconditioning contributes to exertional fatigue comes from studies demonstrating that participation in a home exercise or in a formal rehabilitation program can improve the maximal exercise capacity of patients with heart failure by 15% to 30% (51–53).

The metabolic studies have been conducted using phosphorus-31 NMR, a technique that permits the noninvasive monitoring of phosphocreatine, inorganic phosphate, ATP, and pH in working muscle. Patients with heart failure have a more pronounced increase in the Pi/PCr ratio and a more pronounced decrease in muscle pH than do normal subjects performing comparable workloads (54).

When the uptake of limb substrate has been determined by measuring the arterial-venous (A-V) difference of different metabolites, interesting results have emerged. At rest, the peripheral muscle of patients with heart failure does not extract FFA, but only glucose (55). This suggest an impairment of FFA oxidation that might be due to a lack of carnitine. On the other hand, glucose uptake is enhanced. During moderate exercise, there is an increment of glucose uptake with excessive production of lactate, but no recruitment of FFA (55). All of these observations, and the positive data obtained by the use of propionyl-L-carnitine to improve the walking capacities of patients with peripheral arterial diseases (56), have suggested that propionyl-L-carnitine could specifically improve metabolism and function of skeletal muscle in patients with chronic heart failure.

EFFECTS OF PROPIONYL-L-CARNITINE IN PATIENTS WITH CHRONIC HEART FAILURE

There are several pilot studies in which administration of propionyl-L-carnitine to patients with chronic heart failure has been shown to exert several clinical effects.

Furthermore, there are two current and ongoing large-scale national and international trials, the results of which should be available in a short time (57).

We have studied the effects of acute and chronic administration of propionyl-L-carnitine (1.5 g/d) on hemodynamics, hormonal levels, exercise capacity, and oxygen consumption measurements in 15 patients with chronic heart failure (New York Heart Association [NYHA] classes II and III and left ventricular ejection fraction <40%). There were no changes in the hemodynamics or neurohormonal levels after either acute or chronic administration (22). After 1 month of treatment, however, a significant increase in exercise capacity and peak VO_2 was observed, suggesting a possible improvement of peripheral muscle metabolism.

In a subsequent study, we examined the effects of propionyl-L-carnitine (15g/d for 1 month) on the limb metabolism, both at rest and during exercise (23,58).

Skeletal muscle metabolism was assessed as femoral A-V difference for lactate, pyruvate, and FFA. At rest, propionyl-L-carnitine caused a reduction of arterial and venous blood levels of FFA but did not change overall muscle extraction of FFA, lactate, or pyruvate. After maximal exercise, propionyl-L-carnitine decreased the negative A-V difference for lactate, restored a positive A-V difference for pyruvate, and did not change that for FFA. We concluded that propionyl-L-carnitine improves skeletal muscle metabolism in patients with idiopathic dilated cardiomyopathy by increasing pyruvate flux into the Krebs' cycle and decreasing lactate production. This effect, which occurs in the absence of major hemodynamics and neuroendocrine changes, may underlie the ability of propionyl-L-carnitine to increase exercise performance in patients with heart failure.

Very recently, Caponnetto et al. (59) reported the effects of propionyl-L-carnitine on 50 patients with mild chronic heart failure (NYHA class II), symptomatic despite therapy with digitalis and diuretics, with ejection fraction <45%. They were randomized to receive 1.5 g of propionyl-L-carnitine or placebo as oral treatment for 6 months. Maximal exercise time in the treated group was significantly increased (1 minute longer than placebo), while lactate production was significantly reduced. Left ventricular shortening fraction and left ventricular ejection fraction showed a significant increase in the propionyl-L-carnitine group (respectively, $p<0.0001$), while no difference was apparent in the placebo group. Stroke volume index and cardiac index had significant increments in the treated group ($p<0.05$), and systemic vascular resistance was lowered ($p<0.05$). No hemodynamic variations were observed in the placebo group. The clinical score showed a significant improvement in the propionyl-L-carnitine–treated group. The greatest changes occurred after the first month of treatment and persisted throughout the entire period of treatment. These authors envisage two possible mechanisms of action: an improvement of skeletal muscle function and metabolism as well as a positive effect on cardiac muscle, which explains the enhancement of the hemodynamic parameters.

Finally, it is interesting to note that propionyl-L-carnitine given to patients with severe heart failure (NYHA IV) was able to reduce the increase of soluble receptors of tumor necrosis factor (TNF)-α and, in particular, of the soluble receptor (60).

The specific role of TNF-α and of its soluble receptors in patients with heart failure is not clear and is still under investigation. It is of interest for the present discussion, however, to recall that an increased TNF has been implicated in the skeletal muscle changes of heart failure (61).

SUMMARY

Propionyl-L-carnitine is a naturally occurring component that has been considered for the treatment of heart failure. The rationale for its use in this pathology is related to its effects on cardiac and skeletal muscle. Chronic treatment with propionyl-L-carnitine was shown to improve the contraction of isolated and aerobic perfused rabbit hearts. When administered to open- and closed-chest dogs, propionyl-L-carnitine causes a peripheral vasodilation. The compound was shown to improve energy metabolism and myocardial contractility in different experimental models for heart failure, such as pressure-overloaded rats, infarct model of heart failure, and rabbit with streptozotocin-induced diabetes. Under all of these conditions, the effect of propionyl-L-carnitine was apparent in a situation of high energy demand induced by increased workload. It seems therefore likely that propionyl-L-carnitine is able to correct some metabolic steps of the process that leads to heart failure. In addition, propionyl-L-carnitine could be helpful in heart failure for its specific action on peripheral heart muscles. Administration of propionyl-L-carnitine in patients with chronic heart failure improves skeletal muscle metabolism by increasing pyruvate flux into the Krebs' cycle and decreasing lactate production. These effects occur in the absence of major hemodynamic and neuroendocrinal changes and may underlie the ability of propionyl-L-carnitine to increase exercise performance in patients with heart failure. In a randomized study on 15 patients with mild, chronic heart failure, propionyl-L-carnitine significantly increased the maximal exercise time, reduced lactate production, and improved left ventricular ejection fraction. There are two currently ongoing large-scale national and international trials on the effects of this compound in heart failure, the results of which should be available in a short time.

REFERENCES

1. Bremer J. Carnitine-metabolism and functions. *Physiol Rev* 1983;63:1420–1480.
2. Engel AG, Rebouche CJ. Carnitine metabolism and inborn errors. *J Inherited Metab Dis* 1984;7:38–43.
3. Hulsmann WC, Siliprandi D, Climan M, Siliprandi N. Effect of carnitine on the oxidation of α-oxoglutarate to succinate in the presence of aceto acetate or pyruvate. *Biochim Biophys Acta* 1964;93:166–168.
4. Siliprandi N, Di Lisa F, Rossi CR, Toninello A. Overview of lipid metabolism. In: Ferrari R, Katz AM, Shug A, Visioli O, eds. *Myocardial ischemia and lipid metabolism.* New York: Plenum Press: 1984:1–13.
5. Siliprandi N, Di Lisa F, Pieralisi G, et al. Metabolic changes induced by maximal exercise in human subjects following L-carnitine administration. *Biochim Biophys Acta* 1990;1034:17–21.
6. Thomsen JH, Austin LS, Vincente UY, et al. Improved pacing tolerance of the ischaemic human myocardium after administration of carnitine. *Am J Cardiol* 1979;43:300–306.

7. Cherchi A, Lai C, Angelino F, et al. Effects of L-carnitine on exercise tolerance in chronic stable angina: a multicenter, double-blind, randomized, placebo controlled crossover study. *Int J Clin Pharmacol Ther Toxicol* 1985;23:569–572.
8. Carnitine deficiency [Editorial]. *Lancet* 1990;335:631–632.
9. Brevetti G, Chiariello M, Policchio A, et al. Increases in walking distance in patients with peripheral vascular disease treated with L-carnitine: a double-blind, cross-over study. *Circulation* 1988;77: 767–783.
10. Tripp ME, Katcher ML, Peters HA, et al. Systemic carnitine deficiency presenting as familial endocardial fibroelastosis. A treatable cardiomyopathy. *N Engl J Med* 1981;305:385–390.
11. Waber LJ, Valle D, Neill C, Di Mauro S, Shug A. Carnitine deficiency presenting as familial cardiomyopathy: a treatable defect in carnitine transport. *J Pediatr* 1982;101:700–705.
12. Suzuki Y, Masumuro Y, Kobayashi A, Yamazaki L, Harada Y, Osawa M. Myocardial carnitine deficiency in congestive heart failure. *Lancet* 1982;1:116.
13. Regitz V, Shug AL, Fleck E. Defective myocardial metabolism in congestive heart failure secondary to dilated cardiomyopathy and to coronary, hypertensive and valvular heart disease. *Am J Cardiol* 1990;65:755–760.
14. Regitz V, Shug AL, Schuler S, Yankah AC, Hetze R. Herzinsufficienz bei dilatativer Kardiomyopathie und koronarer Herzerkrankung-beitrag biochemischer Parameter zur Beurteilung der Prognose. *Dtsch Med Wochenschr* 1988;113:781–786.
15. Regitz V, Muller M, Schuler S, et al. Carnitinstoffechsel-veranduregen in Endetadium der dilatativen Kardiomyopathie und der ischamischen Herzmuskeler-krankung. *Z Kardiol* 1987;76:1–8.
16. Figueiredo Ramos ACM, Elian PRP, Barrucand L, Da Silva JAF. The protective effect of carnitine in human diptheric myocarditis. *Pediatr Res* 1984;18:815–819.
17. De Leonardis V, Neri B, Baculli S, Cinelli P. Reduction cardiac toxicity of anthracyclines by L-carnitine preliminary overview of clinical data. *Int J Clin Pharmacol Res* 1985;5:137–142.
18. Ferrari R, Pasini E, Condorelli E, et al. Effect of propionyl-L-carnitine on mechanical function of isolated rabbit heart. *Cardiovasc Drugs Ther* 1991;5:17–24.
19. Ferrari R, Di Lisa F, De Jong JW, et al. Prolonged propionyl-L-carnitine pretreatment of rabbit: biochemical, hemodynamic and electrophysiological effects on myocardium. *J Mol Cell Cardiol* 1992;24:219–232.
20. Pasini E, Comini L, Ferrari R, de Giuli F, Menotti A, Dhalla NS. Effect of propionyl-L-carnitine on experimentally induced cardiomyopathy in rats. *Am J Cardiovasc Pathol* 1992;4:216–222.
21. Pasini E, Cargnoni A, Condorelli E, Marzo A, Lisciani L, Ferrari R. Effect of prolonged treatment with propionyl-L-carnitine on erucic acid-induced myocardial dysfunction in rats. *Mol Cell Biochem* 1992;112:117–123.
22. Anand IS, Chandrashekhar Y, Sarma PR, Ferrari R, Corsi M. Effect of propionyl-L-carnitine on the hemodynamics, peak VO_2 and hormones in CHF. *Chest* 1991;100[Suppl]:110S(abst).
23. Ferrari R, Cargnoni A, de Giuli F, Pasini E, Anand I, Visioli O. Propionyl-L-carnitine improves skeletal muscle metabolism and exercise capacity of patients with congestive heart failure. *Circulation* 1993;88[Supp]:2223 (abst).
24. Cevese A, Schena F, Cerutti G. Short-term hemodynamic effects of intravenous propionyl-l-carnitine in anesthetized dogs. *Cardiologia* 1989;34:95–101.
25. Cevese A, Schena F, Cerutti G. Short-term hemodynamic effects of intravenous propionyl-l-carnitine in anesthetized dogs. *Cardiovasc Drugs Ther* 1991;5[Suppl 1]:45–56.
26. Chiddo A, Musci S, Bortome A, et al. Effetti emodinamici e sul circolo coronarico della propionyl-l-carnitina. *Cardiologia* 1989;54[Suppl 1]:111–117.
27. Chiddo A, Gaglione A, Musci S, et al. Hemodynamic study of intravenous propionyl-L-carnitine in patients with ischemic heart disease and normal left ventricular function. *Cardiovasc Drugs Ther* 1991;5[Suppl 1]:107–112.
28. Tassani V, Cattapan L, Magnanimi L, Peschechera A. Anaplerotic effect of propionyl-L-carnitine in rat heart mitochondria. *Biochem Biophys Res Commun* 1994;199:949–953.
29. Zweier JL, Jacobus E. Substrate-induced alteration of high energy phosphate metabolism and contractile function in the perfused heart. *J Biol Chem* 1987;262:8015–8021.
30. Barbieri M, Carbonin PU, Cerbai E, et al. Lack of correlation between the antiarrhythmic effect of L-propionylcarnitine on reoxygenation-induced arrhythmias and its electrophysiological properties. *Br J Pharmacol* 1991;102:73–78.
31. Noble D. The surprising heart: a review of recent progress in cardiac electrophysiology. *J Physiol (Lond)* 1984;353:1–50.

32. Broderick TL, Quinney HA, Barker CC, Lopaschuk GD. Beneficial effect of carnitine on mechanical recovery of rat hearts reperfused after a transient period of global ischemia is accompanied by a stimulation of glucose oxidation. *Circulation* 1993;87:972–981.
33. Leipala JA, Bhatnagar R, Pineda E, Najibi S, Massoumi K, Packer L. Protection of the reperfused heart by L-propionylcarnitine. *J Appl Physiol* 1991;71(4):1518–1522.
34. Paulson DJ, Traxler J, Schmidt M, Noonan J, Shug AL. Protection of the ischaemic myocardium by L-propionyl-carnitine: effects on the recovery of cardiac output after ischaemia and reperfusion, carnitine transport, and fatty acid oxidation. *Cardiovasc Res* 1986;20:536–541.
35. Micheletti R, Giacalone G, Canepari M, Salardi S, Bianchi G, Reggiani C. Propionyl-L-carnitine prevents myocardial mechanical alterations due to pressure overload in rats. *Am J Physiol* 1994; 266:H2190–2197.
36. Micheletti R, Schiavone A, English E, et al. Propionyl-L-carnitine limits chronic ventricular dilatation after myocardial infarction in rats. *Am J Physiol* 1993;264:H1111–H1117.
37. Pasini E, Comini L, Ferrari R, de Giuli F, Menotti A, Dhalla NS. Effect of propionyl-L-carnitine on experimental induced cardiomyopathy in rats. *Am J Cardiovasc Pathol* 1992;4:216–222.
38. Li P, Micheletti R, Park C, Li BS, Anversa P, Bianchi G. Propionyl-L-carnitine ameliorates myocyte performance after infarction. *Can J Cardiol* 1994;10:85 (abst).
39. Lopaschuk GD, Tahiliani AG, Vadlamudi RVSU, Katz S, McNell JH. Cardiac sarcoplasmic reticulum in insulin- or carnitine-treated diabetic rats. *Am J Physiol* 1983;245:H969–H976.
40. Yang XP, Samaja M, English E, et al. Haemodynamic and metabolic activities of propionyl-L-carnitine in rats with pressure overload cardiac hypertrophy. *J Cardiovasc Pharmacol* 1992;20:88–98.
41. Lipkin DP, Canepa-Anson R, Stephens MR, Poole-Wilson PA. Factors determining symptoms in heart failure: comparison of fast and slow exercise tests. *Br Heart J* 1986;55:439–445.
42. Poole-Wilson PA. Relation of pathophysiologic mechanisms to outcome in heart failure. *J Am Coll Cardiol* 1993;22:22A–29A.
43. Wilson JR, Martin JL, Schwartz D, Ferraro N. Exercise intolerance in patients with chronic heart failure: role of impaired skeletal muscle nutritive flow. *Circulation* 1984;69:1079–1087.
44. Lipkin DP, Poole-Wilson PA. Symptoms limiting exercise in chronic heart failure. *Br Med J* 1986; 292:1030–1031.
45. Wilson JR, Mancini DM. Factors contributing to exercise limitation of heart failure. *J Am Coll Cardiol* 1993;22:93A–98A.
46. Sullivan MJ, Knight JD, Higginbotham MB, Cobb FR. Relation between central and peripheral hemodynamics during exercise in patients with chronic heart failure. *Circulation* 1989;80:769–781.
47. Anand IS, Ferrari R, Kalra GS, Wahi PL, Poole-Wilson PA, Harris P. Edema of cardiac origin, studies of body water and sodium, renal function, hemodynamic indexes, and plasma hormones in untreated congestive cardiac failure. *Circulation* 1989;80:299–305.
48. Wilson JR, Ferraro N, Wiener DH. Effect of the sympathetic nervous system on limb circulation and metabolism during exercise in heart failure. *Circulation* 1985;72:72–81.
49. Gibbons GH, Dzau VJ. The emerging concept of vascular remodeling. *N Engl J Med* 1994;330: 1431–1438.
50. Wiener DH, Fink LI, Maris J, Jones RA, Chance B, Wilson JR. Abnormal skeletal muscle bioenergetics during exercise in patients with heart failure: role of reduced muscle blood flow. *Circulation* 1986;73:1127–1136.
51. Regensteiner JG, Wolfel EE, Brass E, et al. Chronic changes in skeletal muscle histology and function in peripheral arterial disease. *Circulation* 1993;87:413–421.
52. Sullivan MJ, Higginbotham MB, Cobb FR. Exercise training in patients with severe left ventricular dysfunction: hemodynamic and metabolic effects. *Circulation* 1988;78:506–515.
53. Coats A, Adamopoulos S, Radaelli A, et al. Controlled trial of physical training in chronic heart failure. *Circulation* 1992;85:2119–2131.
54. Wilson JR, Fink L, Maris J, et al. Evaluation of skeletal muscle energy metabolism in patients with heart failure using gated phosphorus-31 nuclear magnetic resonance. *Circulation* 1985;71:57–62.
55. Ferrari R, Pasini E, de Giuli F, Opasich C, Cobelli F, Tavazzi L. Limb uptake of substrate in patients with congestive heart failure (CHF). *Can J Cardiol* 1994;10[Suppl A]:73A(abst).
56. Brevetti G, Chiariello M, Ferulano G, et al. Increases in walking distance in patients with peripheral vascular disease treated with L-carnitine: a double-blind, cross-over study. *Circulation* 1988;77: 767–783.
57. Garg R, Yusuf S. Current and ongoing randomized trials in heart failure and left ventricular dysfunction. *J Am Coll Cardiol* 1993;22:194A–197A.

58. de Giuli F, Cargnon A, Pasini E, et al. Effect of propionyl-l-carnitine (PLC) on skeletal muscle metabolism in patients with chronic heart failure (CHF). *Can J Cardiol* 1994;10[Suppl A]: 74A(abst).
59. Caponetto S, Canale C, Masperone MA, Terrachini V, Valentini G, Brunelli C. Efficacy of L-propionyl-carnitine treatment in patients with left ventricular dysfunction. *Can J Cardiol* 1994;10[Suppl A]:66A(abst).
60. Bachetti T, Corti A, Cassani G, Confortini R, Mazzoletti A, Ferrari R. Cytokines in end stage congestive heart failure: effect of propionyl-L-carnitine. *Eur Heart J* 1994;15:1267–1273.
61. Levine B, Kalman J, Mayer L, Fillit HM, Packer M. Elevated circulating level of tumor necrosis factor in severe chronic heart failure. *N Engl J Med* 1991;323:236–241.

The Failing Heart, edited by N. S. Dhalla,
R. E. Beamish, N. Takeda, and M. Nagano.
Lippincott-Raven Publishers, Philadelphia © 1995.

34

Effects of Vitamin E on the Cardiac Function and Contractility in Chronic Volume-Overload Heart Failure

*Kailash Prasad, †J.B. Gupta, ‡Jawahar Kalra,
‡S.V. Mantha, *Paul Lee, and §Baikunth Bharadwaj

*Departments of *Physiology and ‡Pathology, College of Medicine, University of
Saskatchewan, Saskatoon, Saskatchewan, S7N 5E5 Canada; †Cardiovascular Research
Laboratory, Ranbury Research Laboratory, New Delhi, India; and §Division of Thoracic
and Cardiovascular Surgery, Foothills Hospital, Calgary, Alberta T2N 2T9 Canada*

Reactive oxygen metabolites (ROMs) have been reported to depress cardiac function and contractility (1,2). Chronic volume overload is associated with a decrease in the cardiac function and contractility (3–5). The decrease in cardiac function and contractility in chronic volume and pressure overload is associated with an increase in the production of ROMs by polymorphonuclear leukocytes (PMNLs) (6,7). The decrease in cardiac function and contractility could be due to increased levels of ROMs. If this is the case, then an antioxidant (vitamin E) (8,9) should be able to prevent the chronic volume overload–induced depression of cardiac function and contractility concomitant with a decrease in the lipid peroxidation product malondialdehyde (MDA), a finger print for ROMs. We, therefore, investigated the effects of vitamin E on the chronic volume overload–induced changes in cardiac function and contractility and cardiac MDA in dogs.

METHODS

Adult mongrel dogs of either sex, weighing between 14 and 20 kg, were anesthetized initially with pentothal sodium (30 mg/kg) intravenously and intubated with a closed-cuff endotracheal tube. Each animal was ventilated with 95% O_2 and 5% CO_2 via a Harvard respirator (Harvard Apparatus Co., Inc., South Natick, Massachusetts) with a volume of 20 ml/kg and a respiratory rate of 20 breaths/min. Anesthesia was maintained with halothane.

Hemodynamic Measurements

Hemodynamic measurements were made as previously described (1,10). A 7F Cournand catheter was positioned in the left ventricle through the femoral artery to record left ventricular pressure. The first derivative of left ventricular pressure (dp/dt) was recorded with a differentiating device coupled to the left ventricular pressure channel at a frequency of 100 Hz. A similar catheter was positioned at the aortic arch through the common carotid artery to record aortic pressure (Ao). Another Cournand catheter was placed in the right atrium through the external jugular vein to measure mean right atrial pressure (mRAP) and to collect blood samples for biochemical measurements. A Swan-Ganz triple lumen catheter (7F) equipped with a thermistor tip was placed into the pulmonary artery through the right femoral vein to measure cardiac output (CO) and pulmonary arterial wedge pressure (PAW). Cardiac output was measured in triplicate with an Edwards Cardiac Output Computer (COM-1, Edwards Co., Inc., Farmington, Connecticut) using a thermodilution technique. All pressures and lead II ECG were monitored simultaneously. We used dp/dt and the ratio of dp/dt to PAW for assessment of myocardial contractility. Cardiac index (CI) and total systemic vascular resistance (TSVR) were calculated as previously described (1,10). Cardiac index and left ventricular end-diastolic pressure (LVEDP) were used as an index of cardiac function.

Malondialdehyde: Thiobarbituric Acid-Reactive Substances

Malondialdehyde levels in the left ventricular tissue were estimated as thiobarbituric acid (TBA)-reactive substances by the method described earlier (11,12). In short, 1.5 g of left ventricular muscle was washed in cold saline and cut into small pieces. The tissue was immersed in 10 volumes (w/v) of KCl phosphate buffer (pH 7.4) containing 140 mM KCl and 10 mM phosphate buffer, and homogenized with a polytron homogenizer (PT-10, Brinkman Instruments, Rexdale, Ontario, Canada) at a setting of 5 for two periods of 10 seconds each at 0°C to 4°C. A small portion of the homogenate was used for measurement of MDA. One hundred microliters of the homogenate was added in a glass test tube. To four other test tubes, 0, 25, 50, and 100 μl of 10 μM of tetraethoxypropane (TEP) reagent was added; 0.2 ml of 8.1% sodium dodecylsulphate solution was added to each of these tubes. Distilled water was then added to make a final volume of 1.0 ml. Then, 1.5 ml of 20% glacial acetic acid (pH 3.4) and 1.5 ml of 0.67% thiobarbituric acid were added to each tube, mixed, and incubated for 1 hour at 95°C in a polyethylene glycol bath. The tubes were then cooled to room temperature (22°C) and 1.0 ml of distilled water followed by 5 ml of butanol:pyridine (15:1) mixture was added to each tube and vortexed for 2 minutes. The butanol:pyridine layer was separated by centrifugation at 3,000 rpm for 15 minutes. Fluorescence intensity of butanol–pyridine solution was measured at 553 nm with excitation at 513 nm. Malondialdehyde content of cardiac tissue was expressed as nmoles/mg protein. Protein content of the homogenate was measured by using the method of Gornall et al. (13).

Surgical Procedure for Mitral Regurgitation

Volume-overload heart failure was produced by inducing mitral insufficiency by the previously described method (3,4). Briefly, the heart was exposed by opening the chest through the fifth left intercostal space under anesthesia. A small incision was made into the left atrium. The index finger was passed through this incision and through the mitral valve to detach two or more chordae tendineae from the anterior cusp of the valve to raise the mean left atrial pressure (mLAP) to 2.5 to 3 times the normal. The atriotomy was repaired, the lungs were inflated, and the chest was closed. Murmurs and thrill were present throughout the period of observation.

Experimental Protocol

Dogs were assigned to three groups. Group I (control; n = 7) dogs were anesthetized and catheterized for hemodynamic measurements; group II (n = 7), mitral regurgitation (MR) of 4 months' duration; and group III (n = 7), similar to group II but supplemented with vitamin E (40 U/kg/d, orally). Hemodynamic measurements were made before and after 4 months of MR in groups II and III to assess the cardiac function and contractility. At the end of 4 months, the dogs were killed after hemodynamic measurements were made, and a piece of left ventricle was removed for measurement of MDA.

Statistical Analysis

The results were expressed as mean ± SE. Paired Student's *t* test was used to analyze hemodynamic parameters, and unpaired Student's *t* test was used to analyze cardiac MDA. A *p* value of <0.05 was considered significant.

RESULTS

Hemodynamics

The hemodynamic data for control and volume overload with and without vitamin E groups are summarized in Table 1 and Figs. 1 and 2. The values for mean aortic pressure (mAo) and heart rate were similar in the three groups. There were increases in mLAP, LVEDP and TSVR in group II. The index of myocardial contractility [(+) dp/dt, dp/dt/PAW], however, decreased in this group. There was a tendency for a decrease in CI in group II as compared with group I, but the decrease

TABLE 1. *Changes in hemodynamics in control and mitral regurgitation dogs with and without vitamin E supplements*

Group	mAo (mmHg)	TSVR (dynes/sec/cm^{-5})	LVEDP (mmHg)	mLAP (mmHg)	HR (beats/min)	(+)dp/dt (mmHg)
Control	102.00 ± 3.72	2577.28 ± 214.97	13.20 ± 1.52	11.97 ± 0.925	105.80 ± 7.70	2407 ± 315
MR	98.00 ± 8.10	3158.69 ± 315.89*	17.20 ± 1.46*	18.13 ± 3.19*	98.00 ± 8.10	2100 ± 176*
MR + Vitamin E	94.5 ± 3.77	2112.02 ± 375.24†	15.4 ± 1.81	18.75 ± 1.19*	111.80 ± 10.45	2745 ± 328†

The results are expressed as mean ± SEM.
*p <0.05, control versus MR or MR + vitamin E.
†p <0.05 MR versus MR + vitamin E.
MR, mitral regurgitation. mAo, mean aortic pressure; MLAP, mean left atrial pressure; LVEDP, left ventricular end-diastolic pressure; HR, heart rate; TSVR, total systemic vascular resistance.

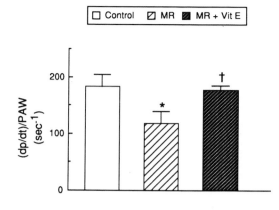

FIG. 1. (dp/dt)/PAW in the three groups. The results are expressed as mean ± SE. PAW, pulmonary arterial wedge pressure; MR, mitral regurgitation. *p<0.05, control vs. MR or MR + vitamin E. †p<0.05, MR vs. MR + vitamin E.

was not significant. The values for index of myocardial contractility were greater in group III than in group II, but similar to those of group I. Left ventricular end-diastolic pressure and TSVR decreased in group III as compared with group II, and the values were similar to those of group I. Mean left atrial pressure in group III remained elevated. Cardiac index increased in group III as compared with group II, but the increase was not significant.

Cardiac Malondialdehyde

Left ventricular MDA levels of the three groups are summarized in Fig. 3. The MDA content of the left ventricle of the control group was 0.0115 ± 0.0013 nmol/mg protein. It increased in groups II and III. The MDA content in group III was lower than that in group II.

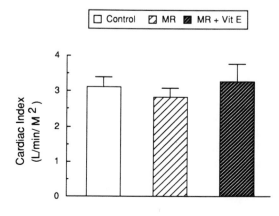

FIG. 2. Changes in the CI of the three groups. Results are expressed as mean ± SE.

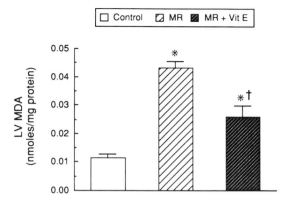

FIG. 3. Left ventricular MDA content in the groups. Results are expressed as mean ± SE. *$p < 0.05$, control vs. MR or MR + vitamin E. †$p < 0.05$, MR vs. MR + vitamin E.

DISCUSSION

In the present study, chronic volume overload of 4 months' duration produced a decrease in the cardiac contractility and cardiac function as indicated by a decrease in (+) dp/dt and (+) dp/dt/PAW and an increase in LVEDP. There was no decrease, however, in CI. A decrease in cardiac contractility without a change in CI in chronic volume overload of 3 months' duration has been observed earlier (5). Volume overload of 6 to 9 months' duration has been shown to depress both cardiac function and contractility (3,6). Cardiac contractility seems to be affected before CI is affected. Maintenance of CI in spite of a decrease in contractility could be due to an increase in end-diastolic volume. A decrease in cardiac contractility may be due to an increase in the levels of ROMs. This is supported by the fact that there was an increase in the cardiac MDA, which is a fingerprint for ROMs. Also, it is known that PMNLs, in chronic volume and pressure overload, produce increased amounts of ROMs (6,7). Reactive oxygen metabolites have been shown to depress cardiac function and contractility (1,2). They are known to depress Ca^{2+} accumulation by sarcoplasmic reticulum and Ca^{2+} ATPase (14,15). Volume overload produced an increase in the TSVR, which could be due to increased levels of ROMs (which are known to constrict the vascular system) (16). Exogenous oxygen free radicals are known to increase systemic and pulmonary vascular resistance (1,2).

Vitamin E treatment prevented the decrease in cardiac contractility in chronic volume overload. The protective effect of vitamin E is probably due to its antioxidant activity (8,9). This is supported by the fact that MDA levels in the left ventricle decreased, suggesting a decrease in the levels of ROMs. Vitamin E treatment also decreased the TSVR, suggesting a decrease in ROMs. An increase in cardiac MDA suggests increased levels of ROMs, which may be due to increased production and/ or decreased metabolism. Polymorphonuclear leukocytes produce an increased amount of ROMs in chronic volume overload (6) and pressure overload (7). Prevention in the rise in cardiac MDA in the vitamin E–treated group could be due to its antioxidant activity. Vitamin E has been shown to prevent hypercholesterolemic atherosclerosis, and this was associated with a decrease in aortic tissue MDA (17).

These results indicate that the decrease in cardiac contractility and function in chronic volume overload is associated with an increase in MDA, a fingerprint for ROMs. Also, vitamin E, an antioxidant, prevented the volume overload–induced decrease in cardiac contractility, and this was associated with a decrease in a volume overload–induced rise in cardiac MDA. These results suggest a role of ROMs in volume-overload heart failure and the effectiveness of vitamin E in prevention of volume-overload heart failure.

SUMMARY

Reactive oxygen metabolites are known to depress cardiac function and contractility. Decreases in cardiac contractility and function in chronic volume overload could be due to increased levels of ROMs. We, therefore, investigated the effects of chronic volume overload in the absence and presence of vitamin E (antioxidant) on cardiac function and contractility and cardiac MDA, a fingerprint for levels of ROMs in dog. Dogs were assigned to three groups of seven dogs each: Group I, control; group II, MR of 4 months' duration; group III, similar to group II but in addition received vitamin E (40 U/kg/d) orally. Volume overload was produced by creating MR by detaching two or more chordae tendineae to raise left atrial pressure to 2.5 to 3 times the normal. Volume overload produced a decrease in myocardial contractility [(+)dp/dt and dp/dt/PAW], and cardiac function manifested by an increase in LVEDP without a significant change in CI. There was an increase in TSVR. These changes were associated with an increase in cardiac MDA. Prevention of a volume overload–induced decrease in cardiac contractility and an increase in TSVR by vitamin E was associated with a decrease in cardiac MDA. These results suggest that a decrease in cardiac contractility and an increase in TSVR in chronic volume overload are associated with an increase in levels of ROMs and that vitamin E, an antioxidant, could be effective in preventing the volume overload–induced cardiac depression.

ACKNOWLEDGMENTS

This study was supported by a grant from the Heart and Stroke Foundation of Saskatchewan. The authors acknowledge the technical assistance of Mr. P.K. Chattopadhyay and Ms. Jackie Andrews.

REFERENCES

1. Prasad K, Kalra J, Chaudhary AK, Debnath D. Effect of polymorphonuclear leukocyte derived–oxygen free radicals and hypochlorous acid on cardiac function and some biochemical parameters. *Am Heart J* 1990;119:538–550.
2. Prasad K, Kalra J, Chan WP, Chaudhary AK. Effect of oxygen free radicals on cardiovascular function at organ and cellular level. *Am Heart J* 1989;117:1196–1202.
3. Prasad K, Khatter JC, Bharadwaj B. Cardiovascular function in experimental mitral insufficiency in dogs. *Jpn Heart J* 1977;18:823–840.

4. Prasad K, O'Neil CL, Bharadwaj B. Effects of chronic digoxin treatment on cardiac function, electrolytes, and sarcolemmal ATPase in the canine failing heart due to chronic mitral regurgitation. *Am Heart J* 1984;108:1487–1494.

5. Prasad K, O'Neil CL, Bharadwaj B. Effect of chronic prazosin treatment on cardiac function and electrolytes in failing heart due to chronic mitral insufficiency. *Can J Cardiol* 1985;2:107–112.

6. Prasad K, Kalra J, Bharadwaj B. Increased chemiluminescence of polymorphonuclear leukocytes in dogs with volume overload heart failure. *Br J Exp Pathol* 1989;70:463–468.

7. Prasad K, Kalra J, Massey KL, Bharadwaj B. Increased production of oxygen free radicals by polymorphonuclear leukocytes in heart failure due to aortic stenosis. *Angiology* 1989;40:472–478.

8. Burton GW, Joyce A, Ingold KU. Is vitamin E the only lipid soluble, chain breaking antioxidant in human blood plasma and erythrocyte membranes? *Arch Biochem Biophys* 1983;221:281–290.

9. Burton GW, Ingold KU. Vitamin E as an in vitro and in vivo antioxidant. *Ann NY Acad Sci* 1989;570:7–22.

10. Prasad K, Lee P, Kalra J. Influence of endothelin on cardiovascular function, oxygen free radicals, and blood chemistry. *Am Heart J* 1991;121:178–187.

11. Kapoor R, Prasad K. Role of oxyradicals in cardiovascular depression and cellular injury in hemorrhagic shock and reinfusion: effect of SOD and catalase. *Circ Shock* 1994;43:79–94.

12. Ohkawa H, Ohishi N, Yagi K. Assay for lipid peroxides in animal tissue by thiobarbituric acid reaction. *Anal Biochem* 1979;95:351–358.

13. Gornall AG, Bardawill CJ, David MM. Determination of serum proteins by means of the biuret reaction. *J Biol Chem* 1949;177:751–766.

14. Hess ML, Okabe E, Kontos HA. Proton and free oxygen radical interaction with the calcium transport system of cardiac sarcoplasmic reticulum. *J Mol Cell Cardiol* 1981;13:767–772.

15. Kaneko M, Elimban V, Dhalla NS. Mechanism for depression of heart sarcolemmal Ca^{++} pump by oxygen free radicals. *Am J Physiol* 1989;257:H804–H811.

16. Lawson DL, Mehta JL, Nichols WW, Mehta P, Donneby WH. Superoxide radical mediated endothelial injury and vasoconstriction of rat thoracic aortic rings. *J Lab Clin Med* 1990;115:541–548.

17. Prasad K, Kalra J. Oxygen free radicals and hypercholesterolemic atherosclerosis: effect of Vitamin E. *Am Heart J* 1993;125:958–973.

The Failing Heart, edited by N. S. Dhalla,
R. E. Beamish, N. Takeda, and M. Nagano.
Lippincott-Raven Publishers, Philadelphia © 1995.

35

Protective Effect of Taurine on the Failing Heart and Its Possible Mechanism of Action

Junichi Azuma and *Stephen W. Schaffer

*Department of Clinical Evaluation of Medicines and Therapeutics, Faculty of Pharmaceutical Sciences, Osaka University, Suita, Osaka 565 Japan; and *Department of Pharmacology, School of Medicine, University of South Alabama, Mobile, AL 36688 United States*

Taurine is a ubiquitous sulfur-containing β-amino acid found in high concentration in the mammalian heart, where its levels exceed those of the plasma by more than 100-fold. Although the intracellular myocardial taurine pool of most species is very large, significant species differences do exist, with the high taurine levels found in species with the highest heart rates. Taurine content of the heart is normally fairly stable; elevated levels have been observed, however, in patients suffering from congestive heart failure (CHF) (1), while decreased taurine content is associated with ischemic heart disease (2).

Taurine was discovered more than 200 years ago. Interest in the role of taurine in the heart, however, has been generated by the recent observations that taurine is beneficial in treating patients with chronic CHF (3,4) and that cats fed a taurine-deficient diet develop a cardiomyopathy that is reversible upon dietary supplementation with taurine (5). Although both humans and cats have a low capacity to synthesize taurine, cats are particularly susceptible to taurine deficiency because of their requirement for taurine in the conjugation of bile acids. Interestingly, rats have high amounts of total body taurine. Hence, it may be providence that cats chase rats.

It has been suggested that the most important function of taurine in the heart is the modulation of Ca^{2+} transport. Depending on the status of the myocardium, taurine is capable of either increasing or decreasing intracellular Ca^{2+} levels (6). This property of taurine is important because Ca^{2+} levels affect myocardial contractile and metabolic function and also because this effect accounts for the ability of taurine to prevent Ca^{2+} overload in a series of heart failure models (7–9). The aim of this chapter is to briefly summarize the effects of taurine on the heart.

MODULATION OF MYOCARDIAL INOTROPIC STATE

A large volume of literature is now available indicating that taurine modulates myocardial contraction, mediating a biphasic response that is dependent on extracellular Ca^{2+}. Hearts made hypodynamic by reductions in medium Ca^{2+} content exhibit improved contractile performance on exposure to pharmacological doses of taurine, while the same concentrations of taurine reduce contractile function in hearts perfused with elevated levels of medium Ca^{2+}.

The inotropic effect of taurine is closely linked to changes in intracellular free Ca^{2+} concentration. We have shown that taurine increases Ca^{2+} flux (I_{Ca}) through the sarcolemmal Ca^{2+} channel. At a concentration of 10 to 20 mM, it produces a small stimulatory effect in myocytes maintained in medium containing low Ca^{2+} concentration (0.8 mM). On the other hand, it exerts a small inhibitory effect at high extracellular Ca^{2+} (3.6 mM) while exhibiting no significant effect on I_{Ca} in normal Ca^{2+} medium (1.8 mM) (10). These multiple effects of taurine on I_{Ca} may partially explain its dual inotropic activity in cardiac muscle, where it can either increase or decrease contraction, depending on extracellular Ca^{2+} concentration. Also, the inhibitory activity of taurine on I_{Ca} may provide some explanation for its protective effect against Ca^{2+} overload.

Using fura-2 as a probe to measure intracellular free Ca^{2+} content, we have demonstrated that addition of taurine to normal medium increased the amplitude of the Ca^{2+} transient of myocytes by 30% while reducing beating rate and having no effect on Ca^{2+} content during diastole. By comparison, raising medium Ca^{2+} concentration resulted in elevations not only in the Ca^{2+} transient amplitude, but also in the free intracellular Ca^{2+} concentration during diastole (11). These differences in the cellular response to taurine and elevated medium Ca^{2+} concentration indicate that the two agents increase intracellular Ca^{2+} content by a different mechanism. Similarly, the positive inotropic action of taurine is different from that of well-known positive inotropic agents, such as catecholamines, phosphodiesterase inhibitors, and digitalis glycosides, because it does not function through changes in cyclic adenosine monophosphate (AMP) levels or by inhibition of Na^+-K^+ ATPase activity. Although several theories have been proposed to explain the positive inotropic effect of taurine, the actual site(s) of taurine action remain to be elucidated.

CARDIOPROTECTIVE ACTIVITY OF TAURINE

Recognition that taurine alters Ca^{2+} movement led to the examination of potential cardioprotective effects of taurine, particularly against Ca^{2+} overload-induced heart failure models, such as the cardiomyopathic hamster (8), cardiotoxicity induced by isoproterenol and doxorubicin (7,9), and calcium paradox–or oxygen paradox–induced myocardial injury (12,13).

Calcium Paradox

The calcium paradox is a "paradoxical" phenomenon that occurs in hearts reperfused with Ca^{2+}-containing medium following a period of Ca^{2+}-free perfusion. During the Ca^{2+}-free perfusion period, intracellular Na^+ concentration rises, predisposing the heart to a massive gain in Ca^{2+} on reperfusion with Ca^{2+}-containing medium. This excessive Ca^{2+} loading via the Na^+-Ca^{2+} exchanger triggers a series of events leading to dramatic cellular damage, characterized by disruption of the electrical and mechanical properties of the heart, a loss of cellular content, a dramatic fall in intracellular high-energy phosphate levels, and the appearance of gross ultrastructural changes. We have found that during the repletion phase of the calcium paradox, taurine is lost from the heart (12). Inclusion of 10 mM taurine in the Ca^{2+} depletion and reperfusion medium with the aim of restoring taurine levels dramatically attenuates the loss of cellular constituents, improves the metabolic state of the heart, enhances recovery of mechanical function, and prevents damage to the cell membrane. Interestingly, we have also reported that not only inclusion of taurine in the perfusion medium, but also daily oral administration of 2 mg taurine/kg to 4-day-old chicks for a period of 4 days prevents ultrastructural and contractile dysfunction during the calcium paradox (13). These actions of taurine have been most closely linked to the modulation of Ca^{2+} homeostasis. Our studies (11) found that myocytes loaded with the Ca^{2+} indicator, fura 2, are unaffected by taurine during the Ca^{2+} depletion phase of the calcium paradox. Taurine-treated myocytes, however, exhibit fewer morphological changes, recover their characteristic beating pattern earlier, and accumulate less Ca^{2+} during the Ca^{2+} restoration phase of the calcium paradox than untreated myocytes (11).

Cardiomyopathic Hamster

The Syrian hamster is genetically predisposed to undergo several discrete phases during its lifetime. Between the ages of 80 and 150 days, the myocardium enters a phase characterized by fibrosis and Ca^{2+} deposition, while in the latter stages of the hamster's cardiomyopathy undesirable metabolic defects are observed. It has been shown that taurine protects against the progression of the lesions in the cardiomyopathic hamster (8). Although studies employing taurine therapy have been restricted to short-term treatment of animals in the early phases of the disease, treatment with taurine has led to a reduction in myocardial Ca^{2+} content. Because the lesions involve defects in Ca^{2+} handling by both the sarcoplasmic reticulum and the sarcolemmal Na^+-Ca^{2+} exchanger, taurine is capable of either preventing the development of the transport abnormalities or somehow neutralizing them.

Isoproterenol Cardiotoxicity

It is well known that a toxic dose of the synthetic catecholamine, isoproterenol, causes massive heart necrosis. We found that administration of a large dose of isoproterenol for 4 days resulted in a substantial accumulation of Ca^{2+} and a profound decrease in myocardial adenosine triphosphate (ATP) content and creatine phosphokinase (CPK) activity. Also, as a measure of lipid peroxidation, a pronounced increase in lipid peroxide and decrease in both reduced glutathione concentration and phospholipid content were observed. Oral administration of taurine partially protected against these isoproterenol-induced changes, suggesting that the beneficial effect of taurine may be related in part to inhibition of lipid peroxide formation and Ca^{2+} accumulation, which in turn prevents loss of membrane phospholipids (9).

Doxorubicin Cardiotoxicity

We have shown that treatment of isolated myocytes, perfused chick hearts, and mice with taurine provides protection against doxorubicin-induced toxicity (7). In the *in vivo* study, we found that a single intraperitoneal injection of mice with doxorubicin produced a significant elevation in lipid peroxidation 72 hours postinjection. Also elevated at this time was cellular Ca^{2+} content, while significant depletions in tissue CPK, glutamic oxaloacetic trausaminase (GOT), and lactic dehydrogenase (LDH) were observed 48 hours postinjection, and glutathione peroxidase activity 25 hours postinjection. Combined oral and intraperitoneal administration of taurine significantly improved the survival rate of mice treated with doxorubicin. Moreover, all of these biochemical alterations, except for the depletion of glutathione peroxidase, were markedly attenuated by taurine treatment.

The effect of chemically induced taurine depletion on doxorubicin cardiotoxicity has also been examined (14). We found that a single intravenous administration of doxorubicin to normal rats led to a 10% increase in myocardial Ca^{2+} content 48 hours after treatment with the anthracycline, while Ca^{2+} levels rose twice as much in doxorubicin-treated rats containing half the normal myocardial taurine content.

PUTATIVE MECHANISMS FOR INOTROPIC ACTION OF TAURINE

Several hypotheses have been introduced as putative mechanisms for the inotropic action of taurine. Many of these relate to the indirect modulation of the Na^+-Ca^{2+} exchanger. It is now recognized that Ca^{2+} entering the myocyte via the Na^+-Ca^{2+} exchanger is coupled to sarcoplasmic reticular Ca^{2+} release, thereby supplying Ca^{2+} to the contractile machinery. Decreases in Na^+-Ca^{2+} exchange, as occurs in hearts exposed to L-methionine, result in a decline in contractile function (15,16). Panagia et al. (15) have shown that L-methionine is metabolized within the myocyte to S-adenosylmethionine, a methyl donor for several enzyme reactions, including the conversion of phosphatidylethanolamine to phosphatidylcholine. Because the Na^+-Ca^{2+} exchanger is very sensitive to changes in the phosphatidylethanolamine and phosphatidylcholine content of the sarcolemma, changes in the activity of the N-methyltransferase enzyme converting phosphatidylethanolamine to phosphatidylcholine will dramatically alter Na^+-Ca^{2+} exchanger activity. Taurine is structurally similar to the phospholipid headgroup of phosphatidylethanolamine and is therefore an effective inhibitor of phospholipid-N-methyltransferase, the enzyme catalyzing the phosphatidylethanolamine to phosphatidylcholine conversion. Consequently, taurine treatment prevents methionine-mediated changes in Na^+-Ca^{2+} exchanger activity, thereby blocking the decline in myocardial contraction noted in hearts exposed to methionine. This effect appears to be physiologically important because chemically induced taurine deficiency leads to a reduction in the capacity of the Na^+-Ca^{2+} exchanger to transport Ca^{2+} (17).

In addition to modulation of Na^+-Ca^{2+} exchanger activity through changes in the phospholipid content of the sarcolemma, taurine also affects flux through the exchanger by altering intracellular levels of Na^+. Sperelakis et al. (18) have reported that taurine stimulates the fast component of the inward Na^+ current, thereby elevating intracellular Na^+ concentration, which in turn promotes Ca^{2+} influx via the Na^+-Ca^{2+} exchanger. Another interesting mechanism for modulation of intracellular Na^+ and Na^+-Ca^{2+} exchanger flux by taurine has been proposed by Suleiman et al. (19). They argue that because taurine transport across the cell membrane occurs by a taurine/Na^+ symport mechanism (20), rapid rates of taurine transport will be associated with Na^+ movement and thus changes in cellular Ca^{2+} content.

Taurine also influences Ca^{2+} transport by the sarcoplasmic reticulum. In accordance with several other Ca^{2+} transporters, the status of the ryanodine-sensitive Ca^{2+} channel is highly dependent on the phospholipid content of the sarcoplasmic reticulum. Perfusion of isolated rat heart with buffer containing L-methionine enhances phospholipid-N-methylation and causes a reduction in Ca^{2+}-induced Ca^{2+} release (21). Because the sarcoplasmic reticulum is located in an environment rich in taurine, activity of sarcoplasmic reticular phospholipid-N-methyltransferase normally will be maintained in a partially inhibited state and Ca^{2+}-induced Ca^{2+} release will consequently be elevated. Thus, taurine ensures effective operation of the Ca^{2+}-induced Ca^{2+} release mechanism, both by promoting Na^+-Ca^{2+} exchange and by modulating ryanodine-sensitive Ca^{2+} channel activity.

Skinned fiber studies reveal that in addition to modulation of Ca^{2+} transport, taurine also increases the sensitivity of the muscle proteins to Ca^{2+} (22,23). Galler et al. (22) have proposed that taurine, because of its dipolar character, weakens charge-dependent protein–protein interactions, in particular interactions involving the various muscle proteins. Because this effect occurs at physiological levels of taurine, it is considered an important physiological mechanism.

PUTATIVE MECHANISMS FOR CARDIOPROTECTIVE ACTION OF TAURINE

The mechanism responsible for the cardioprotective effects of taurine has not been fully established, although several candidates for this phenomenon have been proposed. We have reported that pharmacological concentrations of taurine can suppress Ca^{2+} influx via the L-type Ca^{2+} channel, but only if extracellular Ca^{2+} content is high. This action could lead to a decrease in intracellular Ca^{2+} content, although uncertain is the effect of Ca^{2+} overload on this response. Another mechanism contributing to Ca^{2+} regulation is phospholipid-N-methylation (16,21).

Through modulation of sarcolemmal phospholipid-N-methyltransferase activity, taurine maintains the phospholipid microenvironment of the Na^+-Ca^{2+} exchanger in a less methylated state, thereby ensuring a more active transporter. Because the Na^+-Ca^{2+} exchanger is the major mechanism for the extrusion of Ca^{2+} from the cell, reduction in Na^+-Ca^{2+} exchanger activity can result in intracellular Ca^{2+} accumulation.

Our studies (14,24) have shown that drug-induced taurine depletion renders the heart susceptible to doxorubicin cardiotoxicity and myocardial ischemic injury. Conversely, elevated intracellular taurine is cardioprotective against Ca^{2+}-overload cardiotoxicity. According to the hypothesis advanced by Chapman et al. (25), the cardioprotective activity of taurine is linked to taurine efflux via the taurine/Na^+ symporter. Loss of taurine from the myocyte via this transporter will result in a corresponding reduction in intracellular Na^+ content. The resulting changes in the Na^+ gradient across the cell membrane will favor Ca^{2+} efflux from the cell. Also contributing to the redistribution of Ca^{2+} is taurine-mediated inhibition of both calmodulin-linked phosphorylation and sarcoplasmic reticular phospholipid-N-methyltransferase activity, effects that mediate reductions in sarcoplasmic reticular Ca^{2+} pump activity (21,26). At the same time, taurine-mediated facilitation of Ca^{2+}-induced Ca^{2+} release from the sarcoplasmic reticulum will cause intravesicular Ca^{2+} stores to fall (21).

USE OF TAURINE IN HEART FAILURE

The major goal in the treatment of patients with heart failure is to improve the quality and quantity of life. Presently, the general treatment of overt chronic CHF involves the elimination of excess salt and water, the reduction in workload, the reduction in neurohormonal activity (by angiotensin-converting enzyme [ACE] inhibitors and β-adrenoceptor antagonists), and, presumably, the direct improvement in pumping performance (digitalis glycosides and other inotropic agents). Although several newer inotropic agents have been introduced, they generally have not been shown to consistently improve clinical symptoms. In fact, most of them are associated with increased mortality, presumably because they promote arrhythmias and/or increase energy expenditure secondary to their inotropic activity. Based on these findings, there is a perception that long-term administration of positive inotropic agents that act by increasing intracellular Ca^{2+}, cyclic AMP levels (by β-adrenergic agonists or phosphodiesterase inhibitors), or both, may ultimately be deleterious.

Effect of Taurine in a Heart Failure Model Induced by Aortic Regurgitation

A marked elevation of cardiac taurine content occurs in the heart at autopsy in patients who have died of CHF (1). We therefore examined whether taurine or guanidinoethane sulfonate, a taurine transport inhibitor, could affect the status of heart failure produced by artifically induced aortic regurgitation in rabbits (27). In this study we focused our attention on the ability of taurine to prevent rapid progression of heart failure and hence prolong life expectancy. Daily administration of taurine to the experimental animals prevented a reduction in cardiac function 8 weeks after induction of regurgitation. Left ventricular taurine content of the rabbits with heart failure was significantly increased, with taurine treatment causing a further increase in myocardial taurine levels. The cumulative mortality rate in the taurine-treated heart failure group was 10% at 8 weeks, compared with 53% in the untreated group and 75% in the guanidino-ethane sulfonate–treated group. An important question is whether the increase in myocardial taurine content of the failing heart is a causal factor of heart failure, or whether this is secondary to factors related to the disease process, such as a compensatory mechanism. Interestingly, it has been reported recently that the loss of force development in the taurine-depleted myocardium may be related to a reduction in the number of contractile elements (28).

Clinical Uses of Taurine in Heart Failure

We have performed several clinical studies examining the utility of taurine therapy in the management of CHF. One of the major goals of therapy in CHF is the prolonged relief of symptoms noted with routine daily activity. Generally, taurine therapy has been found effective in treating CHF (3,4,29). Recently, we began a long-term (more than 1 year), randomized but open clinical trial with the aim of determining whether supplementing conventional therapy with oral taurine could improve clinical signs and quality of life measures in patients with chronic symptomatic, but mild CHF.

METHODS

Patients with CHF were randomly enrolled. All the patients had subjective evidence of reduced exercise capacity, as demonstrated by exertional symptoms (New York Heart Association [NYHA] function class II or III) which had been stable despite treatment with digoxin, diuretics, and/or an ACE inhibitor. After initial assessment of the patients, they were randomly assigned to either a group administered additional taurine (3 g/d) for the length of the study period or to a group not receiving taurine therapy. Changes in therapy were allowable if there was evidence of a worsening heart failure condition requiring therapeutic intervention, or of improving symptoms permitting a reduction in the dose of background medication. Information was obtained regarding the studies of all patients at 3, 6, and 12 months. Data were compared by chi-square statistics, Fisher's exact test, or Wilcoxon rank-sum test. All the analyses were two-sided and differences ($p < 0.05$) were considered statistically significant.

RESULTS

Clinical signs and symptoms of the patients were rather mild (mainly in NYHA class II) and fairly stable before entry into the study. The clinical characteristics of the patients in the two study groups were similar on entry. Thirty-eight patients receiving taurine and thirty-three patients without taurine completed the study. Eight patients failed to reach the 1-year endpoint. After the 3- and 6-month assessment, two patients receiving taurine and another two without taurine withdrew because of patient preference. One patient receiving taurine died of a hepatoma. Data from these five patients were not included in the analysis. Two patients who were not administered taurine died from worsening heart failure 3 months and 4 months after initiation of the study, respectively.

During the study, input from patients and physicians were obtained regarding changes in the patients' overall condition. Three months into the study, more patients in the taurine than in the non-taurine group were considered by the investigators to have symptomatic improvement (59% vs. 14%). After 1 year, breathlessness on exertion improved in 32% of the patients receiving taurine, but in only 9% of the patients without taurine ($p<0.01$). Deterioration in NYHA functional class was reported in two patients, one from each therapy group. By contrast, improvement in functional class was reported in 21% of the patients receiving taurine, but in only 6% of those in the non-taurine group; this difference was not statistically significant ($p=0.09$). On completion of the study, 26 patients receiving taurine reported feeling better; that is, either moderately better (18%) or slightly better (49%), compared with 21% who felt slightly better in the non-taurine group ($p<0.01$). When the patients' clinical course was assessed by investigators, the rate of overall improvement was 67% in the taurine group but only 24% in the non-taurine group. Among those without taurine, the clinical status of three patients worsened, while two patients in the taurine group exhibited deterioration of their clinical signs.

DISCUSSION

It has been assumed that depression of cardiac contractility is the primary defect in heart failure and that drug-induced increases in cardiac contractility should have a beneficial effect in patients with heart failure. It is increasingly evident, however, that long-term administration of inotropic agents that increase the intracellular concentration of cyclic AMP through the stimulation of β-adrenoceptors or by inhibiting phosphodiesterase are not necessarily effective in the long-term management of heart failure, and in fact may cause an increase in mortality.

The beneficial effect of taurine supplementation against disease progression in heart failure may be related to its modulation of Ca^{2+} transport by the heart. Impaired diastolic function, possibly caused by abnormal Ca^{2+} handling, is known as one of the potential causes of heart failure and also appears to trigger hypertrophy and progression of left ventricular dysfunction. Taurine supplementation not only improves the heart by altering intracellular Ca^{2+} movement, but lacks many of the adverse side effects of newer inotropic agents, such as increased heart rate and the induction of arrhythmias. It also has an ability either to increase Ca^{2+} availability for contraction or to protect against Ca^{2+}-overload injury. These characteristics of taurine are potentially important therapeutic considerations in the long-term management of patients with CHF.

Recently, Eley et al. (28) reported that taurine depletion may worsen heart failure by causing reduced force generation secondary to a loss of contractile protein. This mechanism has been implicated in the development of taurine-deficient cardiomyopathy in animals, although it remains to be determined if the drug-induced model of taurine-deficiency cardiomyopathy in rats mimics the dietary model of cardiomyopathy in cats and fox (5,30,31). Of more importance clinically is whether humans also develop CHF as a result of taurine deficiency.

A recently developed drug, pimobendan, has been shown to exert its positive inotropic action by enhancing myofilament sensitivity to Ca^{2+}. Interestingly, Galler et al. (22) and Steele and Smith (23) found in skinned heart muscle fibers that part of the positive inotropic effect of taurine can be traced to a dose-dependent enhancement of myofilament sensitivity to Ca^{2+}. It is hoped that this important property to taurine may obviate some of its potentially less favorable effects related to its inotropic action.

Other possible mechanisms by which taurine could benefit heart failure include a reduction in neurohormonal activation, the modulation of sympathetic–parasympathetic autonomic balance, and/or both. Several mechanisms have been proposed explaining the effect of taurine supplementation on the progression of heart failure. It is our contention that resolving the mechanism of taurine action will provide a clue into the fundamental mechanism responsible for the progression of heart failure.

SUMMARY

Taurine is a β-amino acid found in very high concentration in the mammalian heart. In certain species, loss of taurine from the heart leads to the development of a dilated cardiomyopathy. Myocardial taurine loss also potentiates injury to the heart associated with an ischemic-reperfusion insult, doxorubicin toxicity, aortic regurgitation, and Ca^{2+} overload–induced myocardial damage. These adverse effects of taurine depletion are reversible by dietary taurine supplementation. Experimental treatment of animals with pharmacological doses of taurine, as well as exposure of either isolated hearts or myocytes to high extracellular concentrations of taurine, alters cardiac function, including contractile performance, the potential to produce arrhythmias, and the susceptibility to Ca^{2+} overload-mediated myocardial injury. These multiple dietary and pharmacological actions of taurine have largely been attributed to alterations in Ca^{2+} and Na^+ transport, as well as in the function of the muscle proteins. Because taurine is capable of mediating a positive inotropic effect without increasing heart rate or inducing arrhythmias, clinical trials have begun testing its ability to ameliorate the symptoms of CHF. In one such randomized phase 2 study, patients belonging to NYHA functional class II or III were treated with either taurine or placebo for 1 year. Approximately two-thirds of the patients receiving taurine exhibited improvement in their clinical signs compared with only 24% in the placebo group. Thus, taurine shows promise as a new cardiotonic agent for the long-term management of patients with CHF.

ACKNOWLEDGMENTS

The laborious assistance of Dr. Y. Tachi and Ms. E. Tamura is acknowledged.

REFERENCES

1. Huxtable R, Bressler R. Elevation of taurine in human congestive heart failure. *Life Sci* 1994; 14:1353–1359.
2. Crass MF, Lombardini JB. Loss of cardiac muscle taurine after acute left ventricular ischemia. *Life Sci* 1977;21:951–958.
3. Azuma J, Hasegawa H, Sawamura A, et al. Taurine for treatment of congestive heart failure. *Int J Cardiol* 1982;1:303–309.
4. Azuma J, Sawamura A, Awata N, et al. Therapeutic effect of taurine in congestive heart failure: a double blind crossover trial. *Clin Cardiol* 1985;8:276–282.
5. Pion PD, Kittleson MD, Rogers QR, Morris JG. Myocardial failure in cats associated with low plasma taurine: a reversible cardiomyopathy. *Science* 1987;237:764–768.
6. Schaffer SW, Azuma J. Physiological effects of taurine in the heart. In: Lombardini JB, Schaffer SW, Azuma J, eds. *Taurine: nutritional value and mechanisms of action*. New York: Plenum Press; 1992;105–120.
7. Hamaguchi T, Azuma J, Awata N, et al. Reduction of doxorubicin-induced cardiotoxicity in mice by taurine. *Res Commun Chem Pathol Pharmacol* 1988;59:21–30.
8. McBroom MJ, Welty JD. Effects of taurine on heart calcium in the cardiomyopathic hamster. *J Mol Cell Cardiol* 1977;9:853–858.
9. Ohta H, Azuma J, Awata N, et al. Mechanism of the protective action of taurine against isoprenaline induced myocardial damage. *Cardiovasc Res* 1988;22:407–413.
10. Sawamura A, Sada H, Azuma J, Kishimoto S, Sperelakis N. Taurine modulates ion influx through cardiac Ca^{2+} channels. *Cell Calcium* 1990;11:251–259.
11. Takahashi K, Harada H, Schaffer SW, Azuma J. Effect of taurine on intracellular calcium dynamics of cultured myocardial cells during the calcium paradox. In: Lombardini JB, Schaffer SW, Azuma J, eds. *Taurine: nutritional value and mechanisms of action*. New York: Plenum Press; 1992;153–161.
12. Kramer JH, Chovan JP, Schaffer SW. The effect of taurine on calcium paradox and ischemic heart failure. *Am J Physiol* 1981;240:H238–H246.
13. Yamauchi-Takihara K, Azuma J, Kishimoto S, Onishi S, Sperelakis N. Taurine prevention of calcium paradox-related damage in cardiac muscle. *Biochem Pharmacol* 1988;37:2651–2658.
14. Harada H, Cusack BJ, Olson RD, et al. Taurine deficiency and doxorubicin: interaction with the cardiac sarcolemmal calcium pump. *Biochem Pharmacol* 1990;39:745–751.
15. Panagia V, Makino N, Ganguly PK, Dhalla NS. Inhibition of Na^+-Ca^{2+} exchange in heart sarcolemmal vesicles by phosphatidylethanolamine N-methylation. *Eur J Biochem* 1987;166:597–603.
16. Hamaguchi T, Azuma J, Schaffer SW. Interaction of taurine with methionine: inhibition of myocardial phospholipid methyltransferase. *J Cardiovasc Pharmacol* 1991;8:224–230.
17. Harada H, Allo S, Viyuoh N, Azuma J, Takahashi K, Schaffer SW. Regulation of calcium transport in drug-induced taurine-depleted hearts. *Biochim Biophys Acta* 1988;944:273–278.
18. Sperelakis N, Satoh H, Bkaily G. Taurine effects on ionic currents in myocardial cells. In: Lombar-

dini JB, Schaffer SW, Azuma J, eds. *Taurine: nutritional value and mechanisms of action*. New York: Plenum Press; 1992;129–143.
19. Suleiman MS, Rodrigo GC, Chapman RA. Interdependence of intracellular taurine and sodium in guinea pig heart. *Cardiovasc Res* 1992;26:897–905.
20. Schaffer SW, Kulakowski EC, Kramer JH. Taurine transport by reconstituted membrane vesicles. In: Huxtable RJ, Pasantes-Morales H, eds. *Taurine in nutrition and neurology*. New York/London: Plenum Press; 1985:143–160.
21. Punna S, Ballard C, Hamaguchi T, Azuma J, Schaffer SW. Effect of taurine and methionine on sarcoplasmic reticular Ca^{2+} transport and phospholipid methyltransferase activity. *J Cardiovasc Pharmacol* 1994;24:286–292.
22. Galler S, Hutzler C, Haller T. Effects of taurine on Ca^{2+}-dependent force development of skinned muscle fibre preparations. *J Exp Biol* 1990;152:255–264.
23. Steele DS, Smith GL. Intracellular effects of taurine: Studies on skinned cardiac preparations. In: Lombardini JB, Schaffer SW, Azuma J, eds. *Taurine: nutritional value and mechanisms of action*. New York: Plenum Press; 1992:163–172.
24. Schaffer SW, Allo S, Mozaffari M. Potentiation of myocardial ischemic injury by drug-induced taurine depletion. In: Huxtable RJ, Franconi F, Giotti A, eds. *The biology of taurine: methods and mechanisms*. New York/London: Plenum Press; 1987:151–158.
25. Chapman RA, Suleiman MS, Earm YE. Taurine and the heart. *Cardiovasc Res* 1993;27:358–363.
26. Schaffer SW, Allo S, Harada H, Azuma J. Regulation of calcium homeostasis by taurine. In: Pasantes-Morales H, Martin DL, Shain W, DelRio RM, eds. *Taurine: functional neurochemistry, physiology and cardiology*. New York: Wiley-Liss Inc.; 1990:217–225.
27. Takihara K, Azuma J, Awata N, et al. Beneficial effect of taurine in rabbits with chronic congestive heart failure. *Am Heart J* 1986;112:1278–1284.
28. Eley DW, Lake N, ter Keurs HEDJ. Taurine depletion and excitation-contraction coupling in rat myocardium. *Circ Res* 1994;74:1210–1219.
29. Azuma J, Sawamura A, Awata N. Usefulness of taurine in chronic congestive heart failure and its prospective application. *Jpn Circ J* 1992;56:95–99.
30. Lake N, Splawinski JB, Juneau C, Rouleau JL. Effects of taurine depletion on intrinsic contractility of rat ventricular papillary muscles. *Can J Physiol Pharmacol* 1990;68:800–806.
31. Moise NS, Pacioretty LM, Kallflez FA, Stipanuk MH, King JM, Gilmour RF. Dietary taurine deficiency and dilated cardiomyopathy in the fox. *Am Heart J* 1991;121:541–547.

The Failing Heart, edited by N. S. Dhalla,
R. E. Beamish, N. Takeda, and M. Nagano.
Lippincott-Raven Publishers, Philadelphia © 1995.

36

Acute Effects of Thyroid Hormone on the Heart and Cardiovascular System

*Irwin Klein, †John Klemperer, and *Kaie M. Ojamaa

*Division of Medicine and Endocrinology, North Shore University Hospital, Cornell University Medical College, Manhasset, New York 11030; and †Department of Surgery, New York Hospital, Cornell University Medical College, New York, New York 10021

It is well recognized that thyroid hormone has profound effects on the heart and cardiovascular system (1). This relationship was noted in the earliest clinical descriptions of thyrotoxicosis by Caleb Parry and Robert Graves. Thus, the increased cardiac output, widened pulse pressure, tachycardia, and hyperdynamic precordium of hyperthyroidism are frequent clinical findings and stand in marked contrast to the decrease in cardiac work, narrow pulse pressure, and quiet precordium characteristic of myxedema (2).

Thyroid hormone exerts direct cellular effects on almost all tissues of the body, influencing tissue growth and development, cellular differentiation, and metabolism (3). This in part explains the diverse symptoms associated with thyroid disease. The most compelling effect of the thyroid hormones is on basal metabolic rate and tissue oxygen consumption in order to maintain homeostasis and core body temperature (4). To accommodate fluctuations in tissue thermogenesis, a highly regulated system of delivery of substrates to these tissues is required. Therefore, adaptation of the cardiovascular system in response to thyroid hormone–mediated changes in homeostasis is likely to occur both acutely and in the long term (2).

This discussion reviews the possible mechanisms by which thyroid hormone (T_4 and T_3) can effect cardiovascular homeostasis. Understanding the cellular mechanisms of thyroid hormone action and resulting changes in the heart and the systemic vasculature can facilitate a rational approach to the potential use of thyroid hormone in the setting of acute and chronic cardiovascular disease (1–4).

MECHANISMS OF ACTION OF THYROID HORMONE

The cellular actions of T_4 and T_3 hormones are mediated both at the level of the cell nucleus (5) and at extranuclear sites (6). The identification of discrete nuclear T_3

433

binding sites greatly advances our understanding of the mechanism of action of the thyroid hormones. By modulating the transcription rate of target genes, T_3 is able to exert its effects on cellular function. The family of genes responsive to T_3 includes the myosin heavy-chain genes (7) and the sarcoplasmic reticulum ATPase gene of cardiac muscle (8).

EFFECTS OF THYROID HORMONE ON THE CARDIOVASCULAR SYSTEM

As noted, the cardiovascular manifestations of thyroid disease states are some of the most profound clinical changes observed. The effects of thyroid hormone on the heart and circulation constitute a spectrum extending from severe hypothyroidism with myxedema to hyperthyroidism and thyroid storm. In this discussion, we focus on those actions of thyroid hormone that occur rapidly after the parenteral administration of T_3 (Table 1).

Vascular Resistance

One of the earliest cardiovascular responses to thyroid hormone administration is a decrease in peripheral vascular resistance (2,4). This has been observed in both hypothyroid patients as well as in euthyroid animals after acute thyroid hormone administration. Hyperthyroidism may be associated with as much as a 50% decline in systemic vascular resistance (SVR) (9). In animals, beta-adrenergic blockade with propranolol has been shown to reverse the T_3-mediated drop in SVR and to blunt the increase in cardiac output (3). We have observed that chronic propranolol treatment blocks the T_4-induced increase in heart rate, heart work, and cardiac hypertrophy associated with experimental hyperthyroidism, suggesting that these effects of T_4 are indirectly mediated via changes in peripheral hemodynamic parameters (9).

Blood flow to the skin, kidneys, heart, and muscles is increased in hyperthyroidism. This increase in blood flow can be abolished partially by atropine, suggesting a cholinergic-mediated vasodilatory response in hyperthyroidism. Alternatively, the local release of vasodilators in peripheral tissues in response to increased cellular

TABLE 1. *Acute cardiovascular actions of triiodothyronine*

Hemodynamic parameter	Response
Systemic vascular resistance	Decreased
Cardiac output	Increased
Stroke volume	Increased
Heart rate	No change
Blood pressure	No change

respiration associated with hyperthyroidism could cause dilatation of the resistance vessels (3,4).

An alternative hypothesis involves the ability of thyroid hormone to directly affect systemic vascular resistance by regulating arteriolar smooth-muscle tone. This postulate is supported by the studies demonstrating a significant decrease in cardiac output after administration of phenylephrine, an alpha-adrenergic agonist and known vasoconstrictor, in hyperthyroid but not in normal subjects. We have provided direct evidence of a vasodilatory effect of thyroid hormone (4). Addition of T_3 at physiological concentrations to vascular smooth-muscle cells in culture caused visible relaxation of the cells within minutes. This effect was specific to the biologically active hormone T_3 and was not observed with T_4. The vasoreactivity of thyroid hormone may result from a direct effect on the vascular smooth muscle or endothelium, and potentially in conjunction with other vasoactive substances generated by T_3-mediated changes in thermogenesis.

Limited data exist regarding the direct acute effects of triiodothyronine on the coronary vasculature. Acute administration of T_3 decreased coronary vascular resistance, which resulted in increased coronary flow through a range of diastolic loading conditions in the postischemic reperfused canine heart (10).

Increased cardiac contractility and cardiac hypertrophy accompany both spontaneously occurring and experimentally induced hyperthyroidism (1,2,4,8). Treatment of animals with T_4 leads to an increase in heart weight as a result of an increased rate of cardiac protein synthesis. Hyperthyroidism is also characterized by positive cardiac inotropism (1,9). Contractile parameters such as the rate of ventricular pressure development or velocity of contraction are uniformly increased. Hyperthyroid patients may have as much as a 100% increase in cardiac output and resting heart rate (3).

The process of cardiac contraction, mediated via the interdigitation of the two major contractile proteins, actin and myosin, requires myosin-mediated adenosine triphosphate (ATP) hydrolysis and is regulated by the cytosolic concentration of calcium and other myofibrillar proteins. Thyroid hormone can exert effects on cardiac contractility at several discrete points. Myosin ATPase enzymatic activity has been shown to vary with changes in serum levels of both T_4 and T_3 (7). In normal postmortem human heart samples obtained from patients with hyperthyroidism, however, partially purified myosin appeared to be the low enzyme activity beta-myosin-heavy chain (MHC) isoform (2). It therefore appears unlikely that a significant shift in myosin isoenzyme gene expression occurs in humans in response to thyroid hormone.

The acute effects of T_3 administration display several unique features (Table 1). These changes include a decrease in systemic vascular resistance and increases in cardiac output. In animal models, acute T_3 treatment has no effect on the intrinsic contractility of the normal heart; however, an inotropic effect was demonstrated within minutes after the postischemic-reperfused heart was treated with T_3 (11). This acute augmentation of postischemic left ventricular function has been shown previously in models of warm and hypothermic ischemia.

The linear relationship between left ventricular pressure–volume area and myocardial oxygen consumption ($PVA-MVO_2$ relationship) provides a sophisticated method for analyzing the efficiency of myocardial oxygen utilization in response to changes in work. For the chronic hyperthyroid heart, conflicting, though perhaps species-dependent, data have been presented. Isolated rabbit hearts demonstrated a decreased conversion efficiency (12), while isolated canine hearts showed no change compared with the euthyroid state (13). We have recently completed a study in which the effects of acute T_3 treatment on myocardial oxygen utilization efficiency was analyzed using an ex vivo canine heart model of hypothermic global ischemia. Acute T_3 treatment had significant inotropic action that occurred without associated oxygen wasting (10).

Left ventricular diastolic function is influenced by thyroid hormone status (2,4). Hypothyroidism and myxedema are associated with prolonged ventricular relaxation times that are reversible with replacement therapy. In comparison, hyperthyroid patients demonstrate enhanced diastolic relaxation rate as assessed by two-dimensional echocardiographic Doppler (14). Acute effects of T_3 on ventricular diastolic function have been examined in animal models. In a model employing normothermic ischemia-reperfusion injury, improvement in contractility after T_3 treatment was associated with restoration of diastolic function (15).

Intracellular calcium release and re-uptake into the sarcoplasmic reticulum (SR) regulates the rate of ventricular contraction and relaxation (2,8). The cardiac-specific SR calcium ATPase gene, which regulates the sequestration of calcium into the SR during diastole, is activated by thyroid hormone (8) and could in large part, therefore, explain the increased rate of diastolic relaxation observed in the human chronically thyrotoxic heart, and the impaired diastolic function of hypothyroidism (2).

POTENTIAL CLINICAL APPLICATIONS OF THYROID HORMONE THERAPY

In addition to chemical hypothyroidism with low serum T_4 and elevated serum thyroid-stimulating hormone (TSH), other clinical conditions, including various chronic illnesses, cardiac transplantation, cardiopulmonary bypass, heart failure, and sepsis, may lead to reductions in serum T_3 levels that have the potential for altering cardiovascular performance. Currently, accumulating data suggest that supplementation in the form of parenteral T_3 may have salutary effects on the heart and cardiovascular system in specific and identifiable disease states. As a result of the known effects of T_3, both on the heart and on the peripheral circulation, this form of therapy may offer novel benefits and be a useful addition to otherwise standardized forms of therapy (16). We have recently completed a trial in the use of T_3 therapy in high-risk patients undergoing cardiopulmonary bypass. T_3 produced significant improvement in cardiovascular hemodynamics without untoward side effects.

SUMMARY

It is well recognized that thyroid hormone has profound effects on the heart and cardiovascular system. The increased cardiac output, widened pulse pressure, tachycardia, and hyperdynamic precordium of hyperthyroidism are frequent clinical findings and stand in contrast to the decrease in cardiac work, narrow pulse pressure, and quiet precordium characteristic of hypothyroidism. In addition to chemical hypothyroidism with low serum T_4 and elevated serum TSH, other clinical conditions, including various chronic illnesses, cardiac transplantation, cardiopulmonary bypass, heart failure, and sepsis may lead to reductions in serum T_3 levels that have the potential for impairing cardiovascular performance. Accumulating data suggest that supplementation in the form of parenteral T_3 may have salutary effects on the heart and cardiovascular system, including increases in cardiac inotropy and decreases in systemic vascular resistance. As a result of the recently described effects of T_3 on the peripheral circulation, this form of therapy may offer novel benefits to selected patients when used alone or in conjunction with other standard treatment.

ACKNOWLEDGMENT

This research was supported by the Marilyn and Barry Rubenstein Family Foundation.

REFERENCES

1. Klein I. Thyroid hormone and the cardiovascular system. *Am J Med* 1990;88:631–637.
2. Klein I, Ojamaa K. Cardiovascular manifestations of endocrine disease. *J Clin Endocrinol Metab* 1992;75:339–342.
3. Klein I. Thyroid hormone and blood pressure regulation. In: Laragh JH, Brenner BM, eds. *Hypertension: pathophysiology, diagnosis and treatment.* New York: Raven Press; 1989:1661–1674.
4. Ojamaa K, Balkman C, Klein I. Acute effects of triiodothyronine on arterial smooth muscle cells. *Ann Thorac Surg* 1993;56:S61–S67.
5. Samuels HH, Forman BM, Horowitz ZD, Ye ZS. Regulation of gene expression of thyroid hormone. *J Clin Invest* 1988;81:957–967.
6. Davis FB, Davis PJ, Blass SD. Role of calmodulin in thyroid hormone stimulation in vitro of human erythrocyte Ca^{2+}-ATPase activity. *J Clin Invest* 1983;71:579–586.
7. Ojamaa K, Samarel A, Kupfer J, Hong C, Klein I. Thyroid hormone effects on cardiac gene expression independent of cardiac growth and protein synthesis. *Am J Physiol* 1992;263:E534–E540.
8. Dillmann WH. Mechanisms of action of thyroid hormones. *Med Clin North Am* 1985;69:849–861.
9. Klein I, Ojamaa K. Thyroid hormone and the cardiovascular system: from theory to practice. *J Clin Endocrinol Metab* 1994;78:1026–1027.
10. Klemperer JD, Zelano J, Helm RE, et al. Triiodothyronine improves left ventricular function without oxygen wasting effects following global hypothermic ischemia *J Thoracic Cardiovasc Surg* 1994 [*in press*].
11. Dyke CM, Yeh T Jr, Lehman JD, et al. Triiodothyronine-enhanced left ventricular function after ischemic injury. *Ann Thorac Surg* 1991;52:14–19.
12. Goto Y, Slinker BK, LeWinter MM. Decreased contractile efficiency and increased non-mechanical

energy cost in hyperthyroid rabbit heart: relaxation between O_2 consumption and systolic pressure-volume area or force-time integral. *Circ Res* 1990;66:999–1011.

13. Suga H, Tanaka N, Ohgoshi Y, et al. Hyperthyroid dog left ventricle has the same oxygen consumption versus pressure-volume area (PVA) relation as euthyroid dog. *Heart Vessels* 1991;6:71–83.
14. Mintz G, Pizzarello R, Klein I. Enhanced left ventricular diastolic function in hyperthyroidism: noninvasive assessment and response to treatment. *J Clin Endocrinol Metab* 1991;73:146–150.
15. Kadletz M, Mullen PG, Ding M, et al. Effect of triiodothyronine on postischemic myocardial function in the isolated heart. *Ann Thorac Surg* 1994;57:657–663.
16. Klein I, Ojamaa K, Powell S. Potential clinical applications for parenteral thyroid hormone therapy. *Hospital Formulary* 1993;28:848–858.

The Failing Heart, edited by N. S. Dhalla,
R. E. Beamish, N. Takeda, and M. Nagano.
Lippincott-Raven Publishers, Philadelphia © 1995.

37

Implantable Defibrillators in the Management of Malignant Ventricular Arrhythmias in Patients with Left Ventricular Dysfunction

Michael M. Mannino and *Davendra Mehta

*Department of Cardiology, The Mount Sinai Hospital, New York, New York 10029-6574
United States; and *The Mount Sinai School of Medicine of The City University of
New York, New York, New York 10029-6574 United States*

The automatic implantable cardioverter-defibrillator (ICD) has demonstrated the ability to meet the goal set forth by its inventors—specifically, to abort sudden cardiac death caused by ventricular tachyarrhythmias. Numerous studies have shown the sudden-death (SD) rates of patients treated with ICDs to be extremely low. Winkle et al., in an early study of 270 patients over 3 years, found a 4% SD rate (1). A similar result was found by the Cleveland Clinic Foundation and Montefiore Medical Center Experience in their analysis of 377 patients (2). Other authors have noted SD rates in patients with ICDs comparable to these rates as well, ranging from 1% to 5% (3,4). Significant reductions in long-term total cardiac mortality, however, have not been demonstrated. A possible explanation may lie with the fact that a large proportion of the patients with these arrhythmias and receiving such devices suffers from poor left ventricular function. This is not unexpected given the fact that the risk of arrhythmias and SD is higher in patients with chronic heart failure than in any other definable group in medicine. An analysis of the Framingham data revealed an age-adjusted rate of SD of 31.4 per 1,000 for men with heart failure versus 5.7 per 1,000 for men without (9.9/1,000 and 1.8/1,000, respectively, for women) (5).

SUDDEN DEATH AND TOTAL CARDIAC MORTALITY

In regard to sudden cardiac death, survival in patients with poor left ventricular function receiving ICDs is comparable to those with good ventricular function, usually exceeding 90% at 1 year (1–4,6). In the majority of patients, however, much of the survival benefit as a result of the ICD is seen in the first few years after implantation when abortion of a sudden cardiac death results in an extended life. It is following this time that other causes of death are brought out as the natural history of the patients' disease is altered, these deaths being reflected in the total mortality data (Fig. 1). Winkle et al. (1), in a study of 270 patients, reported an SD rate of 4% over 3 years, while total mortality for the same period was 20% (1). Kim et al. (2), in a recent study of 377 patients, showed an actuarial survival rate from SD of 99% at both 1 and 3 years for patients with ejection fractions (EFs) >30%, and 98% 1-year and 92% 3-year survival for those with an EF <30%. With respect to total mortality, the survival rates were 94% at 1 year and 85% at 3 years for patients with an EF >30%, with corresponding values of 84% and 72% for those with EF <30%. Another study by Grimm et al. (7), involving 241 patients, demonstrated a total mortality of 38% at 3 years, with only an 11% SD rate (Table 1).

While significant elimination of sudden cardiac death by ICDs has become accepted, the total cardiac mortality rates remain disappointingly high. The relative survival benefit of the ICD, therefore, is likely to be early after implantation in patients with poor ventricular function and may not be sustained. The overall survival rate will thus be improved in the short-run but will dissipate in the long-run as non-SD assumes the dominant mode of death (Table 1). This phenomenon of altering the rate of sudden cardiac death, but having total mortality remain unchanged, has been termed *conversion* of the mode of death. Patients with advanced (New York Heart Association [NYHA] class III or IV) heart failure therefore, although being saved from sudden unexpected death, are on the average unlikely to experience any significant prolongation of life given their poor 5-year prognosis. It is in the subsequent years of follow-up that other competing causes of death become the more prominent modes of death, and SD, although still significant, becomes less important. New-

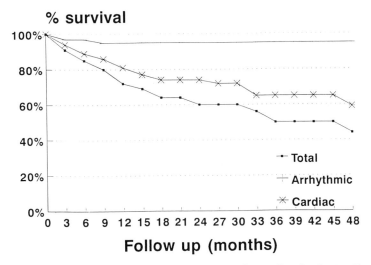

FIG. 1. Actuarial survival from arrhythmic, cardiac, and total mortality of patients with malignant ventricular arrhythmias, LV dysfunction, and implanted cardioverter defibrillators.

TABLE 1. *Benefits of implantable cardioverter-defibrillator therapy on arrhythmic and cardiac mortality in patients with ventricular arrhythmias and left ventricular dysfunction**

Follow-up period (yr)	Arrhythmic mortality (%)	Cardiac mortality (%)	Reference
1	9	—	Myerberg et al. (27)
1	2	16	Kim et al. (2)
3	11	33	Fogoros et al. (6)
3	—	38	Grimm et al. (7)
3	4	20	Winkle et al. (1)
3	8	28	Kim et al. (2)
4	7	40	Mehta et al. (26)

*Left ventricular ejection fraction <30%.

man et al. (8), in their analysis of 60 ICD recipients and 120 historical controls, found that while actuarial survival curves showed a significant difference between the ICD patients and controls (89% vs. 72% at 1 year and 65% vs. 49% at 3 years), the survival advantage afforded by the ICD appeared to dissipate over time with the curves converging at 40 months. In a study of 119 patients by Fogoros et al. (6), cumulative survival at 3 years was 97% for patients with an EF>30% but only 67% for those with an EF<30%.

Several explanations exist for the disappointing reduction in total cardiac mortality as compared with the impressive reduction in SDs in patients receiving ICDs. First, SD comprises only a fraction of the total cardiac deaths in patients with cardiac arrhythmias, accounting for a larger proportion of deaths in patients with better NYHA functional classes. Patients with poorer functional classes and lower EFs tend to suffer more deaths from progressive heart failure than the former group. In fact, despite studies analyzing multiple parameters in patients with poor ventricular function, EF remains the most powerful predictor of cardiac mortality (9). Perhaps an explanation for the large proportion of nonarrhythmic deaths manifested by these patients with ICDs is that their arrhythmias are not necessarily markers for impending sudden cardiac death but are merely a manifestation of poor left ventricular function and impending terminal left ventricular failure (9). A second reason for the discrepancy between the SD and total mortality death rates is that the implantation of defibrillators, especially via a thoracotomy approach, is associated with a small but significant surgical mortality, especially in those patients with poor ventricular function (Table 2). Finally, many patients with heart failure are predisposed to other causes of death, which have been shown to contribute to the overall cardiac mortality to a significant degree. Luu et al. (10) reviewed the terminal rhythms of 21 stable patients with class III congestive heart failure awaiting discharge from the hospital. While all of the arrests can be classified as sudden, only 38% were attributed to ventricular tachycardia or fibrillation (all of which occurred in those with ischemic cardiomyopathy). The most common cause of death, responsible for 62% of the total, was bradycardia or electromechanical dissociation. The latter was responsible for all of the deaths in those patients with idiopathic cardiomyopathy and 35% of the

TABLE 2. *Problems associated with implantable cardioverter-defibrillator implantation in patients with left ventricular dysfunction*

Relatively high defibrillation threshold
   Underlying cardiac disease—ischemia or fibrosis
   Increased left ventricular mass
   Decreased tolerance to induced VF during testing (more likely to have higher threshold with longer time to shock)
   With standard epicardial patches, relatively less myocardium is shocked
Higher perioperative mortality (with epicardial patches)
   Prolonged anesthesia required for thoracotomy[a]
   Perioperative heart failure in hemodynamically compromised patient[a]
   Postoperative infection
   Higher incidence of postoperative atrial and ventricular arrhythmias[a]

[a]Less of a problem with endocardial/nonthoracotomy lead system, with perioperative mortality 0.5% as compared with 2% with epicardial patches (per the PCD Investigators Group [22]).
VF, ventricular fibrillation.

deaths in patients with ischemic heart disease. Two patients died of coronary thrombus, one from a pulmonary embolus, and two from hyperkalemia. Other studies have similarly reported findings of bradyarrhythmias and coronary thrombosis as common causes of death in patients with cardiomyopathy as opposed to those without (11,12). Thus if one were to reasonably assume that 50% of deaths in patients with left ventricular dysfunction are sudden in nature, and that approximately 80% of those are tachyarrhythmic in nature, a 90% reduction in such deaths would calculate into a 36% reduction in total mortality. If one were to add a 3% to 5% surgical mortality for implantation of the ICD to that, the overall reduction is reduced to 31% (13). It remains to be shown if ICDs with antibradycardia pacing, the second generation of devices, improve survival over and above that by shock-only ICDs, especially in patients with impaired left ventricular function.

THE "NOT-SO-SUDDEN" DEATHS AND SURGICAL MORTALITY

While progressive heart failure is understood to be an important cause of nonarrhythmic death in patients with ICDs and poor ventricular function, much discussion has been generated regarding the non-sudden cardiac death rates related to arrhythmias, such as the surgical mortality associated with implantation and the "not-so-sudden" arrhythmic deaths described by Guarnieri et al. (14). The latter term is used to describe those patients with internal defibrillators that were initially successfully defibrillated but who die shortly thereafter from incessant malignant arrhythmias. This phenomenon, as alluded to previously, may be a reflection of the severity of the underlying ventricular disease rather than an indicator of an arrhythmogenic milieu (9). In support of this theory is the fact that the increased presence of complex ventricular arrhythmias on ambulatory monitoring in patients with poor ventricular function has been shown to predict not those dying from SD, but total cardiac mortality (11,15). In addition, as heart failure progresses, the prevalence of nonsustained ventricular tachycardia increases significantly while the rate of SD does not (1,16). Finally, there is the fact that most studies assessing the use of antiarrhythmic agents have found that despite the suppression of arrhythmic activity on ambulatory monitoring, the incidence of SD remains high in this population (17).

In addition to the non-sudden arrhythmic deaths, surgical mortality is an important contributor to mortality in patients receiving ICDs. Kim et al. (18) looked at the influence of left ventricular function on the outcome of patients with implanted defibrillators. Their study of 68 patients, implanted via a thoracotomy approach, found that the incidence of sudden cardiac death was not significantly different between those with EF>30% and those <30% at 1, 2, and 3 years of follow-up. Surgical mortality related to implantation of the defibrillator, however, was 11% for those with poor left ventricular function, compared with 0% for those with an EF>30%. Consequently, the total arrhythmia-related death rate, or those deaths caused by SD, surgical mortality–related arrhythmias, and non-SD (not prevented by automatic internal cardioverter defibrillator [ICD]), was higher for those with low EFs than for those without (30% vs. 3% at 3 years). Concomitant surgery did not influence the surgical mortality; that, however, may just be a reflection of the small amount of patients undergoing concomitant bypass surgery in this study.

A subsequent larger study by Kim et al. (2), reporting the Cleveland Clinic Foundation and Montefiore Medical Center experience, also looked at the influence of left ventricular function on survival and mode of death in patients receiving an ICD. This study of 377 patients compared rates of SD, surgical mortality, total arrhythmia-related death, and total cardiac death in patients with an implanted device and EFs of >30% with those with a device and EFs<30%. Here, the incidence of SD was extremely low in all patients receiving the ICD, survival being 98% for both groups at 1 year, and 95% and 90% at 5 years for patients with EFs>30% and <30%, respectively. Surgical mortality for the groups was improved over their previous study, probably representing improved surgical technique and a larger patient population, thus adding to the statistical power. The surgical mortality was 3.9% in all; 1.8% in patients with EF>30% and 7% in those with EF<30%. Also, unlike their previous report, concomitant bypass surgery did influence the surgical mortality in an unfavorable manner—9% with versus 2.2% without for all patients. Total cardiac mortality, as expected, differed depending on EF—being 19% for patients with EF>30% at 3 years and 28% in those with an EF<30%, with the total arrhythmia-related deaths constituting 63% of all deaths in the latter group.

These findings of surgical mortality in the 7% to 11% range for patients with low EFs appears excessively high compared with other studies that have reported rates of 1.5% to 5.4%, although Gohn et al. found similar elevated mortality rates for patients with low (<30%) EFs compared with those with EFs>30% (19–21). A recent publication, however, comparing the newer transvenous (nonthoracotomy) leads to the traditional thoracotomy approach (epicardial leads), demonstrates an improved survival by the transvenous method (22). The PCD Investigator Group examined the safety of the implantation procedure and clinical outcome of 1,221 patients receiving either a thoracotomy approach with epicardial leads (616 patients) or a nonthoracotomy approach with endocardial leads (605 patients). The nonthoracotomy approach was associated with a significant perioperative survival advantage—0% versus 3.4% for patients with EFs>30%, and 2.1% versus 5.2% for those with EFs<30%. When perioperative events are excluded in their analysis, both cardiac and noncardiac mortality are comparable at 3 years' follow-up.

Interestingly, when one looks at the cause of death immediately following implantation of the transthoracic devices, it appears that arrhythmias account for a significant proportion, although infection and worsening heart failure also contribute. Veltri et al. (23) reported a 50% incidence of death due to "incessant ventricular arrhythmias" during the postoperative period. Similarly, Gohn et al. (21) reported that 58% of postoperative deaths were due to arrhythmic complications. In the study by Kim et al. (24), two-thirds of the early deaths were related to intractable arrhythmias. Unfortunately, the PCD Investigator Group did not elaborate on the early perioperative causes of death. Thus, from the aforementioned data, the reduction in mortality by the transvenous method appears likely, due at least in part to the fact that epicardial electrodes are no longer needed and therefore spare the patient from the risks of a thoracotomy as well as pericardial and myocardial irritation and their potential for arrhythmia provocation. Although this exacerbation, when it occurs, is transient in many patients, in some it may have long-term effects on the natural course of arrhythmia occurrence and may cause more frequent recurrences during the follow-up period than it would have without the ICD implantation (24). Crandall et al. (25), in their study of 194 consecutive patients treated with or without an ICD (thoracotomy approach) for an out-of-hospital SD and non-inducibility by programmed electrical stimulation, suggest such a possibility. Although overall survival rates for the two groups were similar, the arrhythmia event rate of fatal and nonfatal recurrences was significantly higher (30% vs. 12% at 2 years) in those receiving ICDs than in those treated without.

SHOCK OCCURRENCE AND SURVIVAL BENEFIT

In terms of ICD discharge, Mehta et al. (26), in a study of 112 patients with drug refractory ventricular tachycardia or fibrillation, found that the rate of ICD discharge at 4 years was similar for patients with both low (<30%) and high (>30%) left ventricular EFs. The 5-year cardiac mortality in this study, however, was higher in patients with lower EFs (40% vs. 12%), with no difference in mortality between those who received "appropriate" shocks and those who did not (Fig. 2). Grimm et al. (7), in reviewing the rate of discharge of 241 patients with ICDs, found the frequency of administered shocks to increase longitudinally with time—occurring in 15% of patients at 1 year and in up to 76% at 5 years. This observation is in keeping with the findings of other authors and may suggest that the true benefit of these devices may not be apparent for several years; unfortunately for those patients

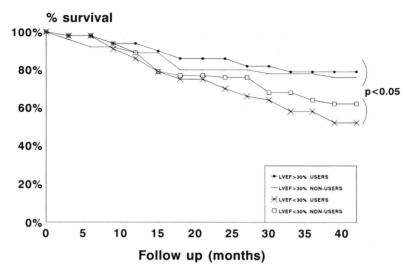

FIG. 2. Comparison of cardiac mortality in patients with good (>30%) and poor (<30%) left ventricular ejection fraction (LVEF) with reference to "appropriate" use of the device. *Users* represents those patients who had appropriate ICD shocks and *non-users* those who did not have any ICD shocks. There was no significant difference in cardiac mortality between the users and non-users in patients with good versus those with poor left ventricular function. Beyond 32 months, however, cardiac mortality was significantly higher in patients with impaired left ventricular function, both in users and non-users of ICD.

with poor ventricular function, this may exceed their life expectancy. In addition, Grimm et al. also found that the survival among patients receiving spontaneous ICD shocks was not significantly different from those not receiving them, the only predictor of total mortality being a low EF. Forgoros et al. (6) analyzed the impact of the ICD on prolongation of life, as measured by time from initial implant to first shock. When comparing results in terms of left ventricular function, a significant difference between the groups was observed, with the <30% EF group surviving a mean of 11 ± 14 months after initial shock, compared with a mean of 42 ± 9 months for those with EFs >30%. Myerberg et al. (27), following 60 patients over 25 months, found that the mean time to death was 14.8 ± 13.1 months for patients receiving any prior shocks and 16.7 ± 11.5 for those not receiving shocks (27). The mean time to first shock for those patients who subsequently died was noted to be 2.3 ± 2 months, thus making the mean time to death following the first shock 11.8 months.

The preceding observations are based mainly on the assumption that a patient with a defibrillator would have died at the time of the first appropriate shock, had the patient been without the ICD. This method of survival analysis, however, has important limitations, as a significant proportion of shocks is not related to potentially fatal arrhythmia. Based on available information, is it possible to determine the appropriateness of delivered ICD therapies? Studies with the aid of the newer third-generation devices exist to suggest that many of the arrhythmias that trigger the ICDs to fire may spontaneously terminate prior to ICD therapy (28). In addition, there exists the possibility that the newly available pacing-capable devices may convert stable, non–life-threatening ventricular or even supraventricular arrhythmias into unstable arrhythmias requiring a discharge from the ICD (29). Controlled studies are currently underway to answer the questions of appropriateness and benefit of ICD therapy when delivered and standardized survival analyses are being encouraged (28). The Multicenter Automatic Defibrillator Implantation Trial (MADIT) aims at comparing conventional therapy with ICD implantation in patients with impaired left ventricular function, coronary artery disease with nonsustained ventricular tachycardia, and inducible sustained ventricular tachycardia. The Coronary Artery Bypass Graft (CABG) Patch trial is investigating the "prophylactic" use of defibrillators in patients with a low EF and positive signal averaged electrocardiogram (SAECG) who are scheduled for bypass surgery. Unlike previous studies, these trials have included patients without a history of sustained tachyarrhythmias.

DEFIBRILLATOR VERSUS MEDICAL THERAPY

While the total cardiac mortality following an ICD implant has not been shown to parallel the impressive early reduction in SD in patients with poor left ventricular function, does medical or antiarrhythmic therapy offer a viable alternative in this population? Large studies such as the Cooperative North Scandinavian Enalapril Survival Study (CONSENSUS) and the Vasadilator Heart Failure Trial (VHEFT) have demonstrated the utility of vasodilators, particularly the angiotensin-converting enzyme inhibitors, in reducing mortality in patients with poor ventricular function (30,31). The results of the Cardiac Arrythmia Suppression Trial (CAST), however, has shed light on the potential harm of the currently available antiarrhythmic agents (32). One antiarrhythmic agent, amiodarone, is currently under much consideration as a possible alternative to ICD therapy in the prevention of sudden cardiac death. Although principally a class-3 antiarrhythmic, amiodarone also possesses properties of beta- and alpha-blockade, as well as calcium channel blockade and, to a small degree, fast sodium channel (class-I) activity. Past studies, performed mainly in Europe, regarding the use of amiodarone have been small or inadequately designed and have thus not produced data implying any significant mortality benefit of the drug. Several large-scale studies, however, are currently underway to assess the utility of amiodarone in terms of preventing sudden cardiac death in patients with malignant ventricular arrhythmias and reduced EF.

In 1987 Neri et al. (33) followed 65 patients with dilated cardiomyopathy and complex ventricular arrhythmias by ambulatory electrocardiographic monitoring, 41 of which received amiodarone (200–400 mg/d). During a mean follow-up of 3 years, there was a total of 18 deaths: ten patients in the group receiving amiodarone, all from progressive congestive heart failure; and eight patients in the group not receiving the agent—four from SD and four from progressive congestive heart failure. Side effects were common (in 23 of 41 patients), but only four patients required discontinuation. A similar small study by Hamer et al. (34) followed 34 patients on low-dose amiodarone or placebo for an average of 2 years. Their findings were not unlike those of the study by Neri et al. in that no episodes of sudden cardiac death were noted in the patients receiving amiodarone (six deaths: two noncardiac and four pump failure), while five of seven deaths in the placebo group were attributed to sudden arrhythmic deaths. In 1988 Cleland et al. (35) reported their study involving 132 patients receiving conventional therapy with or without low-dose (200 mg) amiodarone in a nonrandomized fashion. After 21 months of follow-up, total mortality of the study population was 41% (63 patients), of which 47 (75% of all deaths) were deemed sudden, and only five patients were believed to have died from progressive heart failure. Estimated survival curves of the data revealed that amiodarone reduced the incidence of SD from 45% to 15%. Nicklas et al. (36) studied 101 patients with EFs<30% and nonsustained ventricular tachycardia on ambulatory monitoring receiving either low-dose (200 mg/d) amiodarone or placebo for 1 year. While the frequency of complex arrhythmias on ambulatory monitoring was significantly diminished in those patients receiving active therapy, unlike the aforementioned studies, there was no improvement in mortality or the incidence of sudden cardiac death—26% total mortality on amiodarone versus 19% on placebo. A total of 21 patients died suddenly during the 1-year follow-up, of which 12 were receiving amiodarone and nine placebo. The authors noted in the study that the absence of a beneficial effect might be attributed to the statistical power of their study, but nonetheless argued that any reduction in mortality was likely to be modest (<25%). A recent study by Nul et al. (37) describes a significant reduction in total cardiac mortality over 2 years in patients receiving low-dose (300 mg/d) amiodarone as opposed to a control group (33.5% vs. 41.4%, respectively). Their study of 504 patients, however, only demonstrated a non-significant trend towards a reduction in SD. The aforementioned studies have demonstrated conflicting evidence for a benefit of amiodarone in reducing the incidence of SD. They appear, however, to lack either sufficient power or design to properly evaluate for a significant effect of the medication. Thus, although the above studies have not convincingly demonstrated a benefit of amiodarone in terms of reducing SD, they, as well as others, have provided important data as to the ability of the drug to be fairly well tolerated and associated with significant arrhythmia reduction by ambulatory monitoring (38).

Several large trials are currently underway to answer the question of whether or not amiodarone truly alters the incidence of sudden cardiac death in this population. The Antiarrhythmic Versus Implantable Defibrillator (AVID) study is a National Institutes of Health (NIH)-sponsored multicenter prospective study comparing conventional antiarrhythmic drug therapy with ICDs in patients surviving cardiac arrest or sustained ventricular tachycardia. Drug therapy consists of sotalol (via programmed electrophysiologic stimulation and Holter guidance) or amiodarone. The ICDs used are third generation via a transvenous lead system when possible. The Cardiac Arrest Study in Hamburg (CASH) also is investigating the utility of drug therapy versus ICD implantation. This trial compares amiodarone, metoprolol, or propafenone (latter arm discontinued due to excessive mortality) to an ICD via a transvenous or thoracotomy approach. To date, no differences in total mortality rates have been seen between the ICD and drug groups, or between amiodarone and metoprolol. Sudden death, however, is significantly reduced with the ICD as compared with medical therapy. The Canadian Implantable Defibrillator Study (CIDS) also compares amiodarone with ICD implantation. This latter trial has continued to proceed for more than 2 years without premature termination, thus suggesting that any difference between the two therapies is unlikely to be dramatic. The primary endpoint for all of above studies is total or arrhythmic death and not use of the ICD or recurrence of arrhythmia.

SUMMARY

With regard to SD, the impact of implanted defibrillators is clear. The continued substantial rates of overall mortality, however, especially in patients with reduced ventricular function, call into question the actual ability of these devices to prolong life to a significant degree. Additionally, given the population in which a substantial number of ICDs are likely to be implanted (those with poor ventricular function), a realistic goal as to the benefit in mortality needs to be addressed, given the already compromised survival of this population. Much discussion and literature have been devoted recently to standardizing the mortality analysis and definitions of the causes of death in these studies (39). Because of the high cost of ICDs and the significant risks associated with their implantation, real benefits with regard to both prolongation and quality of life need to be demonstrated. It is hoped that the trials in progress mentioned in this chapter will help to answer these questions.

REFERENCES

1. Winkle RA, Mead RH, Ruder MA, et al. Long term outcome with the automatic implantable cardioverter-defibrillator. *J Am Coll Cardiol* 1989; 16:1353–1361.
2. Kim SG, Maloney JD, Pinski SL, et al. Influence of left ventricular function on survival and mode of death after implantable defibrillator therapy (Cleveland Clinic Foundation and Montefiore Medical Center Experience). *Am J Cardiol* 1993;72:1263–1267.
3. Mirowski M, Reid PR, Winkle RA, et al. Mortality in patients with implanted automatic defibrillators. *Ann Intern Med* 1983;98:585–588.
4. Fogoros RN, Fiedler SB, Elson JJ. The automatic implantable cardioverter-defibrillator in drug refractory ventricular tachyarrhythmias. *Ann Intern Med* 1987;107:635–641.
5. Kannel WB, Plehn JF, Cuppies LA. Cardiac failure and sudden death in the Framingham study. *Am Heart J* 1988;115:869–875.
6. Fogoros RN, Elson JJ, Bonnet CA, Feidler SB, Burkholder JA. Efficacy of the automatic implantable cardioverter-defibrillator in prolonging survival in patients with severe underlying cardiac disease. *J Am Coll Cardiol* 1990;16:381–386.
7. Grimm W, Flores BT, Marchlinski FE. Shock occurrence and survival in 241 patients with implantable cardioverter-defibrillator therapy. *Circulation* 1993;87:1880–1888.

8. Newman D, Suave MJ, Herre J, et al. Survival after implantation of the cardioverter-defibrillator. *Am J Cardiol* 1992;69:889–903.
9. Packer M. Lack of relation between ventricular arrhythmias and sudden death in patients with chronic heart failure. *Circulation* 1992;85[Suppl]:I-50–I-56.
10. Luu M, Stephenson WG, Stephenson LW, Baron K, Walden J. Diverse mechanisms of unexpected cardiac arrest in advanced heart failure. *Circulation* 1990;80:1675–1680.
11. Radhakrishnan S, Kaul U, Bahl VK, Talwar KK, Bhatia ML. Sudden bradyarrhythmic death in dilated cardiomyopathy: a case report. *PACE* 1988;11:1369–1372.
12. Iseri LT, Humphrey SB, Siner EJ. Prehospital bradyasystolic cardiac arrest. *Ann Intern Med* 1978;88:741–745.
13. Sweeney MO, Ruskin JN. Mortality benefits and the implantable-cardioverter defibrillator. *Circulation* 1994;89:1851–1858.
14. Guarnieri T, Levine JH, Griffith LSC, Veltri E. When "sudden cardiac death" is not so sudden: lessons learned from the automatic cardioverter-defibrillator. *Am Heart J* 1988;115:205–207.
15. Packer M. Sudden unexpected death in patients with congestive heart failure: a second frontier. *Circulation* 1985;72:681–685.
16. Calif RM, McKinnis RA, Burke J, et al. Prognostic implications of ventricular arrhythmias during 24 hour ambulatory monitoring in patients undergoing cardiac catheterization for coronary artery disease. *Am J Cardiol* 1982;50:23–31.
17. The Cardiac Arrhythmia Suppression Trial (CAST) Investigators. Effect of encainide and flecainide on mortality in randomized trial of arrhhythmia suppression after myocardial infarction. *N Engl J Med* 1989;321:406–412.
18. Kim SG, Fisher JD, Choue CW, et al. The influence of left ventricular function on outcome of patients treated with implantable defibrillators. *Circulation* 1992;85:1304–1310.
19. Gartman DM, Bardy GH, Allen M, Misbach GA, Ivey TD. Short term morbidity and mortality of implantation of the automatic implantable cardioverter-defibrillator. *J Thorac Cardiovasc Surg* 1990;100:353–359.
20. Mosteller RD, Lehmann MH, Thomas AC, Jackson K. Operative mortality with implantation of the automatic cardioverter-defibrillator. *Am J Cardiol* 1992;68:130–145.
21. Gohn D, Edel T, Pollard C, et al. Determinants of operative mortality in implantable cardioverter-defibrillator. *J Am Coll Cardiol* 1991;17[Suppl]:86A(abst).
22. The PCD Investigator Group. Clinical outcome of patients with malignant ventricular tachyarrhythmias and a multiprogrammable implantable cardioverter-defibrillator implanted with or without thoracotomy: an international multicenter study. *J Am Coll Cardiol* 1994;23:1521–1530.
23. Veltri E, Mower MM, Guarnieri T, et al. Clinical efficacy of the automatic implantable cardioverter-defibrillator: six year cumulative experience. *Circulation* 1986;74[Suppl]:II-109(abst).
24. Kim SG, Fisher JD, Furman S, et al. Exacerbation of ventricular arrhythmias during the postoperative period after implantation of an automatic defibrillator. *J Am Coll Cardiol* 1992;18:1200–1206.
25. Crandall BG, Morris CD, Cutler JE, et al. Implantable cardioverter-defibrillator therapy in survivors of out-of-hospital sudden cardiac death without inducible arrhythmias. *J Am Coll Cardiol* 1993; 21:1186–1192.
26. Mehta D, Saksena S, Krol RB. Survival of implantable cardioverter-defibrillator recipients: role of left ventricular function and relationship to device use. *Am Heart J* 1992;124:1608–1614.
27. Myerberg RJ, Luceri RM, Thurer R, et al. Time to first shock and clinical outcome in patients receiving an automatic implantable cardioverter-defibrillator. *J Am Coll Cardiol* 1989;14:508–514.
28. Ellenbogen K, Luceri R, Dorian P, et al. and Phase-1 Clinical Investigators. Clinical evaluation of implantable cardioverter-defibrillator (ICD) function: importance of data logging to assess device efficacy. *Circulation* 1991;84:II-426.
29. Hook BG, Callans DJ, Kleiman RB, Flores BF, Marchilinski FE. Implantable cardioverter-defibrillator therapy in the absence of significant symptoms: rhythm diagnosis and management aided by stored electrogram analysis. *Circulation* 1993;87:1897–1906.
30. The CONSENSUS Trial Study Group. Effects of enalapril on mortality in severe congestive heart failure: results of the Cooperative North Scandinavian Enalapril Survival Study (CONSENSUS). *N Engl J Med* 1987;316:1429–1435.
31. Cohn JV, Archibald DG, Zeische S, et al. Effect of vasodilator therapy on mortality in chronic congestive heart failure: results of a Veterans Administration cooperative study. *N Engl J Med* 1986;314:1547–1552.

32. The Cardiac Arrhythmia Suppression Trial (CAST) Investigators. Preliminary report: effect of en-cainide and flecainide on mortality in a randomized trial of arrhythmia suppression after myocardial infarction. *N Engl Med* 1989;321:406–412.
33. Neri R, Mestroni L, Salvi A, Pandullo C, Camerini F. Ventricular arrhythmias in dilated cardio-myopathy: efficacy of amiodarone. *Am Heart J* 1987;113:707–712.
34. Hamer AW, Arkles LB, Johns JA. Beneficial effects of low-dose amiodarone in patients with con-gestive cardiac failure: a placebo-controlled trial. *J Am Coll Cardiol* 1989;14:1768–1774.
35. Cleland JG, Dargie HJ, Ford I. Mortality in heart failure: clinical variables of prognostic value. *Br Heart J* 1987;58:572–582.
36. Nicklas JM, McKenna WJ, Stewart RA, et al. Prospective, double-blind, placebo-controlled trial of low-dose amiodarone in patients with severe heart failure and asymptomatic frequent ventricular ectopy. *Am Heart J* 1991;122:1016–1021.
37. Nul DR, Doval HC, and the Grupo de Estudio de Sobrevida en Insuficiecia Cardiaca en Argentina (GESICA). Randomized trial of low-dose amiodarone in severe congestive heart failure. *Lancet* 1994;344:493–498.
38. Kim SG, Mannino MM, Roth SG, et al. Rapid suppression of spontaneous ventricular arrhythmias during oral amiodarone loading. *Ann Intern Med* 1992;117:197–201.
39. Kim SG, Fogoros RN, Furman S, Connolly SJ, Kuck KH, Moss AJ, for the participants of the Policy Conference. Standardized reporting of ICD patient outcome: the report of a North American Society of Pacing and Electrophysiology Policy Conference, February 9–10, *PACE* 1993;16:1–5.

The Failing Heart, edited by N. S. Dhalla,
R. E. Beamish, N. Takeda, and M. Nagano.
Lippincott-Raven Publishers, Philadelphia © 1995.

38

Biomechanical Cardiac Assist for Heart Failure

Yoshio Misawa and *Ray C.-J. Chiu

*Department of Thoracic and Cardiovascular Surgery, Jichi Medical School,
Tochigi, Japan; and *Division of Cardiovascular and Thoracic Surgery,
McGill University, Montreal, Quebec, H3G 1A4 Canada*

Attempts to utilize the contractile power of skeletal muscle to assist a failing heart is currently undergoing various stages of clinical and experimental trials. In this chapter, we review the biological basis of such an approach and provide an overview of how such a muscle has been applied to provide an effective hemodynamic assist in heart failure. The emphasis will be on the system design concepts being explored by various investigators in biomechanical cardiac assist.

BIOLOGICAL BASIS OF BIOMECHANICAL CARDIAC ASSIST

The biological issues that need to be addressed in utilizing skeletal muscle as the power source for cardiac assist include skeletal muscle fatigue upon repetitive stimulation for contraction; the different pattern of response to electrical stimulation between the skeletal muscle and myocardium; and the question of optimal resting tension and blood flow the skeletal muscle should maintain for its performance.

Skeletal Muscle Transformation to Confer Fatigue Resistance

Most skeletal muscles contain types I and II muscle fibers and their subtypes. Type I fibers are fatigue resistant, and have more mitochondria for the oxidative metabolism and less sarcoplasmic reticulum for slow twitch. Type II fibers are more prone to fatigue, have fewer mitochondria, and more sarcoplasmic reticular activity for fast twitch. Salmons and Sreter found that the skeletal muscles can be conditioned to acquire fatigue resistance with low frequency electrical stimulation (1). Such conditioning transforms type II fibers into type I fibers (2). The phenotype transformation of the skeletal muscle enables it to work for a prolonged period of time to provide cardiac assist (3), although the rate of muscle transformation is different among species and individuals and may be influenced by some environmental factors.

Pulse Train (Burst) Stimulation to Summate Muscle Contraction

Myocardium is a syncytium, so that in response to a single electrical impulse, it contracts as a whole in an all-or-none fashion. In contrast, the skeletal muscle, even after transformation, consists of individual motor units, and the contractile strength and duration depend on the number of motor units recruited in response to electrical stimulation. Our group demonstrated (4) that a pulse train stimulator can produce a strong and prolonged skeletal muscle contraction (Fig. 1) (5), and it can be synchronized with the heart beats so that the electrical burst may be delivered to the skeletal muscle during a selected segment of the cardiac cycle. Refinement of such a stimulator resulted in an implantable cardiomyostimulator, which could self-adjust the burst duration automatically in response to changes in heart rate. In a stimulator specially designed to achieve counterpulsation, the sensing-to-burst delay period can also be programmed to change with the heart rate, and arrhythmia-sensing capabilities of such a stimulator can avoid inappropriate firing when irregular heart rhythms are encountered. These stimulators are being employed in the clinical and experimental studies to be described.

Muscle Resting Tension and Conformational Changes

Normally, the skeletal muscle fibers are straight and contract linearly. When the skeletal muscles are wrapped around the heart or mandrels, geometrical and physiological changes may ensue. Geometrically, they become adherent to the heart or to the mandrels and permanently assume a curvilinear shape. Furthermore, in response to altered resting tensions, muscle fibers can add or delete the number of sarcomeres to restore the resting tension. We have called this "conformational change" (6),

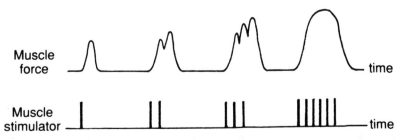

FIG. 1. Schema of pulse train stimulation. Skeletal muscle twitches stimulated by pulse trains show summation of duration and force of contraction. From Hill et al. (5). Copyrighted and reprinted with the permission of Clinical Cardiology Publishing Co., Inc., and/or Foundation for Advances in Medicine and Sciences, Inc.

which reflects the adaptation of the skeletal muscle to a new configuration and length (7) imposed to it when it is being utilized to provide cardiac assist. It has been also shown that loss of resting tension by a skeletal muscle may cause its atrophy and degenerative changes such as fibrosis and fatty infiltration (8). The relationship between conformational changes of the skeletal muscle and degenerative changes, in response to loss of original resting tension in a muscle, needs to be elucidated further.

The Effects of Contraction Pattern on Blood Flow to the Skeletal Muscle

Coronary blood flow to the myocardium is predominantly during the diastolic phase of the cardiac cycle, while skeletal muscle blood flow is greater during systole. Gealow et al. (7) showed that blood flow to the skeletal muscle increased proportionately to the muscle work over a wide range of rate of contractions. Strong skeletal muscle contraction prevents blood from entering the muscle, which can be followed by autoregulatory reactive hyperemia during muscle relaxation. Depending on the rate, strength, and duration of muscle contractions, the autoregulatory mechanism could be overwhelmed, leading to ischemic muscular damage. This is an important consideration in using skeletal muscle as a power source for cardiac assist.

SYSTEM DESIGN CONCEPTS FOR BIOMECHANICAL CARDIAC ASSIST

Utilizing transformed fatigue-resistant skeletal muscle and an appropriately programmed synchronizable burst stimulator, skeletal muscle can be used to directly or indirectly assist a failing heart. The direct approach is to wrap the muscle around the heart and stimulate it to contract in synchrony with cardiac systole. This surgical procedure is now known as "dynamic cardiomyoplasty" and is currently undergoing worldwide clinical trials. The indirect methods are to use the skeletal muscle as a power source to activate cardiac assist devices of various designs. Table 1 shows the biomechanical cardiac assist systems being studied or proposed for investigation at this time.

TABLE 1. *Four system design concepts for biomechanical cardiac assist*

Asynchronized systems
Synchronized systems
co-pulsators
counterpulsators
reciprocal synchronized systems
Hybrid (biomechanical and mechanical) systems
Linear energy converter systems

Asynchronized Systems

In such a system, it is not necessary to synchronize the skeletal muscle contraction with the cardiac cycles. In the skeletal muscle ventricle (SMV) designed by Stephenson's group (9), a single chamber is constructed from a skeletal muscle (Fig. 2). A skeletal muscle, most often a latissimus dorsi muscle, is mobilized as a pedicle graft with intact neurovascular bundle, and electrodes are placed near the thoracodorsal nerve for muscle transformation and stimulation. This muscle is wrapped around a cone-shaped mandrel and transformed according to a conditioning protocol of gradually increasing stimuli. Skeletal muscle ventricle has afferent and efferent limbs, and with appropriate valves, it can be used to provide asynchronous assist, such as from the left ventricle-to-aorta or from the right ventricle-to-pulmonary artery. Such an accessory ventricle can be in parallel or in series with the native circulation and provide right or left cardiac bypass. When an SMV is used as an asynchronized system, it is physiologically similar to the right or left ventricular bypasses provided with a centrifugal pump. The difficulties with SMVs have been thromboembolic complications and rupture of SMVs (10), which need to be resolved before they can be applied clinically.

Our group reported on a dual-chamber device in which one chamber was de-

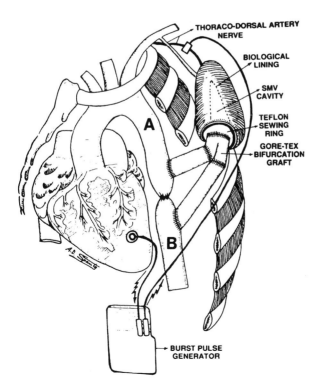

FIG. 2. Single skeletal muscle ventricle (SMV). Stephenson and his associates wrap a skeletal muscle around a pouch to make SMV for counterpulsation. From Anderson et al. (9).

signed to convert muscle contraction energy to hydraulic pressure, which is transmitted to another chamber designed to produce hemodynamic effects (11). A balloon is placed under the latissimus dorsi muscle and the latter stimulated to contract, which compresses the balloon to generate pressure. The balloon contains hydraulic fluid which is not coagulable. The pressure is transmitted through a tube to compress another balloon which is connected to the vascular system. This latter blood-containing chamber also has afferent and efferent limbs, with or without one-way valves. The blood chamber is designed to be located near the desired anatomical position for the specific application, and made to minimize blood turbulence and the associated thromboembolic complications. We feel the advantage of the dual-chamber system is the feasibility of separately designing two chambers optimally for power generation and hemodynamic effects, respectively, which may have different design requirements. In the single-chamber SMV, a compromise may be required, because both functions are performed by the same ventricle.

Synchronized Systems

Co-pulsators

Dynamic cardiomyoplasty is the most widely studied example of a co-pulsator, in which the skeletal muscle is made to contract in synchrony with myocardial contractions (Fig. 3). In cardiomyoplasty (12), the latissimus dorsi muscle graft is wrapped around the heart and transformed by graded electrical stimulation according to a conditioning protocol. Burst stimulation is delivered to the muscle during the systolic phase to provide systolic assist. Although many patients who received cardiomyoplasty did demonstrate improved systolic functions, other patients showed clinical improvement without clear evidence of systolic assist, such as increase in ejection fraction or stroke volume (13). Experimental studies in animals using pressure volume loops and ultrasonography indicate that other more subtle mechanisms may play a role in the observed clinical improvement following cardiomyoplasty (14–16). When a ventricular wall increases in thickness, such as that achieved with cardiomyoplasty, the ventricular wall stress may be reduced in accordance to Laplace's law (ventricular wall stress = pressure × radius/wall thickness) (17,18). In addition to such a stress-sparing effect, the passive presence of muscle itself around the heart, known as *adynamic cardiomyoplasty*, may also affect the natural course of heart failure by providing a "girdling effect" (19), which is likely to be due to modulation of the ventricular remodeling process and delaying of ventricular dilatation in heart failure. There is also experimental evidence that in ischemic cardiomyopathy, stimulated muscle wrap around the heart may be the source of collateral blood flow to the underlying ischemic myocardium (20). The current status of the dynamic cardiomyoplasty clinical trial will be discussed further at the end of this chapter.

Co-pulsation can also be achieved by using SMV or dual-chamber biomechanical

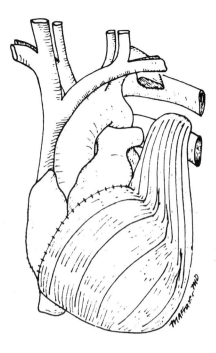

FIG. 3. Dynamic cardiomyoplasty. A left latissimus dorsi muscle is wrapped around the heart in a counterclockwise fashion. The muscle is stimulated to contract in synchrony with the heart. From Hill et al. (5). Copyrighted and reprinted with the permission of Clinical Cardiology Publishing Co., Inc., and/or Foundation for Advances in Medicine and Sciences, Inc.

assist. Skeletal muscle ventricle can be filled during diastole, or during systole when one assist is provided for every second heart beat. Then, during cardiac systole, SMV ejects blood into the circulation, using valves to allow forward flow and prevent retrograde flow. The SMV can thus function as an accessory ventricle, sharing the function of an impaired heart. Such a volume-sparing assist is suitable and effective for advanced heart failure. However, contractile strength of the latissimus dorsi muscle used for present systems is not sufficient to take over the total workload of the left ventricle (21). Geddes et al. showed effectiveness of SMV as a co-pulsator in acute experiments using rectus abdominis muscles in dogs as a power source (22). A twenty-eight percent increase of cardiac output was achieved when SMV contracted once per two heart beats.

The Anstedt pericardial cup is a device derived from the idea of direct mechanical cardiac massage (23). It is composed of an assistor cup and two air systems. The former is a glass housing with an internal silastic diaphragm and is placed around the heart. The latter are a vacuum system and a pulsed pressure system. The device will provide co-pulsation assist and circumvent problems associated with blood-polymer interface and related complications such as thromboembolism. When the device is powered with compressed air, excellent circulatory assist can be achieved and circulation maintained during electrically induced ventricular fibrillation (24). Instead of the compressed air as an energy source, the muscle-powered hydraulic chamber in our dual-chamber system may be utilized as the power source for the Anstedt cup, but its efficacy needs to be proven in future experiments.

Counterpulsators

The SMV and dual-chamber biomechanical cardiac assist systems can both be used as counterpulsators when the skeletal muscle is stimulated to contract during cardiac diastole and relax during cardiac systole. Fietsam and associates showed that SMV can be effective as a counterpulsator, reducing tension time index and increasing endocardial viability ratio in a heart failure model (25). Kochamba et al., from our laboratory, also showed the efficacy of using a dual-chamber muscle-powered pump to achieve counterpulsation (11). Both devices suffer from thromboembolic complications because of the significant turbulence within the chamber and the presence of blood-polymer interface. Stephenson's group has attempted, with some success, to use autogenous pericardium and endothelial seeding in the inner surface of the SMV to prevent thrombus formation (9).

To circumvent such complications associated with blood-polymer interface, the skeletal muscle has also been used to provide periaortic counterpulsation. In aortomyoplasty, studied by Chachques et al. (26), the latissimus dorsi muscle is wrapped around the ascending aorta and stimulated to contract during diastole. In order to obtain sufficient intraaortic volume for compression to achieve effective counterpulsation, however, the ascending aorta had to be enlarged with a patch graft, which has the drawback of creating an iatrogenic aneurysm. Other investigators have tried to perform aortomyoplasty in the descending thoracic aorta, which has more length and volume than the ascending aorta so that patch enlargement is not necessary. Wrapping the descending thoracic aorta, however, requires interruption of many intercostal arteries, which poses the potential risk of paraplegia due to spinal cord ischemia. To avoid such difficulties, we have developed a dual-chambered, periaortic counterpulsation system with a balloon placed between the descending thoracic aorta and a firm hood fixed over it (Fig. 4) (27). Inflation of the balloon would thus compress the descending thoracic aorta against the thoracic vertebra, and this can be achieved without interrupting intercostal arteries. The balloon is powered by a hydraulic system similar to that in the dual-chamber counterpulsator described earlier. The implantable synchronized burst stimulator fires during cardiac diastole to contract the latissimus dorsi muscle, which compresses the hydraulic chamber to generate power. This power is transmitted to the periaortic balloon, which compresses the aorta to produce diastolic augmentation. During systole, the muscle is relaxed, the balloon is deflated, the aorta re-expands, and a measure of systolic afterload reduction can be achieved. Acute experiments showed the efficacy of this system, while long-term experiments are being undertaken in our laboratory.

Reciprocal Synchronized Systems

In a reciprocal synchronized system, co-pulsation assist provided by either dynamic cardiomyoplasty or the Anstadt cup, which are activated during systole, is

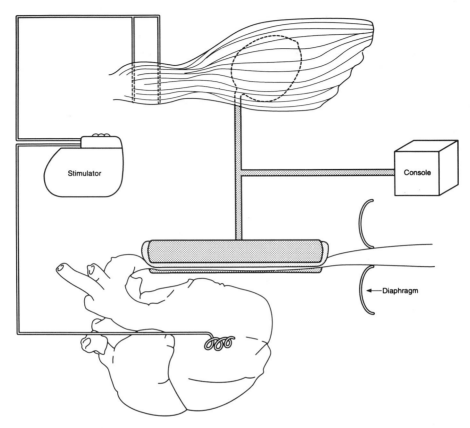

FIG. 4. Periaortic balloon pumping system. A hooded balloon is put around the descending aorta. The balloon is inflated to depress the descending aorta by a contracting skeletal muscle or a console in synchrony with the heart, resulting in increased diastolic pressure and decreased systolic pressure.

coupled with counterpulsation provided by aortomyoplasty or periaortic balloon pumping. We have proposed an integrated system (McGill MCAD) that reciprocally provides both co-pulsation during systole and counterpulsation during diastole for each cardiac cycle (27). Takahashi et al. showed significant systolic and diastolic assist in their combined dynamic cardiomyoplasty and aortomyoplasty model (28). Because both right and left latissimus dorsi muscles will be required for reciprocal synchronized systems, however, it will be more invasive and will require more complex devices.

Hybrid (Biological and Mechanical) Systems

As presently designed, the SMV can generate output approximately one-quarter of that generated by a normal left ventricle, which is sufficient to replace the right ventricular function, but not that of the left ventricle. On the other hand, the mechanical, totally implantable ventricular assist devices being developed require implantation of too much body space–occupying device components, making it difficult to implant two such devices to achieve biventricular assist. Thus, hybrid cardiac assist systems, combining dynamic cardiomyoplasty to assist the right heart and a conventional mechanical left ventricular assist device to assist the left heart, could be an option for the surgical treatment of patients with severe biventricular failure. Acute experiments in our laboratory have demonstrated the feasibility of such an approach (29).

Linear Energy Converter Systems

The skeletal muscle normally contracts in linear fashion. Thus, to obtain power by wrapping the muscle around the heart or an oval SMV is not very efficient because only a smaller vector of contractile force would be utilized. Farrar and Hill described a linear-pull energy converter that can be powered by a linearly contracting latissimus dorsi muscle (Fig. 5) (30). The insertion of this muscle at the humerus is transected and reattached to a small-cylinder hydraulic energy converter, which is fixed to the ribs. Contractile force of the muscle is converted to high-pressure hydraulic energy. The output of this hydraulic energy converter is connected by a small-diameter tube to a hydraulic actuator to drive the pusher plate of the implantable ventricular assist device or another suitable blood pump. Such a muscle-powered energy converter is versatile and can be used to drive a variety of different blood pumps to meet the needs of the full range of patients requiring mechanical circulatory assist, from counterpulsation to total prosthetic ventricular support. It might enable patients to experience a good quality of life free from bulky electric-powered hardware.

CLINICAL TRIALS OF DYNAMIC CARDIOMYOPLASTY

All of the biomechanical muscle-powered cardiac assist systems described are still in the laboratory study phase, except for dynamic cardiomyoplasty, which has undergone worldwide phase I and phase II clinical trials in patients suffering from heart failure. A phase III prospective randomized study was launched in North America in 1993. So far, the cardiomyostimulators and electrodes have functioned as designed (13). Currently, the primary indications for this procedure are patients with heart failure in New York Heart Association (NYHA) functional class III, deteriorating under medical therapy, and not amenable to other conventional surgical procedures (31–36). In terminal heart failure patients in NYHA functional class IV, the operative mortality is considered excessive, while in functional class III patients, the operative mortality has been around 10%. In more than 80% of patients surviving for 3 to 6 months and longer, clinical and functional improvement have been reported. Data from the phase II study also showed small, but statistically significant, improvement in systolic functions following cardiomyoplasty (Chiu

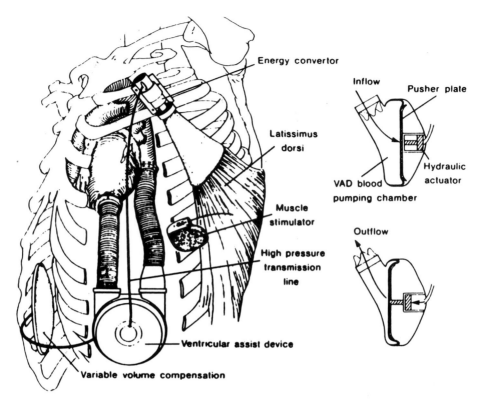

FIG. 5. Linear energy converter system. A latissimus dorsi muscle, which is removed at its insertion from the humerus, is connected to a mechanical-to-hydraulic energy converter. The stimulator causes the muscle to contract, creating high-pressure hydraulic energy that is transmitted to a valved ventricular assist device. This pressurizes a hydraulic actuator attached to the pusher plate of the ventricular assist device, resulting in ejection of blood into the aorta. From Farrar and Hill (30).

RC-J, presented at the American College of Cardiology, Atlanta, GA, March 15, 1994). Further data are required to confirm the survival advantage, if any, of this procedure in patients with severe heart failure.

SUMMARY

Biomechanical cardiac assist devices are at the stage of early development. Although progress has been made, many problems remain to be solved. Nevertheless, this approach appears versatile and highly promising for clinical usage in the future. Of the various biomechanical cardiac assist systems, dynamic cardiomyoplasty is nearest to general clinical application for selected patients with heart failure. Other devices such as SMV, periaortic counterpulsators, and others may also prove useful. A better method to harvest skeletal muscle contractile power for cardiac assist is needed. Thromboembolic complications seen with many devices have not been solved. Other devices may be too bulky and have the risk of structural failure. These issues are the obstacles against their clinical usage at this time. With further development, biomechanical cardiac assist devices, which require no donor organ, no immunosuppression, nor bulky external power source, may be able to provide a unique option for the treatment of patients with intractable heart failure.

ACKNOWLEDGMENT

Supported by an operating grant from the Medical Research Council of Canada.

REFERENCES

1. Salmons S, Sreter FA. Significance of impulse activity in the transformation of skeletal muscle type. *Nature* 1976;263:30–34.
2. Hudlicka O. Anatomical changes in chronically stimulated skeletal muscles. *Semin Thorac Cardiovasc Surg* 1991;3:106–110.
3. Salmons S, Jarvis JC. The working capacity of skeletal muscle transformed for use in a cardiac assist role. In: Chiu RC-J, Bourgeois IM, eds. *Transformed muscle for cardiac assist and repair*. Mount Kisco, NY: Futura; 1990:89–104.
4. Dewar MD, Drinkwater DC, Chiu RC-J. Synchronously stimulated skeletal muscle graft for myocardial repair. *J Thorac Cardiovasc Surg* 1984;87:325–331.
5. Hill A, Chiu RCJ. Dynamic cardiomyoplasty for treatment of heart failure. *Clin Cardiol* 1989; 12:681–688.
6. Chiu RC-J. Biomechanical cardiac assist: quo vadimus? *Semin Thorac Cardiovasc Surg* 1991;43: 160–163.
7. Gealow KK, Solien EE, Bianco RW, Chiu RC-J, Shumway SJ. Conformational adaptation of muscle: implications in cardiomyoplasty and skeletal muscle ventricles. *Ann Thorac Surg* 1993;56:520–526.
8. Oakley RM, Jarvis JC, Barman D, et al. Factors affecting the integrity of latissimus dorsi muscle grafts: implications for cardiac assistance from skeletal muscle. *J Heart Lung Transplant* 1994; 143:S38.
9. Anderson DR, Pochettino A, Hammond RL, et al. Autogenously lined skeletal muscle ventricles in circulation. *J Thorac Cardiovasc Surg* 1991;101:661–670.
10. Nakajima H, Nakajima HO, Thomas GA, et al. Chronic morphologic changes of skeletal muscle ventricles in circulation. *Ann Thorac Surg* 1994;57:912–920.
11. Kochamba G, Desrosiers C, Dewar M, Chiu RC-J. The muscle-powered dual-chamber counterpulsator. Rheologically superior implantable cardiac assist device. *Ann Thorac Surg* 1988;45:620–625.
12. Chachques JC, Grandjean P, Schwartz K, et al. Effect of latissimus dorsi dynamic cardiomyoplasty on ventricular function. *Circulation* 1988;78:III203–III216.
13. Grandjean PA, Austin L, Chan S, Terpstra B, Bourgeois IM. Dynamic cardiomyoplasty: clinical follow-up results. *J Cardiovasc Surg* 1991;6:80–88.
14. Sugiura S, Harada K, Yokoyama H, et al. Analysis of cardiac assistance by latissimus dorsi cardiomyoplasty with a time varying elastance model. *Cardiovasc Res* 1993;27:997–1003.
15. Delahaye F, Jegaden O, Montagna P, et al. Latissimus dorsi cardiomyoplasty in severe congestive heart failure: the Lyon experience. *J Cardiovasc Surg* 1991;6:106–123.
16. Nakajimi H, Niinami H, Hooper TL, et al. Cardiomyoplasty: probable mechanism of effectiveness using the pressure-volume relationship. *Ann Thorac Surg* 1994;57:407–415.
17. Lee KF, Dignan RJ, Parmar JM, et al. Effects of dynamic cardiomyoplasty on left ventricular performance and myocardial mechanics in dilated cardiomyopathy. *J Thorac Cardiovasc Surg* 1991;102:124–131.

18. Lee KF, Dyke CM, Wechsler AS. Theoretical considerations in the use of dynamic cardiomyoplasty to treat dilated cardiomyopathy. *J Cardiovasc Surg* 1991;6:119–123.
19. Capouya ER, Gerber RS, Drinkwater DC, et al. Girdling effect of nonstimulated cardiomyoplasty on left ventricular function. *Ann Thorac Surg* 1993;56:867–871.
20. Bailey WF, Magno MG, Buckman PD, Langan FT, Armenti VT, Mannion JD. Chronic stimulation enhances extramyocardial collateral blood flow after a cardiomyoplasty. *Ann Thorac Surg* 1993;56:1045–1053.
21. Bridges CR, Brown WE, Hammond RL Anderson DR, Anderson WA, Dimeo F. Skeletal muscle ventricles: improved performance at physiologic preloads. *Surgery* 1989;106:275–282.
22. Geddes LA, Janas W, Hinds M, Badylak SF, Cook J. The ventricular-synchronous, skeletal muscle ventricle: preliminary feasibility studies. *PACE* 1993;16:1310–1322.
23. Anstadt GL, Schiff P, Baue AF. Prolonged circulatory support by direct mechanical ventricular assistance. *Trans Am Soc Artif Intern Organs* 1966;12:72–79.
24. Egolov TL, Zimin NK, Kormer AI, Lektorskii BI. Biomedical aspects of cardiac massage in experiments and clinical practice. *Artif Organs* 1983;7:134–138.
25. Fietsam R, Lu H, Hammond RL, et al. Skeletal muscle ventricles with efferent valved homograft. *J Cardiovasc Surg* 1993;8:184–194.
26. Chachques JC, Grandjean PA, Fisher C, et al. Dynamic aortomyoplasty to assist left ventricular failure. *Ann Thorac Surg* 1990;49:225–230.
27. Odim JNK, Li C, Chiu RC-J. Pericardiovascular approach to cardiac assist: acute feasibility study. *Artif Organs* 1992;16:532–542.
28. Takahashi R, Yozu R, Kurosaka Y, Kawada S. Assisted circulation using cardiomyoplasty together with aortomyoplasty. *Artif Organs* 1993;17:914–918.
29. Odim JNK, Li C, Zibaitis A, Desrosiers C, Chiu RC-J. Hybrid biomechanical assist for acute biventricular failure. *J Cardiovasc Surg* 1991;6:164–170.
30. Farrar DJ, Hill JD. A new skeletal linear-pull energy converter as a power source for prosthetic circulatory support devices. *J Heart Lung Transplant* 1992;11:S341–S350.
31. Jatene AD, Moreira LFP, Stolf NAG, et al. Left ventricular function changes after cardiomyoplasty in patients with dilated cardiomyopathy. *J Thorac Cardiovasc Surg* 1993;102:132–139.
32. Belloti G, Moraes A, Bocchi E, et al. Late effects of cardiomyoplasty on left ventricular mechanics and diastolic filling. *Circulation* 1993;88:II304–II308.
33. Magovern JA, Park SE, Cmolik BL, Trumble DR, Christlieb IY, Magovern GJ Sr. Early effects of right latissimus dorsi cardiomyoplasty on left ventricular function. *Circulation* 1993;88:II298–II303.
34. Almada H, Molteni L, Ferreira R, Ortega D. Clinical experience with dynamic cardiomyoplasty. *J Cardiovasc Surg* 1990;5:193–198.
35. Bocchi EA, Moreira LFP, Moraes AV, et al. Effects of dynamic cardiomyoplasty on regional wall motion, ejection fraction, and geometry of left ventricle. *Circulation* 1992;86:II231–II235.
36. Chiu RC-J, Odim JNK, Burgess JH. Responses to dynamic cardiomyoplasty for idiopathic dilated cardiomyopathy. *Am J Cardiol* 1993;72:475–479.

The Failing Heart, edited by N. S. Dhalla,
R. E. Beamish, N. Takeda, and M. Nagano.
Lippincott-Raven Publishers, Philadelphia © 1995.

39

Heart Preservation: Magnetic Resonance Studies of Cardiac Energetics and Ion Homeostasis

Roxanne Deslauriers, Valerie V. Kupriyanov, Ganghong Tian,
John C. Docherty, Laura C. Stewart, *Sylvain Lareau, and
†Tomás A. Salerno

*Department of Biosystems, Institute for Biodiagnostics, National Research Council of
Canada, Winnipeg, Manitoba R3B 1Y6, Canada; *Instruments Anateck, Inc.,
Gatineau, Ontario J8R 1V1 Canada; and †Departments of Cardiothoracic Surgery,
State University of New York at Buffalo, Buffalo, New York 14203 United States*

Magnetic resonance (MR) has become widely accepted as a noninvasive modality for clinical and fundamental research. Our work has focused on the use of magnetic resonance spectroscopy (MRS) to gain a better understanding of the effects of ischemia and reperfusion to improve preservation of hearts for transplantation and during surgery. In addition, we have used MRS as a practical tool to test and develop better strategies for application in the clinical setting.

Much of our research has used the Langendorff perfused rat heart, a practical model for testing fundamental principles and developing new MR techniques. In addition, we have used isolated human atrial tissue removed during cardiac surgery requiring cardiopulmonary bypass as a relevant biochemical and metabolic model of the human heart. We have used the isolated perfused pig heart as a functional model of the intact human heart.

MAGNETIC RESONANCE SPECTROSCOPY

Studies on rat hearts and human atrial tissue were carried out using a Bruker AM-360 (Bruker Instruments, Karlsruhe, Germany) spectrometer equipped with a vertical-bore magnet (8.4 Tesla). Studies of isolated buffer and blood-perfused pig hearts were performed using a Bruker Biospec instrument with either a 30- or 40-cm horizontal-bore 4.7 Tesla magnet.

^{31}P Magnetic Resonance Spectroscopy

^{31}P MR spectra of rat hearts and human atrial appendages were acquired at 145.8 MHz using a broadband probe. The perfusion apparatus for rat hearts was built of nonmagnetic materials to avoid interference with the MR equipment. Field homogeneity was optimized using the Na resonance in the beating heart, with the probe tuned to the Na frequency. Spectra of atrial trabeculae were acquired using a custom-built (Morris Instruments. Inc., Gloucester, Canada) probe incorporating a nonmagnetic, thermostated perifusion system and strain gauge (Instruments Anateck, Gatineau, PQ, Canada). The time resolution was 2.5 to 5.0 minutes for the rat hearts, 30 minutes for the atrial appendages, and 20 to 45 minutes for the human atrial trabeculae.

^{31}P MR spectra of pig hearts was acquired at 81.0 MHz. For studies of the energetics of the whole heart, the organ was suspended in a 10-cm diameter single-turn solenoid coil that encompassed the entire heart and was tuned to the P frequency. The perfusion apparatus was built of nonmagnetic materials to avoid interference with the MR equipment. Field homogeneity was optimized using the Na resonance in the beating heart, with the MR probe tuned to the Na frequency (52.9 MHz). Free induction decays (FIDs) were obtained over a 2-minute sampling period (45° pulses [80 μs], a pulse repetition time of 1.2s). A small glass bead filled with phenylphosphonic acid and inserted into the right ventricle of the heart was used as a chemical shift and peak area standard for the ^{31}P MR spectra.

The area of the β-P peak of adenosine triphosphate (ATP) was used for measuring changes in ATP levels. All spectral data were expressed as a percentage of the initial ATP level, which was set at 100%. In the case of rat hearts, the data were converted to mmol/l intracellular water and reported as mM (1). The intracellular pH was calculated from the chemical shift of inorganic phosphate (P_i) (2). The integral of peak areas was measured using standard Bruker or NMR1 software after removal of the broad baseline component.

Magnetic resonance data were quantified by comparison of final peak areas of ATP and phosphocreatine (PCr), with their respective quantitative measurements made on freeze-clamped human tissue or on needle biopsies taken from pig hearts at the end of the MR experiments. The needle biopsy samples were taken while the pig heart was still being perfused and beating, plunged into liquid nitrogen within 2 seconds, and stored at −70°C. The tissue samples were assayed for ATP and PCr using high-performance liquid chromatography (HPLC) (3). Quantification at the earlier time points in the MR experiments was done by comparing the areas of the experimental peaks with those in the final MR spectrum. The data were further verified by comparing the calculated initial concentrations of ATP and PCr in the beating heart during the control period with data obtained from needle biopsies on normal hearts. In the case of rat hearts, a series was run in parallel with the MR experiments and freeze-clamped for biochemical determination of metabolites.

^{1}H Magnetic Resonance Spectroscopy

^{1}H MR spectra of human atrial appendages and rat hearts were acquired using a broadband probe. For human atrial appendages, interleaved ^{1}H and ^{31}P MR spectra were obtained, with a time resolution of 15 to 30 minutes, to monitor tissue energetics and metabolites (e.g., lactate) in human atrial tissue preserved over periods of up to 24 hours in conjunction with various hypothermic preservation protocols (4–7). For rat hearts, interleaved ^{1}H spectra of lactate and lipids were obtained with a 2-minute time resolution (8). The lactate and lipid levels determined by ^{1}H MR were compared with values obtained biochemically and enzymatically on freeze-clamped tissue at the end of the experimental protocols (8).

^{23}Na Magnetic Resonance Spectroscopy

^{23}Na MR spectra of rat hearts were acquired using a probe at 95.2 MHz with a 2.0- to 2.5-minute time resolution in the presence of 5 mM dysprosium triethylene-tetraminehexaacetate (DyTTHA^{3-}) (shift reagent) to resolve the intracellular and extracellular Na$^+$ signals (9–12). Use of the shift reagent resulted in only minor changes in mechanical function or energetics, determined by ^{31}P MR in a parallel series of hearts.

In studies on isolated pig hearts, ^{23}Na MR spectra were acquired in the presence of shift reagent. For experiments where correlations were drawn between ^{31}P and ^{23}Na data, the spectra were obtained using a 2-cm surface coil applied to the left ventricular wall (13). The surface coil was used (rather than the volume coil described earlier) due to field homogeneity considerations in the ^{23}Na spectra. ^{23}Na and ^{31}P spectra were acquired with a 5-minute time resolution (0.2 s and 1.2 s recycle time, respectively).

^{87}Rb Magnetic Resonance Spectroscopy

^{87}Rb MR spectra were acquired using a broadband probe (Morris Instruments) operating at 117.8 MHz with 2-minute time resolution (90° pulse, 15 ms recycle time). A capillary containing 1M RbCl + 5M KI (10–15 μmol of Rb) was used as a chemical shift and concentration reference. Unlike ^{23}Na, where steady-state levels are determined using ^{87}Rb MR, Rb$^+$ influx and efflux rates are measured which reflect K$^+$ transport because Rb is a biological congener for K$^+$.

MODELS

Langendorff Perfused Rat Heart

Sprague-Dawley rats were anesthetized and the hearts were removed and perfused retrogradely at a constant pressure of 80mm Hg or at a constant flow (15 ml/

min/g wet wt) at 37°C with modified Krebs-Henseleit buffer containing (mM); NaCl (118), NaHCO$_3$ (25), KCl (4.7), CaCl$_2$ (1.75), MgSO$_4$ (1.2), EDTA (0.5), and glucose (11) or pyruvate (5) and oxygenated with a 95% O$_2$/5% CO$_2$ gas mixture. For MR studies, the heart was placed in a 22-mm (O.D.) sample tube and fully immersed in the perfusate. Left ventricular systolic pressure (LVSP), left ventricular end-diastolic pressure (LVEDP), heart rate, and rate-pressure product (RPP; heart rate × [LVSP − LVEDP]) were monitored continuously using a latex balloon placed into the left ventricle and connected to a pressure transducer. Coronary flow was measured with a flow meter. The perfusion (aortic) pressure was measured by means of a side arm on the aortic perfusion line connected to the same pressure transducer as used for measuring left ventricular pressures (constant flow) or from the height of the water column (constant pressure). Oxygen consumption (VO$_2$) was measured from the arteriovenous difference in pO$_2$ × flow rate.

Isolated Human Atrial Tissue

Human atrial appendages removed during cardiac surgery requiring cardiopulmonary bypass were used with patient consent. The samples were placed in buffer or preservation solution immediately upon removal from the patient. The samples were transported without delay to the MR facility. The first MR spectrum was usually acquired within 45 minutes of removal of the tissue from the patient.

Atrial trabeculae (small functional muscles weighing 5–20 mg) isolated from atrial appendages (14) were used in some instances to assess contractility following preservation.

Isolated Perfused Pig Heart

Buffer-perfused Pig Heart

An isolated buffer-perfused pig heart model was developed to study energetics, ion fluxes, and metabolites during long-term (>4 hr) hypothermic preservation and reperfusion (13,15,16). The model was chosen because of its metabolic and coronary architectural similarity to the human heart. In this model, MR was used both on the arrested heart during preservation and on the beating heart during normothermic reperfusion.

Functional and metabolic assessments were performed while the heart was within the bore of the MR magnet. In addition to measurement of the RPP and ± dp/dt, functional assessment included left ventricular elastance, which was obtained by filling the left ventricular balloon with known quantities of saline or water. End-diastolic and peak systolic pressure readings were obtained corresponding to preloads of known volume. Regression analysis was performed to generate end-diastolic elastance and peak systolic elastance values. Elastance data were calculated as percent changes.

Blood-perfused Pig Heart

Classical isolated heart preparations used for MR studies require cardiac arrest (hypothermic ischemic and/or cardioplegic arrest) during excision of the organ from the animal. We developed a new model of the isolated blood-perfused mammalian heart suitable for MR studies in a horizontal bore magnet, which is useful for studies of myocardial protection (17,18). The model does not require ischemia, cardioplegia, or hypothermia during excision of the heart and prior to the MR experiment. It was chosen over single-animal bypass and cross-circulated heart preparations temporarily supported by a second animal, in an effort to remove unwanted secondary neural and humoral influences on myocardial metabolism and function (18,19).

RESULTS

Fundamental Studies

Potassium and Sodium Transport Mechanisms

Changes in the average extra- and intracellular K^+ and Na^+ levels caused by perturbations such as ischemia can be assessed noninvasively in the intact heart using shift reagent–aided MRS (20). Other methods either provide information on small portions of the heart (microelectrodes, fluorescent probes), are invasive (flame photometry, atomic absorption), or do not distinguish between extra- and intracellular compartments (radioisotopes). Under steady-state conditions, when $[K^+]$ and $[Na^+]$ are constant, their fluxes across the sarcolemma of cardiac cells can be estimated by tracer techniques, which use radioactive isotopes of these ions, ^{42}K and ^{22}Na (21). For measurements of K^+ fluxes, the radioactive isotope of Rb^+, $^{86}Rb^+$, has been used (22) because rubidium is a well-established congener for potassium (23). The relatively high natural abundance (28%), low biological abundance, and high MR sensitivity of ^{87}Rb make it a good tracer for K^+ influx and efflux studies by MR (24). In addition, in an open system when coronary flow is high and extracellular $[Rb^+]$ is constant, Rb^+ influx and Rb^+ efflux from Rb^+-loaded cells can be measured in the absence of shift reagent.

^{23}Na and ^{87}Rb MRS have been used to characterize the routes of influx of Rb^+ into cardiac cells and to evaluate their links to the intracellular Na^+ concentration ($[Na^+]_i$). It is known from studies using radioisotopes, atomic absorption, and MRS that Rb^+ is transported via the Na^+/K^+-ATPase (24,25). However, potential pathways of Rb^+ influx in cardiac cells could also involve $Na^+/K^+/2Cl^-$ cotransport (26) and K^+ channels. Under steady-state conditions, Rb^+ influx mediated by Na^+/K^+-ATPase is proportional to the rate of efflux of Na^+ (Fig. 1) if the contribution of Na^+/Ca^{2+} exchange to Na^+ efflux is small (27). Therefore Rb^+ influx reflects the rate of Na^+ influx rather than Na^+/K^+ pump activity per se because Na^+ influx and efflux rates are equal at steady state.

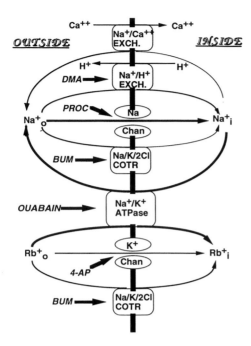

FIG. 1. Coupling between Rb^+ and Na^+ fluxes in cardiomyocytes. DMA, dimethylamiloride; PROC, procaine; BUM, bumetanide; 4-AP, 4-aminopyridine.

Magnetic resonance spectroscopy studies showed that initial rates of Rb^+ accumulation in the heart were linear. Rubidium efflux was a linear function of the total Rb^+ content, indicating the passive nature of this process (28,29). Both Rb^+ influx and intracellular Na^+ were sensitive to the Na^+/K^+-ATPase inhibitor, ouabain (0.2–0.5 mM) (Fig. 2), the Na^+ ionophore, monensin (1 μM) (Fig. 2), and the Na^+ (and Ca^{2+}) channel blockers, procaine (5 mM) (Fig. 2) and lidocaine (1 mM) (28,29). Rubidium transport was insensitive to the inhibitor of $Na^+/K^+/2Cl^-$ co-

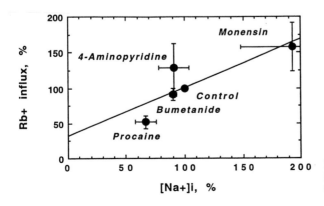

FIG. 2. Dependence of the rate of influx of Rb^+ on intracellular Na^+.

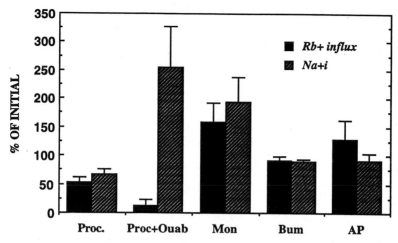

FIG. 3. The effect of some drugs on the intracellular Na^+ content and the Rb^+ influx rate measured by MRS. Ouab, ouabain; Mon, monensin; AP, 4-aminopyridine; Proc, procaine; Bum, bumetanide.

transport, bumetanide (30 μM) (Fig. 2), the K^+ channel blocker, 4-aminopyridine (1 mM) (Fig. 2), and the Na^+/H^+ exchange inhibitor, dimethylamiloride (15 μM) (28,29). In addition, Rb^+ influx was dependent on intracellular $[Na^+]$ (Fig. 3): The rate of Rb^+ influx increased when Na^+ influx was activated by monensin and decreased when Na^+ entry was inhibited by procaine or lidocaine (28,29). These data show that under normal physiological conditions, Rb^+ influx occurs mainly via Na^+/K^+-ATPase; the contribution of the $Na^+/K^+/2Cl^-$ cotransporter and K^+ channels is minimal. Therefore in rat hearts, under steady-state conditions, Rb^+ influx can serve as a measure of Na^+ influx when the contribution of Na^+/Ca^{2+} exchange to Na^+ efflux is relatively small. This suggests that the rate of Rb^+ accumulation can be used as an index of the Na^+ influx rate and therefore of ionic metabolism in excitable tissues in vivo where the aforementioned assumptions are valid. The Na^+ channels are estimated to represent more than 50% of the total Na^+ influx into beating rat cardiomyocytes; the remainder can be ascribed to the Na^+/H^+ exchanger, the $Na^+/K^+/2Cl^-$ cotransporter, and nonspecific Na^+ permeability.

Cardiac Energetics and Sodium Fluxes

A number of pathological situations (ischemia, anoxia, metabolic inhibition) lead to breakdown of PCr and adenine nucleotides and to accumulation of metabolic products, such as P_i, lactate, and H^+. The combination of decreased substrate (ATP) and accumulation of inhibitors (P_i, H^+, ADP) leads to inhibition of Na^+/K^+-ATPase, which, in combination with activation of Na^+ influx via the Na^+/H^+, is followed by accumulation of intracellular Na^+ and subsequently Ca^{2+} due to reversal of Na^+/Ca^{2+} exchange. The resultant intracellular Ca^{2+} overload may contribute to cell death. Because decreases in PCr and [ATP]/[ADP] are inevitably related to accumulation of P_i, it is difficult to discriminate between the relative importance of inhibitory effects of reduced [ATP]/[ADP] and increased P_i.

We used the phosphate trap 2-deoxyglucose to deplete ATP and decrease [ATP]/[ADP] without affecting [P_i] or pH in order to assess the effect of these changes on Na^+/K^+ ATPase activity in isolated rat hearts.

[ATP]/[ADP] was calculated using the creatine kinase (CK) equilibrium:

$$[ATP]/[ADP] = K_{CK^{app}} \times [PCr] \ [H^+]/[Cr]$$

assuming the equilibrium constant for the CK reaction, $K_{CK^{app}}$ (30):

$$K_{CK^{app}} = 1.66 \times 10^9 \ M^{-1} \ \text{at} \ [Mg^{2+}]\text{free} = 1 \ mM$$

Adenosine triphosphate affinity, A(ATP), was calculated from [ATP]/[ADP] and [P_i] using:

$$A(ATP) = -\Delta G° + RT\ln[ATP]/[ADP]\cdot[P_i]$$

where $\Delta G°$ is the standard free energy of ATP hydrolysis taken to be equal to 30.5 kJ/mol.

A 30-minute infusion of 2-deoxyglucose (2 mM) with insulin resulted in accumulation of 2-deoxyglucose-6-phosphate (to 25 mM, as observed by ^{31}P MR) and caused an irreversible decrease in [ATP] (to 25% of the initial level) due to the hydrolysis of ATP and subsequent loss of adenosine and inosine and a reversible decrease in [PCr]. The MR spectra also showed that P_i and intracellular pH remained nearly constant (1). The calculated [ATP]/[ADP] decreased 25-fold, A(ATP) decreased by 10 kJ/mol, free [ADP] rose 13-fold, and free [AMP] increased 240-fold. These results were the consequence of trapping a phosphoryl group from the fixed pool of metabolizable phosphate into the slowly metabolized 2-deoxyglucose-6-phosphate. Under these conditions, the hearts kept beating spontaneously; the RPP, however, was reduced by half.

^{23}Na MR measurements showed that intracellular [Na^+] did not change during the low-energy state induced by the 2-deoxyglucose treatment. The lack of change in intracellular [Na^+] could result from either unchanged Na^+ influx and efflux rates, or from parallel changes in the opposing fluxes. Magnetic resonance studies performed with ^{87}Rb, a congener of K^+, showed no alteration in the Rb^+ influx, which is proportional to Na^+ efflux, thus implying that the Na^+ influx and efflux rates remained unchanged. These data show that the kinetic parameters of the Na^+/K^+ ATPase (V_{max}, K_m for Na) were unaffected by unfavorable thermodynamic (low A[ATP]) and kinetic (low [ATP], high [ADP]) conditions.

These studies support the hypothesis that during anoxia the observed rise in intracellular [Na^+] is not due to inhibition of the Na^+/K^+-ATPase by decreased [ATP]/[ADP], but by other mechanisms such as increased [P_i] or long-chain acyl-carnitine derivatives.

Na$^+$ Fluxes in Ischemia-Reperfusion

^{23}Na and ^{31}P MRS data obtained from rat and pig hearts have been useful in elucidating the relationships between intracellular [Na$^+$], [H$^+$], and energetic state during cardioplegic ischemia and reperfusion (31). It is known that Na$^+$ overload during cardiac ischemia and reperfusion is considered as one of the key events contributing to cell damage. The increase in intracellular Na$^+$ during ischemia in rapidly beating rodent hearts is well documented (32). It has been suggested that intracellular acidosis activates Na$^+$ entry via the Na$^+$/H$^+$ exchanger, while ATP depletion and ADP and P$_i$ accumulation inhibit Na$^+$ efflux via Na$^+$/K$^+$-ATPase. Consequently, intracellular [Ca^{2+}] increases due to activation of Na$^+$/Ca^{2+} exchange, resulting in cell damage. Information on the contribution of Na$^+$ to ischemic damage in large, slowly beating hearts, which are more similar to the human heart, is scarce. In addition, little is known regarding [Na$^+$]$_i$ during cardioplegic ischemia (i.e., ischemia preceded and followed by KCl infusion) in either type of heart. In our studies, isolated hearts of both Sprague-Dawley rats and domestic pigs were used in MR experiments designed to assess the importance of changes in intracellular [Na$^+$] in ischemic damage under hyperkalemic conditions.

Comparable decreases in ATP content and intracellular pH were observed after 90 minutes of normothermic cardioplegic ischemia in pig hearts and after 20 minutes in rat hearts. The increase of intracellular (Na^+_i) in the rat heart at the same level of energy depletion, however, was much larger than in the pig heart. In addition, the increase of Na$^+$ in the rat heart subjected to 30-minute ischemia preceded the development of ischemic contracture, which occurred at approximately 23 minutes, whereas no signs of contracture were observed in the pig heart after 90 minutes of ischemia. Metabolic and functional recovery after 20 minutes of reperfusion with Krebs-Henseleit buffer of the rat heart subjected to 30 minutes of ischemia was poorer than that of the pig heart at 20-minute reperfusion following 90-minute ischemia. These data showed that Na$^+$ balance is less sensitive to cardioplegic ischemic stress in the pig heart than in the rat heart. The lower level of [Na$^+$]$_i$ in the ischemic pig heart at comparable pH$_i$ and ATP levels can be related to a number of factors, including (a) the sensitivity of Na$^+$/K$^+$-ATPase to ischemic inhibition; (b) a higher glycolytic capacity relative to ATPase activity in the pig heart; and/or (c) different ratios of the maximal rates of Na$^+$ carriers responsible for Na$^+$ entry (Na$^+$ channels, Na$^+$/H$^+$ exchanger, Na$^+$/K$^+$/2Cl$^-$ cotransporter) and Na$^+$ efflux (Na$^+$/K$^+$-ATPase).

Contribution of Na$^+$/H$^+$ Exchange to Intracellular pH Balance

Total global ischemia in the perfused rat heart is characterized by profound intracellular acidosis resulting from ATP degradation and accumulation of end products of anaerobic glycolysis. On reperfusion, the intracellular pH normalizes rapidly. Likely contributors to this process are thought to be metabolite washout, activation of Na^+/H^+ exchange, and activation of bicarbonate-dependent systems. It is not known whether activation of the Na^+/H^+ exchanger in the presence of bicarbonate occurs during ischemia, reperfusion, or both. The contribution of the Na^+/H^+ exchanger to the transsarcolemmal pH gradient during ischemia-reperfusion has been estimated using ^{31}P MRS in the isolated rat heart (33). β-aminoethyl phosphonate and P_i were used as extracellular and intracellular pH markers, respectively. Dimethylamiloride (10–15 μM) was used as a specific inhibitor of Na^+/H^+ exchange in the test group. Prior to ischemia, the intracellular pH was 7.1 and the extracellular pH was 7.3. In both the test and control groups, the difference between intracellular and extracellular pH (ΔpH) increased during the first 2.5 minutes of a 20-minute ischemic period, due to the faster decrease in intracellular pH. Thereafter, the difference decreased and approached zero. The normal physiological pH gradient was quickly restored during the first few minutes of reperfusion. Compared with the control group, the intracellular pH in the presence of dimethylamiloride was lower in the early stages of ischemia and reperfusion, while the extracellular pH was identical in both groups. These data suggest that the Na^+/H^+ exchange markedly contributes to H^+ extrusion from the myocytes at the beginning of ischemia as well as reperfusion under conditions where HCO^{3-}-dependent transporters are likely to be active.

Amiloride (0.5 mM), an inhibitor of Na^+/H^+ and Na^+/Ca^{2+} exchange, when present during ischemia and reperfusion in the pig heart at 36°C, did not affect functional recovery. The absence of ischemic or reperfusion contracture and the lack of a protective effect of amiloride agree with the relatively small increase in $[Na^+]_i$ during ischemia and reperfusion in this species. These data suggest a relatively small contribution of Na^+/H^+ exchange to Na^+ accumulation in the presence of bicarbonate buffer in pig hearts.

Metabolic Effects of Ischemia-Reperfusion on Lactate and Lipid Accumulation

Myocardial lipid and lactate levels are sensitive indicators of biochemical status. Lipid levels have been shown to respond to high-fat diets, disease, and metabolic stress. Elevated lactate levels are indicative of a reduced oxygen supply. Selective ^1H MRS measurement of lactate and lipids is not straightforward because the methyl resonances commonly used to measure lactate (1.3 ppm) overlap with the lipid methylene groups. Using a spectral editing technique (8), it is possible to observe both lipid methylene and lactate methyl resonances in the perfused rat heart under a variety of conditions with 2-minute time resolution. In agreement with previous biochemical measurements, ^1H MRS has shown that lactate levels increase during 28-minute ischemia and decrease during reperfusion. The increase in lactate during ischemia was prevented by iodoacetate (8), an inhibitor of one of the key regulatory enzymes in glycolysis, glyceraldehyde-3-phosphate dehydrogenase. In contrast, lipid levels observed by MR increased during ischemia and remained elevated during reperfusion. Hearts from rats fed high-fat diets showed elevated lipid levels during control perfusion (8).

The MR spectra provide no information regarding the source of the lipid in the ischemic heart; in the absence of exogenous lipid sources (the hearts are perfused with Krebs-Henseleit buffer containing 11 mM glucose as the energy source), however, the accumulation of lipid must arise from a change in the MR visibility of lipids rather than in the absolute amount of lipid in the heart (8).

Applications

Effect of Hypothermia

Porcine Heart

Energetics, Sodium, and Contractility. The aim of this study was to compare the effects of hypothermic and normothermic cardioplegic (using 16 mM KCl) ischemia on myocellular homeostasis and function. Initial work focused on determining whether intracellular Na^+ accumulation during normothermic (36°C) and hypothermic (18°C) cardioplegic ischemia is involved in ischemic damage to the buffer-perfused pig heart.

^{31}P and ^{23}Na MRS showed that normothermic (45-min) and hypothermic (210-min) cardioplegic ischemia resulted in comparable decreases in high-energy phosphates and pH_i with no change in LVEDP. The increase in $[Na^+]_i$, however, was greater after 210 minutes of ischemia at 18°C (180%) than after 45 minutes at 36°C (67%) (13). The larger increase in Na^+_i at 18°C than at 36°C may reflect the longer ischemic time and a more significant inhibition by temperature of the Na^+ pump relative to Na^+/H^+ exchange and passive Na^+ permeability. On reperfusion, Na^+_i and PCr returned to the initial levels, whereas both ATP and VO_2 recovered to approximately 70% of the initial levels at both temperatures. Functional recovery, as measured by the RPP, was much higher after hypothermic ischemia (67% of initial) than after normothermic ischemia (25% of initial). In addition, the efficiency of energy use, RPP/VO_2, and coronary resistance returned to their initial values after hypothermic ischemia but decreased after normothermic ischemia.

Another dissimilarity between the effects of normothermic and hypothermic ischemia is the larger decrease in contractile function relative to that in VO_2, after normothermic ischemia and the proportional decreases in RPP and VO_2 after hypothermic ischemia. This can be ascribed to energy-wasting effects (34) during normothermic ischemia and inhibition of this process under hypothermic conditions. These data also show that functional recovery of the pig heart after cardioplegic ischemia does not correlate directly with either ischemic H^+ and Na^+_i accumulation or depletion of high-energy phosphates.

Human Tissue

Energy Homeostasis. Magnetic resonance provides a unique opportunity to study the time course of energetic changes during preservation of small pieces of human tissue, such as atrial appendages ($\cong 0.5$ g) (4–6) or even atrial trabeculae (5–20 mg) (7,14). Atrial appendages provide a practical model of ischemically preserved tissue. Magnetic resonance spectroscopy of isolated human atrial tissue has been used to evaluate the energy balance in tissue preserved in hypothermic saline solution (which is used in some institutions for transportation of donor hearts). We have measured the temperature dependence of energy production via glycolysis (^{1}H measurement of lactate production) and total energy consumption (^{31}P measurement of ATP levels) by interleaving ^{1}H and ^{31}P data acquisition within a single MR experiment. We have shown that between 1°C and 20°C, the rate of energy consumption exceeds its production and the imbalance increases with increasing temperature. Based on these observations, it can be concluded that energy reserves are best preserved at low (1°C–4°C) temperature. Trabeculae can be isolated from atrial appendages and be perifused to provide sufficient oxygen delivery to maintain aerobic metabolism and to allow manipulation of experimental conditions. Magnetic resonance studies of these tissues have shown that metabolic stores within the tissue allow preservation of energy levels for more than 18 hours at 4°C and 12°C when the tissue is provided with O_2 and waste products are removed.

Magnetic resonance spectroscopy has shown that the optimal temperature for long-term (hours) ischemic preservation of energy stores varies with the length of the preservation time. For instance, after 5 hours preservation in an extracellular-type crystalloid cardioplegic solution, ATP stores were best preserved at 12°C rather than 4°C. For longer periods, up to 24 hours, ATP stores were best preserved at the lower temperature. The reason for this behavior is that the shape of decay curves of ATP at the two temperatures are different. At 12°C, the high-energy stores decrease linearly over the 24-hour preservation period, whereas at 4°C, there is an initial rapid decrease followed by a plateau. The MR data have been verified using HPLC on samples quick-frozen at specific time points (5,6).

Effect of Buffer. Using human atrial appendages, we showed that increasing the buffering capacity of preservation solutions at 12°C can decrease the rate of intracellular acidification and allow glycolysis to proceed longer than in saline solution. The data support the hypothesis that the higher buffer capacity of the medium allows proton transport mechanisms (such as lactate-proton cotransport) to proceed by providing an extracellular "sink" for the protons (5).

In addition, measurements of lactate production at 12°C showed that the presence of high extracellular buffering capacity is associated with greater rates of lactate production (5). The phenomenon is highly temperature-dependent. Studies repeated at 4°C showed no increase in lactate production with increasing extracellular buffer concentration, which is consistent with the temperature dependence of glycolysis (5,6).

Development of Cardioplegic Solutions

Crystalloid Solutions

Importance of Calcium in Preservation Solutions. The relative merits of cardioplegic solutions that simulate the composition of either the intracellular or the extracellular milieu have been the subject of many investigations. We have recently compared the efficacies of St-Thomas II solution (an extracellular-type solution) and the University of Wisconsin Cold Storage Solution (UW, an intracellular-type solution) for 8-hour ischemic hypothermic preservation of porcine hearts. Preservation at 4°C with either solution resulted in equally good recovery of cardiac function following reperfusion. A large difference between the solutions, however, was observed for hearts preserved at 12°C. With UW solution, there was total loss of high-energy phosphates upon reperfusion, and lack of cardiac functional recovery in 50% of the hearts, as well as "stone heart" formation in others. In contrast, with St-Thomas II solution, all hearts recovered high-energy phosphates and contractile function. The "calcium paradox" was postulated to be the cause of the dysfunction observed with UW solution at 12°C because the solution contains no Ca^{2+}, and the paradox is known to be temperature-dependent (16). These studies highlight the importance of stringent control of temperature when using Ca^{2+}-free cardioplegic or preservation solutions.

If the calcium paradox is a major factor in the failure of UW solution to protect the ischemic myocardium preserved at 12°C, it can be postulated that addition of Ca^{2+} to the solution would be beneficial to the reperfused heart. Studies using pig hearts were repeated in which 0.5 mM Ca^{2+} was added to UW solution used for 8-hour ischemic preservation at 12°C. The hearts were subsequently reperfused using a blood perfusate (blood:Krebs–Henseleit solution, 1:1, v/v). Again, hearts subjected to UW solution without Ca^{2+} performed poorly, whereas those preserved with the Ca^{2+}-supplemented UW solution showed no loss of ATP or PCr during reperfusion, and achieved the same level of function as did the hearts preserved with UW at 4°C or with St-Thomas II solution at either temperature (35). In addition, the hearts preserved in Ca^{2+}-supplemented UW solution showed an increase in diastolic pressure and accelerated breakdown of PCr during ischemia relative to the Ca^{2+}-free UW solution, suggesting that the presence of Ca^{2+} may result in a significant increase in intracellular Ca^{2+}, which does not, however, offset its beneficial effects and may be attenuated by modifying the $[Na^+]$ in the solution (35).

Effect of Calcium on the Postischemic Heart. Contractile dysfunction induced by ischemia and reperfusion in the heart can be due to disturbances in (a) energy transduction including substrate/oxygen supply, oxidative phosphorylation, energy transfer, contraction, and ion pumping; and (b) energy regulation, which involves electromechanical coupling/Ca^{2+} handling. The relative importance of each of these systems in contractile failure depends on the experimental conditions. For example, in the case of short-term reversible ischemia when heart "stunning" takes place, moderate contractile dysfunction is reversed by inotropic agents such as catecholamines and increased Ca^{2+}, implying limitations in excitation-contraction coupling.

We have investigated the mechanism of contractile dysfunction induced by KCl arrest and normothermic ischemia in the perfused pig heart. Normothermic (36°C) total global cardioplegic ischemia (45 min) resulted in a severe decrease in PCr and an increase in P_i, a moderate decrease in ATP, and a significant drop in intracellular pH that did not affect LVEDP. Subsequent reperfusion for 20 minutes with a high K^+ solution (secondary cardioplegia) was followed by complete recovery of PCr and pH and partial recovery of ATP levels. When perfusion was subsequently switched to normal KH buffer and pacing started, the heart recovered only 25% of its initial RPP, and 67% of its initial oxygen consumption rate, VO_2. In addition, the RPP/VO_2 was reduced, diastolic stiffness increased, and coronary resistance decreased. Lastly, stimulation of cardiac function by increased coronary flow or balloon volume was poor (13).

During reperfusion, the hearts were allowed to reach a stable level of function and then stimulated using isoproterenol (0.1 μM) or by increasing $[Ca^{2+}]$ in the prefusate in order to assess contractile and metabolic reserves. Following isoproterenol washout, the perfusate $[Ca^{2+}]$ was increased from 1 to 1.66 mM. Isoproterenol treatment increased RPP, VO_2, and RPP/VO_2 by 400%, 85%, and 190%, respectively, while the $[Ca^{2+}]$ increase produced less stimulation (by 95%, 38%, and 46%, respectively). Preischemic hearts showed less relative stimulation with isoproterenol and a comparable level of stimulation with Ca^{2+}. The absolute values of RPP and VO_2 remained lower in the postischemic hearts, however, and were 60% and 90% of the isoproterenol-stimulated level of normal hearts, respectively. Postischemic hearts responded differently to an increase in heart rate compared with normal hearts: The increase in heart rate did not affect LVDP in the postischemic heart, whereas it decreased LVDP by 29% in the preischemic heart. The addition of alternative substrates during reperfusion, such as pyruvate (5 mM), lactate (3 mM), or acetate (5 mM), did not affect the functional parameters of the postischemic hearts.

These data show that there are two major causes for the severe contractile dysfunction caused by cardioplegic ischemia in pig hearts. First, uncoupling of mitochondrial electron transport and myofibrillar mechanical work takes place as shown by a twofold decrease in the RPP/VO_2 ratio. This could be due to either uncoupling of oxidative phosphorylation or activation of extramitochondrial futile cycles. The former seems to be less probable because the basal VO_2 in KCl-arrested hearts did not increase after ischemia and PCr returned to its initial level. Second, the observed deficit in activating Ca^{2+} or the decrease in Ca^{2+} sensitivity of the myofibrils was caused by the ischemia, as demonstrated by the observation that isoproterenol greatly improved contractile function and increased VO_2. The increase in RPP (fivefold) was larger than the increase in VO_2 (twofold), such that the efficiency of energy utilization, RPP/VO_2, returned to the initial preischemic level. This may imply that myofibrillar ATPase activated by isoproterenol effectively competes with futile cycles for ATP and redirects energy flux to mechanical work. We cannot exclude that myofibrillar activity could form a futile cycle as a consequence of chemomechanical uncoupling. Disturbances in Ca^{2+} handling were also demonstrated by a change in the relation between LVDP and heart rate: LVDP was independent of heart rate (in the range 110–180 bpm).

Effect of Magnesium during Cardioplegia and Reperfusion. A number of studies have demonstrated a beneficial effect of Mg^{2+} in the reperfused heart. The beneficial effects of Mg^{2+} are dependent on both the species used as well as on the conditions under which it is administered (36–41). Studies were performed on rat hearts subjected to 30 minutes of normothermic *perfusion* with St-Thomas II cardioplegic solution containing either 0 mM $MgCl_2$ or 16 mM $MgCl_2$. A third group of hearts was perfused at 10°C with St-Thomas II cardioplegic solution containing 0 mM $MgCl_2$ for the same period. The hearts were subsequently reperfused with Krebs-Henseleit solution and contractile function evaluated. The data showed a lesser increase in resting LVEDP and a lesser decrease in LVDP, RPP, and RPP/VO$_2$ in the hearts exposed to normothermic St-Thomas II cardioplegia containing 16 mM $MgCl_2$. Furthermore, hypothermia produced the same level of beneficial effects as did 16 mM $MgCl_2$ in this model.

In another series of experiments, rat hearts were subjected to 30-minute normothermic ischemia following a 2-minute infusion of St-Thomas II cardioplegia containing either 0 mM $MgCl_2$ or 16 mM $MgCl_2$. When the hearts were subsequently reperfused with Krebs-Henseleit solution and contractile function assessed, no beneficial effect of Mg^{2+} could be demonstrated on functional recovery.

These studies show that the effect of Mg^{2+} was limited to hearts that had been perfused continuously with St-Thomas II solution at normothermia. One hypothesis is that the continuous perfusion with high KCl (St-Thomas contains 16 mM KCl) led to Ca^{2+} overload (evidenced by high LVEDP), which was prevented by high Mg^{2+}.

The studies were extended to the porcine heart; we verified that, similar to results obtained in the rat but not the rabbit, Mg^{2+} acts as a negative inotrope in the pig (39). Our studies then focused on the effect of Mg^{2+} in St-Thomas II solution used for hypothermic preservation of the heart. The hearts were rendered ischemic for 4 hours at 12°C following the infusion of a single dose of St-Thomas II solution containing either 0 mM or 16 mM $MgCl_2$. Magnetic resonance and functional studies on the reperfused hearts showed complete recovery of initial levels of ATP, PCr, and RPP using either solution (40).

In order to enhance the possibility of observing any potential protective effects of Mg^{2+}, pig hearts were stressed with normothermic hypoxia (60 min, 37°C) under a *continuous flow* of St-Thomas II cardioplegic solution containing either 0 mM or 16 mM $MgCl_2$. The hearts were then reperfused with Krebs-Henseleit solution and tested functionally. The treatment resulted in only 50% recovery of contractile function and 90% to 95% recovery of ATP and PCr. There were no differences between the hearts preserved with or without Mg^{2+} (38).

Lastly, to test the effect of Mg^{2+} added to secondary cardioplegic solution, pig hearts were subjected to 4-hour ischemia at 12°C, rewarmed for 20 minutes by perfusion with cardioplegic solution (secondary cardioplegia) containing either 0 mM MgCl$_2$ or 16 mM MgCl$_2$, and then reperfused with KH solution at 37°C. Records of mechanical function showed that Mg^{2+} in the secondary cardioplegic solution did not provide additional benefit to the reperfused myocardium (36). The major beneficial effects of secondary cardioplegia, improved LVDP, and absence of ventricular fibrillation were due primarily to the presence of high (16 mM) K$^+$, because similar results were obtained using KH buffer containing 16 mM KCl as the secondary cardioplegic solution. These beneficial effects may have resulted from the mechanical arrest that allowed the heart to reestablish ionic and energetic homeostasis prior to resuming mechanical activity.

The ensemble of data show that, under our experimental conditions in pig hearts, there is no major effect of a high concentration of Mg^{2+} (16 mM) added to a high K$^+$ (16 mM) extracellular-type cardioplegic solution. The differences between the data obtained with the rat heart may be related to the larger Na$^+$ and Ca^{2+} overload that occurs in the rat heart compared with the pig heart at similar levels of energy depletion (*vide supra*).

Effect of Potassium in Cardioplegia. The high [K$^+$] used in cardioplegic solutions can produce not only protective but also deleterious effects on cardiac function. Such effects of hyperkalemia on the vascular endothelium (42) and contractility (43) have been demonstrated. We therefore tested the effect of prolonged exposure to high [K$^+$] on cardiac function. Preliminary experiments showed that 115-minutes' arrest using a constant flow of high-potassium (16 mM K$^+$) cardioplegic solution resulted in a 50% decrease in RPP, which returned to the initial level following addition of isoproterenol (44). One of the possible explanations for this observation is the depletion of endogenous stores of noradrenaline during long-term exposure to high K$^+$ and loss of natural inotropic stimulation. Alternatively, accumulation of noradrenaline in the recirculating perfusate could lead to cytotoxic effects (45,46).

Blood Cardioplegia

Continuous Normothermic Blood Cardioplegia. The blood-perfused pig heart model was developed (17,18) to assess the efficacy and limits of the relatively new technique of normothermic blood cardioplegia for surgery. The model is being used in conjunction with MR techniques to assess the time limits and the consequences of interrupting blood cardioplegia during surgery, to determine the optimal route of delivery of cardioplegia (antegrade versus retrograde), and to optimize the flow rate and hematocrit of cardioplegia. Normal blood-perfused pig hearts have been used to model the human heart subjected to a coronary artery bypass graft (CABG) procedure.

During preliminary studies to evaluate the usefulness of the MR methodology, normal blood-perfused hearts were subjected to 20 minutes of controlled normothermic ischemia during which MR was used to monitor energetics and intracellular pH. A group of hearts was rendered ischemic by stopping the flow of blood cardioplegia for 20 minutes in the middle of a 1-hour cardioplegic arrest period. The hearts were subsequently reperfused and mechanical function assessed. ^{31}P MR spectra obtained during ischemia showed that after 14 minutes of normothermic ischemia, PCr decreased to unobservable levels and P_i increased accordingly. After 20-min normothermic ischemia, the intracellular pH determined from the chemical shift of P_i decreased to 6.8. Within 3 minutes of reperfusion with high-potassium blood cardioplegic solution, PCr, P_i and pH returned to initial values. End-systolic and end-diastolic elastance returned to 88% and 136% of their pre-arrest values, respectively (19). For needle biopsies taken at the end of the experiments, HPLC assays demonstrated no significant differences in PCr and ATP (49 and 21 μmol/g dry wt, respectively) (19), as compared with controls (54 and 21 μmol/g dry wt, respectively) which underwent a 1-hour period of arrest with continuous normothermic blood cardioplegia (CNBC).

Intermittent Normothermic Blood Cardioplegia. Magnetic resonance provides a unique opportunity to measure, on a minute-to-minute basis, the effects of interrupting cardioplegia and to determine whether successive periods of cardioplegic ischemia produce a cumulative, detrimental effect on metabolic parameters. We have recently completed the first of a series of experiments to determine whether safe limits exist for interrupting normothermic blood cardioplegia (47) during surgery.

Initial parameters were chosen based on the study just described in which we determined that PCr becomes undetectable (i.e., <10% of its initial value) within 15 minutes of interrupting normothermic blood cardioplegia. It is also known that when PCr reserves are depleted, ATP is used as the primary source of high-energy phosphates (48). When ATP is metabolized to ADP, AMP, and further breakdown products (adenosine, inosine, hypoxanthine), the latter are lost from the cell (49). Following reperfusion, it may require a number of days to restore the initial ATP levels. We chose 10 minutes as the ischemic interval in order not to decrease ATP levels measurably during ischemia. A reflow period of 5 minutes was chosen based on MR results showing that PCr and pH returned to normal values within 3 minutes of reperfusion following 20 minutes of ischemia. Six cycles of ischemia-reperfusion were chosen to mimic a clinically relevant situation.

Three groups of isolated blood-perfused pig hearts were studied: Group 1 underwent 90 minutes of CNBC; group 2 was subjected to six 10-minute episodes of ischemia interleaved with six 5-minute periods of continuous reflow of normothermic blood cardioplegia; and group 3 was continuously perfused with normokalemic blood for the same total time. The entire protocol required 150 minutes and included a 30-minute period of control perfusion and a 30-minute reperfusion period with normokalemic blood during which contractile function was assessed.

Interruption of cardioplegia resulted in a significant decrease in the PCr peak (by 45%) and an increase in the P_i peak (88%). Both PCr and P_i levels returned to baseline during subsequent 5-minute cardioplegic reflow periods. Adenosine triphosphate decreased slightly during the 90 minutes of intermittent cardioplegia and recovered completely during reperfusion. The changes in ATP, PCr, and P_i observed in the course of the experiments are summarized in Fig. 4. Statistical analysis of the data confirmed that intermittent warm-blood cardioplegia resulted in a significant drop in PCr ($p<0.01$, one-way ANOVA). There were, however, no significant differences between PCr values measured during the six interruptions ($p>0.05$, one-way ANOVA). Moreover, although P_i increased significantly ($p<0.01$) during each interruption, the differences at the end of each of the six interruptions were not statistically significant ($p>0.05$) (47). These results suggest that, under our experimental conditions, intermittent warm-blood cardioplegia does not result in a cumulative loss of PCr or gain in P_i.

The levels of PCr and ATP measured at the end of reperfusion in the hearts subjected to either control perfusion, continuous, or intermittent warm-blood cardioplegia were not significantly different among the three groups. The level of inorganic phosphate in the hearts that underwent CNBC was significantly higher than in the hearts subjected to intermittent warm-blood cardioplegia and may be a consequence of the edema that occurs when hearts are perfused at a hematocrit value lower than normal (because the blood perfusate contained P_i).

Intracellular pH during both control perfusion and reperfusion was 7.2. A 10-minute interruption of warm-blood cardioplegia resulted in an average decrease in intracellular pH of 0.1 unit. During the subsequent interruptions, pH_i did not de-

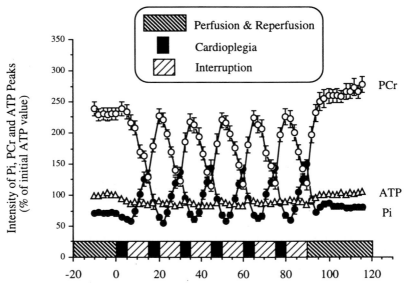

FIG. 4. Time course of myocardial ATP, PCr, and P_i in isolated pig hearts during control perfusion with normokalemic blood, intermittent warm-blood cardioplegia, and reperfusion with normokalemic blood. Data are presented as means $\pm$ SE of the mean (n = 9).

crease to any greater extent than during the first interruption ($p>0.05$) (i.e., there was no cumulative effect of the ischemia with each period of interruption) (47).

Comparison of RPP and $+$ dp/dt during reperfusion of the hearts receiving continuous and intermittent cardioplegia showed no significant differences between the groups, suggesting that intermittent warm-blood cardioplegia did not worsen myocardial contractile function compared with continuous cardioplegia (47).

In contrast, a single 60-minute period of normothermic ischemia initiated with St-Thomas II solution in isolated pig hearts resulted in complete depletion of observable PCr, an 80% decrease in ATP, a 370% increase in P_i, and a decrease in intracellular pH from a control value of 7.2 to 6.1, which suggests that this length of normothermic cardioplegic ischemia can cause severe or irreversible myocardial damage (GH Tian et al., *unpublished data*). In our study of intermittent normothermic blood cardioplegia, we found that a total ischemic time of 60 minutes consisting of six 10-minute ischemic periods interleaved with six 5-minute periods of continuous cardioplegic reperfusion caused very mild changes in myocardial energy metabolites, pH_i, and contractile function. This suggests that warm-blood cardioplegia may be safely interrupted in the *normal heart* for surgical precision without causing myocardial ischemic injury.

Blood Cardioplegia in the Damaged Heart. To assess the potential of CNBC to metabolically "resuscitate" (e.g., restore ATP) the damaged heart, we performed a series of MR experiments on hearts that were subjected to a 20-minute period of normothermic ischemia prior to reperfusion with normokalemic blood or cardioplegia (18). The studies addressed the clinical situation in which surgery is performed on severely energy-depleted hearts.

Isolated blood-perfused pig hearts were subjected to a control perfusion period, in the MR magnet, during which elastance measurements were performed. The beating hearts were then subjected to 20 minutes of normothermic ischemia by interrupting the flow of normokalemic blood perfusate. Three groups of hearts were studied: (a) immediately reperfused for 1 hour with normothermic, normokalemic blood; (b) subjected to intermittent hypothermic blood cardioplegia consisting of a 5-minute infusion at 14°C, every 20 minutes, repeated 3 times; and (c) perfused for 1 hour with continuous normothermic blood cardioplegia. Following cardioplegia, the hearts were reperfused with normokalemic blood and elastance measurements performed in conjunction with MR data acquisition. Needle biopsies were obtained from the beating hearts for quantitative measurements of high-energy phosphates by HPLC.

Magnetic resonance data showed that within 5 to 10 minutes of normothermic ischemia in the beating heart, PCr became unobservable. After 20 minutes, the intracellular pH decreased to 6.7. All of the hearts lost 23% to 31% of their ATP during the initial normothermic ischemic period. Upon reperfusion with either normokalemic blood (group 1) or blood cardioplegia (groups 2 and 3), PCr and pH returned to preischemic levels, but ATP did not return to preischemic levels in any of the groups. The qualitative MR data were consistent with the HPLC data, which showed a loss of 29% to 40% of initial ATP levels (Table 1). The average ATP value

TABLE 1. *High-energy phosphates and function in ischemically stressed blood-perfused porcine hearts*

	MR (n)	HPLC (n)	Function (n)
Control	71 ± 7 (6)	60 ± 5 (6)	86 ± 18 (5)
ICBC	77 ± 13 (6)	69 ± 6 (6)	88 ± 9 (5)
CNBC	69 ± 13 (6)	71 ± 10 (6)	115 ± 30 (5)

All data are presented as % of the initial value measured in the beating blood-perfused heart. MR and HPLC were used to measure ATP at the end of the reperfusion period. Function was measured as end-systolic elastance.

ICBC, intermittent normothermic blood cardioplegia; CNBC, continuous normothermic blood cardioplegia.

for the reperfused hearts was 18 μmol/g dry wt, compared with 24 μmol/g dry wt in fresh controls. Function upon reperfusion with normokalemic blood in the three groups varied between 86% and 115% of baseline values (Table 1). There were no statistically significant differences between any of the treatments, possibly due to the relatively large standard deviations of the data (ca. 10–20%) and the small number of hearts studied (six in each group). The data, however, do indicate that blood cardioplegia prevents exacerbation of ischemic injury, but does not restore depleted ATP levels.

PERSPECTIVES

The research described herein has focused primarily on the use of ^{31}P, ^{23}Na, ^{1}H, and ^{87}Rb MR to follow energetics and ion fluxes in isolated perfused hearts and in human atrial tissue. A wealth of information could also be obtained from the use of ^{13}C MR to follow the fate of ^{13}C-labeled substrates in hearts (50) that have been subjected to preservation. This MR modality would be particularly useful in assessing the metabolic utility of substrate enhancement (e.g., aspartate, glutamate) of solutions used to reperfuse the heart following cardioplegic arrest for surgery. In addition, less sensitive nuclei such as ^{39}K have been measured directly by MR in cardiovascular tissue (20). ^{7}Li, a congener of Na, has been monitored by MR to measure fluxes of Na^{+} (51,52).

The data reported herein have been obtained either from the whole heart or from single, localized regions of the heart using a surface MR coil. Techniques such as spectroscopic imaging when applied to the heart (53) can provide information from a number of localized regions simultaneously. In addition, techniques have been developed that allow MR spectra to be obtained from a number of sections across the left ventricular wall (54). Differences in response of the epicardial and endocardial layers of the heart can be monitored separately during and following metabolic stresses.

SUMMARY

Our MR studies have focused on monitoring changes in energetics, pH, and intracellular Na^+ concentrations in both normal and ischemic rat and pig hearts and correlating these data with contractile function. Magnetic resonance has been used to assess the contributions of different ion transporters to cellular ion homeostasis under normal and ischemic conditions to determine how these ion transporters are regulated in vivo. We have shown that ^{87}Rb MRS is a valuable tool for noninvasive measurements of K^+ fluxes in the isolated heart, which allows quantitative evaluation of the contributions of different ion transporting systems to K^+ fluxes as well as of the effects of various drugs on these systems. In addition, under appropriate conditions (steady-state) in tissues where Na^+/K^+-ATPase is the major route for K^+ entry and Na^+ efflux, Rb^+ influx may serve as a measure of Na^+ influx.

The combination of ^{31}P and cation (^{23}Na, ^{87}Rb) MR provides a unique opportunity to study the relation between ionic transport and energetics under normal and pathological conditions. We have found that severe decreases in cytoplasmic [ATP] and [ATP]/[ADP] in rat hearts caused by trapping phosphate with 2-deoxyglucose, and similar to those observed in anoxic/hypoxic hearts, did not affect Na^+ homeostasis or Na^+/K^+-ATPase activity. The resulting hypothesis is that inhibition of the Na^+ pump under anoxic conditions may occur as a consequence of accumulation of P_i or other metabolic products of anoxia.

Comparison of the metabolic, ionic, and functional effects of cardioplegic ischemia in small rat (fast heart rate) and large human-sized pig (slow heart rate) hearts showed striking species differences. In addition to the anticipated slower rate of degradation (three- to fourfold) of high-energy phosphates in pig hearts compared with rat hearts, we observed less accumulation of intracellular Na^+ in the pig hearts at similar levels of ATP, and pH_i decreases for both species. This was followed by better functional and metabolic recovery in the pig hearts. These findings may be related to a higher glycolytic relative to aerobic capacity and total ATPase activity of the pig hearts, which facilitates maintainance of Na^+ homeostasis under ischemic conditions. Furthermore, the pig hearts did not show any correlation between Na^+ accumulation during ischemia and subsequent functional recovery: Hypothermic ischemia resulted in a larger increase in Na^+_i than did normothermic ischemia; hypothermic ischemia, however, was associated with better postischemic functional recovery.

Our experiments in the pig heart showed that hyperkalemia, which is frequently used for cardiac arrest and protection, may cause contractile dysfunction. This effect may be related to noradrenaline release from sympathetic nerve endings occurring as a result of K^+-induced membrane depolarization. Noradrenaline release can have a dual effect on contractile function: It may cause loss of natural inotropic stimulation; conversely, there may be toxic effects related to its accumulation during long-term recirculating perfusion.

Pig hearts showed a large contractile reserve following 45 and 90 minutes of normothermic high-K^+ cardioplegic ischemia, as revealed by isoproterenol and Ca^{2+}

stimulation. This phenomenon resembles cardiac stunning with, however, greater contractile dysfunction (up to 25% of the initial RPP value). The mechanism of the contractile dysfunction is suggested to involve chemomechanical uncoupling associated with abnormalities in Ca^{2+} handling. We speculate that interventions preventing or limiting cardiac stunning may be useful in cardioplegic protection.

Work on the practical, applied aspects of cardioplegia in the pig heart has shown the importance of incorporating Ca^{2+} into intracellular-type cardioplegic solutions where strict hypothermia (ca. 4°C) cannot be maintained, in order to avoid the so-called calcium paradox. ^{31}P and ^{1}H MR experiments performed using human atrial tissue have shown the importance of high buffer capacity and temperature (>12°C) in maintaining glycolytic energy production in ischemic tissue. These data support the use of blood as the basis of a cardioplegic solution.

^{31}P MR has shown that continuous normothermic blood cardioplegia can maintain energy reserves and intracellular pH in the arrested heart. Combined ^{31}P MR and contractility studies have showed that repeated short interruptions (<10 min) of normothermic blood cardioplegia do not result in cumulative decreases in either intracellular pH or high-energy phosphates and may even limit the edema and contractile dysfunction associated with the use of a continuous flow of high-$[K^{+}]$ cardioplegia. Normothermic blood cardioplegia, however, should be used with caution because it cannot metabolically resuscitate (restore depleted ATP levels) the ischemically damaged heart, and, as demonstrated earlier, the contractile dysfunction associated with a given level of energy depletion is greater following normothermic than hypothermic ischemia.

In the future, a larger number of studies should be devoted to damaged hearts (e.g., hypertrophied) under conditions that approximate clinically relevant situations in order to develop better strategies for treatment and preservation.

ACKNOWLEDGMENT

This work was supported in part by the Heart and Stroke Foundation of Ontario, the Heart and Stroke Foundation of Manitoba, and the Medical Research Council of Canada.

REFERENCES

1. Stewart LC, Deslauriers R, Kupriyanov VV. Relationships between cytosolic [ATP], [ATP]/[ADP] and ionic fluxes in the perfused rat heart: A ^{31}P, ^{23}Na and ^{87}Rb NMR study. *J Mol Cell Cardiol* 1994;26:1377–1392.
2. Moon RB, Richards JH. Determination of intracellular pH by ^{31}P magnetic resonance. *J Biol Chem* 1973;260:7276–7278.
3. Lareau S, Boyle A, Deslauriers R, Keon WJ, Kroft T, Labow RS. Magnesium enhances function of postischemic human myocardial tissue. *Cardiovasc Res* 1993;27:1009–1014.
4. Deslauriers R, Keon WJ, Lareau S, et al. Preservation of high energy phosphates in human myocardium: a ^{31}P NMR study of the effect of temperature on atrial appendages. *J Thorac Cardiovasc Surg* 1989;98:402–412.

5. Lareau S, Keon WJ, Wallace JC, Whitehead K, Mainwood GW, Deslauriers R. Cardiac hypothermia: ^{31}P and ^{1}H NMR spectroscopic studies of the effect of buffer on preservation of human heart atrial appendages. *Can J Physiol Pharmacol* 1991;69:1726–1732.
6. Mainwood GW, Lareau S, Whitehead K, et al. The effect of temperature and buffer concentration on the metabolism of human atrial appendages measured by ^{31}P NMR and ^{1}H NMR. In: Rakusan K, et al., eds. *Oxygen transport to tissue XI*. New York: Plenum Press; 1989:611–619.
7. Lareau S, Labow RS, Keon WJ, Deslauriers R. Metabolism in isolated human cardiac tissue preserved at low temperature: A ^{31}P NMR study. *Proceedings of the Tenth Annual Meeting of the Society of Magnetic Resonance in Medicine*, San Francisco, 1991, p. 1096.
8. Stewart LC, Saunders JK, Deslauriers R, Bourgeois D, Nédélec JFJ. Simultaneous measurement of both lipid and lactate in isolated rat hearts by ^{1}H NMR spectroscopy. *Magn Reson Med* 1993; 30:655–660.
9. Springer CS. Transmembrane ion pumping: high resolution cation NMR spectroscopy from isolated cells to man. *Ann NY Acad Sci* 1987;506:130–148.
10. Boulanger Y. Nuclear magnetic resonance monitoring of sodium in biological tissues. *Can J Physiol Pharmacol* 1989;67:820–828.
11. Malloy CR, Buster DC, Margarida M, et al. Influence of global ischemia on intracellular sodium in the perfused rat heart. *Magn Reson Med* 1990;15:33–44.
12. Ingwall JS. Measurement of sodium movements across the myocardial wall using ^{23}Na NMR spectroscopy and shift reagents. In: Schaefer S, Balaban RS, eds. *Cardiovascular magnetic resonance spectroscopy*. Boston: Kluwer Academic, 1993:195–213.
13. Kupriyanov VV, Butler KW, Xiang B, St-Jean M, Deslauriers R. ^{31}P and ^{23}Na NMR spectroscopic studies of the mechanism of ischemic damage during preservation of the isolated pig heart. *Bull Magn Res* 1995 [*in press*].
14. Lareau S, Mainwood GW, Labow RS, Keon WJ, Deslauriers R. A NMR probe to study function and metabolism in isolated human cardiac tissue. *Magn Reson Med* 1991;20:312–318.
15. Tian GH, Mainwood GW, Biro GP, et al. The effect of high buffer cardioplegia and secondary cardioplegia on cardiac preservation and postischemic functional recovery: a ^{31}P NMR and functional study in Langendorff perfused pig hearts. *Can J Physiol Pharmacol* 1991;69:1760–1768.
16. Tian GH, Smith KE, Biro GP, et al. A comparison of University of Wisconsin cold storage solution and St Thomas solution II for hypothermic cardiac preservation: a ^{31}P NMR and functional study of isolated porcine hearts. *J Heart Transplant* 1991;10:975–985.
17. Deslauriers R, Panos A, Barrozo CAM, et al. Myocardial protection: energy profile during continuous normothermic blood cardioplegia. *Proceedings of the Tenth Annual Meeting of the Society of Magnetic Resonance in Medicine*, San Francisco, 1991, p. 1098.
18. Deslauriers R, Tian G, Aronov A, Salerno TA. The isolated pig heart as a model for basic research on cardioplegia using ^{31}P magnetic resonance spectroscopy. In: Calafiore AM, ed. *Proceedings of the Workshop on Blood Cardioplegia Techniques* 1994 [*in press*].
19. Ali IS, Al-Nowaiser O, Barrozo CAM, Panos A, Deslauriers R, Salerno TA. Continuous normothermic blood cardioplegia: experimental evaluation and future considerations. *J Saudi Heart Assoc* 1992;4:116–120.
20. Pike MM, Frazer JC, Dedrick DF, et al. ^{23}Na and ^{39}K NMR studies of perfused rat hearts. *Biophys J* 1985;48:159–183.
21. Horres CR, Wheeler DM, Piwnica-Worms D, Lieberman M. Ion transport in cultured heart cells. In: Pinson A, ed. *The heart cell in culture*. Vol. 1. Boca Raton: CRC Press; 1987:77–108.
22. Ponce-Hornos JE, Marquez MT, Bonazzola P. Influence of extracellular potassium on energetics of resting heart muscle. *Am J Physiol* 1992;262;H1081–H1087.
23. Beauge LA, Ortiz O. Rubidium, sodium and ouabain interactions on the influx of rubidium in rat red blood cells. *J Physiol (Lond)* 1970;210:519–532.
24. Allis JL, Snaith CD, Seymour AML, Radda GK. ^{87}Rb NMR studies of the perfused rat heart. *FEBS Lett* 1989;242:215–217.
25. Haworth RA, Goknur AB, Berkoff HA. Inhibition of ATP-sensitive potassium channels of adult rat heart cells by antiarrhythmic drugs. *Circ Res* 1989;65:1157–1160.
26. Haas M. Properties and diversity of (Na-K-Cl) cotransporters. *Annu Rev Physiol* 1989;51:443–457.
27. Eisner DA, Smith TW. The Na-K pump and its effectors in cardiac muscle. In: Fozzard HA, Haber H, Jennings RB, Katz AM, Morgan HE, eds. *The heart and cardiovascular system*. 2nd ed. 1992:863–902.
28. Stewart LC, Xiang B, Kwak J, Deslauriers R, Kupryianov VV. Pathways of Rb$^+$ influx and their

relation to intracellular [Na$^+$] in the perfused rat heart: ^{87}Rb and ^{23}Na NMR Study. *Proceedings of the 12th Annual Meeting of the Society for Magnetic Resonance in Medicine.* New York, 1993, p.1064.

29. Kupriyanov VV, Stewart LC, Xiang Bo, Kwak J, Deslauriers R. Pathways of Rb$^+$ influx and their relation to intracellular [Na$^+$] in the perfused rat heart: a ^{87}Rb and ^{23}Na NMR study. *Circ Res* 1995;76:839–857.

30. Lawson JWR, Veech RL. Effects of pH and free Mg2$^+$ on the Keq of the creatine kinase reaction and other phosphate transfer reactions. *J Biol Chem* 1979;247:667–674.

31. Kupriyanov VV, Xiang B, Butler KW, St-Jean M, Deslauriers R. Energy metabolism, intracellular Na$^+$ and contractile function in isolated pig and rat hearts during cardioplegic ischemia and reperfusion: ^{23}Na and ^{31}P NMR studies. *Basic Res Cardiol* 1995 [*in press*].

32. Tani M. Mechanisms of Ca^{2+} overload in reperfused ischemic myocardium. *Annu Rev Physiol* 1990;52:543–559.

33. Kupryianov VV, Docherty JC, Xiang B, Deslauriers R. The contribution of Na$^+$/H$^+$ exchange to the transsarcolemmal pH gradient during ischemia-reperfusion of the isolated rat heart: a ^{31}P-NMR study. Abstract at the *Scientific Conference on the Application of Magnetic Resonance to the Cardiovascular System.* Atlanta, Dec. 15–18, 1993.

34. Liedtke AJ, Nellis SH, Neely JR. Effects of excess free fatty acids on mechanical and metabolic function in normal and ischemic myocardium in swine. *Circ Res* 1978;43:652–661.

35. Tian GH, Biro GP, Butler KW, Xiang B, Vu C, Deslauriers R. The effects of Ca^{++} on the preservation of myocardial energy and function with University of Wisconsin solution: a ^{31}P nuclear magnetic resonance study of isolated blood perfused Langendorff pig hearts. *J Heart Lung Transplant* 1993;12:81–88.

36. Tian GH, Biro GP, Xiang B, Butler KW, Deslauriers R. The effect of magnesium added to secondary cardioplegia on postischemic myocardial metabolism and contractile function—a ^{31}P NMR spectroscopy and functional study in the isolated pig heart. *Basic Res Cardiol* 1992;87:356–365.

37. Lareau S, Boyle A, Deslauriers R, Keon WJ, Kroft T, Labow RS, Magnesium enhances function of postischemic human myocardial tissue. *Cardiovasc Res* 1993;27:1009–1014.

38. Tian GH, Xiang B, Butler KW, Ghomeshi HR, Biro GP, Deslauriers R. Magnesium in St-Thomas cardioplegia solution: a ^{31}P NMR and functional study in isolated rat and pig hearts. *Can J Appl Spectrosc* 1994;39:68–75.

39. Tian GH, Butler KW, Xiang B, Biro GP, Deslauriers R. Magnesium depresses excitation and contraction in isolated pig hearts. *J Mol Cell Cardiol* 1993;25[Suppl III]:S23.

40. Tian GH, Butler KW, Xiang B, Ghomeshi HR, Biro GP, Deslauriers R. A ^{31}P NMR study of the effect of Mg^{++} in cardioplegia in the isolated pig heart. *J Mol Cell Cardiol* 1993;25[Suppl III]:S22.

41. Tian GH, Xiang B, Butler KW, Ghomeshi HR, Biro GP, Deslauriers R. Addition of magnesium to St-Thomas solution does not improve myocardial recovery in the isolated pig heart. *J Mol Cell Cardiol* 1993;25[Suppl III]:S23.

42. Leicher FG, Magarasse P, LaRaja PJ, Derkac WM, Backley MJ, Austen WG. Blood cardioplegia delivery. *Ann Surg* 1983;198:266–272.

43. Handy JR, Spinale FG, Mukherjee R, Crawford FA. Hypothermic potassium cardioplegia impairs myocyte recovery of contractility and inotropy. *J Thorac Cardiovasc Surg* 1994;107:1050–1058.

44. Kupriyanov VV, St-Jean M, Xiang B, Butler KW, Deslauriers R. Contractile dysfunction caused by normothermic ischemia and KCl arrest in the isolated pig heart: a ^{31}P NMR study. *J Mol Cell Cardiol* 1995 [*in press*].

45. Schomig A, Kurz T, Richardt G, Schoming E. Neuronal sodium homeostasis and axoplasmic amine concentration determine calcium-independent noradrenaline release in normoxic and ischemic rat heart. *Circ Res* 1988;63:214–226.

46. Rump AFE, Klaus W. Evidence for norepinephrine cardiotoxicity mediated by superoxide anion radicals in isolated rabbit hearts. *Naunyn Schmiedebergs Arch Pharmacol* 1994;349:295–300.

47. Tian GH, Xiang B, Butler KW, et al. Effects of intermittent warm blood cardioplegia on myocardial high energy phosphates, intracellular pH and contractile function—a ^{31}P NMR study in isolated rat and pig hearts. *J Thorac Cardiovasc Surg* 1994 [*in press*].

48. Connett RJ. Analysis of metabolic control: new insights using scaled creatine kinase model. *Am J Physiol* 1988;254:R949–R959.

49. Jennings RB, Reimer KA, Hill ML, Mayer SE. Total ischemia in dog hearts in vitro. 1. Comparison of high energy phosphate production, utilization, and depletion, and adenine nucleotide catabolism in total ischemia in vitro vs. severe ischemia in vivo. *Circ Res* 1981;49:892–900.

50. Sherry DA, Malloy CR, Zhao P, Thompson JR. Alterations in substrate utilization in the reperfused myocardium: a direct analysis by ^{13}C NMR. *Biochemistry* 1992;31:4833–4837.
51. Keon C, Nédélec JF, Rokosh E, Clarke K. Lithium as a probe in the study of transsarcolemmal sodium in heart: ^{7}Li and ^{31}P NMR spectroscopic studies. *Proceedings of the Eleventh Annual Meeting of the Society of Magnetic Resonance in Medicine.* Berlin, 1992, p. 2207.
52. Keon C, Nédélec JF, Clarke K. Characteristics of lithium relaxation in the perfused heart. *Proceedings of the Eleventh Annual Meeting of the Society of Magnetic Resonance in Medicine.* Berlin, 1992, p. 2206.
53. Bourgeois D, Deslauriers R. Phasing spin-echo acquired ^{31}P spectroscopic images using complex conjugate data reversal. *Magn Reson Med* 1992;28:122–128.
54. Menon RS, Hendrich K, Hu X, Ugurbil K. ^{31}P NMR spectroscopy of the human heart at 4 Tesla; detection of uncontaminated cardiac spectra and differentiation of subepicardium and subendocardium. *Proceedings of the Eleventh Annual Meeting of the Society for Magnetic Resonance.* Berlin, 1992, p. 342.

Subject Index

Subject Index